W9-APK-022

Small Animal
ULTRASOUND

Small Animal ULTRASOUND

EDITED BY

Ronald W. Green, ***DVM, MS***

WITH 10 CONTRIBUTORS

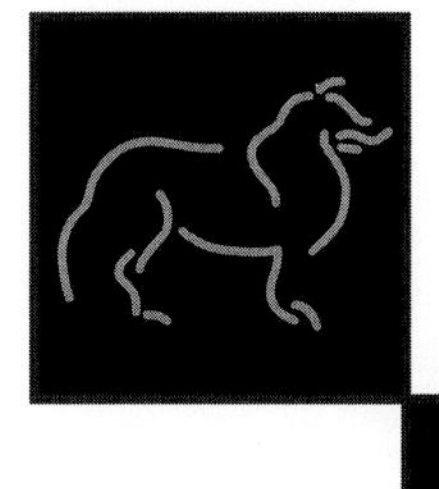

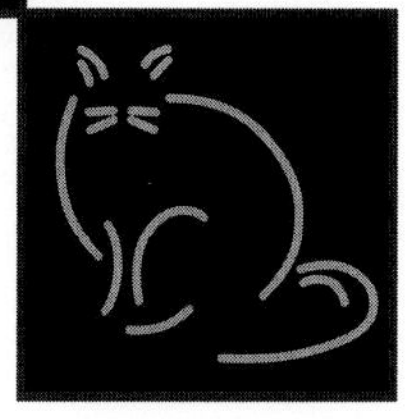

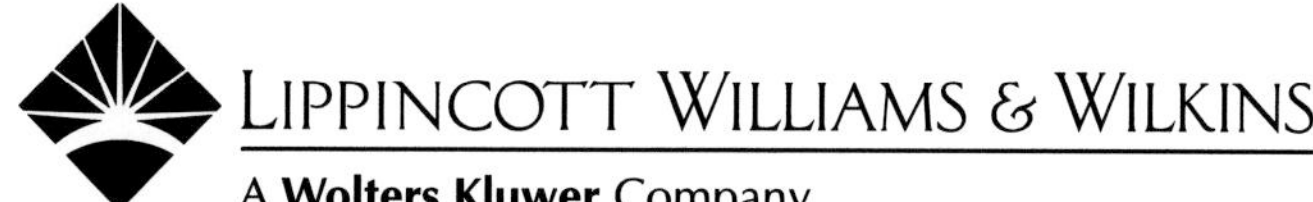

Philadelphia • Baltimore • New York • London
Buenos Aires • Hong Kong • Sydney • Tokyo

Acquisitions Editor: Paula Callaghan
Sponsoring Editor: Melissa J. James
Associate Managing Editor: Elizabeth A. Durand
Production Manager: Caren Erlichman
Production Coordinator: MaryClare Malady
Design Coordinator: Doug Smock
Interior Designer: Elizabeth Rudder
Cover Designer: Marty Malone
Indexer: Marjorie Cohen
Compositor: Circle Graphics
Printer/Binder: Quebecor / Kingsport

Small animal ultrasound / edited by Ronald W. Green.
p. cm.
Includes bibliographical references and index.
ISBN 0-397-51387-9 (hc : paper)
1. Dogs—Diseases—Diagnosis. 2. Cats—Diseases—Diagnosis.
3. Veterinary ultrasonography. I. Green, Ronald W.
SF991.S5956 1996 95-31392
636.7'08960743—dc20 CIP

The material contained in this volume was submitted as previously unpublished material, except in the instances in which credit has been given to the source from which some of the illustrative material was derived.

Great care has been taken to maintain the accuracy of the information contained in the volume. However, neither Lippincott Williams & Wilkins nor the editors can be held responsible for errors or for any consequences arising from the use of the information herein.

The authors and publisher have exerted every effort to ensure that drug selection and dosage set forth in this text are in accord with current recommendations and practice at the time of publication. However, in view of ongoing research, changes in government regulation, and the constant flow of information relating to drug therapy and drug reactions, the reader is urged to check the package insert for each drug for any change in indications and dosage and for added warnings and precautions. This is particularly important when the recommended agent is a new or infrequently employed drug.

9 8 7 6 5 4 3 2

To my wife, Judy,
and our children, Ryan and Nicole,
for making everything worthwhile.

Contributors

Robert J. Bahr, DVM
Diplomate, American College of Veterinary Radiology
Associate Professor of Veterinary Radiology
College of Veterinary Medicine
Oklahoma State University
Stillwater, Oklahoma

David S. Biller, DVM
Diplomate, American College of Veterinary Radiology
Associate Professor and Head of Radiology
College of Veterinary Medicine
Kansas State University
Manhattan, Kansas

Patrick W. Concannon, PhD
Senior Research Associate
College of Veterinary Medicine
Cornell University
Ithaca, New York

Charles S. Farrow, DVM
Diplomate, American College of Veterinary Radiology
Professor of Radiology
Western College of Veterinary Medicine
University of Saskatchewan
Saskatoon, Saskatchewan
Canada

Ronald W. Green, DVM, MS
Diplomate, American College of Veterinary Radiology
Associate Professor of Radiology and Ultrasound
College of Veterinary Medicine
Texas A&M University
College Station, Texas

Linda D. Homco, DVM
Diplomate, American College of Veterinary Radiology
Assistant Professor of Radiology and Ultrasound
College of Veterinary Medicine
Texas A&M University
College Station, Texas

Beth Paugh Partington, DVM, MS
Diplomate, American College of Veterinary Radiology
Assistant Professor of Radiology
School of Veterinary Medicine
Louisiana State University
Baton Rouge, Louisiana

Charles R. Pugh, DVM
Diplomate, American College of Veterinary Radiology
Assistant Professor of Radiology
School of Veterinary Medicine
University of Pennsylvania
Philadelphia, Pennsylvania

Philip F. Steyn, DVM, BVSc, MRCVS, MS
Diplomate, American College of Veterinary Radiology
Associate Professor of Radiology
College of Veterinary Medicine and Biomedical Sciences
Colorado State University
Fort Collins, Colorado

Michael A. Walker, DVM
Diplomate, American College of Veterinary Radiology
Diplomate, American College of Veterinary Radiology–Affiliate Radiation Oncology
Professor and Chief of Radiology
College of Veterinary Medicine
Texas A&M University
College Station, Texas

Amy E. Yeager, DVM
Diplomate, American College of Veterinary Radiology
Staff Veterinarian
New York State College of Veterinary Medicine
Cornell University
Ithaca, New York

FOREWORD

It is a distinct pleasure to write the forward for this important textbook of diagnostic ultrasonography. Veterinary sonography has expanded rapidly over the last two decades on a worldwide basis. Despite the explosive growth of this field, the extensive applications of sonographic techniques, and the need, few comprehensive veterinary sonographic reference texts are available.

As both an art and a science, ultrasound is a challenging subject to teach. This book is intended to give basic knowledge of veterinary diagnostic ultrasound to practicing ultrasonologists, students, and residents. It fills a void in the current veterinary ultrasound literature, as no comprehensive textbook on abdominal ultrasound has hitherto been available. Teaching beginning sonologists, residents, and students early in their careers in ultrasonography has proven frustrating until now because of the lack of a comprehensive textbook. This textbook is useful not only as a textbook for the beginner, but also as a resource for those more experienced to learn of other ideas and methods.

The task of compiling all the material necessary to complete a textbook is enormous and one that could not be done without the direction and encouragement of a dedicated and focused editor and the cooperation of excellent contributors. The authors who contributed chapters to this book are recognized experts in their fields. This textbook represents a culmination of information published by contributing sonologists and personal experience. As such it is useful as both a reference and a teaching text.

The book is organized into 20 chapters. It includes sections on the historical perspective of veterinary ultrasound, knobology, explanation of ultrasound terms, physics, and artifacts. One chapter is dedicated to the particulars of scanning techniques, and another to comparison of normal sonographic anatomy with similar sections on MRI. Sixteen chapters cover specific organs. Each chapter is organized with a preliminary discussion on sonographic technique and pertinent normal anatomy, followed by a review of abnormalities. Each chapter includes an extensive reference list. The book is completed with a glossary of ultrasound terms.

Diagnostic ultrasound involves both a physical and mental skill that is developed with practice. This book, either as a textbook or as a reference book, will be an asset for the emerging sonologist.

Kathy Spaulding, DVM
Associate Professor of Ultrasound
College of Veterinary Medicine
North Carolina State University
Raleigh, North Carolina

Preface

After graduating from veterinary college, I had the pleasure of working with Dr. W.C. Banks, a pioneer in veterinary radiology and a founding father in the American College of Veterinary Radiology. He told me that after Texas A&M obtained its first x-ray machine only one or two radiographs were made a week. Radiographs were such a novelty that clinicians would carry them around to show to the students and other veterinarians in the clinics. Some scoffed that radiology would never be used much in veterinary medicine; however, these critics were wrong. Today, it would be hard to imagine practicing veterinary medicine without radiography.

In 1981 Texas A&M purchased its first ultrasound machine for the small animal clinic. One or two sonograms were made a week, and they, too, were taken around the clinics as novelties. Again, some scoffed and said ultrasound would not be used much in veterinary medicine. Remarks such as "... and we thought before that radiologists had a great imagination" or "It looks like a thunderstorm located over Dallas to me," were heard. History repeated itself, and the skeptics were proved wrong. As with radiography, it would now be hard to imagine practicing veterinary medicine without ultrasound.

In 1988 diagnostic ultrasound was added to the radiology course taught to third-year veterinary students. In 1992, an elective diagnostic ultrasound course was added to the fourth-year curriculum. Also in 1992, Texas A&M had its first annual ultrasound short course for practicing veterinarians.

This book attempts to provide basic information about diagnostic ultrasound for the small animal practitioner. It is my sincere wish that this book present the complex field of small animal ultrasonography in a comprehensive and clinically relevant manner for both veterinary students and veterinarians alike.

Ronald W. Green, DVM

ACKNOWLEDGMENTS

This book required the efforts of many people. I would like to express my gratitude to Drs. Linda Homco, Mike Walker, and Earl Morris, and Mrs. Diane Bowen for reviewing the manuscripts.

The preparation of the manuscript has been difficult and at times tedious. I would like to thank Lauren Smith and Kristi Yancy for typing (and retyping) the manuscripts.

The photographers in Media Resource Services did a wonderful job in preparing photographs. I would like to express my gratitude to Tony Rydzewski, Beth Morgan, and Jan Worley for their photographic skills, as well as to Marty Malone for her work in graphic design.

I would like to thank Vicki Weir, Jane Thoos, Betsy McCauley, Joni Watkins, and Trisha Campbell for their excellent technical support.

Dr. Bill Moyer, head of the Department of Large Animal Medicine and Surgery, has been a real friend and I would like to express my gratitude for his support.

Thanks also go to Dr. Gary Norsworthy for constantly reminding me to produce something practical.

I am appreciative of the enthusiasm and patience of the people at Lippincott, especially Melissa James, Wendy Greenberger, and Mary K. Smith.

A very special thanks to Dr. Linda Homco, whose attention to detail, willingness to put in long hours, and constant encouragement made this book possible.

Contents

1

The Veterinarian and Ultrasound 1

Ronald W. Green

2

How Ultrasound Works 7

Charles S. Farrow

3

Ultrasound Scanning Techniques 29

Linda D. Homco

4

Heart 59

Charles S. Farrow

5

Thorax 89

Robert J. Bahr

6

Liver 105

Beth Paugh Partington and David S. Biller

7

Spleen 131

Beth Paugh Partington and David S. Biller

8
Gastrointestinal Tract 149
Linda D. Homco

9
Pancreas 177
Linda D. Homco

10
Kidneys 197
Ronald W. Green

11
Adrenal Glands 211
Linda D. Homco

12
Urinary Bladder 227
Ronald W. Green

13
Prostate Gland 237
Ronald W. Green and Linda D. Homco

14
Testes 251
Charles R. Pugh

15
Uterus 265
Amy E. Yeager and Patrick W. Concannon

16
Ovaries 293
Amy E. Yeager and Patrick W. Concannon

17
Lymph Nodes 305
Linda D. Homco

18
Eye 323
Phillip F. Steyn

19
Musculoskeletal System 335
Charles S. Farrow

20
Gross Anatomy of the Abdomen for the Ultrasonologist 353
Michael A. Walker

Glossary of Ultrasound Terms 363

Index 369

Small Animal Ultrasound, edited by Ronald W. Green.
Lippincott-Raven Publishers, Philadelphia © 1996.

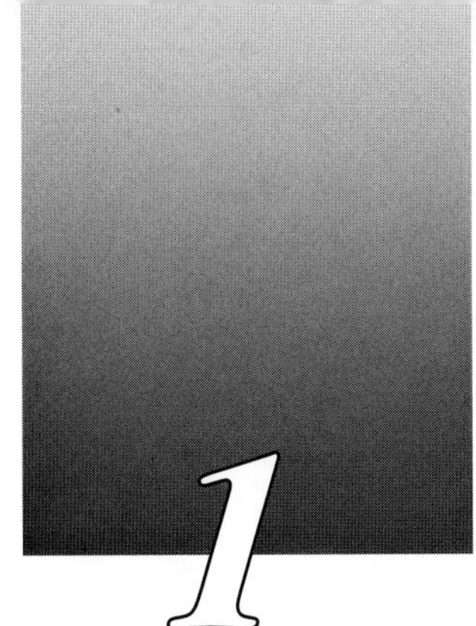

THE VETERINARIAN AND ULTRASOUND

Ronald W. Green

Ian Donald developed the first contact scanner or diagnostic ultrasound machine in 1957, and he pioneered its application in human obstetrics and gynecology.[1] The potential of this new imaging modality was quickly recognized. As image quality rapidly improved, the equipment became easier to operate, and ultrasonography became a common diagnostic tool in human medicine.

Animals were studied in ultrasound research as early as 1949, but it was not until the mid-1970s that a few veterinarians at academic institutions began using sonography on clinical patients.[2] Early reports showed that sonography had important diagnostic applications in veterinary medicine.[3–5] Sonography has become an important and popular diagnostic tool in veterinary medicine. Even the name of the official journal of the American College of Veterinary Radiology and the International Veterinary Radiology Association was changed in 1992 from *Veterinary Radiology* to *Veterinary Radiology & Ultrasound* to reflect ultrasound's increasing popularity. Part of ultrasound's popularity in veterinary medicine is because sonography is a simple, noninvasive diagnostic procedure that seldom requires the use of tranquilizers or anesthetics, and equipment that is affordable and easy to operate has become available. What began as a diagnostic tool available only at veterinary colleges is now used by veterinarians all across the country.

ADVANTAGES OF ULTRASOUND

As an imaging modality, ultrasound has many benefits. Diagnostic ultrasound is a nonionizing form of energy that has no known health risks. Shielding, lead gloves and aprons, film badges, special licensing, and government inspections are not required. Ultrasound images are the result of the acoustic properties of the object being imaged rather than its electron density, which is the basis for x-ray imaging. X-ray films can only differentiate five major densities in the body (ie, metal, bone, water or muscle, fat, and gas), but ultrasound can differentiate numerous types of tissues.

The way in which images are produced explains some of the advantages and disadvantages of ultrasound. Ultrasound is able to image radiolucent objects, such as urate and cystine uroliths, and foreign bodies, such as wood and string. The pancreas, adrenal glands, ovaries, lymph nodes, and internal structures of the eye are not normally recognized radiographically, but they are routinely evaluated sonographically. Free fluid (eg, pleural effusion, ascites) is easily penetrated by ultrasound, but it absorbs x-rays and blocks them from reaching the x-ray film. Gases are easily penetrated by x-ray but reflect ultrasound, which creates artifacts on the sonogram. Sonography can be used to detect pregnancy earlier than radiography. By day 21, canine and feline fetuses are easily detected with ultrasound, but radiography cannot detect a fetus until mineralization of the skeleton occurs at about day 38 of the pregnancy. Because the fetal heart can be monitored by using real-time ultrasound, fetal death is readily detected sonographically, but fetal death cannot be detected radiographically until major changes such as gas formation in the fetus or reabsorption of the fetal skeleton occurs. Real-time ultrasound allows the clinician to evaluate the movement of organs such as the heart and bowel. Organ movement can also be evaluated radiographically, but a fluoroscope is required. Another advantage of ultrasound over radiography is that it can be used to guide needles or biopsy instruments into an organ or mass.

Many special radiographic procedures such as cardioangiography, excretory urography, cystography, and upper gastrointestinal contrast studies can be replaced with sonography. Ultrasound often yields more diagnostic information with less effort on the part of the clinician, less stress to the patient, and less expense to the client. Abdominal sonography and ultrasound-guided biopsies often eliminate the need for exploratory laparotomies.

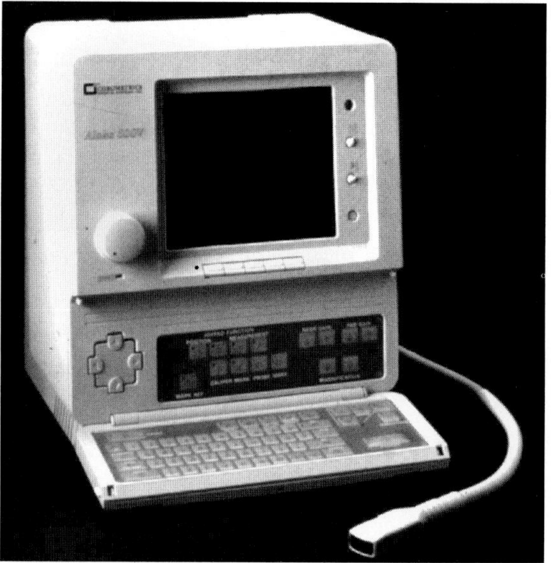

Figure 1-1. Portable ultrasound machine designed for veterinary use. (Courtesy of Corometrics Medical Systems, Incorporated, Wallingford, CT.)

CONSIDERATIONS BEFORE PURCHASE

Points to consider before purchasing a diagnostic ultrasound machine include cost, necessary education, and cost effectiveness.

How Much Will It Cost?

A new ultrasound machine equipped with a 5-MHz or 7.5-MHz transducer or both transducers costs between $14,000 and $35,000 (Figs. 1-1 and 1-2). This is a considerable investment for most veterinarians, and leasing is an option that should be considered. Leasing allows the veterinarian the use of new equipment without a substantial down payment. Because of the rapid technological advances in ultrasound equipment, a diagnostic ultrasound machine may become outdated rather quickly. Leasing is one way to maintain state-of-the-art technology in the clinic. Lease agreements vary, and the purchaser should fully understand the terms of the lease before entering into a contract.

Many physicians and hospitals replace their ultrasound machines when newer models become available. These used machines are usually available for resale. The purchase price of used equipment depends on the type, age, and condition of the equipment. Some of these units can be a real bargain, but the veterinarian should be aware that some machines are not well suited for veterinary use. A large motorized "portable" unit may not be considered portable in the average veterinary hospital. Transducers used for human patients often have a surface area or "footprint" that is too large and a frequency that is too low for small animal patients. Because service availability, especially on discontinued models, may also be a problem, a veterinarian should be very cautious when purchasing used equipment.

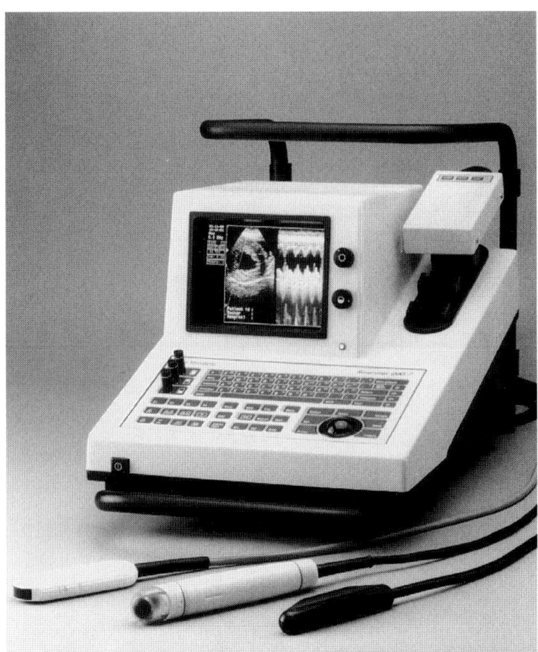

Figure 1-2. Portable ultrasound machine designed for veterinary use with sector, linear, and convex probes. (Courtesy of Classic Medical Supply, Inc., Tequesta, Florida.)

How Long Will It Take to Learn?

The training time is different for each individual, but learning how to use the ultrasound machine does require an investment of time and effort. Attending an ultrasound short course is a good starting place. Ideally, these courses provide individual experience with ultrasonography and often with a variety of machines. Reading the current issues of journals such as *Veterinary Radiology & Ultrasound* is also highly recommended. To be successful with ultrasound, the veterinarian must learn to use the ultrasound machine, scan the patient, and interpret the sonogram.

Understanding the Ultrasound Machine

The ultrasound machine with its computer keyboard, monitor, trackball, buttons, and knobs can be intimidating (Fig. 1-3). The first step in producing a sonographic image is to learn to use the machine properly. The first step is to study the owner's manual to learn the function of each button, switch, and knob. This is often referred to as "knobology." Knowledge of basic ultrasound physics facilitates understanding the function and use of the time-gain compensation control, the power control, and the depth control (see Chap. 2). When the veterinarian is comfortable with his or her ability to operate the ultrasound machine, the next step is to scan the patient.

Scanning the Patient

A good sonographer (one who makes sonograms) must be able to locate the organs of interest through an *acoustic window* (see Chap. 3). This requires a good working knowledge of anatomy (see Chap. 20). Sonographic anatomy is cross-sectional anatomy similar to that seen with computed tomography (CT) and magnetic resonance imaging (MRI). Because the sonogram is a two-dimensional display of a three-dimensional object, the sonographer must think in three dimensions while he or she is scanning the patient. Sonography is operator dependent. To view the image on the monitor and move the transducer on the patient in the desired direction requires good eye-hand coordination. To find an appropriate acoustic window for scanning demands a knowledge of anatomy and ultrasound and requires problem solving skills. Scanning is a physical skill and a mental skill that is developed by practice. In producing a high-quality sonogram, the sonographer's ability to scan the patient is equally important to his or her ability to use the ultrasound machine.

Interpreting the Sonogram

The sonologist (one who interprets sonograms) has to have the knowledge of a sonographer (ie, anatomy and ultrasound physics) plus the skills of a diagnostician. The patient history, clinical signs, laboratory findings, and radiographic findings must be incorporated into the final interpretation of the sonogram. Sonograms are sensitive but often nonspecific for the diagnosis of tissue abnormalities. Some diseases

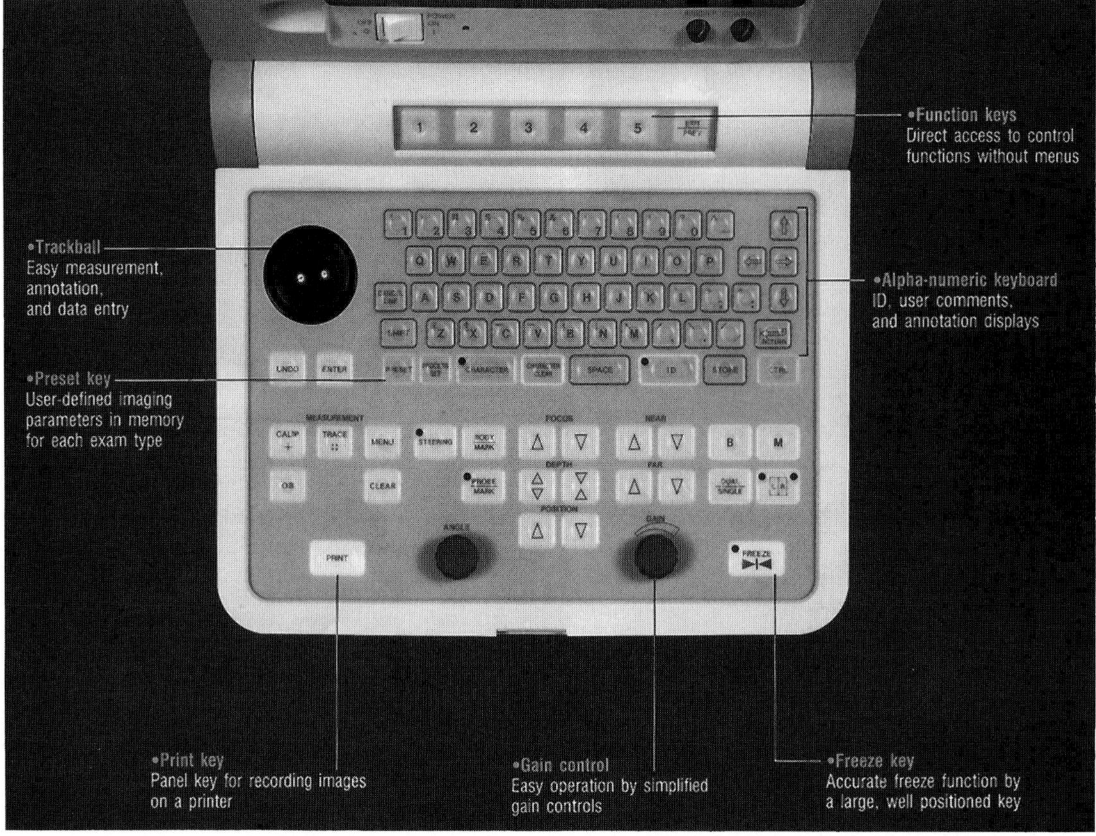

Figure 1-3. Keyboard of ultrasound machine. (Courtesy of Hitachi Corporation, Tarrytown, NY.)

generate no sonographic changes, some produce the same sonographic changes as other diseases, and some diseases cause a variety of sonographic changes. Fine-needle aspirates and biopsies are often employed in conjunction with sonography to make a specific diagnosis.

Will It Be Cost Effective?

In most cases, ultrasound is cost effective. Clients typically want the best affordable care for their pets. When compared with other diagnostic procedures, such as exploratory surgery, special radiographic procedures, nuclear medicine, CT, or MRI, ultrasound often provides the most diagnostic information for the least expenditure. There is minimal patient preparation and no patient aftercare for ultrasound.

CONCLUSION

Sonography is an important diagnostic tool available to the veterinarian. Because a concerted effort is required to become proficient in its use, it is important to attend seminars and workshops, study the literature, and practice with the machine.

REFERENCES

1. Donald I, MacVicar J, Brown TG. Investigation of abdominal masses by pulsed ultrasound. Lancet 1958;1:1189.
2. Ludwig GD. Report of the 81st meeting of the Society of Clinical Surgery, Boston, MA, November 1, 1949.

3. Pipers FS, Hamlin RL. Clinical use of echocardiography in the domestic cat. J Am Vet Med Assoc 1980;176:57.
4. Nyland TG, Park RD, Lattimer JC, et al. Gray scale ultrasonography of the canine abdomen. Vet Radiol 1981;22:220.
5. Cartee RE. Diagnostic real-time ultrasonography of the liver of the dog and cat. J Am Anim Hosp Assoc 1981;17:731.

Small Animal Ultrasound, edited by Ronald W. Green.
Lippincott-Raven Publishers, Philadelphia © 1996.

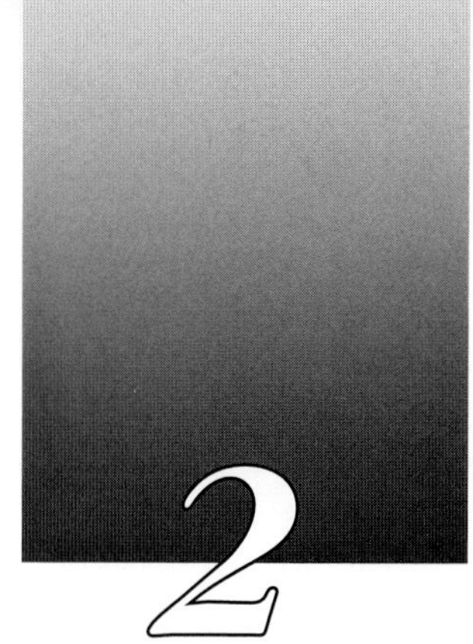

HOW ULTRASOUND WORKS

Charles S. Farrow

Ultrasonography is used to produce two-dimensional, gray-scale anatomic images, principally of internal organs, for the purpose of medical diagnosis. Images are obtained by placing a hand-held scanner on the surface of an animal and pulsing high-frequency sound waves into an area of interest. Portions of these waves are returned to the scanner, where they are detected and processed electronically for near-instantaneous viewing on a television screen. The resultant images may be displayed continuously (ie, real time) or individually as freeze frames. The appearance of the image may be modified by the operator using a series of electronic controls, variable scanning angles, and different transducer frequencies.

Most organs are well suited to ultrasound diagnosis, but there are exceptions. Air-containing structures, such as the lung, stomach, and bowel, reflect most of the ultrasound beam at their surfaces because of their extremely low relative density compared with adjacent soft tissue. The interior of these organs cannot be imaged, nor can anything beyond be seen. Bone causes the same problems because of its high relative density compared with surrounding tissues.

THE BEHAVIOR OF SOUND WAVES INSIDE THE BODY

As the sound beam departs the scanner and enters the body on its journey to the area of interest, it momentarily vibrates the tissue through which it passes, after which the tissue relaxes and returns to its original form. This process of vibration and relaxation is repeated over and over again as the ultrasound beam travels deeper into the body, with each individual cycle initiating the next.[1] An ultrasound beam may be characterized by its frequency, the number of times per second that it vibrates a particular point within a tissue. A typical ultrasound scanner emits a beam that vibrates millions of times per second; the most commonly used frequencies are 5 and 7.5 MHz. A megahertz is equal to one million vibrations per second. Imagined in ultraslow motion, the described events loosely resemble "the wave" performed by exuberant fans in a football stadium. Eventually, the energy of the beam is exhausted or attenuated as a result of various types of tissue interactions, and it is incapable of producing any further images. These interactions between the ultrasound beam and the tissues through which it passes include reflection, refraction, and absorption.[1]

Reflection

The most important ultrasound beam interaction with tissue is reflection, which is responsible for the return of a portion of the sound beam to the scanner, where it is processed for display. It is this reflection process that creates the echoes that eventually are represented as an image on the television screen.

Echoes are created as sound waves pass from one tissue interface to the next and are strongly dependent on the difference in the sound-transmission qualities of the two tissues. The greater this difference, the greater is the resultant echo.

The rate at which a particular tissue transmits ultrasound depends on its density, which determines the speed of ultrasound in that particular tissue. Together, the two qualities of density and speed are used to calculate the acoustic impedance of a tissue.[1] Among the various body organs, the lung exhibits the poorest sound transmission because of the very low density of its large air content. Bone transmits sound readily because of its high density. The heart, vasculature, kidneys, liver, spleen, muscles, tendons, ligaments, and fat possess intermediate sound-transmission qualities.

The strongest echoes are produced between tissues having the greatest difference in acoustic impedance.[1] Strong echoes, however, are not always desirable. The stomach, because it usually contains air, reflects most of the ultrasound beam, and as a consequence, nothing is seen beyond the soft tissue–air interface. The same is true of interfaces involving bone or extensively mineralized tissue.

The echoes generated by the reflections of the ultrasound beam at the tissue interfaces within the body are what eventually form the sonographic image that appears on the television monitor. Using a conventional white-on-black image format, a strong echo appears white; an intermediate-strength echo shows as a light or medium shade of gray; a weak echo is represented by dark gray; and the absence of an echo is expressed as black. These sonographic appearances are called, respectively, hyperechoic, echoic, hypoechoic, and anechoic, and they comprise in part the descriptive language of ultrasound.[2]

Refraction

When an ultrasound beam passes from one tissue to another in a nonperpendicular plane, it is said to be bent or angled. This bending or change in direction of the beam is called refraction, and it causes a loss of image clarity (ie, decreased resolution).[1] If severe, refraction can make structures appear to be in the wrong location on the television monitor. Like reflection, refraction dissipates the energy of the ultrasound beam.

Absorption

Absorption of the ultrasound beam (sonic energy) refers to its conversion to heat (thermal energy). The rate of absorption is affected by three factors: the frequency of the sound beam, tissue viscosity, and the amount of time required by a tissue to return to its undisturbed state after the sound wave has passed (ie, relaxation time).[1] Only one of these factors, the transducer frequency, can be manipulated by the examiner. Like reflection and refraction, tissue absorption reduces beam strength.

INSIDE AN ULTRASOUND MACHINE

Although they vary in appearance, ultrasound machines share many of the same electronic components. These may include a scanner containing one or more transducers, a pulser, a receiver, a pair of signal converters, preprocessors and postprocessors, memory storage, an image recorder and photography unit, and a monitor. The pathway traveled by a reflected sound wave through an ultrasound machine to its eventual destination as a screen image is shown in Figure 2-1.

The Scanner

Contemporary scanners contain one or more specialized crystals that are designed to produce bursts of high-frequency sound when momentarily deformed by an electric current. They are

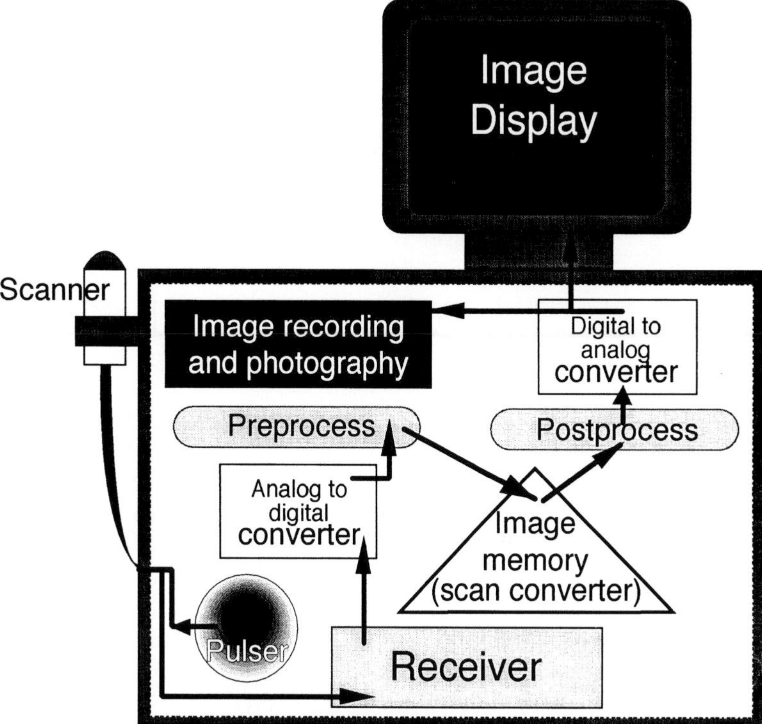

Figure 2-1. Diagram of the major internal components of an ultrasound machine. Interconnecting arrows show the pathway traveled by reflected sound waves as they negotiate the circuitry on their way to becoming a screen image.

called transducers because of their capacity to convert one form of energy to another (ie, electrical to sound and vice versa). These crystals are also able to detect and change the reflected sound waves, called echoes, emanating from the patient into electrical signals that are required for television viewing. Single crystals or crystalline composites are usually mechanically operated, and multiple crystals arranged in various configurations, called arrays, are typically controlled electronically.[3]

The Pulser

The pulser sends electric signals to the transducer located inside the scanner, causing the crystal to vibrate and emit ultrasound pulses. The number of electrical pulses generated per second is the pulse repetition frequency (PRF).[4] When the pulse frequency is multiplied by the pulse duration, the duty factor (ie, percentage of total operational time that the scanner is emitting sound) is determined. For most automatic scanners, the duty factor is about 5%.[5] The scanner spends most of its time detecting incoming echoes and only a comparatively brief period in the sending mode.

The acoustic power, which is the strength of the electrical signal produced by the pulser, can be adjusted by the operator using the power output control. Increasing the power increases the sensitivity of the scanner, enabling it to detect and display weaker echoes. Increasing the pulse intensity also increases the amount of heat produced in the tissues by the ultrasound beam.

The Receiver

The receiver initiates the electrical processing of the echo signals obtained from the scanner for their eventual display on the television monitor. The receiver increases the strength of the incoming echoes by amplifying their electrical signals.[4] The amount of signal amplification is called the gain of the receiver. Typically expressed in sound units called decibels, receiver gain may be calculated by dividing the strength

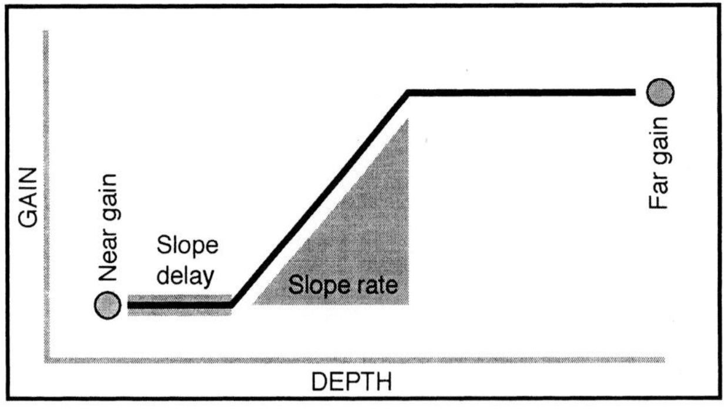

Figure 2-2. Graph of the four principal time-gain compensation controls: near gain, slope delay, slope rate, and far gain.

of the amplified electrical signal by the strength of the nonamplified signal.

Because of tissue attenuation, distant echoes are weak compared with echoes originating close to the scanner. The receiver evens out these differences in signal strengths through a process known as time-gain compensation. In a commonly used form of time-gain compensation, receiver amplification is increased with time after the transmitted pulse so that the echoes produced by distant tissues are amplified more than those arriving from nearby structures.

The receiver is also responsible for signal compression, a process that reduces the difference between large and small amplitude signals so that components handling the signals after the receiver may do so with greater selectivity.[4]

Like home stereo receivers, ultrasound receivers may be electronically evaluated by their specifications. For example, dynamic range indicates the spectrum of electrical signals that the receiver can respond to without distortion.

Signal Conversion and Signal Processing

The first signal conversion after amplification by the receiver is by the analog-to-digital converter. The electrical signal is transformed into a numeric or digital format before being preprocessed.

Signal processing refers to the manipulation of digitized echo signals before and after being stored in memory. If the signals are adjusted before memory storage, it is called preprocessing.[4] Preprocessing is exemplified by the gain settings employed by the ultrasound machine at start-up and before the controls have been adjusted by the operator. Postprocessing is performed on the image after it has been placed into memory and preceding its display on the monitor.[4] For example, the values of stored digital echoes may be altered to change their appearance on the monitor.

Memory Storage

Echo signals from the receiver are stored in a scan converter as digital memory corresponding to the location and strength of the echo. The contents of the memory are read out on a television monitor, forming a sonogram. In the case of motion-mode ultrasound, the data are also processed in memory and displayed on the monitor as a continuous trace of echo location versus time.

Image Viewing and Recording

Television monitors, which are cathode ray tubes, display information from memory as a pair of interwoven gray-scale fields composed of 256 lines each. Together, the fields combine to create a 512-line image that is changed (ie, refreshed) every 0.033 of a second. Increased resolution may be achieved by increasing the number of lines in the image, which is a function of monitor design.

The screen images may be recorded on videotape, individually photographed from the screen on Polaroid film, printed on thermal paper, or placed on x-ray film with a multiformat camera.

KNOBOLOGY: ULTRASOUND CONTROLS AND HOW TO USE THEM

There are numerous and variably appearing controls on different ultrasound machines. The most influential of these are designed to regulate the strength of the echoes originating from the underlying tissues. Because these structures are located at different depths, the echoes they generate vary greatly in intensity, sometimes by a factor of over a million. If the weak distant echoes are not strengthened (ie, amplified) to match the stronger superficial signals, they become invisible on the television monitor. This electronic enhancement or evening-out process is called time-gain compensation, which is regulated by four controls: near gain, slope delay, slope rate, and far gain (Fig. 2-2). There also are controls for beam power, depth, and image enlargement, and numerous secondary adjustments are available through a touch pad located on the scanner deck.

Time-Gain Compensation

Let us begin by seeing what happens when each of the four time-gain compensation controls are adjusted and then consider the basis for the observed changes.

Figure 2-3 shows a cross-sectional image of a dog's liver in which the time-gain compensation controls have been preset by the ultrasound machine. These selections are called the *default settings*. Compare this sonogram with the appearance of the following images in which the various time-gain compensation settings have been increased or decreased by the sonographer.

The *near gain* control is often used to decrease the strength of echoes originating close to the scanner when more distant organs are being examined.[6] When superficial structures are being studied, the near gain may be increased or left in the default position (Figs. 2-4 and 2-5).

An increase in *slope delay* increases the depth at which the time-gain compensation controls begin to take effect on weaker echoes; a decease in delay has the opposite effect (Fig. 2-6).

Perhaps the easiest way to understand *slope rate* is to picture it as a diagonal line representing the relative amounts of amplification applied to echoes located at increasingly distant

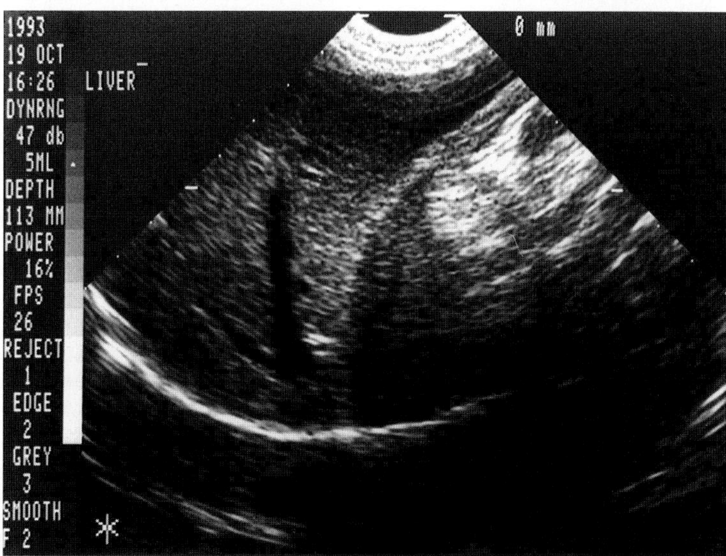

Figure 2-3. Sector scan of a dog's liver in which the time-gain compensation (TGC) controls have been preset by the ultrasound machine.

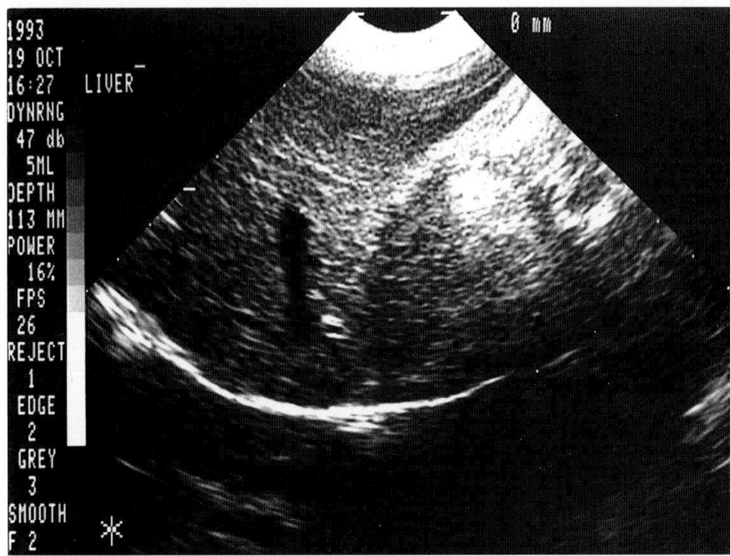

Figure 2-4. Sector scan of a dog's liver in which the near gain has been increased.

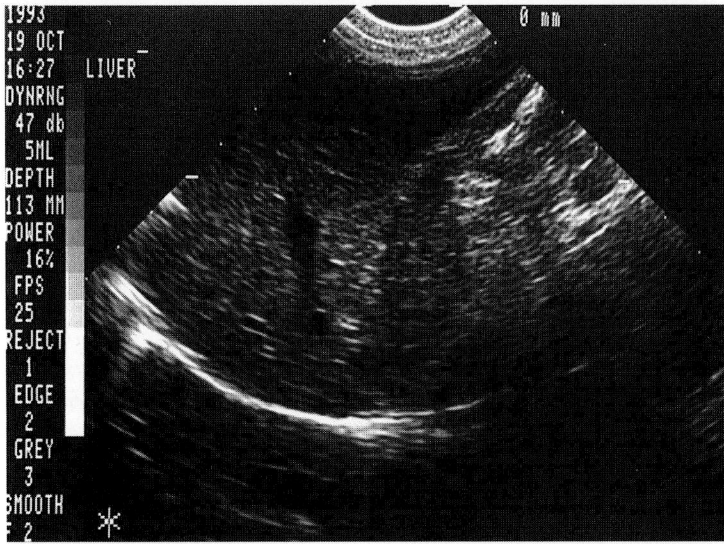

Figure 2-5. Sector scan of a dog's liver in which the near gain has been reduced.

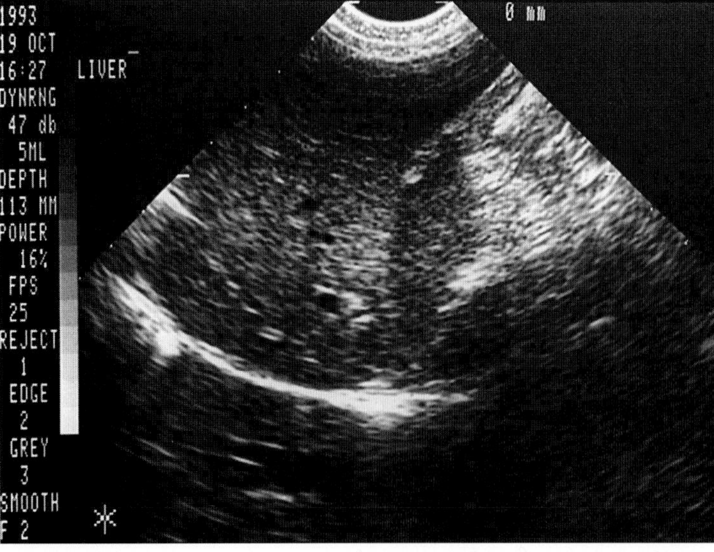

Figure 2-6. Sector scan of a dog's liver in which the slope delay has been increased.

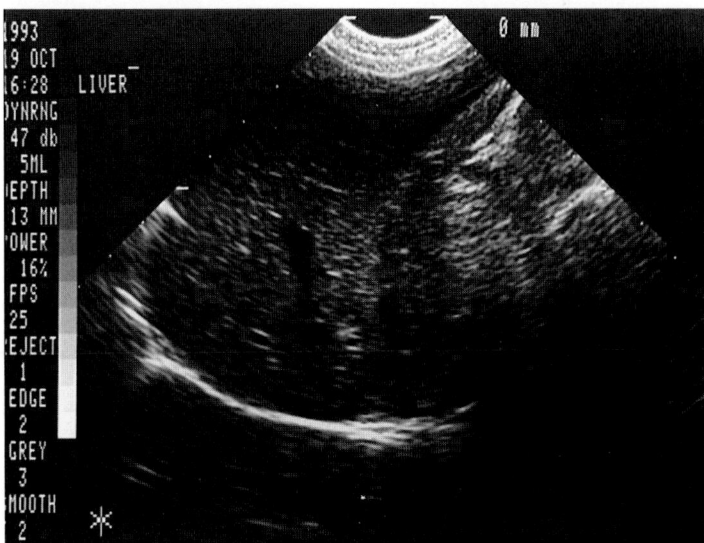

Figure 2-7. Sector scan of a dog's liver in which the slope rate has been increased.

points from the scanner.[6] Conceiving of slope rate in this manner enables the examiner to understand how echo strength may be equalized regardless of depth (Figs. 2-7 and 2-8).

Deep or distant echoes may be enhanced by increasing the *far gain* (Figs. 2-9 and 2-10).

Power, Depth, and Zoom Controls

Increasing the *power setting* increases the energy of the ultrasound beam, which boosts echo strength. Unlike the time-gain compensation controls, which affect echoes at a particular depth, changes in power affect echoes at all levels (Figs. 2-11 and 2-12).[6]

The *depth control* increases or decreases the depth at which the tissues are optimally displayed.[6] The lower the transducer frequency, the greater is the depth that can be imaged (Figs. 2-13 and 2-14).

The *zoom* or image magnification control is typically trackball activated. It places a "box" on the screen, which can be moved to a region of interest and which may be enlarged using another

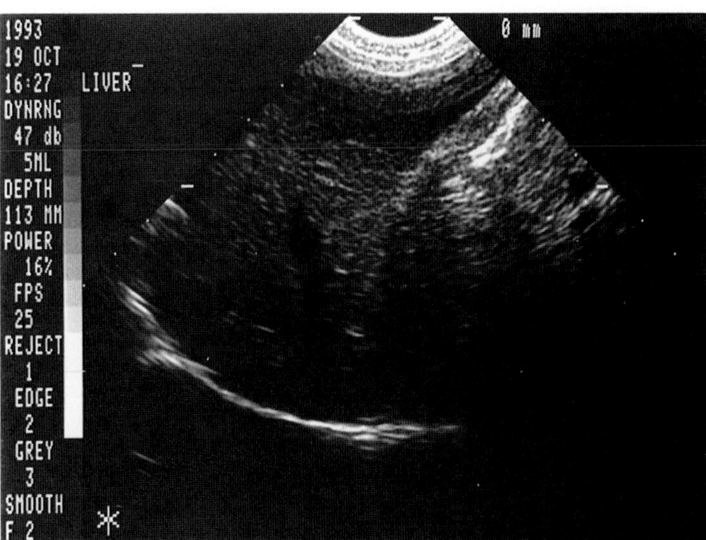

Figure 2-8. Sector scan of a dog's liver in which the slope rate has been decreased.

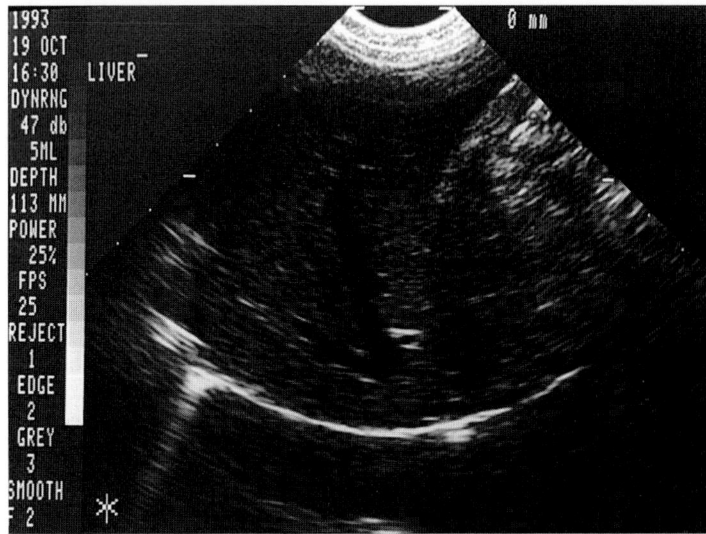

Figure 2-9. Sector scan of a dog's liver in which the far gain has been increased.

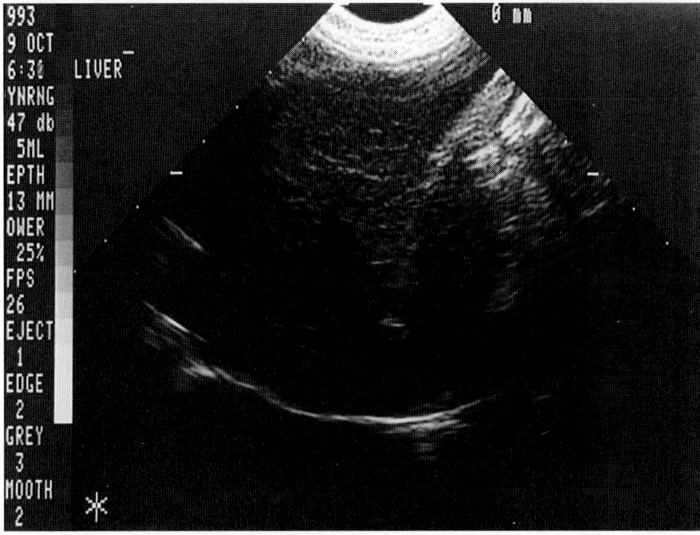

Figure 2-10. Sector scan of a dog's liver in which the far gain has been decreased.

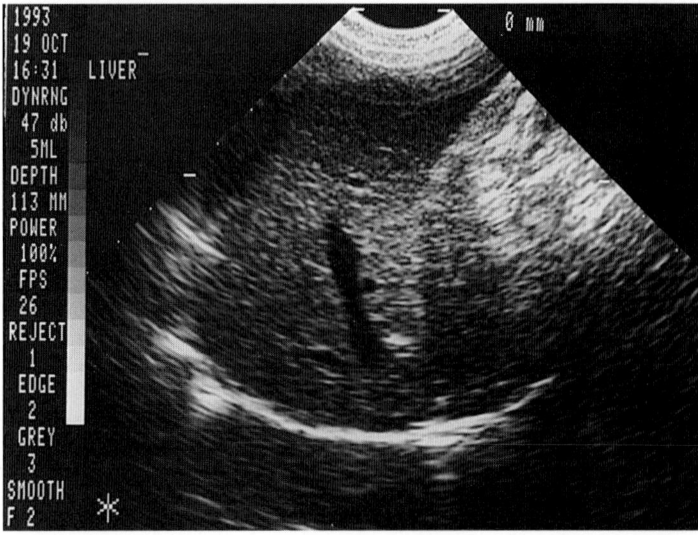

Figure 2-11. Sector scan of a dog's liver in which the power has been increased.

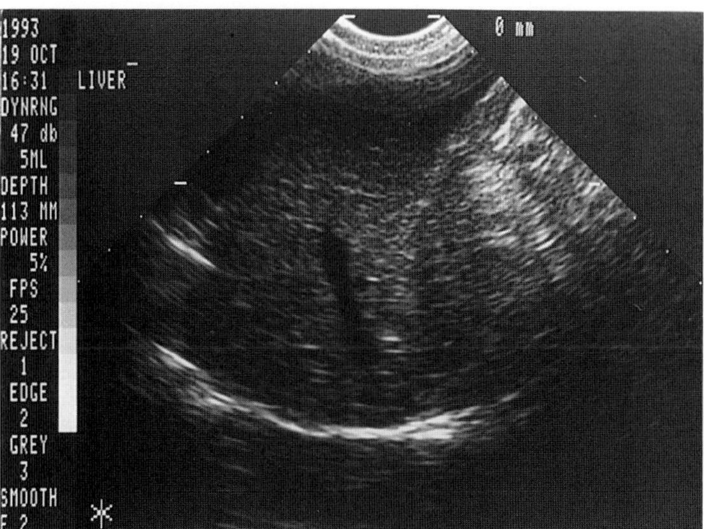

Figure 2-12. Sector scan of a dog's liver in which the power has been decreased.

control. As the screen image is enlarged, its sharpness is reduced.[6]

Secondary Controls

Transducer Selection

Some ultrasound scanners contain multiple transducers, each of which emits a different ultrasound frequency. The most common combination is 3, 5, and 7.5 MHz. The desired frequency is selected by the sonographer before starting the examination.

Dual Image

In addition to being viewed in real time or as a single freeze frame, the ultrasound image may be divided into two individual images. This viewing format is called a split or dual image.[6] Splitting is useful for comparing different phases of the cardiac cycle, the relative

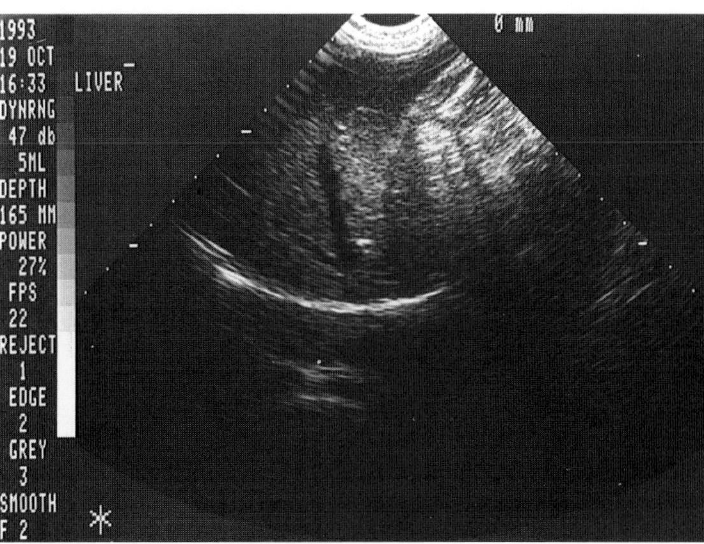

Figure 2-13. Sector scan of a dog's liver in which the depth has been increased to the maximum.

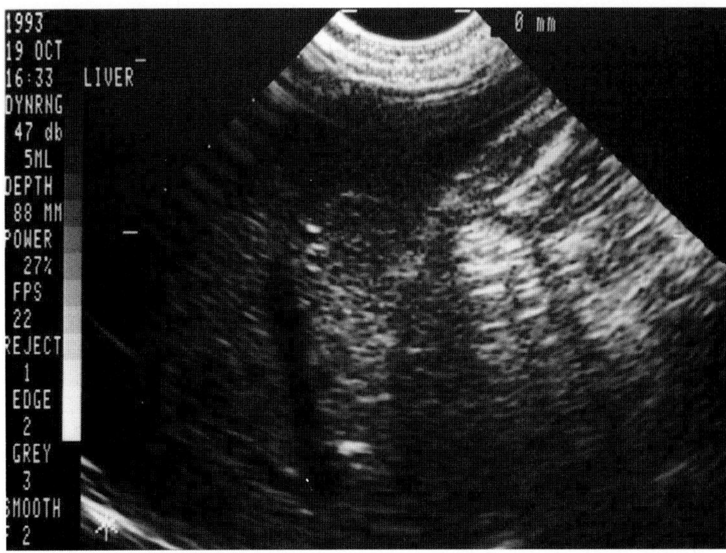

Figure 2-14. Sector scan of a dog's liver in which the depth has been reduced to better see the large vein located in the middle and far fields.

echogenicity of different organs, or parts of an organ (Fig. 2-15).

Mode Selection

Most ultrasound machines default to *regular mode,* consisting of a two-dimensional sector scan. This mode may be modified by selecting a broad or narrow display, the former providing greater resolution but a smaller field of view. *Motion mode* (M-mode) is employed when specific aspects of cardiac function are calculated from time-motion tracings (Fig. 2-16). *Biopsy mode* is used when organ or lesion samples are obtained with sonographic guidance. A *Doppler ultrasound* machine may operate in different modes as well: continuous wave, pulsed wave, and color flow.

Video Invert

Image background and foreground selection may be controlled using the invert control. In negative video mode, which is the most common viewing format, the image is displayed in various shades of gray against a black background

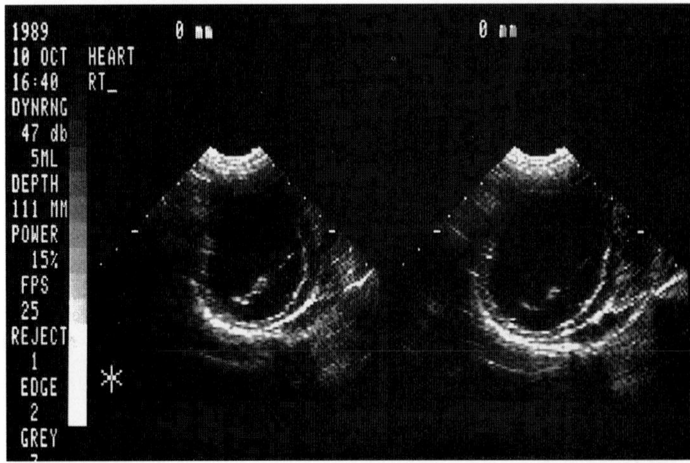

Figure 2-15. Dual cross-sectional images of a dog's dilated left ventricle made at different times during the cardiac cycle.

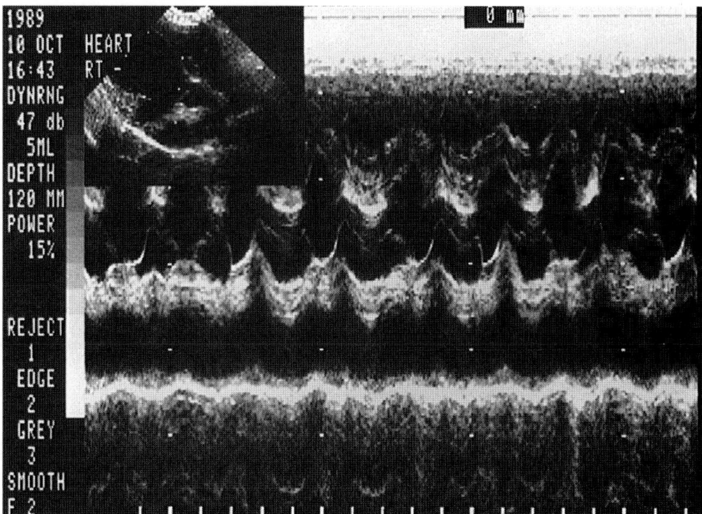

Figure 2-16. M-mode image of a dog's heart. A miniature sector scan appears in the upper left corner showing the direction of the ultrasound beam (*dotted line*) relative to a long-axis view of the heart.

(Fig. 2-17). This format is best for viewing textural detail in the sonographic image. Structural outline may sometimes be better appreciated as a dark image on a white background, also called a positive video mode (Fig. 2-18).

Recording Screen Images

Screen images may be recorded in a number of different ways. Individual freeze frames are usually printed on thermal paper or Polaroid positive film, and cardiac studies are typically videotaped. Individual screen images may also be put on x-ray film in various configurations, usually six images on an 8 × 10 inch film.

Adjusting the Television Picture

The television image may be adjusted with the contrast and brightness controls located on the monitor. Although in part subjective, these controls may be objectively set by using the gray-scale bar located on the margin of the image. The contrast and brightness settings are

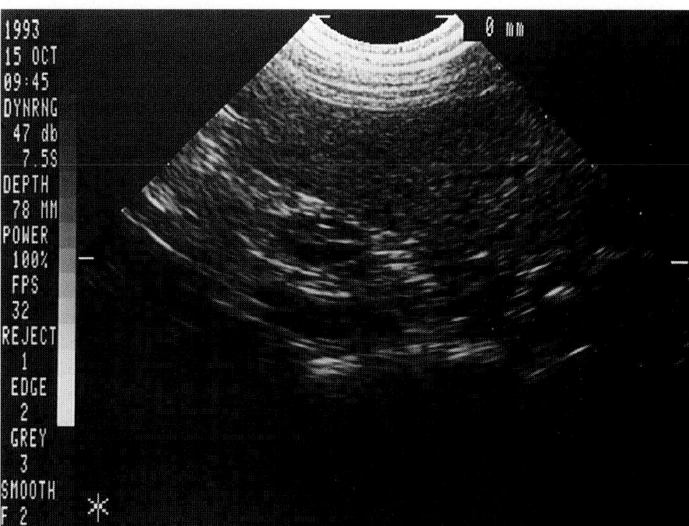

Figure 2-17. Sector scan of a dog's spleen displayed in negative video mode (ie, white echoes on a black background).

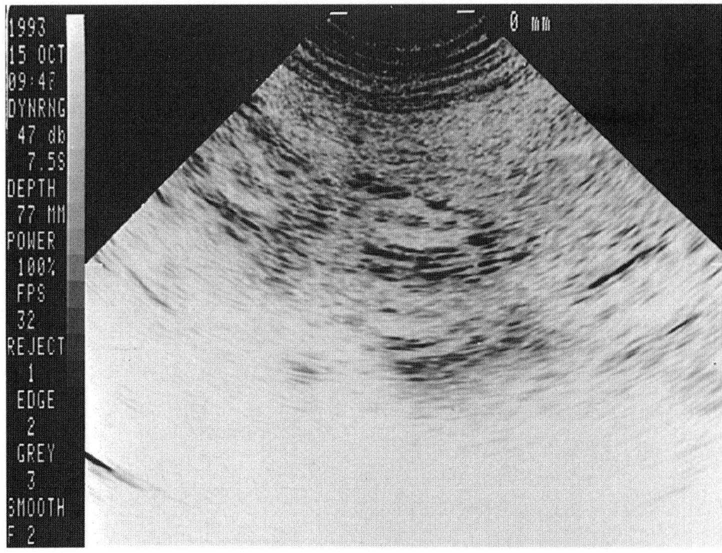

Figure 2-18. Sector scan of a dog's spleen displayed in positive video mode (ie, black echoes on a white background).

optimal when all of the elements on the gray-scale bar are discernible.

Measuring Screen Images and Their Depth

Structural height and width may be measured with electronic calipers on the screen image (Fig. 2-19). Some machines also are capable of calculating circumference and area from a broken line placed around an area of interest with the trackball.

TYPES OF ULTRASOUND MACHINES

Real-Time Ultrasound

Contemporary ultrasound machines operate electronically in what is called real time. The

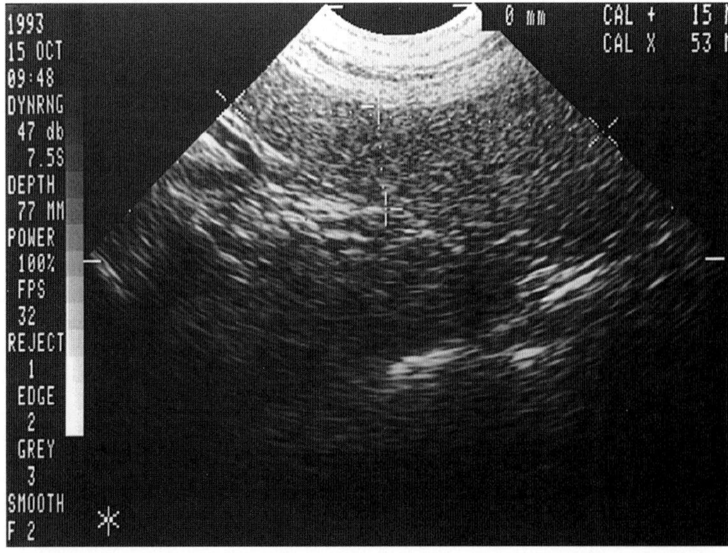

Figure 2-19. Sector scan of a dog's spleen shows paired electronic calipers positioned for height and width measurements, which appear in the upper right corner.

image displayed on the television monitor appears to be "live" by virtue of its movement. In reality, the examiner views a series of rapidly changing still images that only simulate motion. Another way to conceptualize real-time imagery is to think of it as information that is being displayed at about the same rate as it is being obtained.

Depending on the number and arrangement of transducers, screen images appear to be rectangular or triangular. Ultrasound machines producing a rectangular image are called linear array or rectilinear scanners, and those displaying a triangular image are called sector scanners.[3] Linear units employ a series of stationary transducers that are electronically controlled, and sector scanners may be mechanically operated from a point source or electronically controlled.

All modern scanners use gray-scale imaging. This means that the individual echoes that produce the screen image are assigned specific shades of gray according to their signal strength. Weak echoes appear dark gray, and stronger echoes appear light gray. Maximum-strength echoes such as those generated from soft tissue–air and soft tissue–bone interfaces appear white, and fluid typically generates almost no echoes and appears black.

Motion-Mode Sonography

M-mode sonography, a form of echocardiography, displays the various surfaces of the heart as a series of irregular lines oriented horizontally on the image (see Fig. 2-16).[7] The distances between these lines are used to measure the thickness of the heart at different points, the chamber sizes, and motion over time.

Doppler Ultrasound

Doppler ultrasound is used to detect motion, specifically within blood vessels. There are four types of Doppler ultrasound machines: continuous wave, pulsed wave, duplex, and color flow.[1] The simplest of these is continuous wave Doppler, in which the scanner contains a pair of transducers, one to emit ultrasound and another to detect the returning echoes. The frequency difference between the outgoing and incoming signals is the *Doppler shift*, and when amplified, it may be recorded and used to obtain velocity information.[8]

Pulsed wave Doppler is superior to continuous wave technology because it includes depth and velocity information. Both continuous wave and pulsed wave information are typically presented as a jagged line, representing the plot of Doppler shift versus time.

Duplex scanners couple a Doppler unit (usually pulsed wave type) with real-time sector imaging. Such combinations allow the operator to locate and identify correctly the area of interest and then freeze it on the screen. The Doppler unit is then activated and electronic calipers are used to mark more precisely the sampling area within the frozen screen image.

Color flow Doppler superimposes a color Doppler image on a gray-scale real-time image, and in this respect, is like a duplex scanner.[8] Unlike duplex scanners, which obtain flow information from only a small part of the total image, Doppler color flow provides imaging of flow throughout the entire real-time image. Color flow scans are obtained using a pulse-echo technique similar to that for gray scale imaging. However, instead of displaying the returning echoes in gray scale according to signal strength, echoes are shown in different colors that correspond to flow directions. The brightness of the color represents the intensity of the echoes. Although many colors may be selected by the operator, red is usually assigned to arteries and blue to veins.

ULTRASOUND ARTIFACTS

Sonographic artifacts are any unintended information on an image that does not represent the object. Artifacts may be caused by equipment deficiencies, peculiar patient structural features, or image processing. Recognition of characteristic artifacts is important in interpreting images and for reducing diagnostic errors. Artifacts in sonography occur as structures that are not real, missing, improperly located, or of improper brightness, shape, or size.[9]

Although considered as errors, some artifacts are beneficial in understanding the characteristics of a lesion or structure. Distant enhancement and acoustic shadowing are two such artifacts.

Distant enhancement (ie, enhanced through transmission) occurs because the ultrasound machine anticipates that there will be attenuation of the sound beam as it penetrates soft tissue. To maintain uniform brightness, the machine adjusts echoes from deep structures to provide uniform intensity.[10] When the sound travels through a fluid-filled structure, the expected attenuation does not occur. The machine falsely amplifies the signal, which results in the appearance of an enhanced signal.[11] Tissues distal to a fluid-filled structure are enhanced or made brighter (Fig. 2-20). This artifact is useful in detecting abscesses, cysts, and effusions.

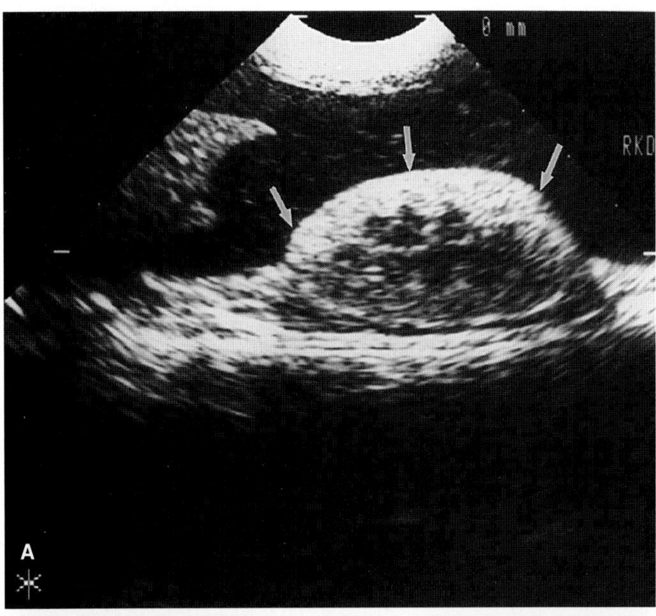

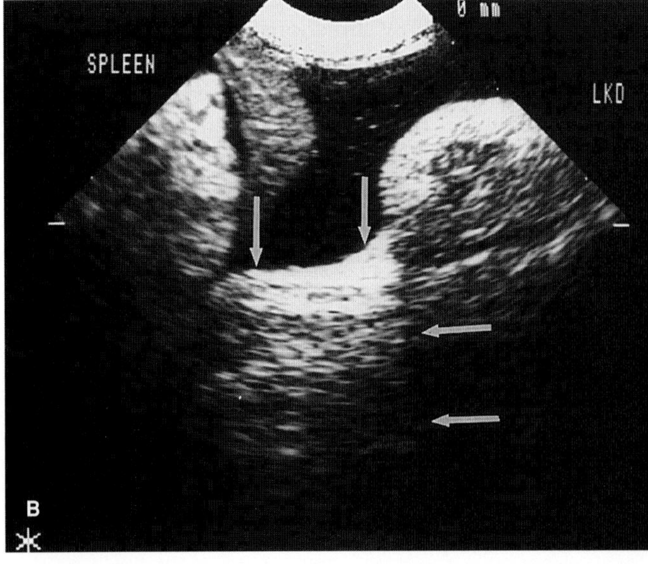

Figure 2-20. Sagittal sonograms of the cranial portion of an abdomen with ascites. (**A**) Notice the bright echoes (*arrows*) from the right renal cortex (*RKD*) and (**B**) the bright echoes (*arrows*) from the dorsal musculature between the spleen and left kidney (*LKD*). These echoes are caused by distant enhancement.

Acoustic shadowing occurs when the ultrasound beam strikes highly attenuating tissues such as compact bone or calcified masses. Because of the high attenuation of ultrasound in these tissues, no sound travels beyond the structure, and an anechoic or hypoechoic "shadow" is seen distal to the ultrasound-tissue interface (Fig. 2-21).[10,12] This artifact is useful in detecting cystic and renal calculi, choleliths, dystrophic mineralization, and mineralizing tumors. Acoustic shadowing is also helpful in monitoring the development of the fetal skeleton.

Reverberation occurs when the sound beam is perpendicular to a highly reflective object such as gas or metal.[10] Sound reflection from such an interface strikes the transducer and reenters the patient. When this echo returns to the transducer, it receives a spatial assignment twice as deep as the original reflector. This "round trip" of the sound may be repeated several times, resulting in an image characterized by repetitive interfaces occurring at regular intervals and decreasing in intensity with depth (Fig. 2-22).[13]

A *ring-down artifact* is a particular type of reverberation artifact in which numerous parallel lines are seen for a considerable distance, frequently observed behind each of the higher-amplitude linear reverberation echoes.[11,12] This type of artifact is usually the result of a small but strong reflector, such as gas bubbles or metal (Fig. 2-23).

A *comet tail* appears as a trail of dense continuous echoes resulting from multiple internal reverberations within a small reflector such as gas or metal.[12] Because the echo bands are closely spaced and very intense, they appear to merge and create a comet tail that rapidly diminishes in intensity on the image (Fig. 2-24).[10]

A *refraction* or *edge shadow* artifact occurs when the incident beam interacts with a curved surface. The sound beam is bent and diverges, resulting in a narrow or broad shadow deep to the curved surface.[12,13] Typically, this artifact is created by the gallbladder, kidneys, cysts, and fetal skull (Fig. 2-25).

A *mirror-image artifact* may occur adjacent to highly reflective acoustic interfaces such as the diaphragm or pleura.[10] Reverberations develop between a mass or structure such as the gallbladder and the reflective surface. This phenomenon doubles the round-trip time for the returning echo from each point within the structure and registers the echoes created by this structure equidistant from and on the opposite side of the reflector.[12,13] This artifact is most frequently seen with hepatic sonography during which a duplicate gallbladder appears on the opposite side of the diaphragm (Fig. 2-26), but it

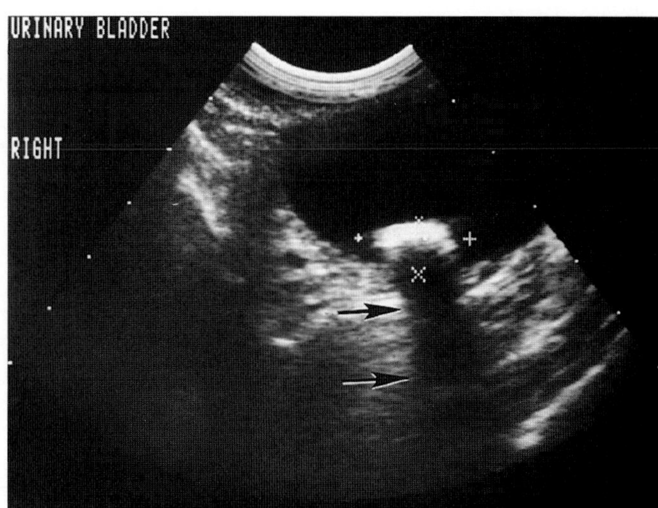

Figure 2-21. Transverse sonogram of the urinary bladder with acoustic shadowing (*arrows*) resulting from a cystic calculus (+ and x calipers).

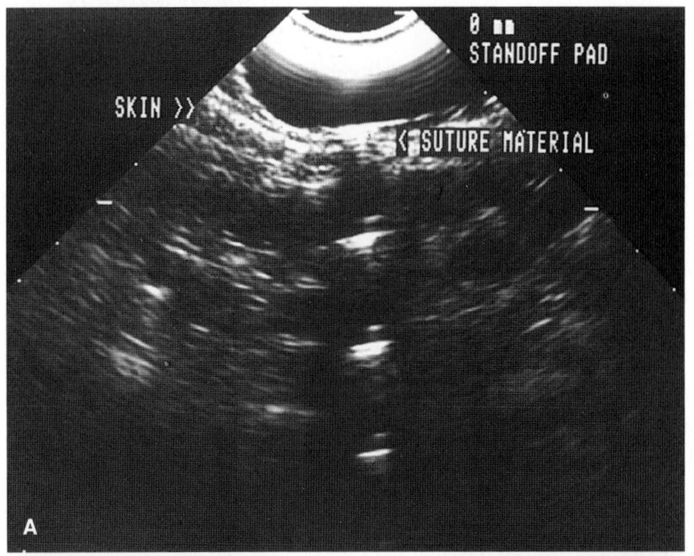

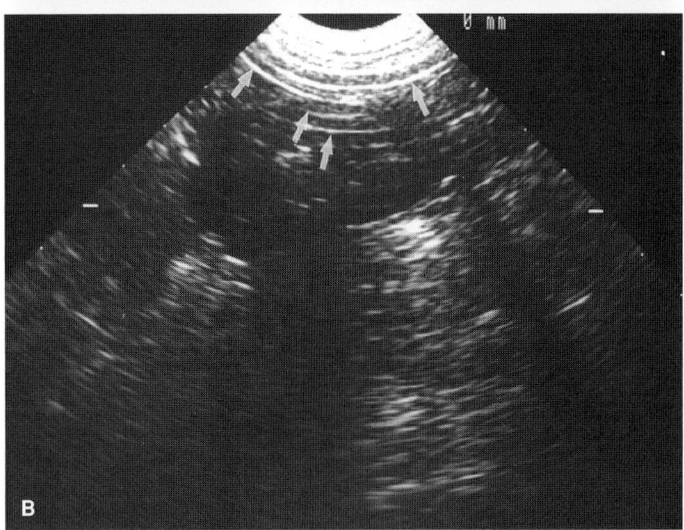

Figure 2-22. (**A**) Reverberation artifact created by a stainless steel skin suture. (**B**) Reverberation artifacts (*arrows*) resulting from insufficient gel and poor coupling of the transducer with the patient.

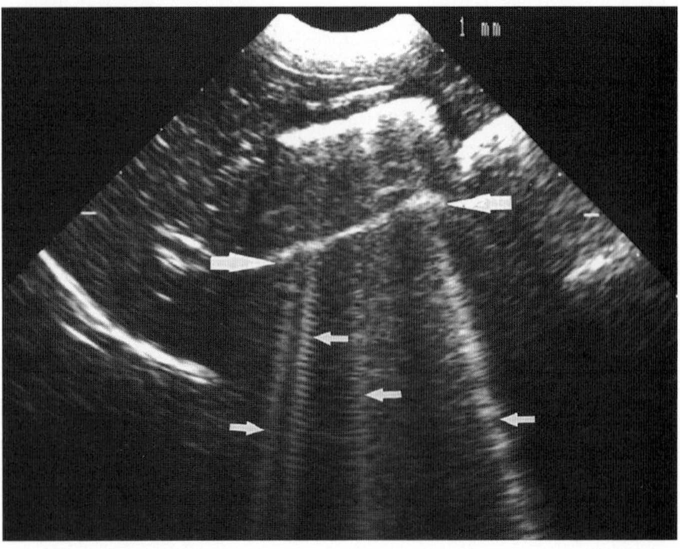

Figure 2-23. Ring-down artifacts (*small arrows*) behind linear reverberation artifacts (*large arrows*) that were generated by gas within the stomach.

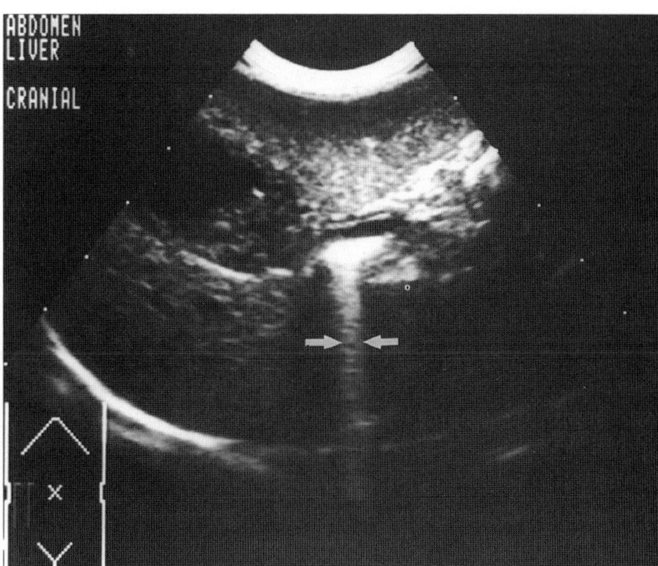

Figure 2-24. A comet tail artifact (*arrows*) resulting from gas within the duodenum.

can also occur when scanning the urinary bladder and an air-filled descending colon acts as a strong reflector, creating a cystic mass deep to the colon.

Beam-width artifacts occur as a result of the width of the ultrasound beam. If the beam is too wide, one portion of the ultrasound beam may be interacting with a fluid-filled structure, and another portion of the beam interacts with the adjacent tissue.[12,13] The result is the registration of echoes within the fluid-filled structure (Fig. 2-27).[14] Beam-width artifacts can also cause

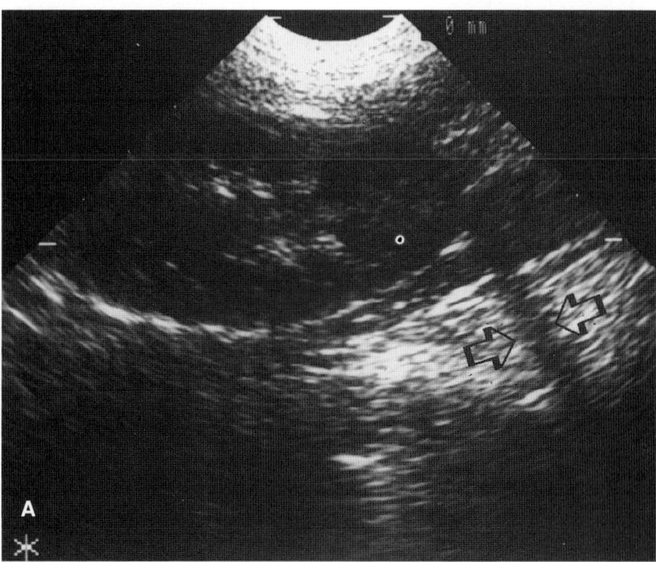

Figure 2-25. Refraction artifacts (*arrows*) created by bending of the sound beam as it encounters the curved surfaces of (**A**) the kidney and (**B**) the gallbladder. Also notice the distant enhancement deep to the gallbladder.

(*continued*)

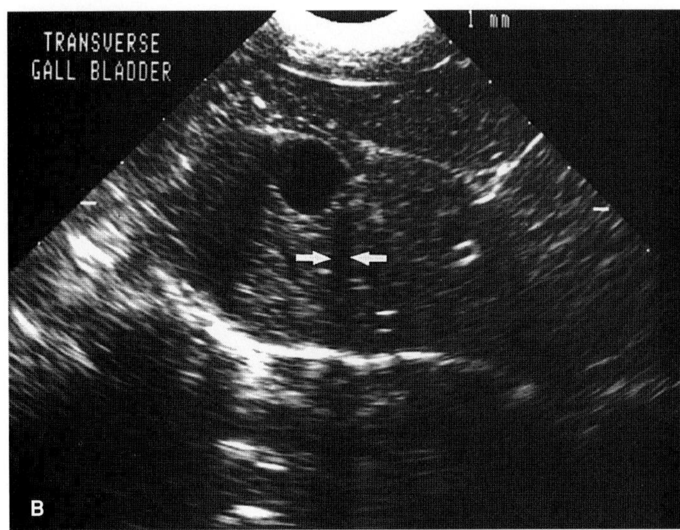

Figure 2-25. *(Continued)*

masses of low contrast to be less apparent or missed entirely because of reduced contrast at the borders.[13]

Side-lobe artifacts are a result of lower-intensity beams that are emitted off the central axis of the ultrasound beam.[12] These peripheral beams produce a reflection from a "side view" rather than from points along the transducer's axis. However, because the ultrasound instrument assumes that the primary beam is the only one that exists, it displays all of these peripheral reflections in the image at the proper depth, just as if they originated from the central beam.[14] Side lobes can occur adjacent to highly reflective surfaces, such as the diaphragm, gallbladder, and urinary bladder, or when highly reflective

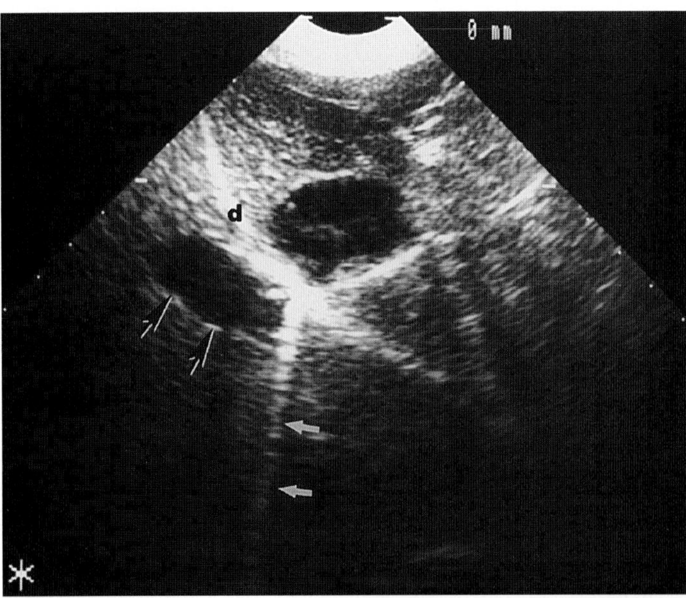

Figure 2-26. Mirror image artifact (*black arrows*) of the gallbladder on the opposite side of the diaphragm (*d*). A comet tail artifact is also present (*white arrows*).

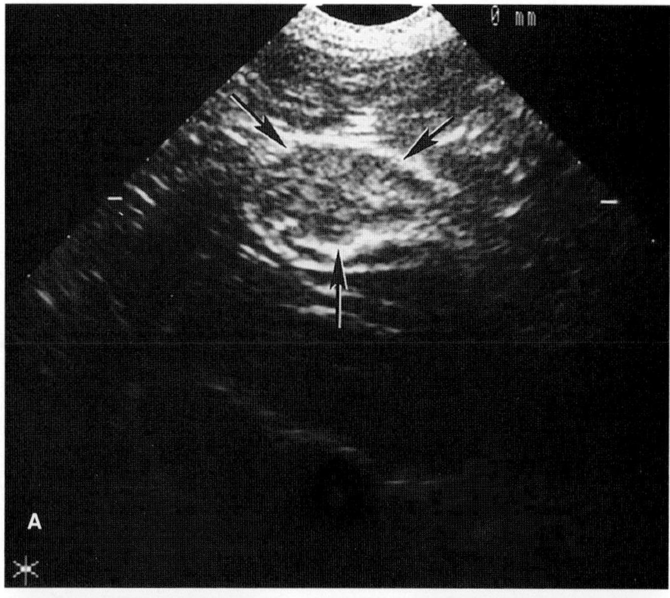

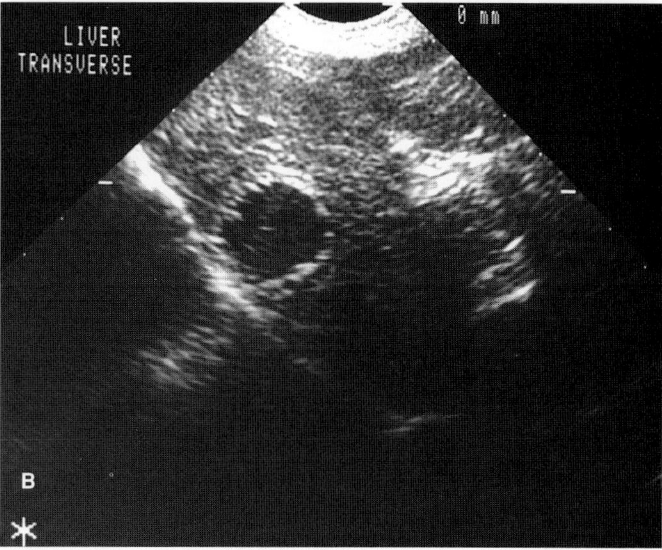

Figure 2-27. Beam width artifact. (**A**) Sagittal sonogram of the gallbladder (*arrows*) that appears uniformly echogenic due to the sound beam interacting with liver and gallbladder, erroneously registering parenchymal echoes within the gallbladder. (**B**) Transverse sonogram of the same gallbladder, showing hypoechoic rather than echogenic fluid within.

bowel gas is adjacent to a fluid-filled structure, such as the urinary bladder (Fig. 2-28).

Grating lobe artifacts are a type of side-lobe artifact peculiar to array transducers, particularly a linear array.[9] The artifacts are the result of the periodic spacing of the transducer's elements, which creates echoes that travel at an angle outside the central axis of the beam.[9,14] Depending on whether these peripheral beams encounter the reflector before or after the central axis beam, a small, curvilinear echo may be displayed above or below the actual reflector.[14] This type of artifact is associated with cystic structures (Fig. 2-29) but it can also originate at the diaphragm.

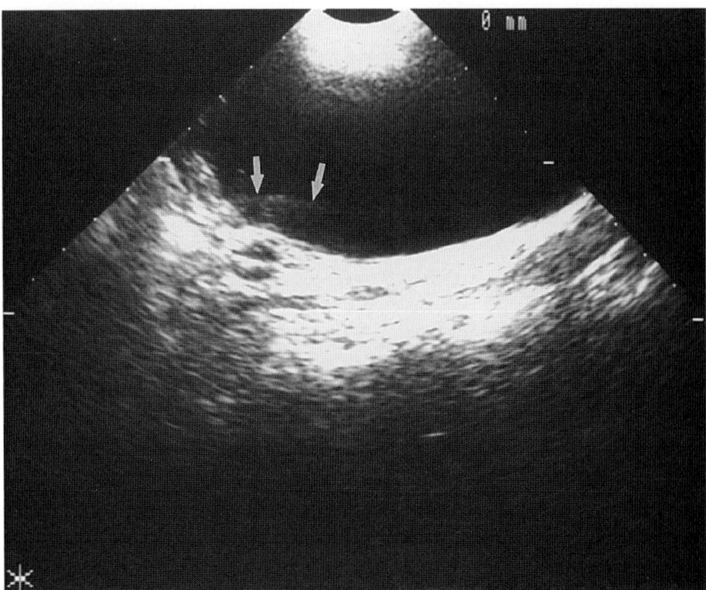

Figure 2-28. Side lobe artifact (*arrows*) within the urinary bladder created by adjacent gas-filled bowel.

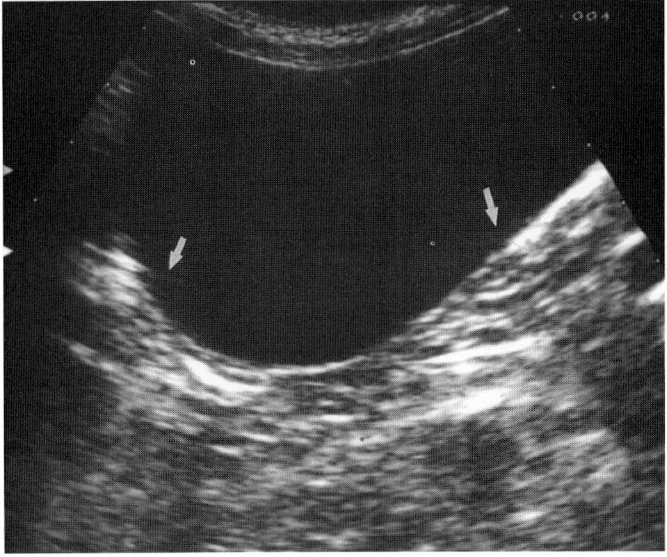

Figure 2-29. Grating lobe artifacts (*arrows*) generated by peripheral ultrasound beams, displaying small curvilinear echoes above the actual reflector (bladder wall).

REFERENCES

1. Curry TS, Dowdey JE, Murry RC. Christensen's physics of diagnostic radiology. 4th ed. Philadelphia: Lea & Febiger, 1990:323.
2. Farrow CS. UltraTalk: beginners guide to the language of ultrasound. Vet Radiol Ultrasound 1992:33:31.
3. Powis RL, Powis WJ. A thinker's guide to ultrasonic imaging. Baltimore: Urban & Schwarzenberg, 1984:299.
4. Kremkau FW. Diagnostic ultrasound: principles and instruments. 4th ed. Philadelphia: WB Saunders, 1993:129.
5. Zagzebski JA. Pulse-echo ultrasound instrumentation. In: Hagen-Ansert SL, ed. Textbook of diagnostic ultrasonography.

3rd ed. Philadelphia: Mosby Year Book, 1989:34.

6. Maggio M, Sanders RC. Knobology. In: Sanders RC, ed. Clinical sonography: a practical guide. 2nd ed. Philadelphia: WB Saunders, 1991:17.
7. Feigenbaum H. Echocardiography. 3rd ed. Philadelphia: Lea & Febiger, 1981:1.
8. Zwiebel WJ. Color duplex imaging and Doppler spectrum analysis: principles, capabilities, and limitations. Semin Ultrasound CT MR 1990;11:84.
9. Kremkau FW. Diagnostic ultrasound: principles and instruments. 4th ed. Philadelphia: WB Saunders, 1993:221.
10. Bushong SC, Archer BR. Diagnostic ultrasound: physics, biology, and instrumentation. St. Louis: Mosby Year Book, 1991:133.
11. Waldrop LD, Kremkau FW. Artifacts in ultrasound imaging. In: Goldberg BB, ed. Textbook of abdominal ultrasound. Baltimore: Williams & Wilkins, 1993:50.
12. Laing FC. Commonly encountered artifacts in clinical ultrasound. Semin Ultrasound 1983;4:27.
13. Scanlan KA. Sonographic artifacts and their origins. Am J Roentgenol 1991; 156:1267.
14. Sanders RC, Maggio M. Artifacts. In: Sanders RC, ed. Clinical sonography: a practical guide. 2nd ed. Boston: Little, Brown & Co, 1991:459.

Small Animal Ultrasound, edited by Ronald W. Green.
Lippincott-Raven Publishers, Philadelphia © 1996.

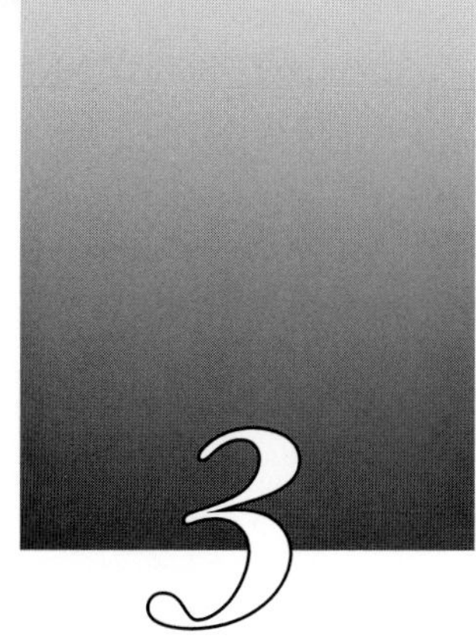

Ultrasound Scanning Techniques

Linda D. Homco

Ultrasound imaging is operator dependent. The sonographer has complete control over the study by controlling the power, gain, time-gain control, and gray scale. The sonographer can dictate and even change the appearance of any organ or tissue by how he or she holds and moves the transducer across the patient. Learning how to control the image with the transducer in hand is a skill similar to playing a musical instrument. Although some may have an "ear" for music, all must practice, and the more they practice, the better they will become.

As a starting point, the veterinary sonographer must intimately know the anatomy of the patient, including the organ locations, shapes, and sizes and how each may differ between patients. The best sonographers are those who know anatomy and also can think in three dimensions while performing a sonogram. This chapter is designed to give some important basic information on how to become a good sonographer.

TRANSDUCER MOVEMENTS

The scanning of an abdomen, thorax, or individual organ is accomplished with a few simple hand movements. These maneuvers are accomplished by moving the transducer across the skin surface or, while keeping the transducer's skin contact point or "footprint" the same, rotating or angling the transducer in place. Four simple maneuvers with the transducer have been described in the veterinary literature and are discussed as they apply to the abdomen.[1]

Sliding is done with the transducer held perpendicular to the skin surface, and movement occurs in a longitudinal, transverse, or oblique direction across the surface (Fig. 3-1*A*, *B*). This is the simplest maneuver, allowing the operator to move from one area of the abdomen to another to scan an entire organ, to find another organ, or to locate an acoustic window (Fig. 3-1*C*, *D*).

In *rotating* the transducer, the footprint is kept in contact with and in a fixed position on the skin's surface. The area of interest remains centered while the transducer is turned 90° about its axis, usually in a counterclockwise direction (Fig. 3-2*A*, *B*). This maneuver is common, because every organ should be evaluated in longitudinal and transverse planes (Fig. 3-2*C*, *D*). Slight rotation in either direction may be needed to obtain true sagittal or transverse views of individual organs.

Fanning is similar to peeking through a keyhole of a door. The transducer is held in a fixed position on the skin surface while the hand and wrist lean the transducer from side to side so that the image on real time is a sweeping view of the organ below (Fig. 3-3*A*, *B*). This move-

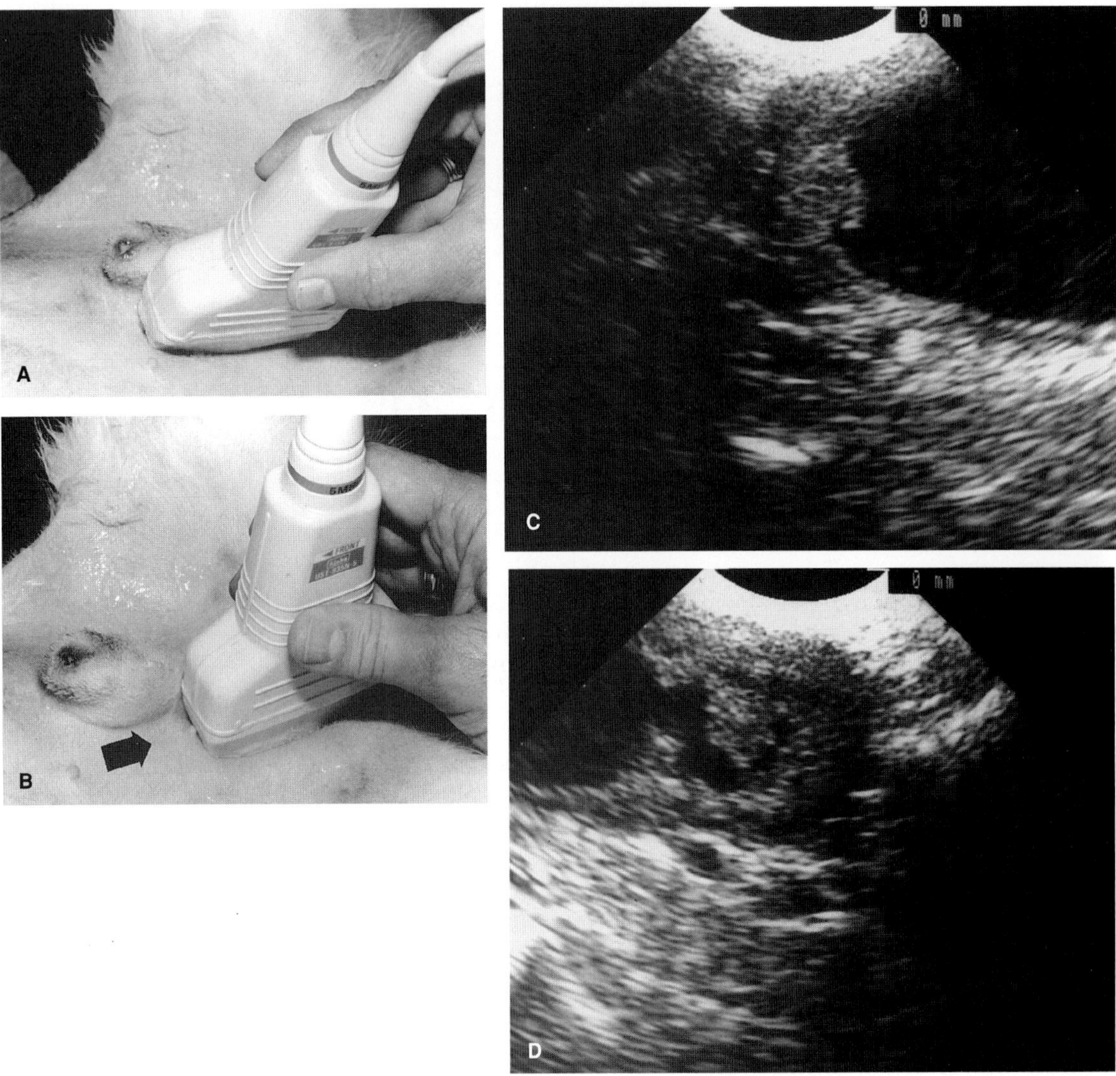

Figure 3-1. (**A and B**) Slide maneuver performed to view the urinary bladder in a longitudinal plane. The arrow indicates the direction of movement of the transducer. This maneuver allows the operator to move from (**C**) the bladder apex to (**D**) the bladder neck to evaluate the entire structure. Cranial is to the left, and caudal is to the right on all longitudinal images.

ment is helpful if only a small window is available but the organ to be viewed is much larger (Fig. 3-3*C, D*). A classic example of fanning is cardiac scanning in short-axis planes from apex to base (see Chap. 4).

Rocking or *rolling* the transducer can be performed only with a transducer with a curved surface, such as a sector or a convex phased-array transducer. The transducer is kept in contact with the skin at all times and, by applying added pressure to the front or back of the transducer (Fig. 3-4*A, B*), the apparent depth of tissues or parts of organs to one side of the real-time image can be altered (Fig. 3-4*C, D*). This maneuver also allows the operator to aim the beam at objects just beyond reach, such as a prostate gland that is partially hidden by the acoustic shadow created by the pubis.

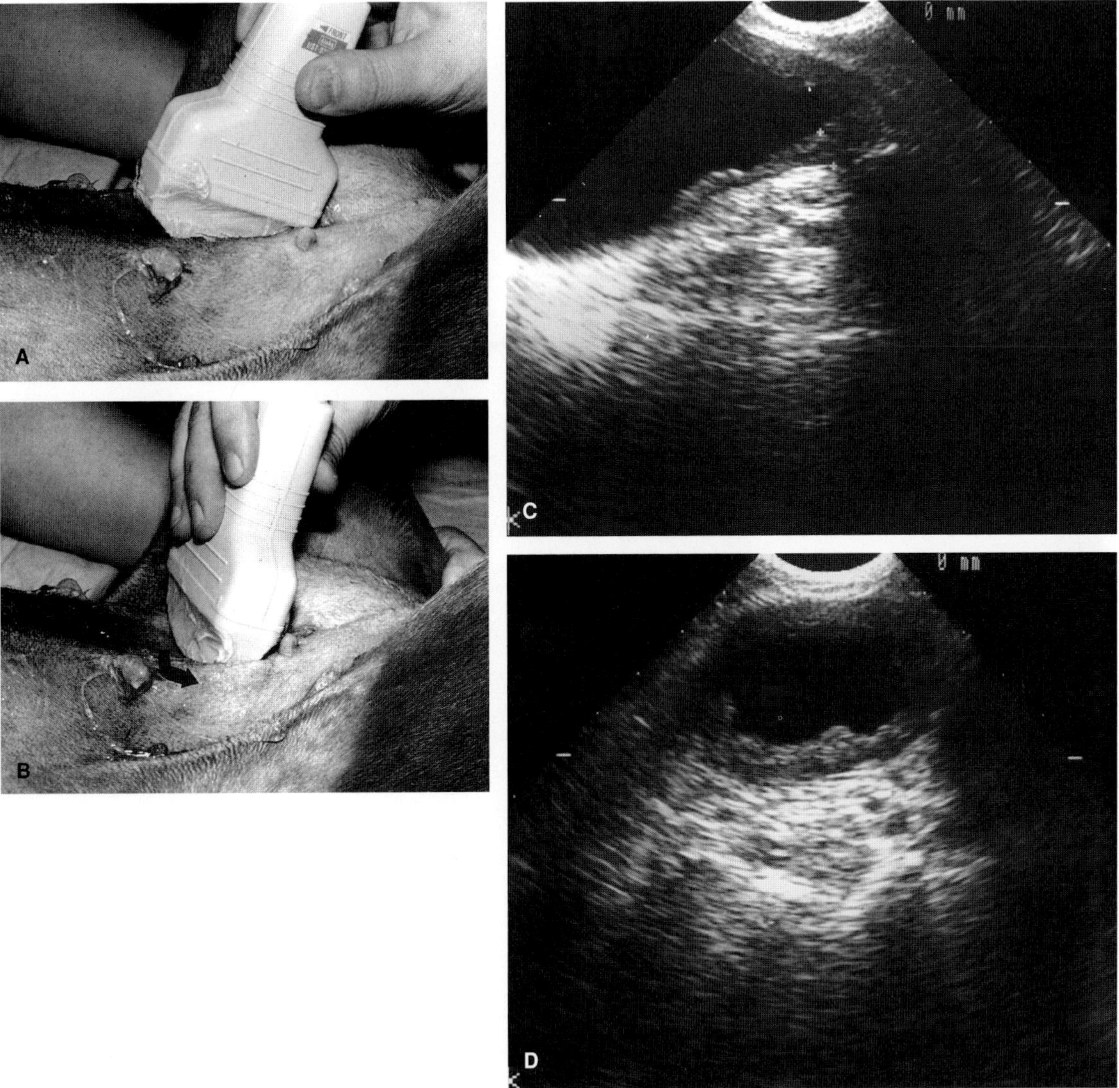

Figure 3-2. (**A and B**) Rotate maneuver performed to evaluate the urinary bladder trigone in (**C**) longitudinal and (**D**) transverse planes. The arrow indicates the direction of movement of the transducer. The patient's right is to the reader's left on all transverse images.

SCANNING PLANES AND IMAGE ORIENTATION

Various anatomic imaging planes are used in ultrasonography to provide a reference for the spatial associations of organs with each other and to facilitate image interpretation. Each one of these is primarily used to describe the image plane used on the patient during scanning, but each may also be used to describe the image plane through an individual organ, which may vary from the animal's axis planes.

Sagittal and *parasagittal* image planes are oriented with the *longitudinal* axis of the body (Fig. 3-5*A*). A parasagittal ultrasound image slice of an organ parallels the long axis of that organ (Fig. 3-5*B*, *C*), and a *midsagittal* plane divides that organ into right and left halves (Fig. 3-5*D*).

Transverse image planes pass through the body perpendicular to the long axis and divide

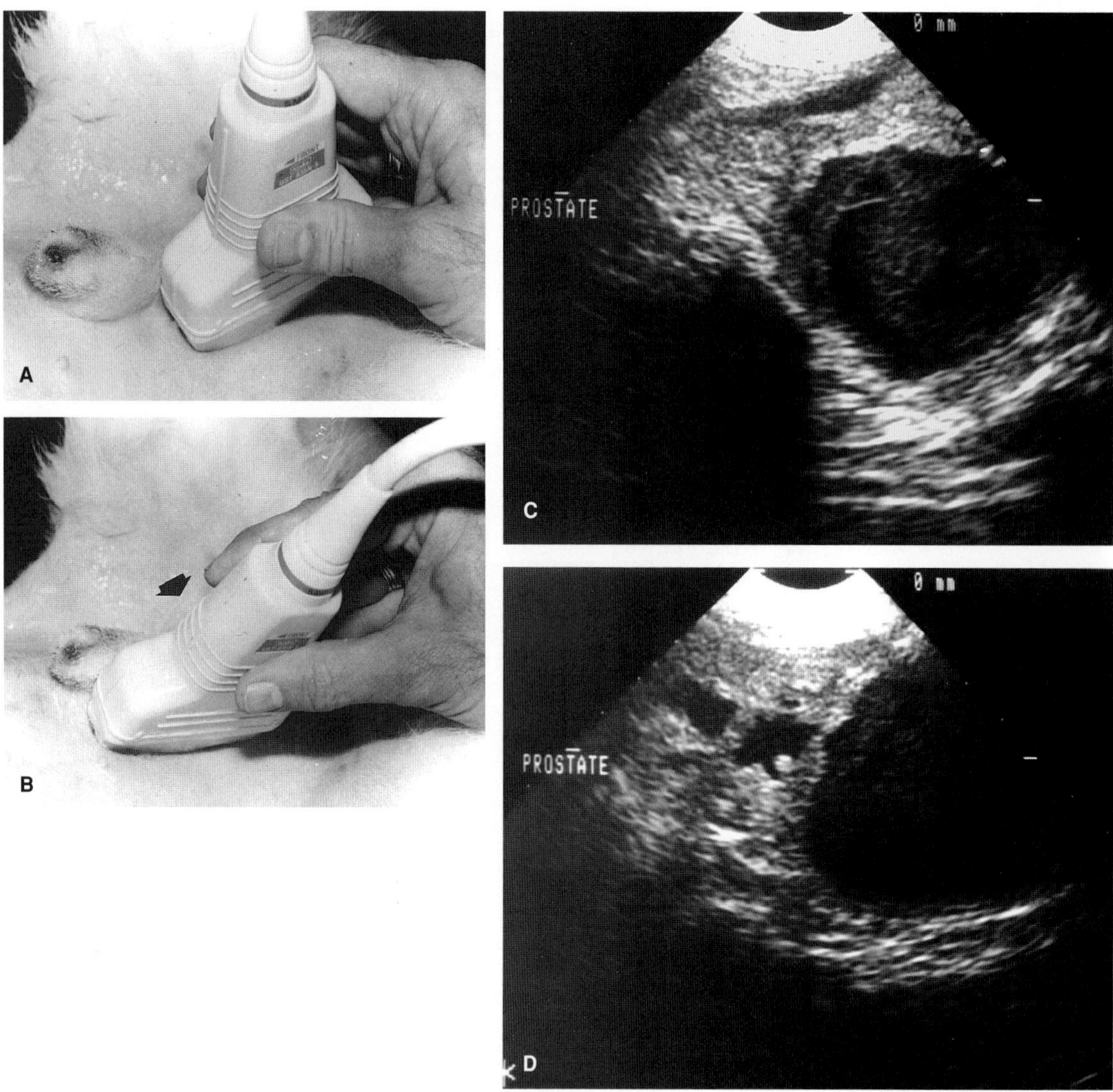

Figure 3-3. (**A and B**) Fan maneuver performed to view both lobes of the prostate gland in a longitudinal plane. The arrow indicates the direction of movement of the transducer. (**C**) is a long-axis sonogram of the right lobe, and (**D**) fans to show a long-axis sonogram of the left lobe.

the body or a specific organ into cranial and caudal segments (Fig. 3-6*A–C, E*).

Frontal, dorsal, or *coronal* image planes are perpendicular to the sagittal and transverse planes and divide the body longitudinally into dorsal and ventral segments (Fig. 3-6*A, B, D, F*). Many veterinary anatomy texts favor the words frontal or dorsal, but coronal is preferred in human imaging.[2,3] Frontal or dorsal scans are performed from the patient's side in the decubitus (ie, laterally recumbent) position.

Ultrasound, unlike computed tomography, is flexible in regard to scanning planes. Any oblique plane can be used as long as bone and gas do not interfere with the sound beam.[4]

For the purposes of uniformity and to aid in interpretation, ultrasound images (except in echocardiography) are displayed on the screen in an orientation similar to that conventionally used for radiography. Sagittal, parasagittal, and long-axis frontal or dorsal planes are displayed with the cranial portion of the organ to the left

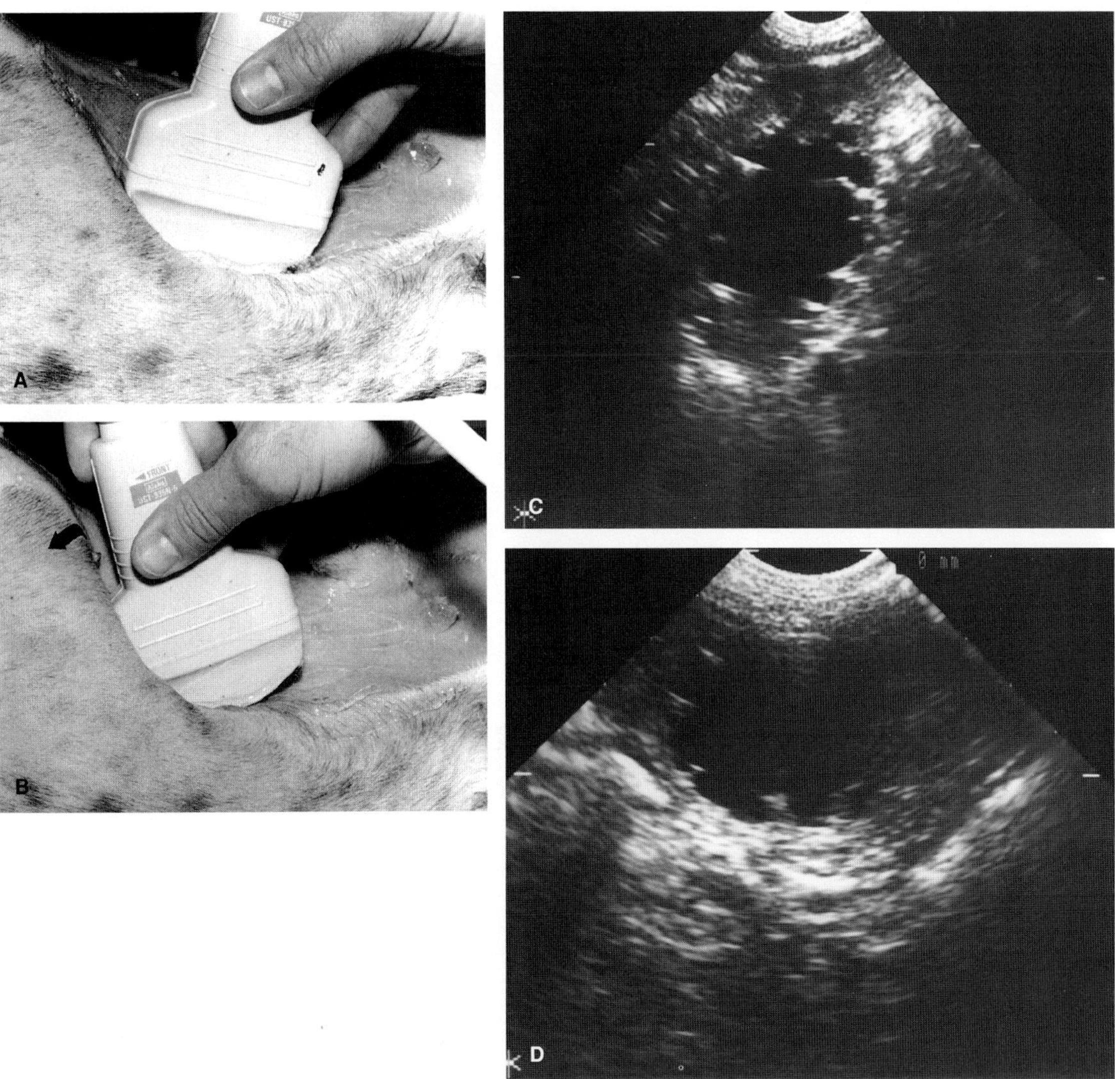

Figure 3-4. (**A and B**) Rock (or roll) maneuver performed to view the right kidney in a perpendicular long-axis plane. The arrow indicates the direction of movement of the transducer. (**C**) The position of the right kidney in a deep-chested dog relative to the neutral transducer placement. (**D**) The right kidney after the rock maneuver is perpendicular to the transducer and the ultrasound beam.

and the caudal aspect to the right of the screen. Transverse image planes are displayed with the animal's right to the viewer's left, similar to the way a ventrodorsal thoracic radiograph would be placed on a viewbox. Many ultrasound machines come equipped with icons, which are body position marks that can be used to indicate the placement and orientation of the transducer with the body (see Fig. 3-15*B*). The near field of the image in most cases is displayed at the top, and the far field is placed at the bottom of the screen.

PATIENT PREPARATION

To have an acoustic window to the body, it is necessary to clip the hair of most animals. Even with the use of copious amounts of ultrasound gel, hair traps some air between the transducer

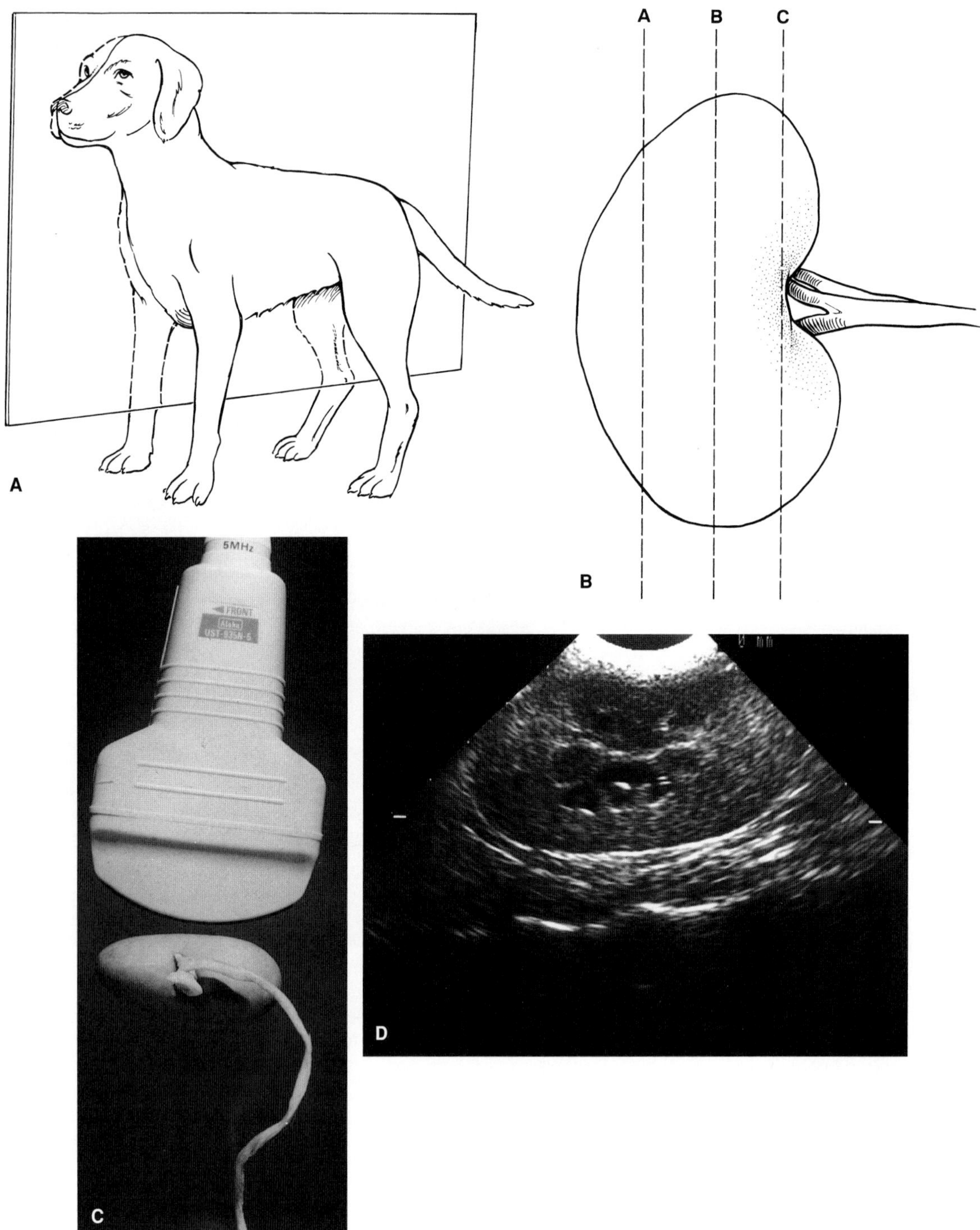

Figure 3-5. (**A**) Line drawing of a midsagittal plane through the body of a dog. (**B**) Line drawing of sagittal planes through the kidney. (**C**) Anatomic demonstration of the relation of the transducer to the kidney during a sagittal image. (**D**) Sagittal sonogram of the kidney in a cat that corresponds to plane B in **B**.

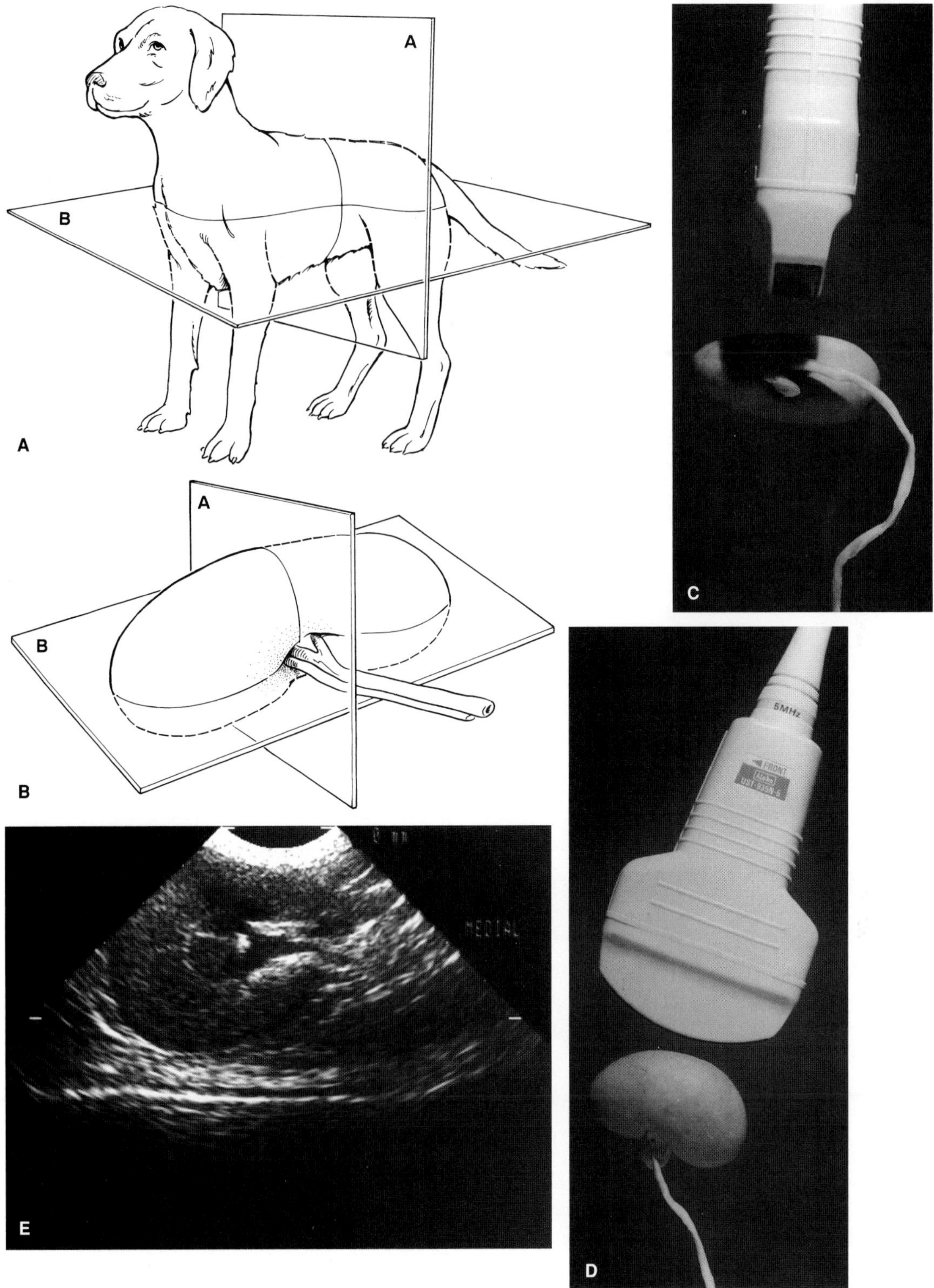

Figure 3-6. (**A**) Line drawing of transverse (A) and frontal or dorsal (B) planes through the body of a dog. (**B**) Line drawing of transverse (A) and frontal or dorsal (B) planes through the kidney. (**C**) Anatomic demonstration of the relationship of the transducer to the kidney during a transverse image. (**D**) Anatomic demonstration of the relationship of the transducer to the kidney during a frontal or dorsal image. (**E**) Transverse sonogram of the right kidney in a cat. *(continued)*

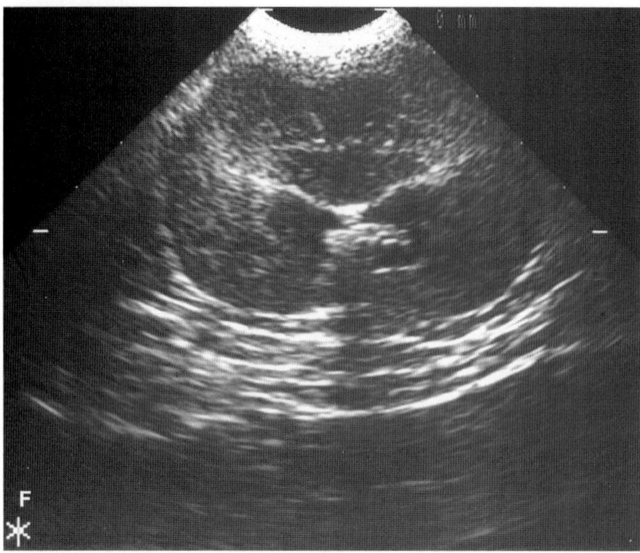

Figure 3-6. *(Continued)* (**F**) Frontal or dorsal plane sonogram of the kidney in a cat.

and the skin surface, which degrades the quality of the ultrasound image. Very fine, sparse hair, such as that seen in dogs with Cushing's disease, may not be an impediment.

The entire area of interest should be clipped with a #40 clipper blade. For general abdominal imaging, the clip should resemble the type the surgeon would perform for an exploratory laparotomy (Fig. 3-7). If only one organ, such as the urinary bladder, is to be evaluated, the area clipped may be reduced. For echocardiography, a small intercostal window of hair should be removed from both sides of the chest to include the third through fifth intercostal spaces. Cranial mediastinal imaging windows are the ventral aspects of the first three intercostal spaces

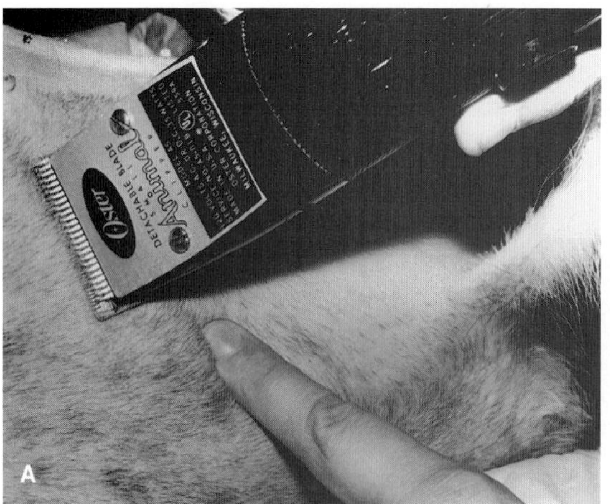

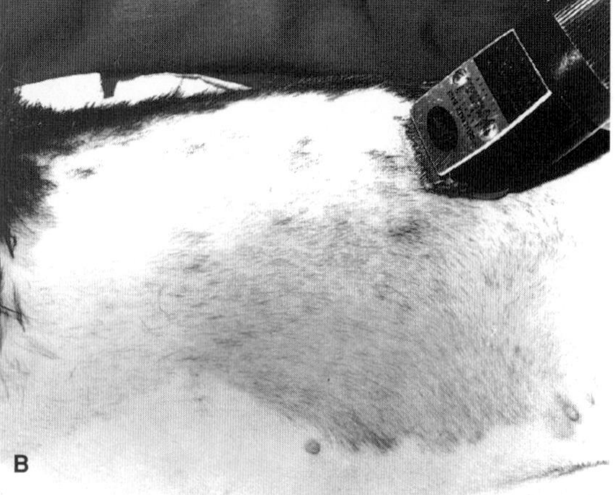

Figure 3-7. (**A**) Clipping the patient for a routine abdominal ultrasound examination requires removal of the hair with a #40 clipper blade to at least the level of the costal arch (indicated by finger). (**B**) The clipped area may need to be extended dorsally if the animal is to be examined in lateral recumbency and cranial to the costal arch if the liver is small or the diaphragm is to be examined.

and the ventral neck at the thoracic inlet. Musculoskeletal imaging requires that hair is clipped over the joint or entire tendon or muscle of interest. Clipping the hair from the contralateral limb provides a normal specimen for comparison. For superficial and other small-parts imaging, a small area is clipped, making sure that the margins extend beyond the palpable borders of the lesion. Brain imaging requires only a tiny area of hair to be removed over the open fontanelle. Hair is not routinely clipped for ocular sonography unless there is interference from excess hair with transpalpebral imaging.

After the hair has been removed, surface dirt or debris should be removed with soap and water. The ultrasound coupling gel is then applied liberally to the skin and should be "massaged" with the transducer to eliminate any small air pockets (Fig. 3-8*A*). Ultrasound gel is manufactured by many companies and is supplied in a wide variety of sizes of containers (Fig. 3-8*B*). Although the viscosity and texture vary slightly among brands, all are acoustically inert media that permit maximum transmission of the sound beam across the transducer-patient interface without attenuation (ie, loss of sound). Mineral oil can be used as a coupling medium, but it has not gained wide acceptance in small animal sonography because of the potential need to bathe the patient after an examination.

Sterile individual gel packets are available for ocular sonography and biopsy procedures (see Fig. 3-8*B*). Rubbing alcohol can be substituted for sterile gel during biopsy procedures, but it is not ideal because it evaporates quickly and may not deliver a good image.

Sedation or anesthesia is rarely required for routine ultrasonography. Tranquilizing the animal may be indicated for some intractable patients, and heavy sedation or general anesthesia is recommended for many ultrasound-guided biopsy procedures. With the animal intubated and under general anesthesia, respirations can be controlled and breath-holding maneuvers can be mimicked for stabilization of small biopsy targets.

PATIENT POSITIONING AND ULTRASOUND APPROACHES

For general ultrasonography, a variety of patient positions is acceptable. There are advantages and disadvantages to each.

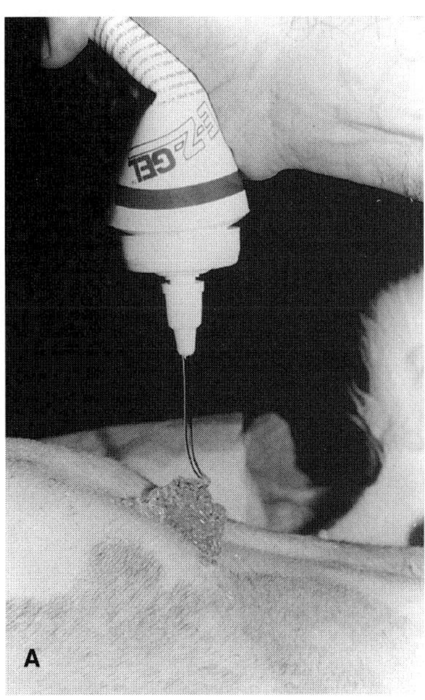

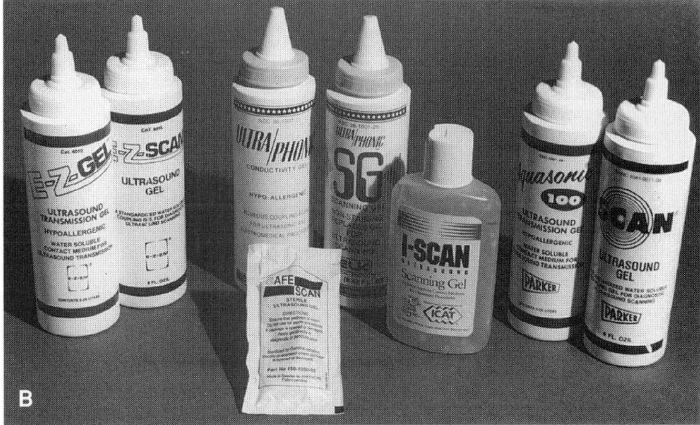

Figure 3-8. (**A**) Ultrasound gel should be applied liberally to the clipped area and massaged to provide adequate coupling of the transducer with the patient. (**B**) Some of the many ultrasound gels and coupling media available for use in diagnostic ultrasonography.

Dorsal Recumbency

Dorsal recumbency is a common patient position for abdominal ultrasound examinations (Fig. 3-9). Many sonographers find they are more comfortable with the abdominal anatomy with the animal in dorsal recumbency, because it is the patient position chosen most often for abdominal surgery. Most are familiar with the predictable location of organs seen through a ventral midline approach, because this view is often chosen by anatomy texts to display organs and their orientations. Veterinarians are also familiar with this orientation when viewing a ventrodorsal abdominal radiograph. Some organs fall into a predictable location with the animal on its back: kidneys, urinary bladder, and portions of the spleen. The urinary bladder with the animal in dorsal recumbency can be used as an imaging window for the gravid uterus, the iliac vessels, and lymph nodes.

For ventral imaging of the abdomen, the animal is placed on its back in a low positioning trough like that used for radiography or on a V-troughed surgery table. Some padding added to the table makes this position quite comfortable for most patients. The disadvantages of this imaging position are poor tolerance by animals with severe cardiopulmonary disease and aerophagia in some patients, which creates additional gas interference. The use of a deep trough or V-troughed table may interfere with lateral oblique or frontal scan planes, and this position is not ideal for cardiac, thoracic, or transrectal imaging or for imaging some deep abdominal structures.

Lateral Recumbency

Many trained sonographers are comfortable with scanning the abdomen with the animal in right or left lateral recumbencies (Fig. 3-10). These positions are also referred to as right decubitus (ie, left side up) and left decubitus (ie, right side up). In lateral recumbency, the position of various organs such as the kidneys, spleen, and gastrointestinal viscera changes. This position is helpful in altering the orientation of fluid and gas within the stomach or intestines. Gravitational effects on fluid in the pleural or peritoneal cavities can benefit scanning of some organs by surrounding them with fluid (see Fig. 3-10). The urinary bladder and spleen can be used as acoustic windows. For oblique and frontal scanning planes, the transducer is placed dorsolaterally or laterally. For complete examination of some organs, the patient may need to be scanned in both lateral recumbencies.

Lateral recumbency is preferred for cardiac and pleural imaging, particularly if a cardiac

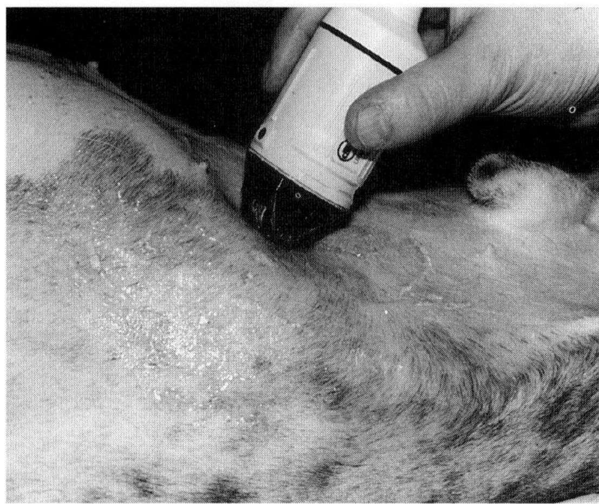

Figure 3-9. Abdominal sonography with the patient in dorsal recumbency.

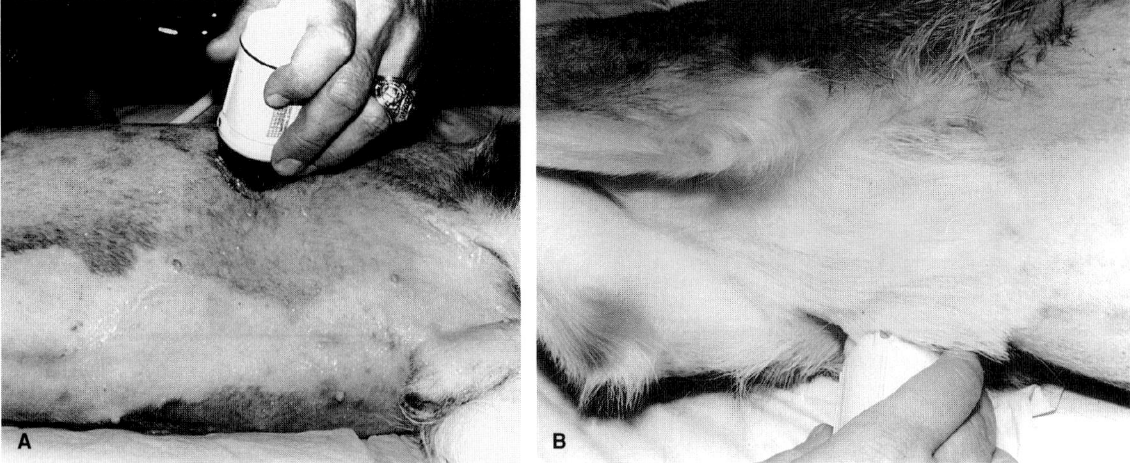

Figure 3-10. (**A**) Abdominal sonography with the patient in right lateral recumbency (ie, right decubitus position). (**B**) Sonography of the cranial mediastinum with the patient in lateral recumbency to position thoracic fluid for an acoustic window.

table is available (Fig. 3-11). This type of table has specially designed cut-outs to allow transducer placement on the dependent chest wall, avoiding artifacts created by air-filled lung. Musculoskeletal ultrasound is often performed with the animal in lateral recumbency and may be repeated with the animal bearing weight on the limb.

Sternal Recumbency

This patient position is ideal for scanning the eye, brain, and the cranial mediastinum and pleural space when they contain fluid (Fig. 3-12). Many animals allow transrectal imaging in a sternally recumbent position with minimal additional restraint. This position has limita-

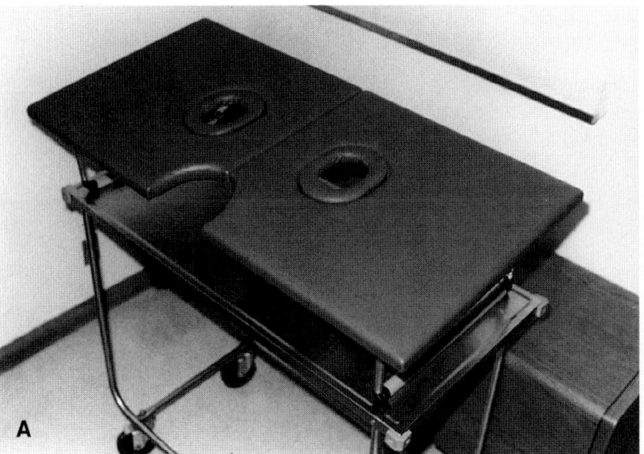

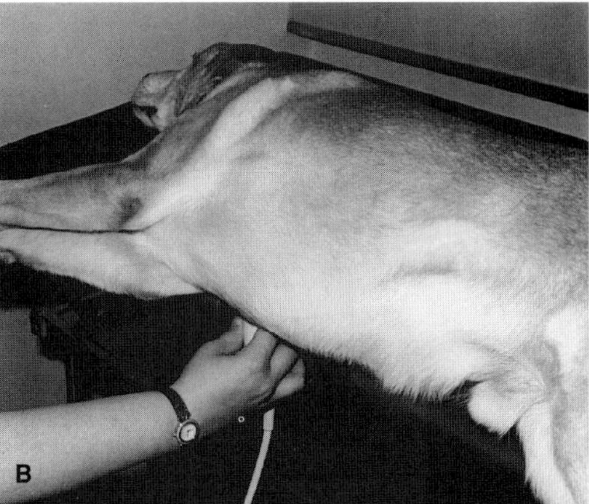

Figure 3-11. (**A**) A specially designed cardiac imaging table (Longman Enterprises) with multiple removable cut-outs to provide easy access to the heart without interference from aerated lung. (**B**) Right parasternal echocardiography performed with the aid of cardiac table (compare with Figure 3-10B).

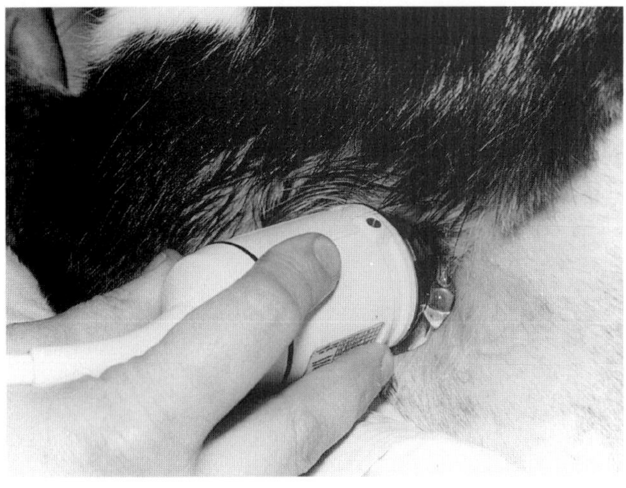

Figure 3-12. Sonography of the cranial mediastinum of a dog in sternal recumbency with the forelimb in extension. This position shifts fluid ventrally and is tolerated well in compromised patients.

tions for abdominal imaging, but is ideal for thoracic imaging of a compromised patient.

Standing

Imaging of the standing animal is recommended by many sonographers as a way to avoid interference from bowel gas during abdominal sonography (Fig. 3-13).[5,6] This position is ideal in a compromised patient if lateral or dorsal recumbency with the necessary restraint would add undue stress. This position is good for cardiac, thoracic, transrectal, and musculoskeletal imaging and for evaluating trauma to the ventral abdominal wall and diaphragm.

Miscellaneous Techniques

Intracavitary Scanning

Newer generations of transducers have been designed for *intracavitary* or *endoluminal* scanning. Specialized transducers, with diameters often the size of a pencil, can be inserted into the rectum, vagina, or esophagus (Fig. 3-14).[7] These transducers are useful in evaluating these and adjacent organs with higher frequencies with-

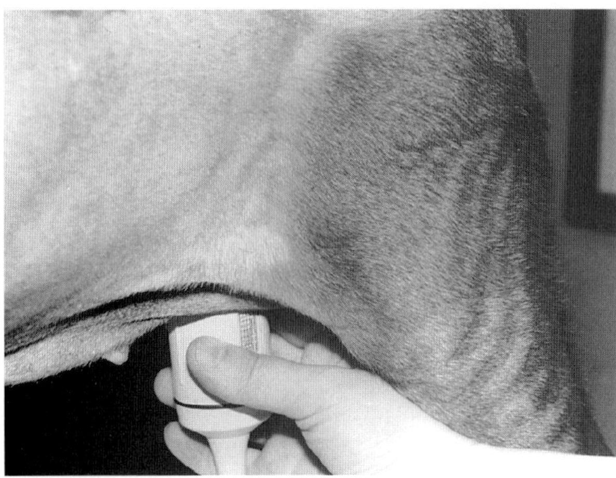

Figure 3-13. Sonography of the caudal abdomen in a standing patient.

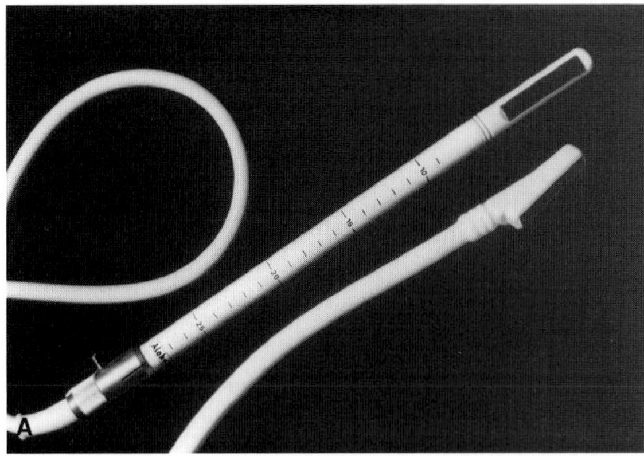

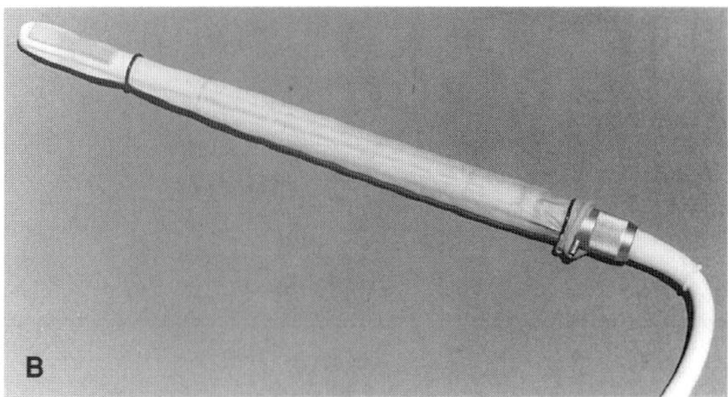

Figure 3-14. (**A**) Examples of transducers that can be used for transrectal sonography in small animals. Both are 7.5-MHz linear array transducers with insertional diameters of less than 2 cm. (**B**) A rigid transrectal transducer fitted with a probe cover for endocavity scanning.

out the interference of gas or attenuation from the body wall. Although transrectal sonography has been widely used in large animal obstetrics, its use in small animals has been limited. The most frequent application of intracavitary scanning in small animals is transrectal sonography of the canine prostate gland. Transrectal scanning can be performed with the animal standing or in sternal or lateral recumbency, and sedation is often unnecessary.

Acoustic Standoff Pads

Fluid offsets or *standoff pads* (Fig. 3-15*A*) are used for evaluating superficial structures or lesions that lie outside the focal zone of the transducer (Fig. 3-15*B*). Optimal focal zone placement is important, because mistakes can be made when an object lies outside the focal zone. A cyst in the near field may contain false echoes and appear to be filled in or solid. The acoustic shadow from a mineral-dense structure may be lost if the structure is outside the focal zone. Imaging within the focal zone also defines margins better because of improved lateral resolution.

A standoff may be made of any echolucent material that does not attenuate the sound beam.[6] Many commercially manufactured standoff devices or gel pads are available (Fig. 3-15*C*). A fluid offset can also be made out of a surgical glove filled with degassed water, saline, or ultrasound gel (Fig. 3-15*D*). Some transducers have a built-in fluid offset to bring the object within the focal zone of the beam (Fig. 3-15*E*).

ORGAN ECHOTEXTURES AND ECHOGENICITIES

Ultrasound is an imaging modality with its own vocabulary. Many terms are used to describe a particular lesion and to describe the appearance of one organ or structure relative to another. *Hyperechoic* describes a structure that produces more echoes than it normally does (implying pathology) or more echoes than another comparative organ. *Hypoechoic* implies there are fewer than normal echoes from that organ or fewer echoes than an adjacent or comparative tissue. *Isoechoic* implies that two organs or tissues are equal in echogenicity. An *anechoic* structure is without internal echoes.

One drawback in ultrasound is the broad range of organ echotexture. Each animal's tissues and each acoustic interface within that animal responds to the ultrasound beam in a subtly unique way. Because of this variability and the wide range of machine settings, it is not possible to compare a kidney of one dog to the corresponding kidney of another. A control within each patient by which changes in echogenicity

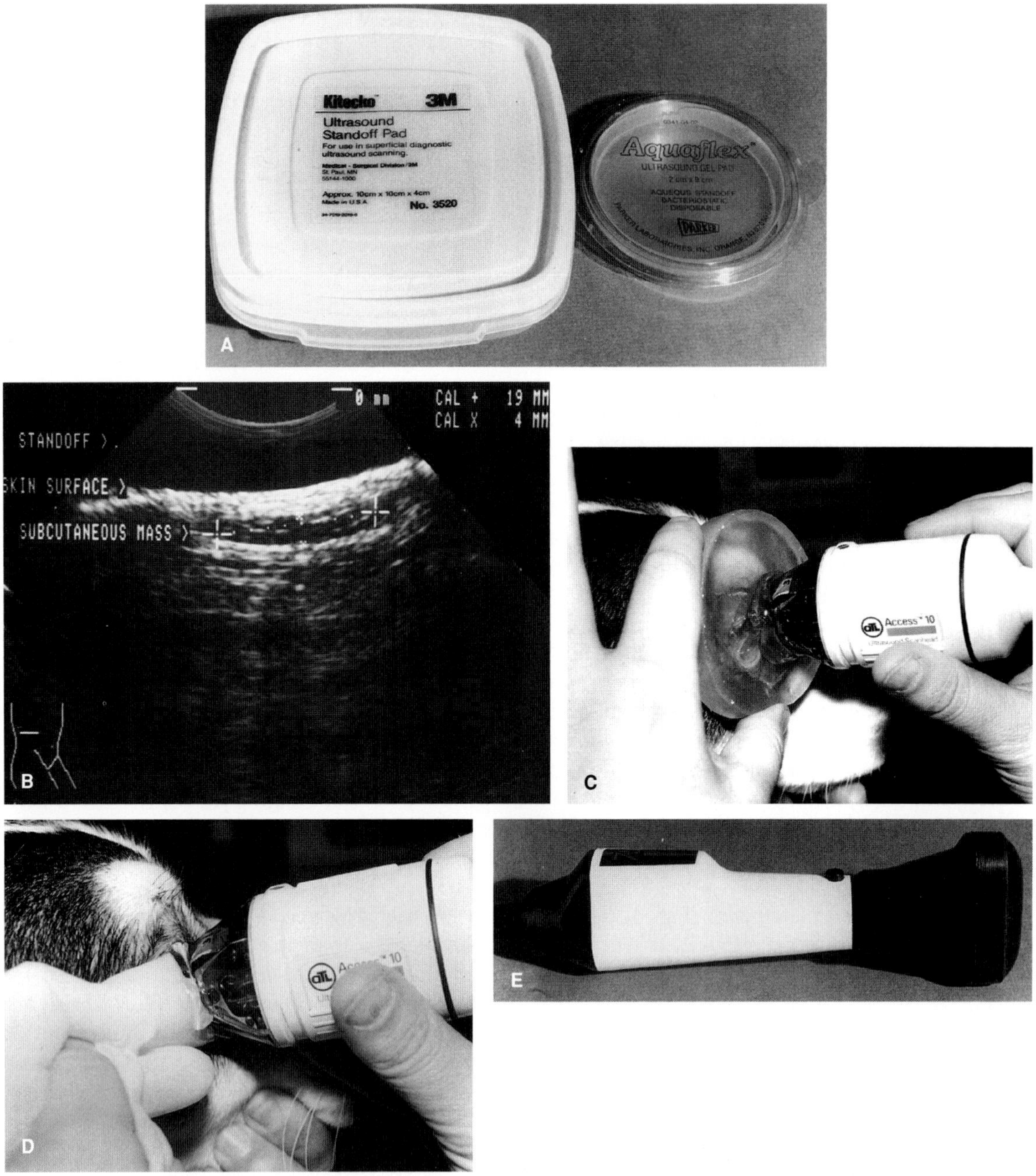

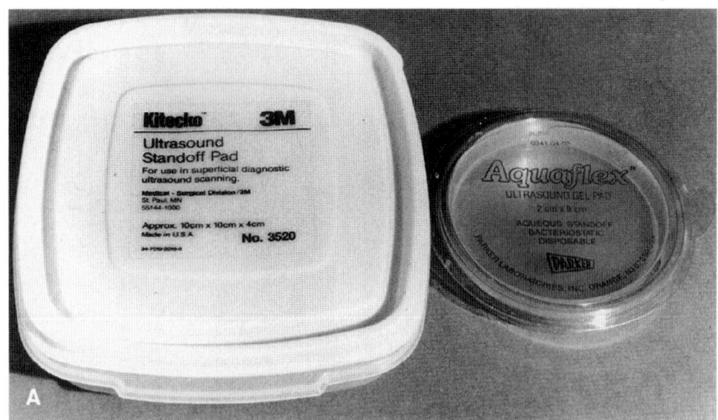

Figure 3-15. (**A**) Commercially available standoff pads for use in diagnostic ultrasonography. (**B**) Sonogram of a subcutaneous mass imaged with the aid of a standoff pad. Notice the black space in the near field and the definition of the skin surface and mass, which now lie within the focal zone of this transducer. The body position mark or icon in the lower left of the image indicates the location of the mass and the orientation of the transducer relative to the body. (**C**) Use of a standoff for ocular imaging. Gel must be applied to both surfaces for acoustic coupling. (**D**) A home-made standoff device for ocular sonography using a fluid-filled surgical glove. (**E**) A 7.5-MHz sector transducer with a built-in fluid offset.

can be measured is a key in determining organ pathology.

The relative echogenicities of normal abdominal organs from least echogenic (ie, relatively hypoechoic) to most echogenic (ie, relatively hyperechoic) are renal medulla, renal cortex, liver, spleen, and prostate gland. The normal spleen is hyperechoic relative to the kidney and to the liver (Fig. 3-16*A, C*), and the kidney is hypoechoic relative to the liver (Fig. 3-16*B*). The renal cortex and liver in some normal animals may appear isoechoic. It is important to be able to locate and identify two of these organs or tissues together in one real-time image plane and at the same depth to be able to assess changes in parenchymal echogenicity.

Scanning of individual organs relies on the sonographer's knowledge of the organ's anatomy and its location and on his or her ability to find an acoustic window for imaging. The appropriate patient positioning and good scanning techniques are imperative for a high-quality ultrasound examination.

Scanning of commonly imaged organs is described and accompanied by examples with the patient in dorsal recumbency. The reader is referred to specific chapters of this text for tips from other sonographers on scanning techniques that may be unique to that particular organ.

ABDOMINAL SONOGRAPHY

The order used to scan organs within the abdomen is dictated by a priority concern or by personal preference. Regardless of the order used, it must be done in a systematic fashion so that no organ or part of an organ is left unscanned. Scanning is also considered incomplete or inadequate if interrogated in only one image plane. Scanning in at least two planes permits the differentiation between spherical and tubular structures and provides the opportunity to recognize detrimental artifacts.

The *liver* is the largest and perhaps the most difficult organ in the abdomen to scan completely. It consists of six lobes that occupy large portions of the right and left cranial abdominal quadrants. If parts of the liver cannot be evaluated from a ventral approach caudal to the costal arch, intercostal scanning must be done to complete the examination. I scan the liver from the patient's right (Fig. 3-17*A*) to left (Fig. 3-17*B*) in parasagittal planes and then return to the patient's right to scan in transverse planes across the entire liver (Fig. 3-17*C*). Because the gallbladder in the dog tends to lie in an oblique plane, scanning in its long-axis plane requires a slight rotation of the transducer for better visualization of the gallbladder neck. This is usually accomplished by rotating the front of the transducer toward 11 o'clock if 12 o'clock represents a sagittal plane (Fig. 3-17*D*).

The location of the *spleen* varies within the abdomen. The triangular head is located in the left cranial quadrant, and it is fixed with a portion of the splenic body to the greater curvature of the stomach by the gastrosplenic ligament. The tail of the spleen may be located in the left cranial quadrant of the abdomen caudal to the stomach or it may cross over the midline to lie near the right kidney. A distended stomach displaces the spleen caudally and often into the left lateral midabdomen. The spleen changes its size dramatically in many physiologic states and in response to many drugs. Because the head of the spleen most often lies deep to the last few ribs, it may not be possible to image in two planes from a ventral approach, and intercostal imaging must be done. The body and tail of the spleen are imaged along the organ's long- and short-axis planes by maneuvering the transducer in any oblique plane necessary relative to the body's imaging planes (Fig. 3-18).

The *kidneys* lie in the retroperitoneal space ventrolateral to the vertebrae. In the dog, the right kidney is located at the level of the thoracolumbar junction with the cranial pole in contact with the renal fossa of the caudate lobe of the liver, an excellent site to compare the echogenicity of these two organs (Fig. 3-19). The left kidney, lying at the level of the first three lumbar vertebrae, is more caudal and variable in its location (Fig. 3-20). Because the left kidney is often dorsomedial to the spleen, the spleen can be used as an imaging window and can provide the opportunity to compare the relative echogenicities of these two organs. In the cat, both kidneys are more caudal than in the dog

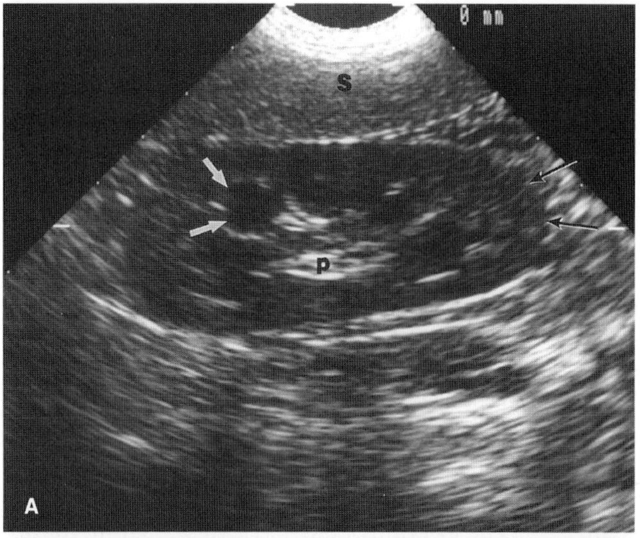

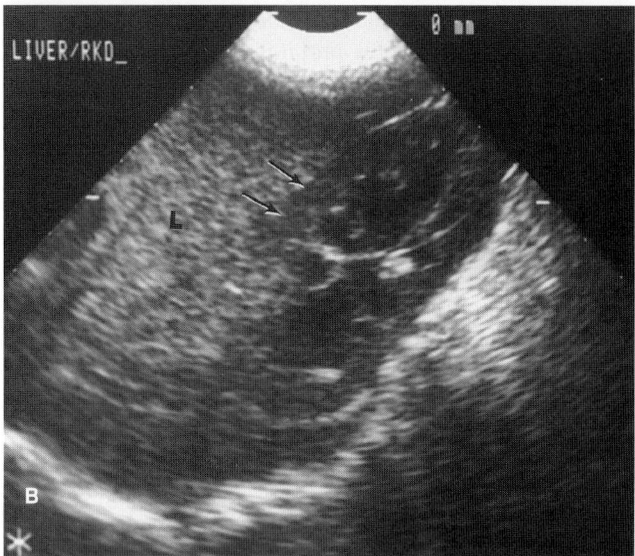

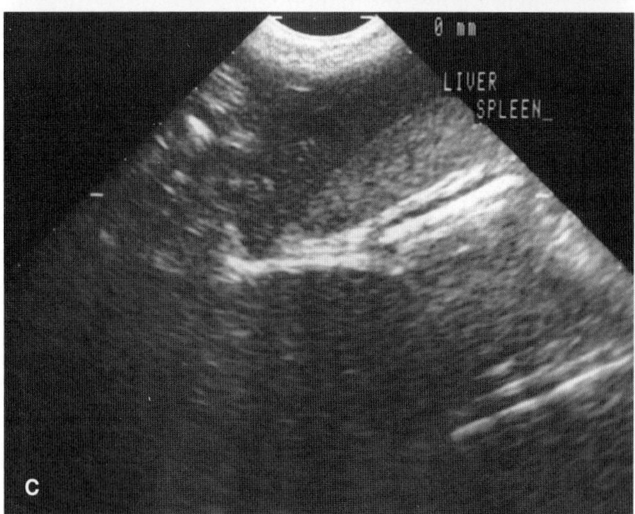

Figure 3-16. (**A**) Sonogram of the left kidney and spleen in a dog shows the normal relative echogenicities. The renal medulla (*white arrows*) is hypoechoic relative to the renal cortex (*black arrows*), which is hypoechoic relative to the spleen (*s*). Notice also that the peripelvic fat (*p*) is very echogenic. (**B**) Sonogram of the right kidney and liver (*L*) in a dog shows that the renal cortex (*arrows*) is hypoechoic relative to the liver parenchyma. (**C**) Sonogram of the normal relative echogenicities of the liver and spleen in a dog.

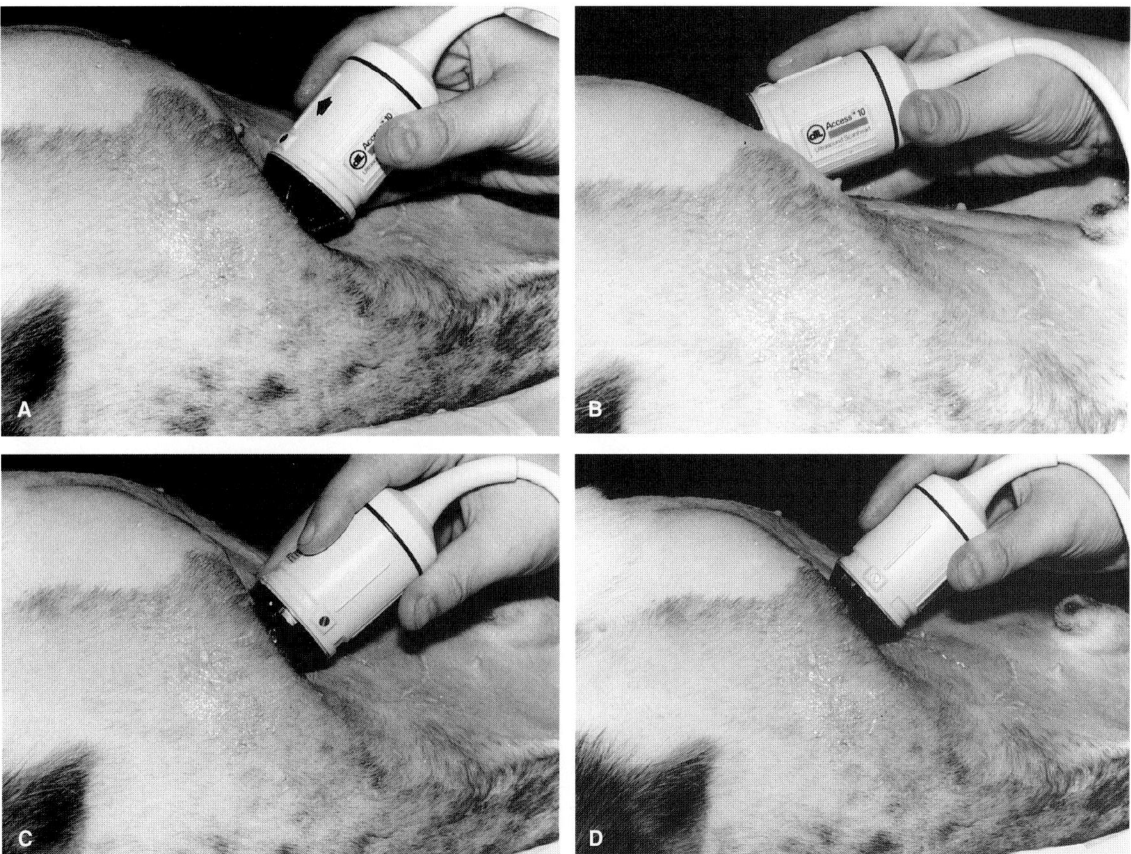

Figure 3-17. (**A**) Scanning the right liver lobes in a longitudinal or parasagittal plane with the patient in dorsal recumbency. The raised ridge on the transducer housing (*arrow*) is used as an aid in transducer orientation. The transducer should be held so that this ridge, which indicates the front of the transducer, points toward the patient's head to place the cranial aspect of the long-axis scan plane on the left of the screen on the monitor. (**B**) Parasagittal long-axis scanning of the left liver lobes. Notice the rocking of the transducer necessary in this dog to avoid interference from gas within the stomach. (**C**) Transverse scanning of the right liver lobes. Notice that the ridge on the transducer has been rotated to the patient's right. The transducer should always be positioned this way for transverse scan planes so that the right side of the patient is consistently displayed on the left of the screen. (**D**) Oblique scan plane used to evaluate the gallbladder.

and are also more variable in their position. The long axis of each kidney in the cat is often parallel to the midsagittal or median plane of the body, but canine kidneys may be parallel or slightly oblique in position, with the cranial poles closer to the midline.

Each kidney should be scanned in multiple longitudinal planes to include the area between the pelvis and the lateral cortex and scanned again in transverse planes to include the area from the cranial pole to the caudal pole. When scanning from the lateral body wall with the animal in a lateral or decubitus position, a frontal or dorsal long-axis view of the kidney can be obtained. With the patient in dorsal recumbency, the right kidney lies farther away from the transducer than the left kidney, particularly in deep-chested dogs, and often the cranial pole is seated deeper in the abdomen than the caudal pole. To minimize distortion and attenuation differences between the two poles, the sonographer must rock the transducer forward in the long-axis

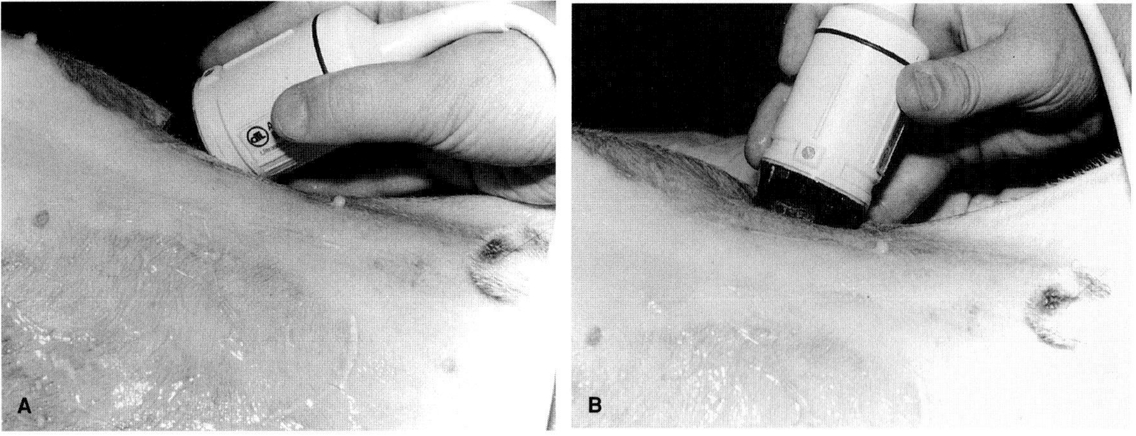

Figure 3-18. (**A**) Long-axis plane of the head of the spleen. (**B**) Short-axis or transverse scanning of the body or tail of the spleen.

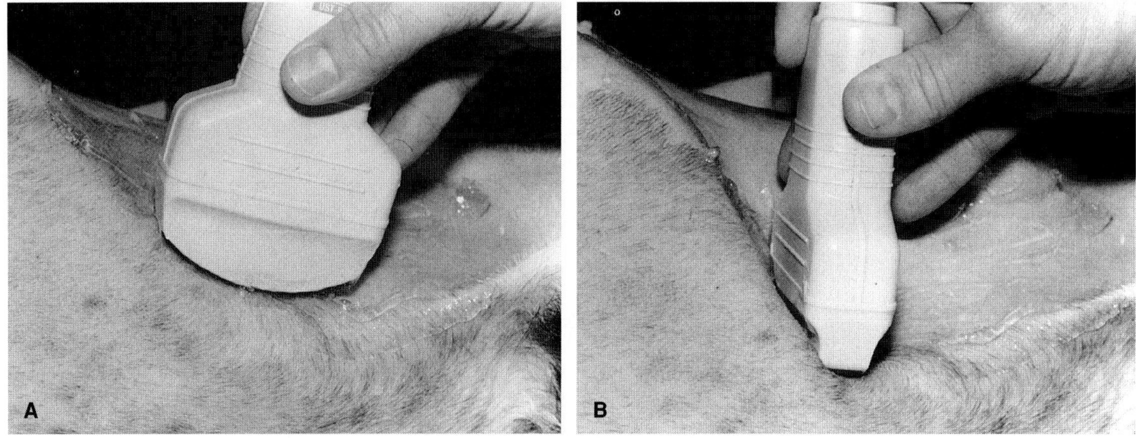

Figure 3-19. (**A**) Sagittal and (**B**) transverse scanning of the right kidney.

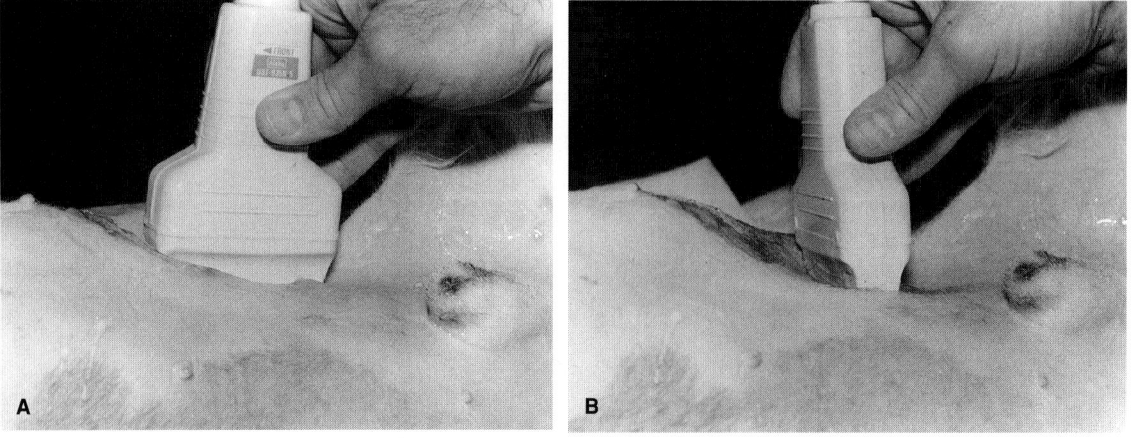

Figure 3-20. (**A**) Sagittal and (**B**) transverse scanning of the left kidney.

view to keep the kidney perpendicular to the ultrasound beam (see Fig. 3-4).

The *urinary bladder* can be the easiest or the most difficult organ for a novice sonographer to evaluate. When first learning to scan, the operator has the tendency to press too hard. This can compress a nearly empty bladder, which can make it unidentifiable or can create false calculi from an acoustic shadow artifact created by the colon. To scan the urinary bladder, the transducer is placed on midline just cranial to the pubis in a female dog (Fig. 3-21*A*) and on either side of the sheath and fanned toward midline in a male dog (Fig. 3-21*B*). The bladder should be scanned in multiple parasagittal planes, making sure to include all areas between the apex and the neck. The transducer is rotated 90° to scan the bladder in transverse planes from the apex to the neck (Fig. 3-21*C*).

The *prostate gland* is most successfully imaged transabdominally when the urinary bladder is distended. The prostate gland lies caudal to the neck of the urinary bladder at or near the brim of the pubis. The sonographer typically has to rock or fan the transducer in sagittal or transverse planes, respectively, to avoid an acoustic shadow from the pubis over the caudal aspect of the gland (Figs. 3-3 and 3-22).

The *uterus* is imaged by using the distended urinary bladder as an imaging window (Fig. 3-23). Many sonographers find success by scanning first in a transverse plane to identify the two horns in cross section ventral to the aorta and vena cava or iliac vessels. Because of interference from visceral gas, the horns usually cannot be followed cranially and laterally to the level of the ovaries unless they are distended and diseased.

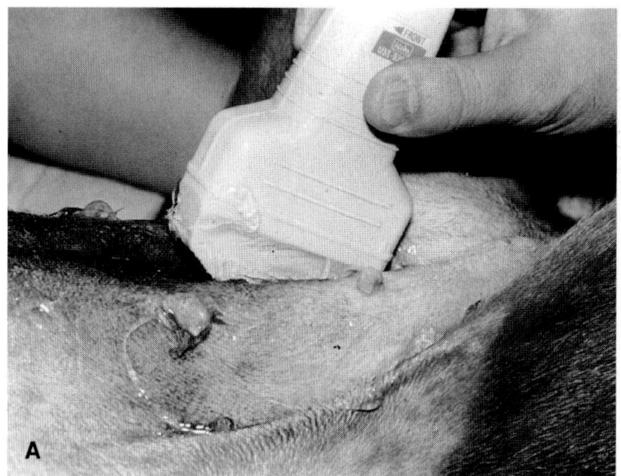

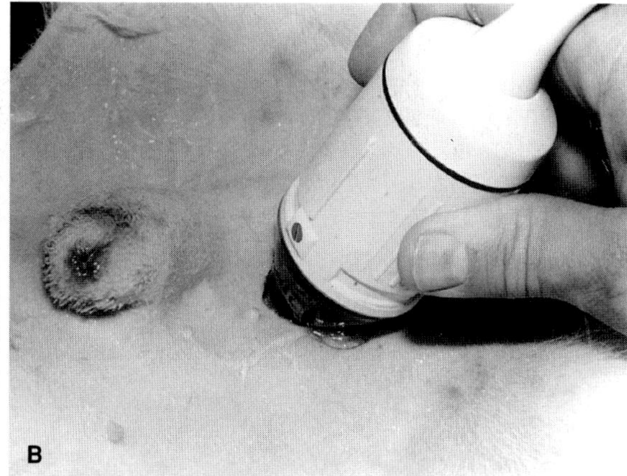

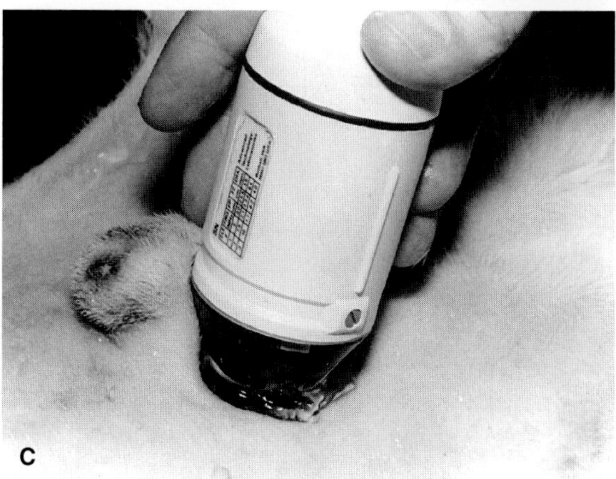

Figure 3-21. (**A**) Sagittal scanning of the urinary bladder in a female dog. (**B**) Sagittal scanning of the urinary bladder in a male dog. (**C**) Transverse scanning of the urinary bladder in a male dog.

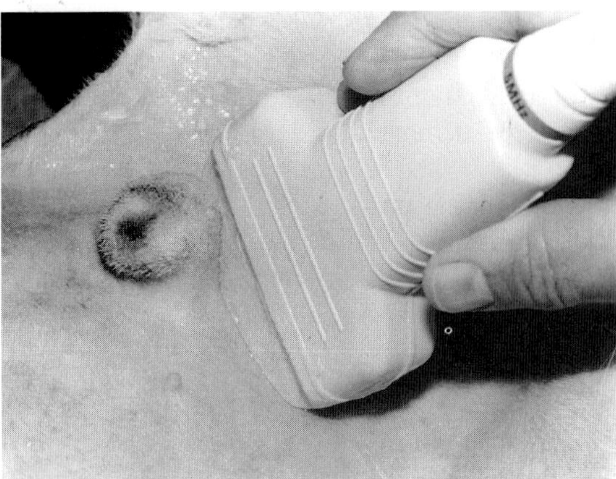

Figure 3-22. Transverse scanning of the prostate gland in a dog. Sagittal scanning is shown in Figure 3-3.

The *ovaries* are caudal and lateral to each kidney and appear much shallower during ultrasound than they appear in surgery.

The *testes* in the dog are easy to locate and can be manually stabilized for imaging in sagittal and transverse planes (Fig. 3-24*A*). To facilitate the imaging of a testicle, it can be displaced into the subcutaneous tissues cranial to the scrotum as the surgeon would do during a routine castration (Fig. 3-24*B*). This prevents movement of the testicle during scanning and provides a tissue background in the far field to aid in the recognition of enhancement or shadowing artifacts.

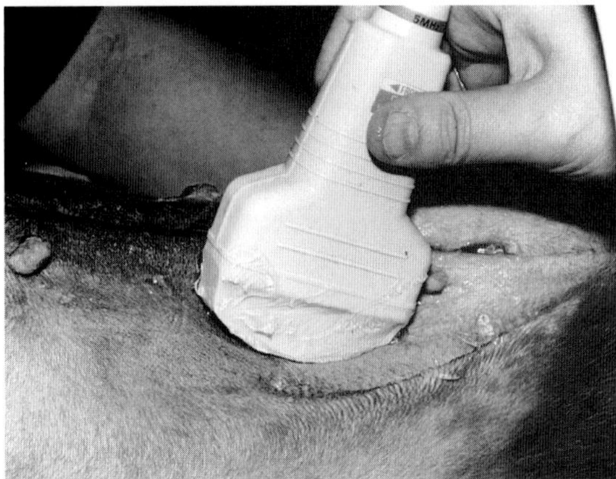

Figure 3-23. Sagittal scanning of the right uterine horn. The normal uterine horns cannot usually be identified, but in pregnancy or disease, they can be found lateral and slightly cranial to the urinary bladder.

The *gastrointestinal tract* is difficult to image in a complete and systematic manner because the small intestines cannot be "run," as in surgery. The stomach and some of the fixed bowel structures, such as the descending duodenum and descending colon, can be identified, but other portions of the tract are too variable in location to consistently permit identification. Each segment of intestine can be seen in long axis and transverse planes, and it is often easiest to follow a particular segment over a greater distance in a transverse plane (Fig. 3-25).

The *pancreas* lies in the right and left cranial abdominal quadrants, with a portion of the right limb extending into the right midabdomen. The left limb lies caudal to the greater curvature of the stomach, and in a long-axis view of this limb, the transducer is actually transverse to the median sagittal plane of the body. The right limb is typically parallel to the long axis of the patient when the descending duodenum also follows this path (Fig. 3-26). Transverse views of the right limb are obtained by following the descending duodenum in a transverse plane from the pylorus to the duodenal loop. The stomach is usually in the field of view when transversely scanning the left limb.

The *adrenal glands* are craniomedial to the kidneys and are retroperitoneal, located deep within the right and left cranial quadrants (Fig. 3-27). The long axis of each gland is not necessarily parallel to the midsagittal plane nor does it follow the same sagittal plane as the kidney. The right adrenal in the dog is often in contact with the right kidney.

The *lymph nodes*, when they can be seen, are found in various locations within the abdomen, depending on the type of node. Many are clustered around or lie adjacent to major blood vessels (Fig. 3-28).

THORACIC SONOGRAPHY

The standards for *cardiac imaging* have been described.[8] The reader is referred to this reference and to Chapter 4 in this text.

The *cranial mediastinum* and its associated structures can be interrogated by an intercostal approach (Fig. 3-29*A*) or by imaging through the

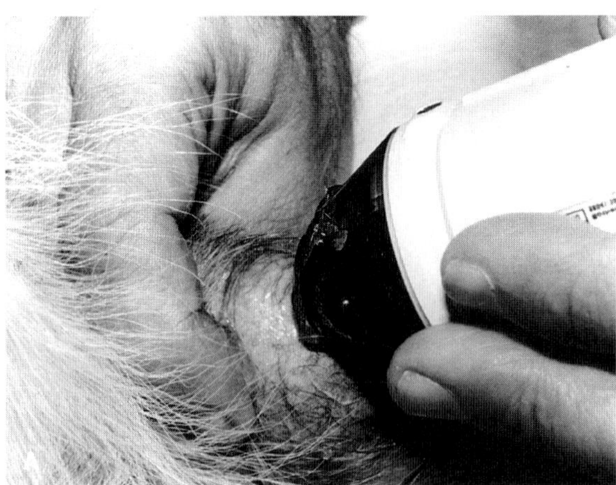

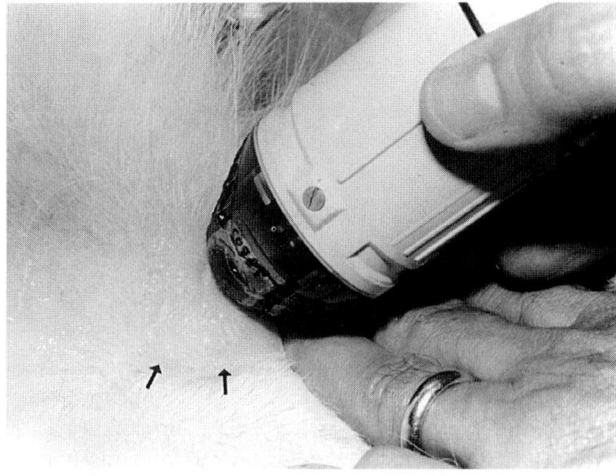

Figure 3-24. (**A**) Manual stabilization of the testes and scrotum for sonography. (**B**) Cranial displacement of the testis (*arrows*) into the subcutaneous space along the prepuce to stabilize it for ultrasonography.

thoracic inlet in the caudal cervical region (Fig. 3-29*B*). When intercostal imaging is performed, the resulting image planes are frontal and transverse. The transducer is placed between the ribs. The length of the frontal plane on the screen is limited by the size of the transducer and its ability to fit between the ribs. Scans performed from the thoracic inlet can yield sagittal and transverse images by fanning the transducer to image through the tissues of the caudal cervical region ventral to the trachea.

Imaging of the *lung* and *pleura* is accomplished by scanning between the ribs with the transducer imaging frontal and transverse planes. Oblique planes are possible when imaging from the more dorsal or ventral aspects of the intercostal spaces or can be accomplished by fanning the transducer. *(text continues on p. 52)*

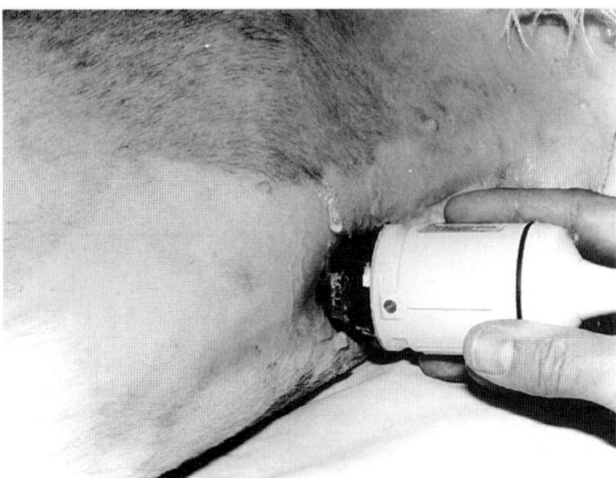

Figure 3-25. Scanning of the gastrointestinal tract with the patient in right lateral recumbency (animal's head is toward the reader's left). This allows gas-filled viscera to be displaced into the left lateral abdomen out of the ventral image plane.

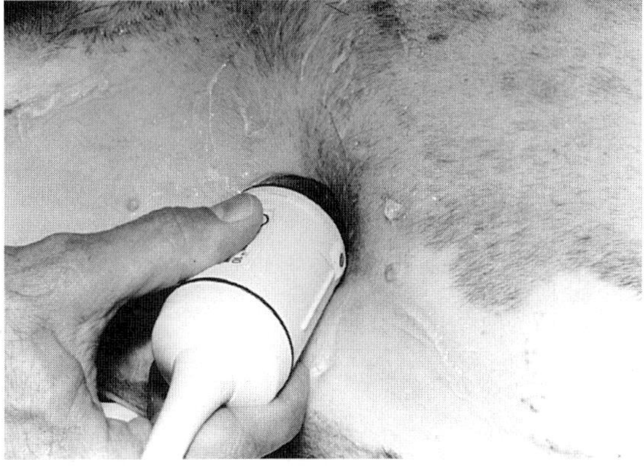

Figure 3-26. Scanning of the right limb of the pancreas with the animal in left lateral recumbency (animal's head is toward the reader's right). This position permits the duodenum to fill with gas and "drift up" into the right lateral abdomen, a technique that may assist the sonographer in locating the pancreas.

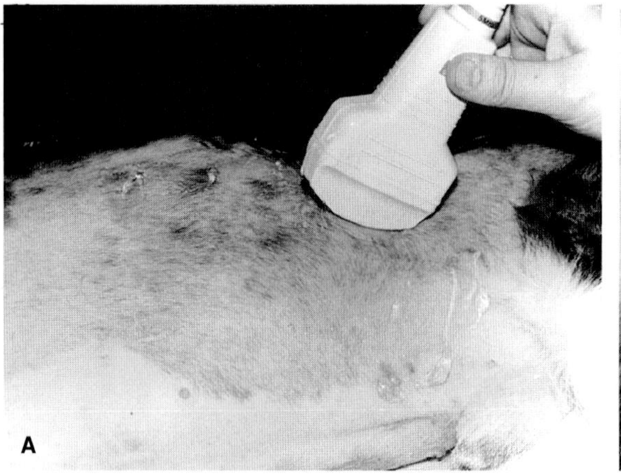

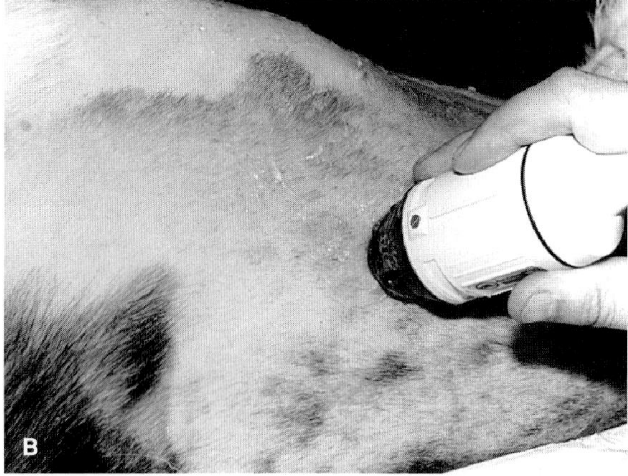

Figure 3-27. (**A**) Scanning of the left adrenal gland with the patient in right lateral recumbency. (**B**) Scanning of the right adrenal gland through a long-axis dorsal image plane with the patient in dorsal recumbency.

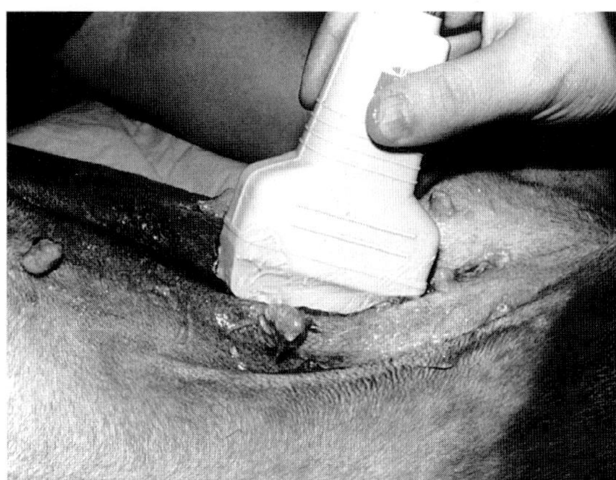

Figure 3-28. Scanning of the medial iliac lymph nodes by using the urinary bladder as an imaging window.

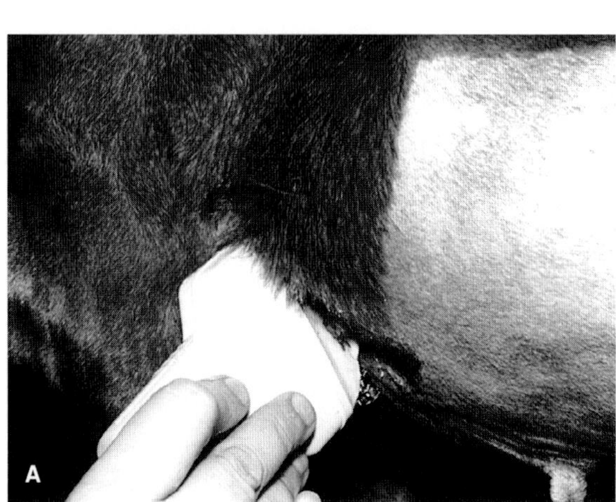

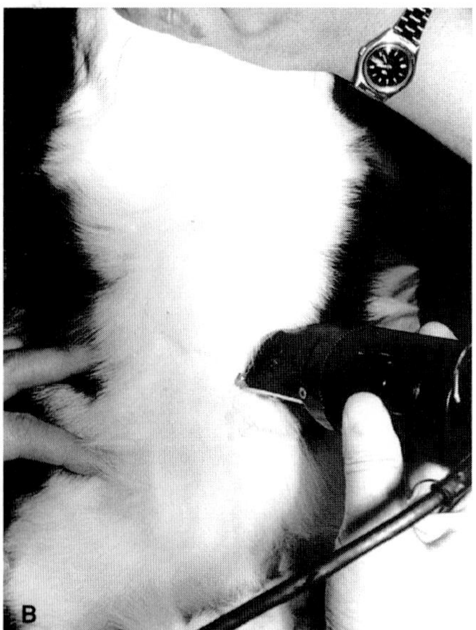

Figure 3-29. (**A**) Scanning of the cranial mediastinum using an intercostal approach with the animal standing. (**B**) Clipping the hair from the caudal cervical region for scanning of the cranial mediastinum through a thoracic inlet approach.

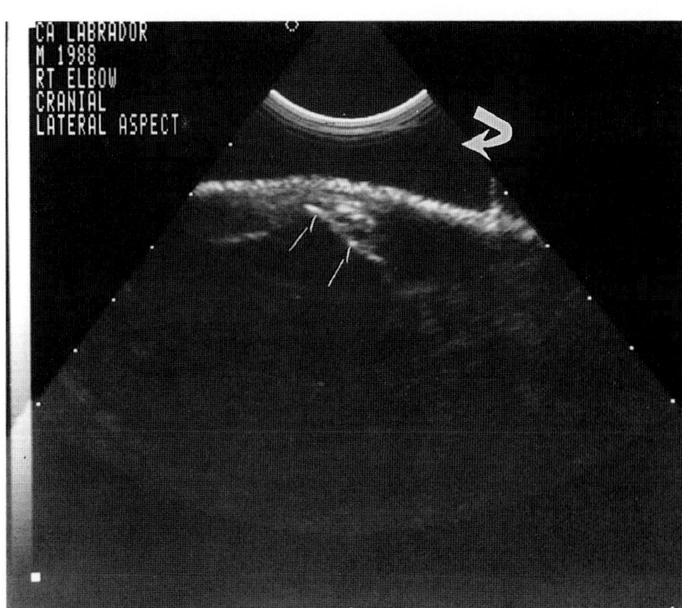

Figure 3-30. Sonogram of the lateral collateral ligaments of the elbow joint in a dog. A standoff pad has been used (*white arrow*). The echogenic surface of the lateral humeral condyle is seen (*black arrows*).

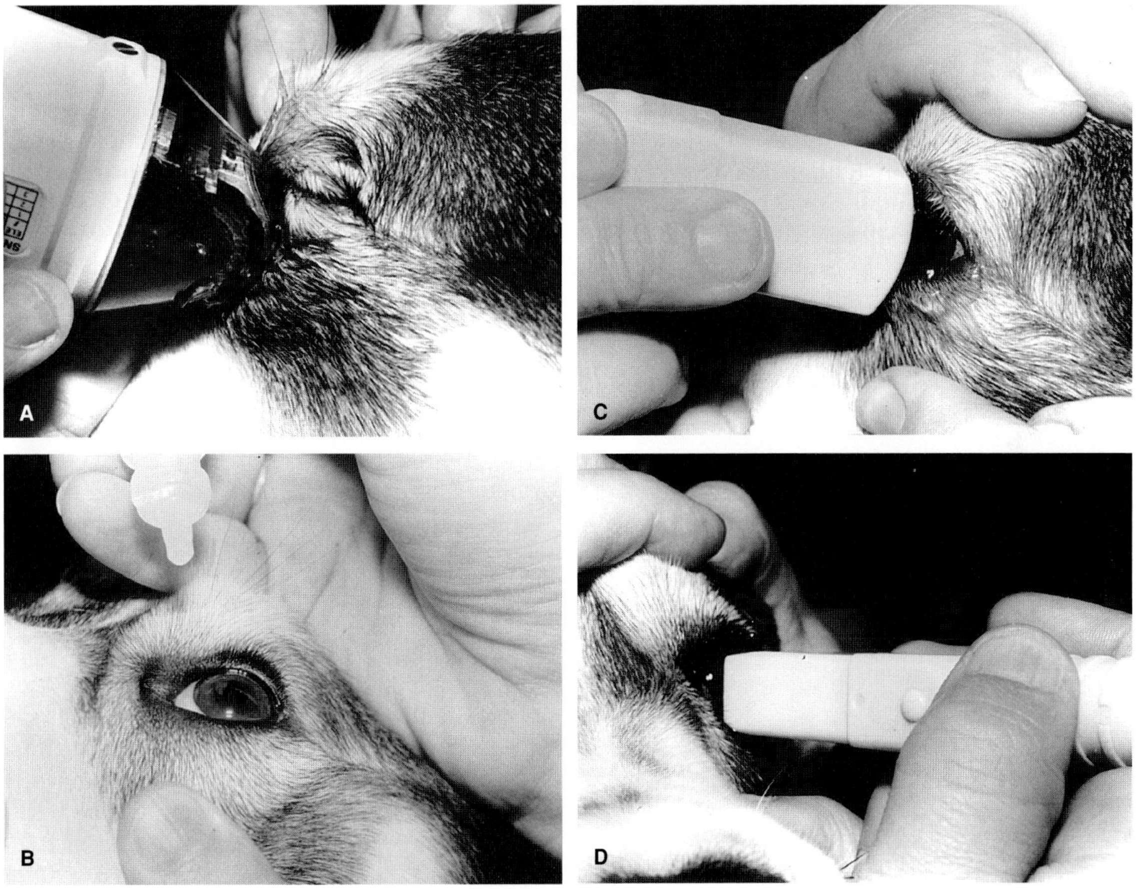

Figure 3-31. (**A**) Ocular sonography with the transpalpebral technique. It may be necessary to clip the hair from the eyelids. (**B**) Topical ophthalmic anesthetic drops are used before ocular sonography with the direct corneal contact technique. This method is tolerated very well and tranquilization is rarely needed. (**C**) Sagittal or vertical and (**D**) frontal or horizontal scanning of the eye. Sterile gel has been applied to the transducer's surface and to the eye.

MISCELLANEOUS STRUCTURES

Musculoskeletal imaging typically is accomplished in two imaging planes. With tendon scanning, for example, the long axis of the tendon follows the long axis of the limb, and transverse scanning is performed with a 90° rotation of the transducer. Joint imaging is more complex because of the variety of bony prominences and collateral ligaments encountered (Fig. 3-30).

Ocular sonography, which can be performed through the lids or with direct corneal contact, is done in sagittal and frontal image planes that many operators refer to as vertical and horizontal sections through the eye (Fig. 3-31).

Brain sonography can only be performed through open fontanelles, which are usually located between the frontal and parietal bones in the middorsal or bilateral dorsal oblique aspects of the cranial vault (Fig. 3-32). The cranial sutures are typically not wide enough to permit passage of the sound beam. Sagittal and transverse image planes are possible when scanning through open fontanelles. By lateral fanning of the sagittally oriented transducer, parasagittal oblique planes through the brain are obtained. Rostral to caudal fanning of the transversely oriented transducer yields oblique transverse planes from the rostral brain through the brain stem.

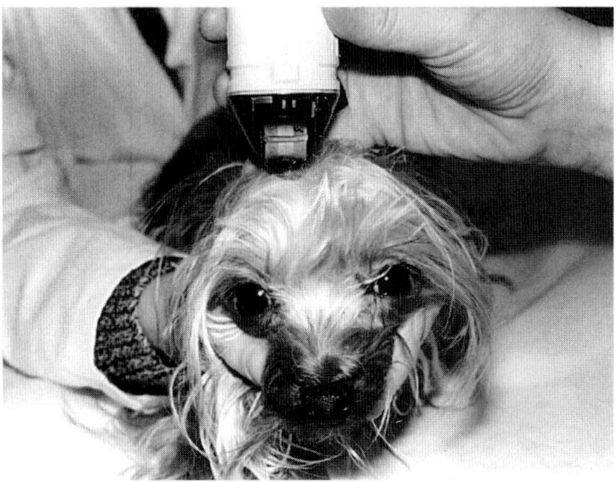

Figure 3-32. Sagittal scanning of the brain through an open fontanelle in a dog with hydrocephalus. Only a small amount of hair needs to be clipped over the defect in the cranium.

ULTRASOUND-GUIDED BIOPSY

Although ultrasound can be used to detect organ or tissue abnormalities, it can not differentiate benign from malignant disease based on sonographic appearance. A biopsy or fine-needle aspirate is often necessary to arrive at a diagnosis. Many lesions are focal, and many tumors are heterogenous, making "blind" percutaneous biopsies or aspirations of organs inaccurate or nondiagnostic. Ultrasound can be used during an aspiration or biopsy procedure to guide the needle tip into the area of greatest sampling accuracy.

Two types of ultrasound-guided biopsies are possible: mechanically guided and free-hand procedures. In the mechanically guided method, a ring or clamp device that contains a sterile guide or port through which the needle is passed is attached to the transducer (Fig. 3-33*A*, *B*). The path the needle will take is indicated by a track guide, which appears on the monitor superimposed over the real-time image (Fig. 3-33*C*). This method improves the sampling accuracy by allowing the operator to position the lesion within the biopsy track with transducer manipulation before the needle is inserted. In free-hand biopsies, the needle is inserted at an angle relative to the transducer, so that it will pass lengthwise through the beam path (Fig. 3-33*D*). The operator has complete control of the needle's movement in all planes and must coordinate both hands so that the transducer and the needle move in unison. If the operator understands the geometry of the ultrasound beam relative to the lesion and the patient, this method of sampling can be just as accurate as sampling done with the aid of a needle guide.

Whether mechanically guided or free-hand, biopsy samples may be obtained with manual or automated devices. Manual biopsies use sampling needles that require operation of a trocar and cannula with both hands. The ultrasound-guided tissue biopsies with manual needles will require two people: one to hold the transducer while the other operates the needle. Several automated biopsy devices allow quick and accurate sampling by a single operator (Fig. 3-34*A*–*C*). These are spring-loaded devices that can be fired with the touch of a button,

(text continues on p. 56)

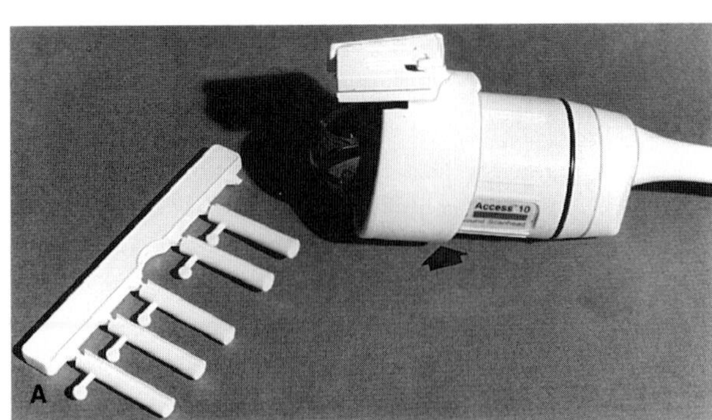

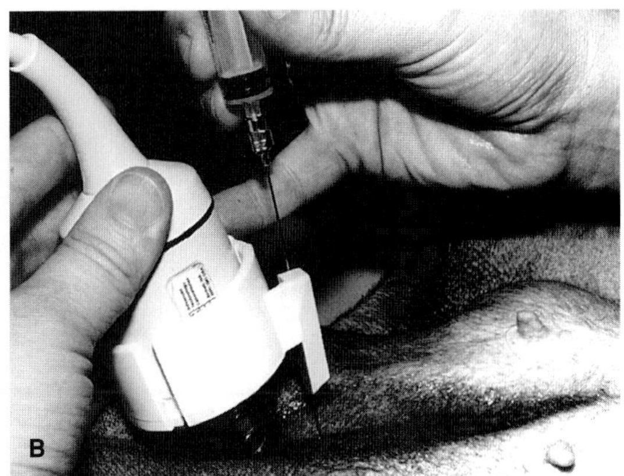

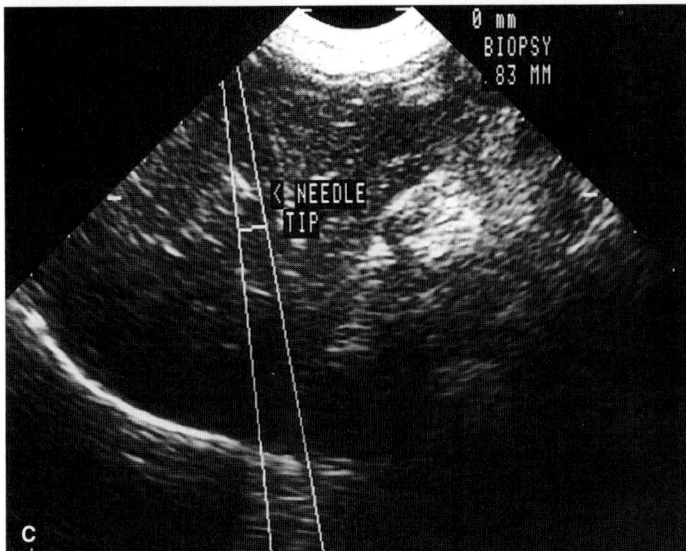

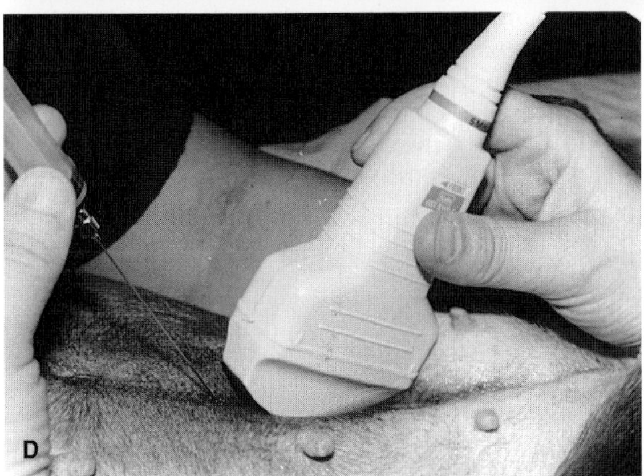

Figure 3-33. (**A**) Biopsy guide (*arrow*) attached to the transducer. Needle ports come in various sizes to accommodate all gauges. (**B**) Biopsy guide and needle in place for ultrasound-guided needle aspiration. (**C**) Biopsy track guide on the screen showing the expected path of the needle as it passes through the guide. The depth of the lesion can be premeasured so that the proper needle length can be chosen. The tip of this needle is at 8.3 cm. (**D**) Free-hand technique for ultrasound-guided fine-needle aspiration.

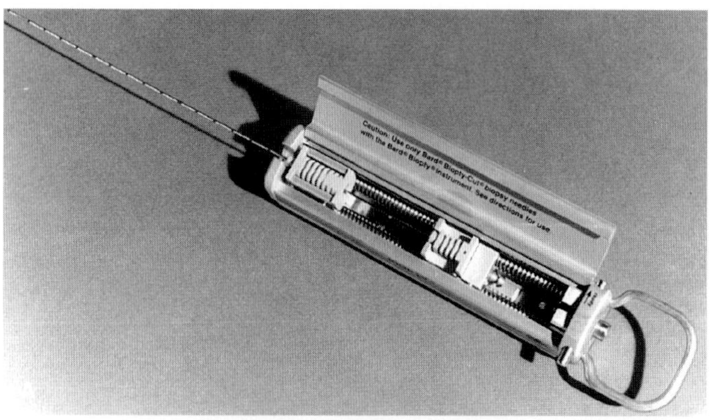

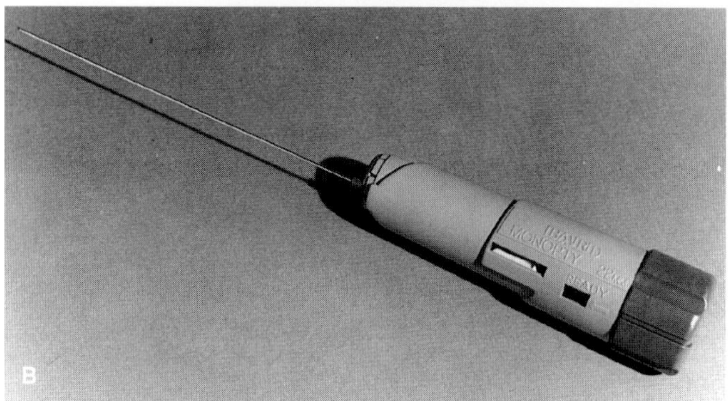

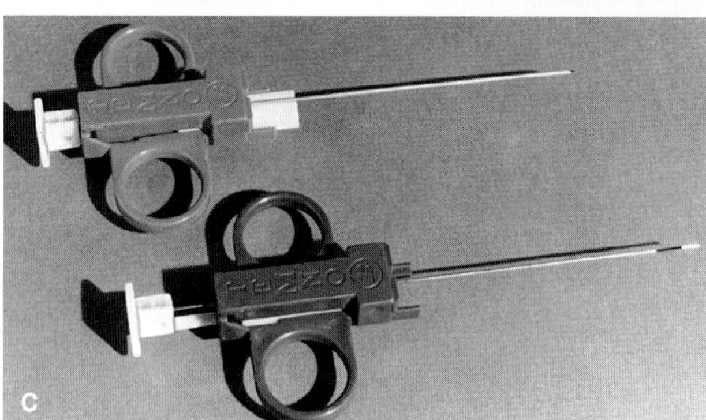

Figure 3-34. Automated biopsy devices for ultrasound-guided biopsy procedures. (**A**) The Bard Biopty brand biopsy instrument opened to show the spring mechanism and a Tru-cut–type biopsy needle in place. (**B**) The Bard Monopty instrument, which is a disposable version of the biopsy "gun." (**C**) Temno brand biopsy needles, another disposable automated biopsy device.

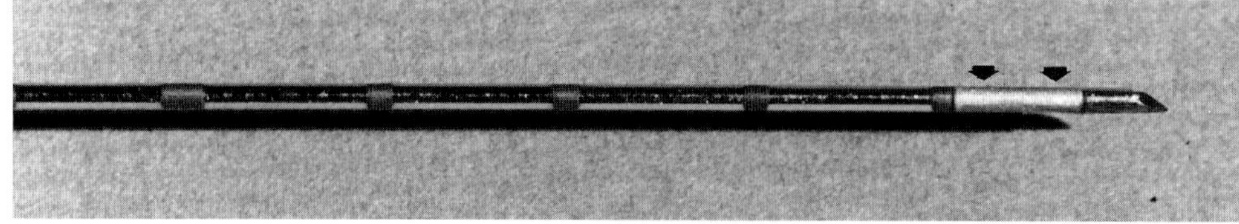

Figure 3-35. Tru-Cut–type biopsy needle, showing the treated surface near the needle tip (*arrow*) to enhance needle visualization within the tissues. Other marks are visual depth indicators spaced at 1-cm intervals.

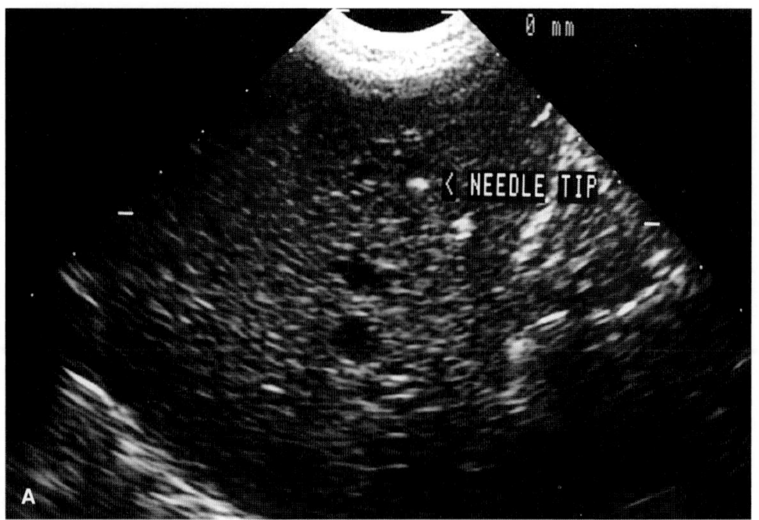

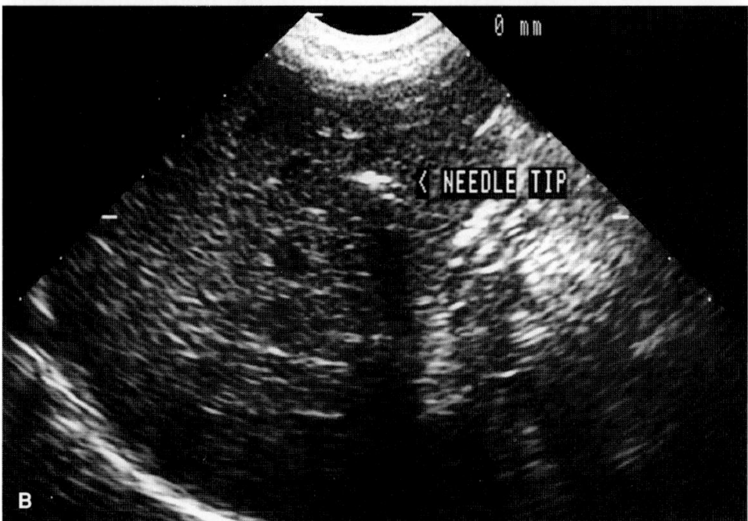

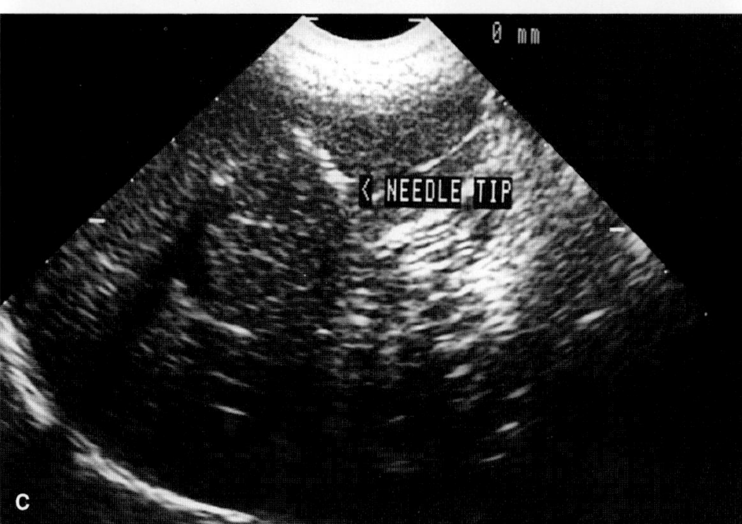

Figure 3-36. (**A**) Echogenic focus within the liver parenchyma generated by a spinal needle to be used for fine-needle aspiration. This needle was introduced using a free-hand technique. (**B**) Increased echogenicity of this spinal needle tip was created by scoring the shaft of the needle near the tip with a sterile scalpel blade. Compare with Figure 3-26A. (**C**) Enhanced visualization of the spinal needle created with the pump maneuver. Compare with Figure 3-36A.

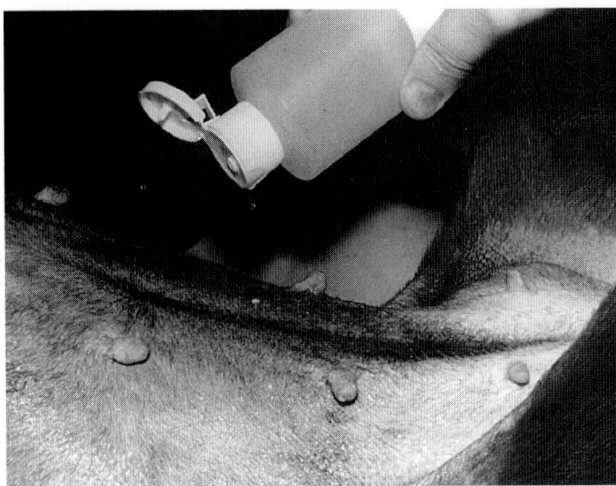

Figure 3-37. After the area has been surgically prepped, alcohol or sterile ultrasound gel is applied to provide coupling between the transducer and the patient.

advancing the needle, obtaining the sample, and sheathing the trocar all in one swift maneuver. The sonographer can hold the transducer in one hand and operate the automated biopsy gun with the other.

Ultrasound-guided biopsies and fine-needle aspirates are more accurate than blind sampling of focal lesions. However, sampling problems do occur. The most common reason for poor sampling is inadequate visualization of the needle tip. For the entire needle to be visible at all times during ultrasound-guided biopsies, the needle must travel parallel to the beam path. If the needle varies from the beam path, the apparent tip on the ultrasound image could be a portion of the shaft, with the tip a few centimeters deeper than desired.

The type and size of needle also control its visibility in the ultrasound image. Large-gauge needles are more easily detected than small ones. Manufacturers make sampling needles of all types and sizes, with echogenic tips to enhance visualization within the tissues (Fig. 3-35). These needles have a special echogenic coating or a roughened surface near the tip to scatter the ultrasound beam, which creates a bright spot on the image display to indicate the exact location of the needle tip. A similar effect can be created by scoring the shaft of the needle near the tip with a sterile scalpel before sampling (Fig. 3-36*A, B*). Another technique to enhance needle tip localization is the pump maneuver, in which pumping the stylet in and out of the stationary needle shaft increases the echogenicity of the needle shaft and tip (Fig. 3-36*C*).[9] This works well with spinal needles, which are often used for fine-needle aspirates.

Most biopsy or aspiration procedures are best performed with the animal sedated or anesthetized. Local anesthetic can also be used. An initial ultrasound examination of the organ or area to be sampled should be performed first.

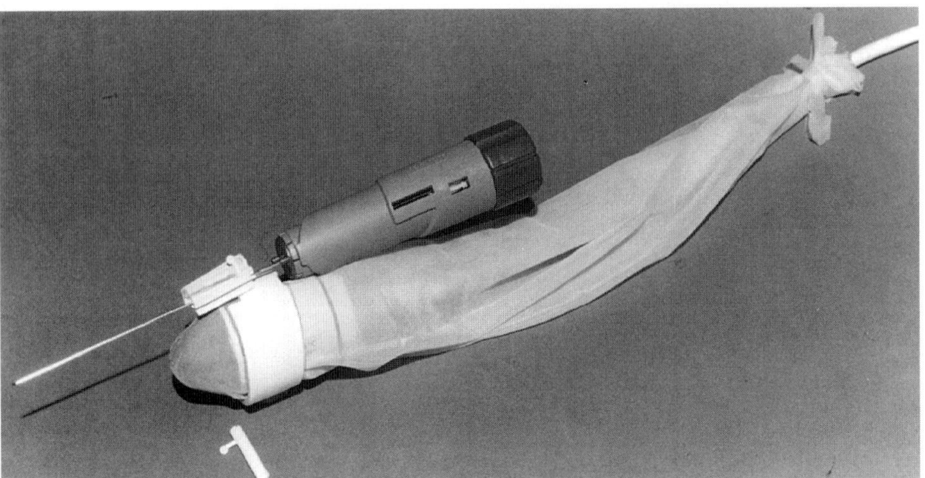

Figure 3-38. Ultrasound transducer covered with a sterile sleeve. The sterilized biopsy guide has been attached over the sleeve, and an automated biopsy device has been positioned within the needle guide.

The patient's skin is then prepared using a standard presurgical preparation technique. Sterile gel or alcohol is used on the skin to provide coupling for the ultrasound beam (Fig. 3-37). The ultrasound transducer may be covered with a commercially available sterile sleeve with sterile gel or other coupling medium inside and sterile gel placed on the skin (Fig. 3-38). As an alternative to covering the probe, the transducer surface can be disinfected topically and the procedure performed without a probe cover. (Transducers should never be autoclaved, because the piezoelectric crystal is heat sensitive.) A stab incision with a scalpel blade is recommended to prevent dulling the needle. After any aspirate or biopsy procedure, the area sampled should be monitored for hemorrhage for at least 5 minutes. An article in the veterinary literature serves as an excellent reference on ultrasound-guided percutaneous needle biopsies.[10]

CONCLUSION

Ultrasound is not only a science but an art. Many techniques and helpful suggestions have been presented in this chapter to make investigations into the world of veterinary ultrasound as easy and as enjoyable as possible. Although some preparation is necessary to learn a new skill, no amount or reading or studying can teach someone to be a good sonographer. The best teacher is practice.

REFERENCES

1. Blevins WE. Scanning technique. In: Blevins WE, Widmer WR, Jakovljevic S, Peter AT. Veterinary diagnostic ultrasound: a course for those new to diagnostic ultrasound. West Lafayette: Purdue University, 1990:22.
2. Rosenzweig LJ. Introduction to the cat. In: Rosenzweig LJ, ed. Anatomy of the cat: text and dissection guide. Dubuque: William C Brown, 1990:2.
3. Adams DR. Directional terminology. In: Adams DR. Canine anatomy: a systemic study. Ames: The Iowa State University Press, 1986:7.
4. Miner NS. Basic principles. In: Sanders RC, ed. Clinical sonography: a practical guide. 2nd ed. Boston: Little, Brown and Co, 1991:38.
5. Herring DS. Abdominal ultrasound: theory and practice. Semin Vet Med Surg (Small Anim) 1986;1:102.
6. Barr F. Imaging of the liver and spleen. In: Barr F, ed. Diagnostic ultrasound in the dog and cat. Oxford: Blackwell Scientific Publications, 1990:21.
7. Bushong SC, Archer BR. Diagnostic ultrasound: physics, biology, and instrumentation. St. Louis: Mosby Year Book, 1991:88.
8. Thomas WP, Gaber CE, Jacobs GJ, et al. Recommendations for standards in transthoracic two-dimensional echocardiography in the dog and cat. J Vet Intern Med 1993;7:247.
9. Bisceglia M, Matalon TAS, Silver B. The pump maneuver: an atraumatic adjunct to enhance US needle tip localization. Radiology 1990;176:867.
10. Finn-Bodner ST, Hathcock JT. Image-guided percutaneous needle biopsy: ultrasound, computed tomography, and magnetic resonance imaging. Semin Vet Med Surg (Small Anim) 1993;8:258.

Small Animal Ultrasound, edited by Ronald W. Green.
Lippincott-Raven Publishers, Philadelphia © 1996.

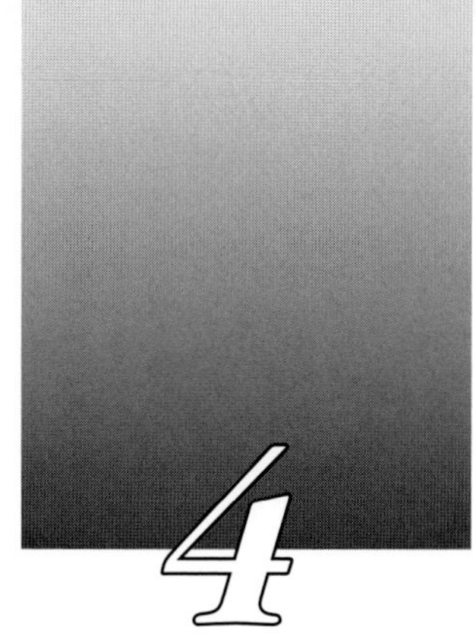

HEART

Charles S. Farrow

In contemporary clinical echocardiography, two modes of sonographic investigation predominate: long- or cross-sectional anatomic imaging and blood flow assessment.

Sectional cardiac scanning, also known as cross-sectional or two-dimensional echocardiography, is used to evaluate the anatomy of the heart. It also is capable of doing so dynamically, providing a measure of physiologic data with the anatomic information.

Intracardiac blood flow is assessed using Doppler-based sonography, including continuous-wave, pulsed-wave, and color-mapping methods. Doppler enables the examiner to determine several features of blood flow: direction, disturbed or undisturbed character (also called laminar or turbulent), and velocity (v).[1] Using the modified Bernoulli equation ($\Delta P = 4v^2$), Doppler can also be employed to calculate transvalvular pressure gradients (Δ).[2]

Although this chapter focuses on the basics of sectional cardiac imaging, the subsequent learning and integration of Doppler blood flow evaluation is strongly encouraged. Introductory articles on Doppler echocardiography are included in the references.[3,4]

THE RADIOGRAPHIC IMPERATIVE

The veterinarian should obtain and analyze thoracic radiographs before performing echocardiography. Radiography and sonography are complementary, not alternative or competing diagnostics. A radiograph is the superior method of assessing heart size and shape, and sonography is unsurpassed in depicting the internal cardiac anatomy. Radiography often infers the presence of an intracardiac shunt based on reduced (oligemic) or increased (hyperemic) pulmonary vasculature, but sonography is capable of confirming such anomalies.

Before Scanning

A few steps are necessary before scanning:

- The veterinarian should make a tentative diagnosis and a list of alternative possibilities.
- The typical and atypical sonographic features of the diseases being considered should be reviewed.
- Use of an anatomic check list can ensure that nothing is omitted during the sonographic examination (Fig. 4-1).
- Recent thoracic radiographs should be displayed in the examination area.
- Sufficient time should be allowed for a careful and unhurried examination.
- An animal that will not remain still should be tranquilized or sedated.
- An examination may be continued at a later time, especially in cases of complex congenital anomalies.

Echocardiography Worksheet

Examiner : CSF JWP RStV RB *Case Number :* *Date :*

Left Inflow

Left Atrial Size: normal / enlarged

Left Atrial Content/ Structure
- thrombus
- mass
- septal defect
- membrane

Mitral Valve Appearance: normal / abnormal
- endocardiosis
- endocarditis
- dysplasia

Mitral Valve Motion: normal / abnormal
- doming
- inverting

Left Ventricular Size: normal / enlarged

Left Ventricular Thickness: normal / enlarged

Interventricular Septum: normal / thickened
- septal defect
- motion + / -

FLOW

Mitral Regurgitation + / - (mild • mod • severe)

Mitral Stenosis + / - (mild • mod • severe)

Right Inflow

Right Atrial Size: normal / enlarged

Right Atrial Content / Structure
- thrombus
- mass
- septal defect
- membrane

Tricuspid Valve Appearance: normal / abnormal
- endocardiosis
- endocarditis
- dysplasia

Tricuspid Valve Motion: normal / abnormal

Right Ventricular Size: normal / enlarged

Right Ventricular Thickness: normal / enlarged

FLOW

Tricuspid Regurgitation + / - (mild • mod • severe)

Tricuspid Stenosis + / - (mild • mod • severe)

Left Outflow

Left Ventricular Outflow Tract: normal / narrowed
- mitral obstruction - / + (*Venturi effect*)

Aortic Valve Appearance: normal / abnormal
- stenotic (sub-/ aortic/ supra-)
- endocarditis
- dysplasia

Aortic Root: normal / dilated
narrowed / displaced

FLOW

Aortic Stenosis + / - (mild • mod • severe)

Aortic Regurgitation + / - (mild • mod • severe)

Transvalvular Gradient

Right Outflow

Right Ventricular Outflow Tract: normal / narrowed

Pulmonic Valve Appearance: normal / abnormal
- stenotic (sub-/ aortic/ supra-)
- endocarditis
- dysplasia

Pulmonic Root: normal / dilated
narrowed / displaced

FLOW

Pulmonic Stenosis + / - (mild • mod • severe)

Pulmonic Regurgitation + / - (mild • mod • severe)

Transvalvular Gradient

Provisional Diagnosis Endocardiosis (L • R• L/R), Endocarditis, Dysplasia (MV•TV•AV•PV), PS, AS Myopathy (TIM• Hyper• Dilated), ASD, VSD, PDA, Eisenmenger, TofF, HWD Combined Anom's

Designed & developed by C.S. Farrow DVM D-3 11-4-94

Figure 4-1. Echocardiography worksheet. This scheme divides the heart into four flow regions: left and right *inflows*, and left and right *outflows*. The cross-sectional anatomy and flow characteristics of each region are assessed independently as normal or abnormal, and in the case of the latter, the specific abnormality is selected from the listed diseases. If Doppler is available, associated flow characteristics and gradients (where appropriate) are also recorded. The obtained information is then integrated into a provisional diagnosis and chosen from the disorders listed at the bottom of the page. *Worksheet entries may be made by circling or checking off the desired choices.*

The veterinarian should learn to expect the unexpected; diagnostic bias can be the strongest ally and the most treacherous enemy.

Functionally Conceptualizing the Heart

The internal workings of the heart may be conceptualized anatomically and physiologically. Anatomically, the heart has been likened to a pair of pumps working side by side to satisfy the circulatory needs of the body (Fig. 4-2). The right pump is the weaker of the two, needing only to overcome the relatively low vascular resistance of the lung, and it is composed of an upper thin-walled chamber (ie, right atrium), an intervening one-way valve (ie, tricuspid or right atrioventricular valve), and a much larger, thicker, lower chamber (ie, right ventricle). The left pump is organized in a similar fashion—left atrium, mitral valve, left ventricle—but has a more muscular wall to meet the prodigious demands of driving the systemic circulation.[5]

Two additional one-way valves control the external movement of blood from the heart: the pulmonic valve leading from the right side of the heart to the lung and the aortic valve providing an exit from the left hand side of the heart to the remainder of the body.

From a functional perspective, the heart may be viewed in terms of its blood flow. In such a scheme, there are four divisions: the left and right inflows and the left and right outflows (Fig. 4-3). The *left inflow* is composed of the left atrium, mitral valve, chordae, papillary muscles, and the main chamber of the left ventricle. The *left outflow* is made up of the muscular tunnel leading from the main chamber of the left ventricle (ie, ventricular outflow tract) to the aortic valve, the aortic valve, and aortic sinus and proximal aortic trunk. The *right inflow* is composed of the right atrium, tricuspid valve and chordae, papillary muscles, and most of the right ventricle. The *right outflow* consists of the muscular tunnel leading from the main chamber of the right ventricle to the pulmonic valve (ie, pulmonic outflow tract), the pulmonic valve, and proximal aspect of the main pulmonary artery.

Scanning Technique

A dog or cat may be scanned in a variety of positions: standing, on its sternum, or lying laterally recumbent (Fig. 4-4). In the lateral recumbent position, the scanner (ie, transducer, probe) may be placed on the upper or lowermost sides of the thorax, which in the case of the latter, requires a cut-out examination table (see Figs. 3-11 and 4-4D), raised platform, or slotted pad. A modified lowermost scanning position may be achieved using a conventional table top by extending the animal's sternum beyond the

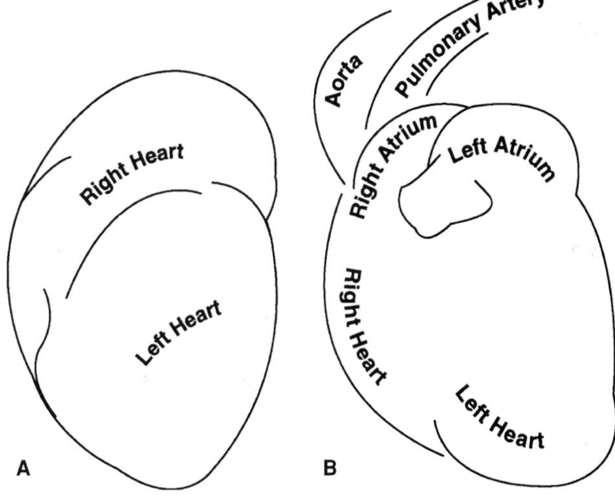

Figure 4-2. Two-pump concept. Although a highly integrated, single organ, the heart may be conceptualized mechanically as a pair of pumps: a right pump to oxygenate the blood and dispel carbon dioxide through the lung and a left pump to distribute the reconstituted blood to the remainder of the body. **(A)** Right and left sides of the heart viewed from the ventral aspect. **(B)** Right and left sides of the heart viewed from left lateral aspects.

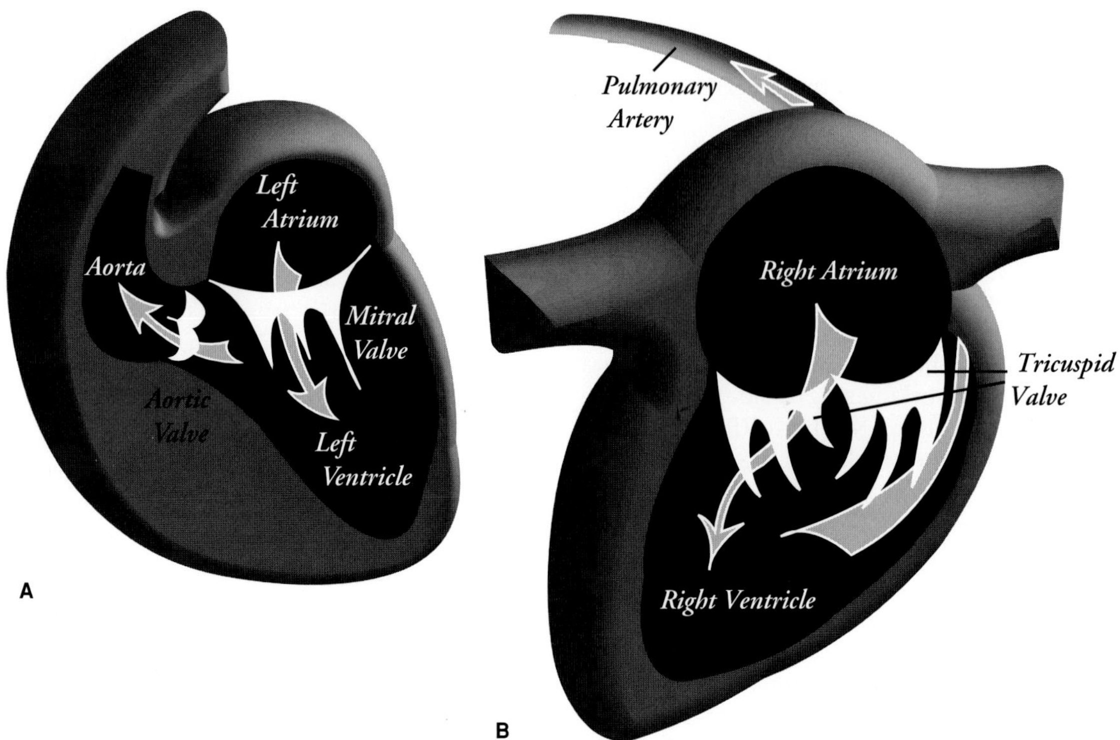

Figure 4-3. Cardiac flow regions. Functionally, the heart may be thought of as having four *flow regions* (ie, left inflow, left outflow, right inflow, right outflow), blood pathways to and from the left and right sides of the heart. (**A**) Left inflow and outflow (cutaway left lateral perspective). (**B**) Right inflow and outflow (cutaway right lateral perspective). Flow tracts are indicated by arrows (the discontinuity in the upper part of the right outflow arrow reflects the crossing of the outflow tract from the right to the left sides of the heart).

table edge sufficiently far to allow for ventral scanner placement.

The scanner is placed on the lateroventral aspect of the thoracic wall, adjacent to the sternum and caudal to the axilla. The optimal scanner placement varies with the breed of animal, its particular heart disease, and the amount of postural atelectasis present, but it usually coincides with the point of maximum palpable cardiac intensity.

It is useful for the beginner to imagine the relative positions of the heart valves in terms of the one-way, side-by-side entrance and exit doors found in many stores. Although this analogy is more appropriate to the left side of the heart, it nevertheless provides the examiner with a sense of relative valvular position that is not easily developed otherwise.

Precise, standardized scan planes are often difficult to achieve in dogs and cats. A group of veterinary cardiologists have proposed a standard examination protocol for cross-sectional echocardiography in dogs and cats.[6] I recommend that the reader learn and adopt this method after the more simplified version described subsequently has been mastered.

Simplified Scanning Protocol

Basics

After locating the heart, the examiner picks a standardized plane, holds the scanner still, and becomes accustomed to the surroundings. Because the sonographic environment is unique, it

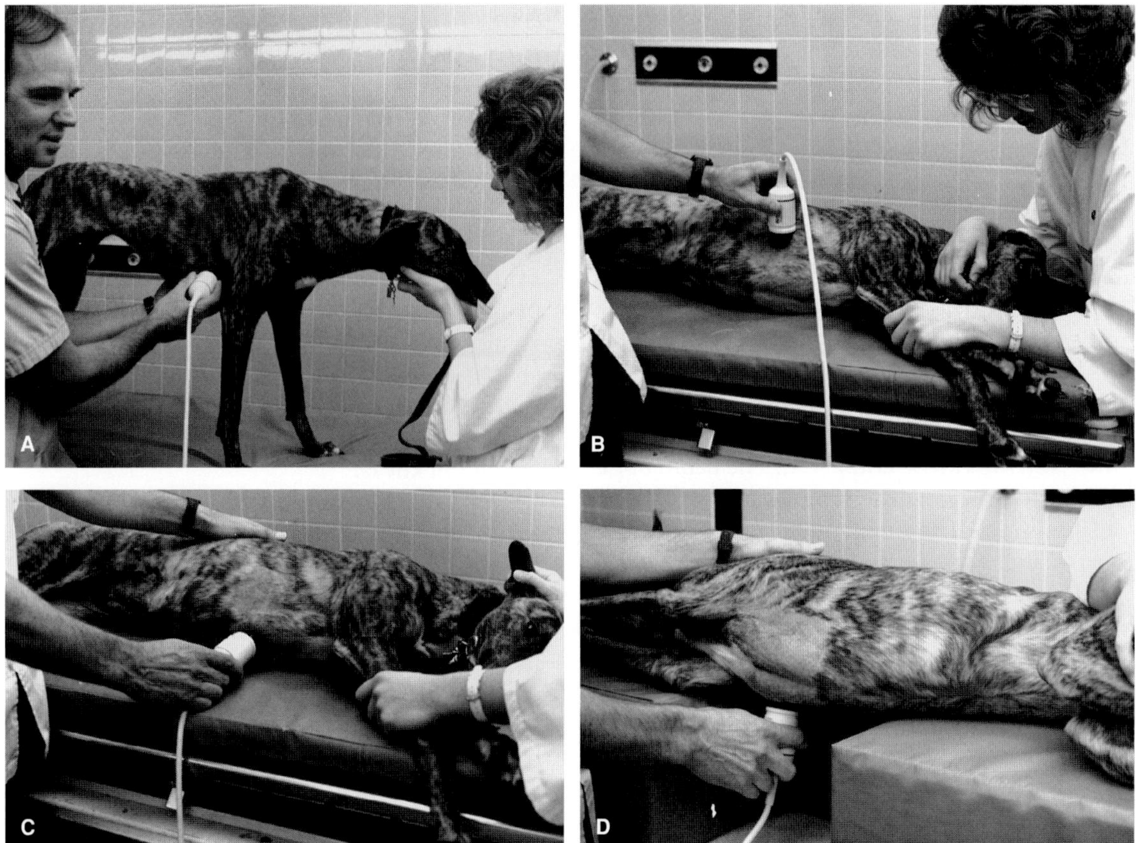

Figure 4-4. Scanning positions. The heart may be scanned with the animal in a variety of positions: (**A**) standing; (**B**) on its left (or right) side, with the scanner positioned above the sternum; (**C**) with scanner positioned below the sternum; (**D**) from the lowermost aspect of the thorax using a slotted pad or table.

requires some getting used to, especially for beginners. This is also the ideal time to adjust the controls.

After becoming acclimated to the sonographic surroundings and optimizing the image, the operator begins the examination by rotating or rocking the scanner through the initial contact point on the thoracic wall. Only after these planes have been investigated should the scan head be moved to a new location to begin the process anew. Bear in mind that the surest indication of an inexperienced examiner is perpetual scanner motion.

The examiner should always be aware of the position in the heart and what structures are being imaged. It is impossible to detect the abnormal without first learning to recognize the normal. In the case of the heart, this means normal variations, because the heart is constantly in motion.

Examining From the Right Parasternal Position

The initial scanner placement can be estimated by studying the heart position on survey radiographs. The examiner grips the scanner like a pistol, with the thumb uppermost on the index ridge, button, or mark. The forefinger of the scanning hand is extended to the chest wall to determine the point of maximum cardiac intensity, and the examiner positions the scanner accordingly. Observing the monitor for characteristic heart motion, the examiner manipulates the scanner to bring the heart into the center of the screen and makes the necessary angular corrections to visualize the left inflow tract in long section, with left atrium to the right side of the screen.

The examiner continues to adjust beam angle until the length and width of the left ventricle has been maximized. The area can be evaluated with a cineloop if available; otherwise, freeze frames, thermal prints, or videotape and real-time viewing can be employed. The beam angle is adjusted to view the long section of the left outflow tract. The image is optimized and the area evaluated.

The scanner is directed toward the estimated distal third of the heart and rotated approximately 90°. This provides a cross-sectional image of the ventricles. Stepwise fanning of the ultrasound beam dorsally provides cross-sectional views of the ventricles, the mitral and aortic valves, and the right outflow tract, including the pulmonic valve.

Examining From the Left Parasternal Position

The examiner estimates the initial scanner placement by studying the heart position on survey radiographs. The scanner is gripped like a pistol, with the thumb uppermost on the index ridge, button, or mark. The examiner extends a forefinger of the scanning hand to the chest wall and determines the point of maximum cardiac intensity, positioning the scanner accordingly.

He or she observes the monitor for characteristic heart motion, manipulates the scanner to bring the heart into the center of the screen, and makes the necessary angular corrections to visualize the entire heart (right and left sides) in long section. This is called a four-chamber view. With a small adjustment in the rotational angle of the scanner, the aorta may also be included in the four-chamber view, in which case it is called a five-chamber view. Either of these views provides a superior overview of the heart.

Normal Sonographic Anatomy and Pitfalls

The normal sonographic anatomy of the dog and cat heart are shown in Figures 4-5 and 4-6. Normal, breed-associated sonographic variability coincides well with reported normal radiographic variations. In general, a tall, thin breed of dog, such as an Afghan hound, has a more oval left ventricle, and the ventricle of a bulldog is more spherically configured. The ventricle shapes of most other breeds lie somewhere between. The heart chambers of most breeds are comparable in shape but not in size or in wall or septal thickness.

In addition to the more traditional transthoracic imaging planes, the heart may also be scanned from the abdomen, using the liver as an acoustic window (Fig. 4-7).

One of the most important observations that may be made in echocardiography concerns the contractility or force of contraction of the heart. Weak contraction is for the most part a reliable indicator of heart disease, but there are exceptions. Many medium-sized and most large breeds of dogs have slower heart rates and weaker-appearing contractility. The veterinarian should exercise caution in assessing reduced contractility in such animals.

Note to the Novice

Because this chapter is written for the beginner, the process has been made as simple as possible and some selected disorders have been omitted. However, what was left out is not essential to entry-level sonology, and overly detailed instructions may actually impede the learning process for some.

I have attempted to simplify the descriptive sonographic terminology or "ultra talk," as it has been called. For example, because most cardiac ultrasound examinations are performed from the parasternal position (right or left), I omitted this descriptor from the figure legends. I also dropped the term "apical," because all cardiac examinations in animals are performed from at or near the cardiac apex on the lateroventral aspect of the thoracic wall. I omitted

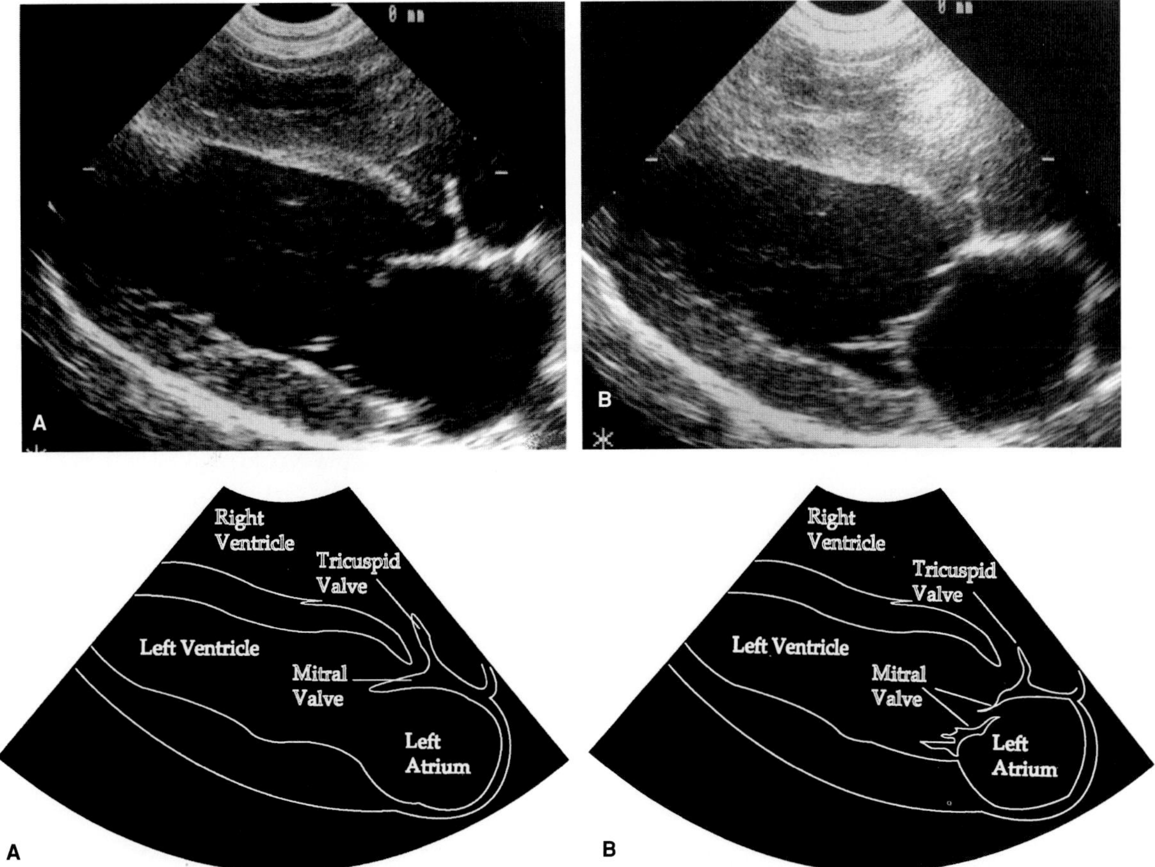

Figure 4-5. Normal dog. (**A**) Long-sectional image and diagram of the left inflow with the mitral valve open. (**B**) Long-sectional image and diagram of the left inflow with the mitral valve closed. *(continued)*

unnecessary encumbrances such as "two dimensional" or "real time."

I chose the descriptors cross and long section over short and long axis because the former seemed more intuitive. I accept anterior and posterior with reference to a human heart wall, but for dogs and cats, cranial and caudal seem more appropriate.

COMMON CONGENITAL HEART DISEASES

Patent Ductus Arteriosus

Radiographic Features

Radiographically, patent ductus arteriosus (ie, persistent arterial duct) is characterized by cardiomegaly with left-sided emphasis, enlarged aortic trunk and main pulmonary artery, and pulmonary overcirculation. In some patients, localized convexities appear on the left margin of the heart at the 1, 2, and 3 o'clock positions, representing the aortic trunk, main pulmonary artery, and left auricular appendage (viewed in the dorsoventral projection), respectively.

Sonographic Features

Sonographically, a patent ductus arteriosus may sometimes be identified as a small vessel joining the aortic root and main pulmonary artery (Fig. 4-8). However, the ductus is usually first located using color Doppler (Fig. 4-9).

More commonly, especially by the novice, a patent ductus is diagnosed on the basis of cir-

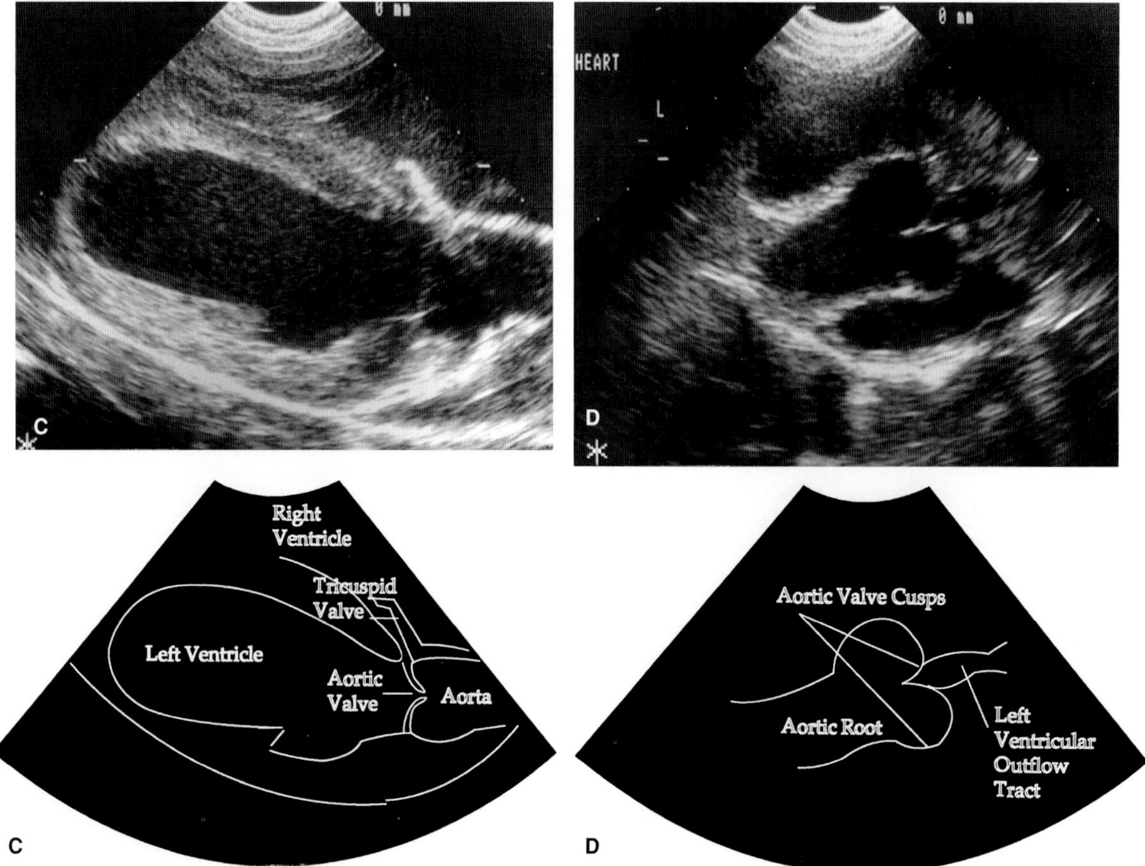

Figure 4-5. *(Continued)* (**C**) Long-sectional image and diagram of the left outflow. (**D**) Long-sectional close-up image and diagram of the aortic region.

cumstantial sonographic evidence (Fig. 4-10). Such evidence may include dilation of the left inflow tract, dilation of the aortic trunk to the extent that a discrete aortic sinus is no longer appreciable, or dilation of the main pulmonary artery.

Aortic Stenosis

Radiographic Features

Radiographically, aortic stenosis is characterized by cardiomegaly with left-sided emphasis, enlarged aortic trunk, and normal pulmonary vasculature. The enlarged aorta gives the heart an abnormally elongated appearance in the ventrodorsal projection.

Sonographic Features

Sonographically, aortic stenosis is characterized by an abnormal left heart (Figs. 4-11 and 4-12). The left inflow tract shows a dilated left atrium and ventricle. The left ventricular wall is variably thickened.

The left outflow tract often shows narrowing with one or more small, variably shaped tissue mounds proximal to the aortic valves. Occasionally, a subvalvular collar or membrane is present. In my experience, the most common ab-

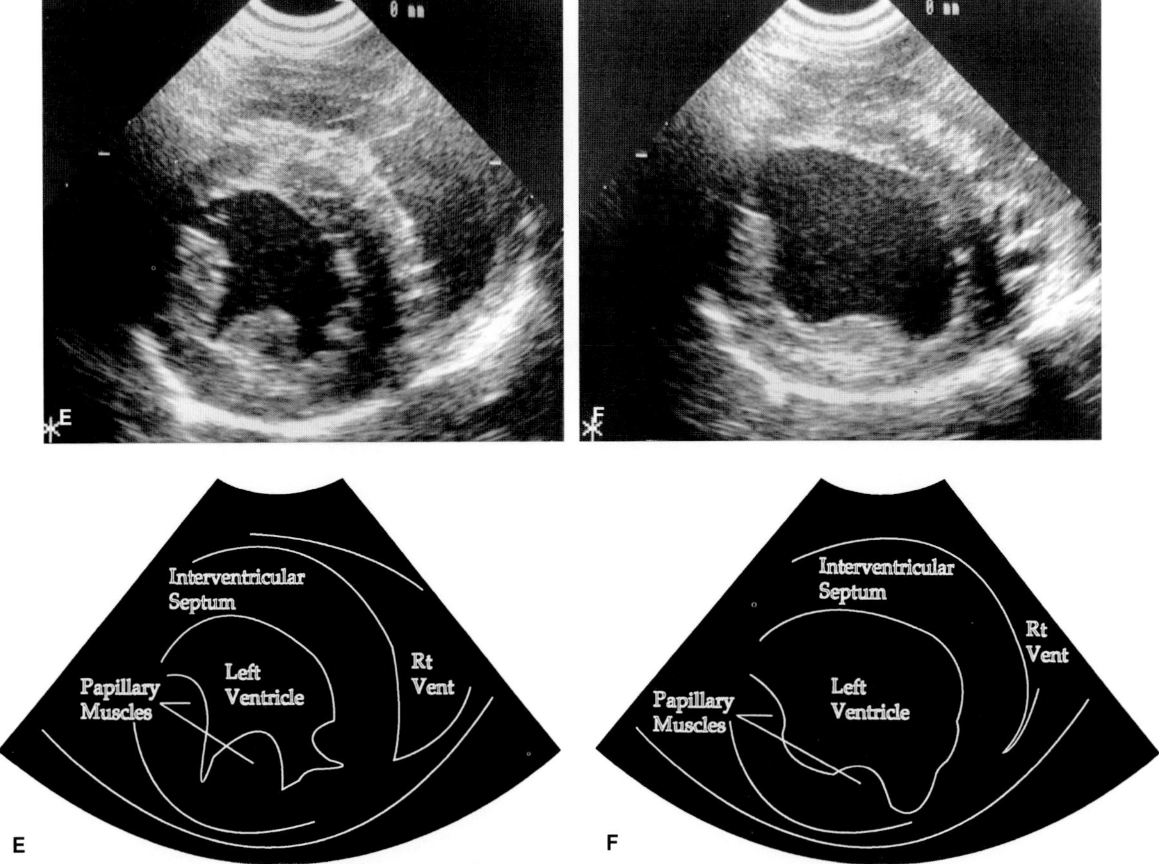

Figure 4-5. *(Continued)* (**E**) Cross-sectional image and diagram of the left inflow and midlumen of the left ventricle (during systole) (**F**) Cross-sectional image and diagram of the left inflow and midlumen of the left ventricle (during diastole). *(continued)*

normal septal configuration consists of an angular projection immediately proximal to the septal cusp that is most pronounced during systole.

One or more aortic valve cusps may move abnormally, and they occasionally appear thickened. The aortic root is usually dilated, often to the extent that it is comparable in diameter to the aortic sinus.

Pulmonic Stenosis

Radiographic Features

Radiographically, pulmonic stenosis is characterized by cardiomegaly with right-sided emphasis, enlarged pulmonic trunk, and normal or small pulmonary vasculature.

Sonographic Features

Sonographically, pulmonic stenosis is characterized by an abnormal right heart (Figs. 4-13 and 4-14). The right inflow tract shows a dilated right atrium and ventricle. The right ventricular wall is thickened. The right outflow may or may not appear narrowed.

The pulmonic valve is usually more visible than normal because of increased echogenicity, thickening, or deformity. One or more pulmonic valve cusps may move abnormally. The pulmonic trunk appears dilated.

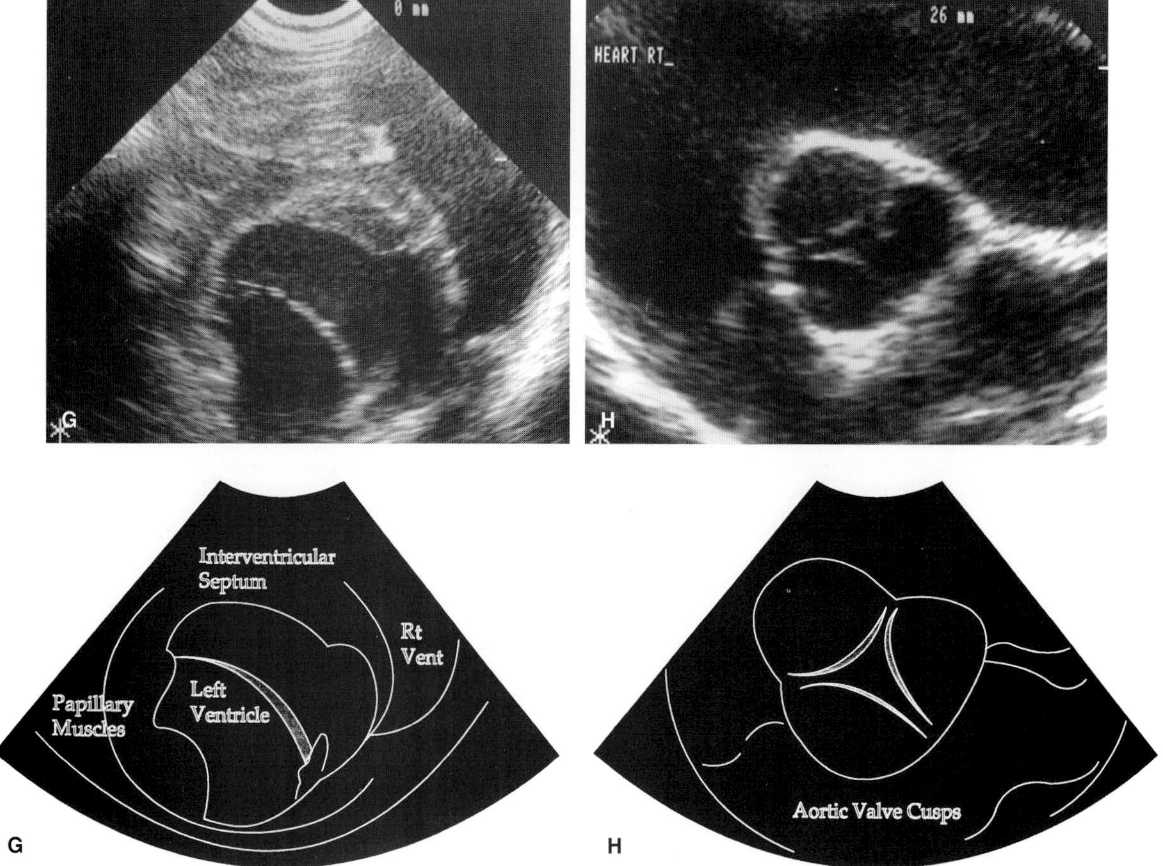

Figure 4-5. *(Continued)* (**G**) Cross-sectional image and diagram of the left inflow and mitral valve. (**H**) Cross-sctional image and diagram of the left outflow and aortic valve.

Ventricular Septal Defect

Radiographic Features

Radiographically, a medium or large, left-to-right septal defect is characterized by cardiomegaly with right-sided emphasis, enlargement of the main pulmonary artery, and pulmonary overcirculation. A long-standing ventricular septal defect associated with increased pulmonary resistance may lead to right-to-left interventricular blood flow. This condition is referred to as an Eisenmenger syndrome or Eisenmenger physiology. In some of these reverse shunts, there are large, tortuous lung vessels, reflecting chronic pulmonary hypertension.

Sonographic Features

Sonographically, a ventricular septal defect is characterized by an enlarged right heart. Ventricular septal defects are usually best seen in the long-sectional image of the left cardiac outflow tract at the level of the atrioventricular valves (Figs. 4-15 and 4-16).

The right inflow tract shows varying degrees of dilation and hypertrophy and, depending on the size of the ventricular septal defect, an incomplete septum. The right outflow tract may be smaller than normal due to hypertrophy.

The main pulmonary vessel is dilated. The left heart may also be dilated, although not typically to the same extent as the right.

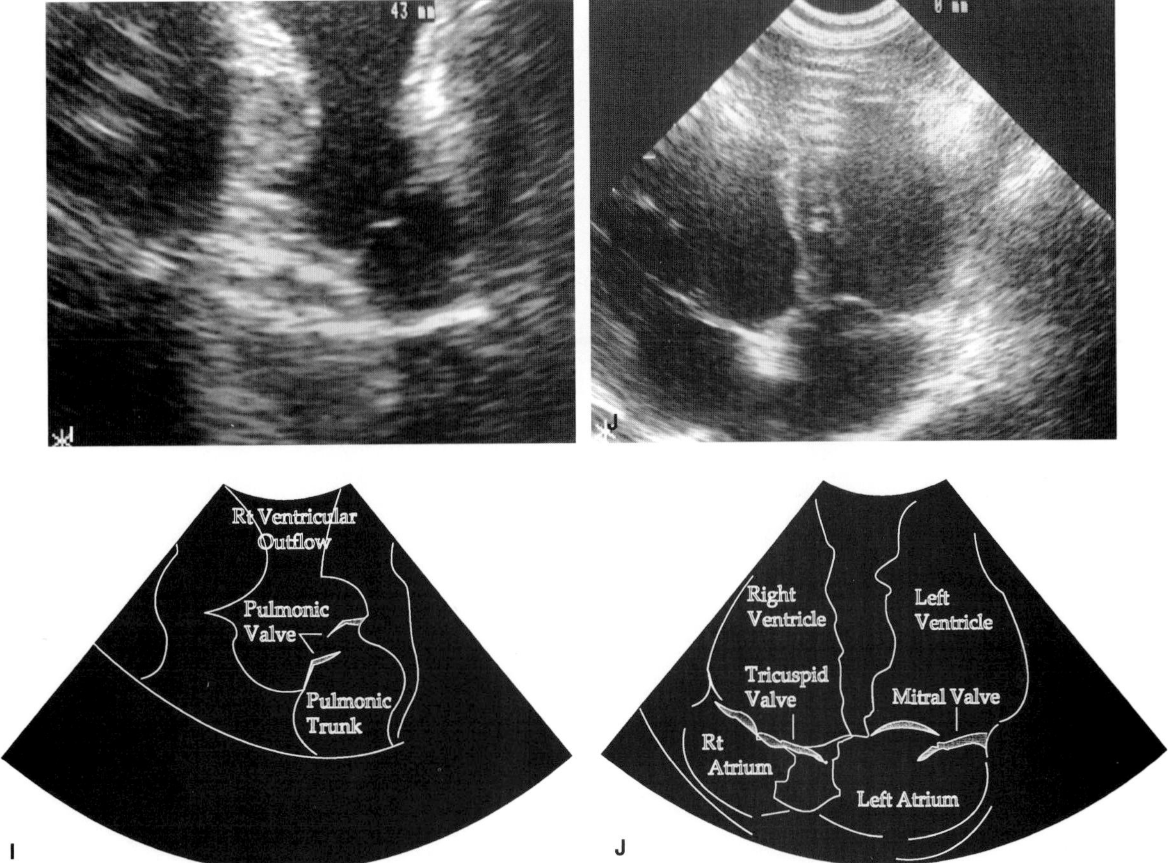

Figure 4-5. *(Continued)* (**I**) Cross-sectional image and diagram of the right outflow and pulmonic valve. (**J**) Four-chamber image and diagram of the heart.

The most proximal part of the ventricular septum commonly appears hypoechoic or even anechoic in long section, falsely suggesting a ventricular septal defect.

UNCOMMON CONGENITAL HEART DISEASES

Atrial Septal Defect

Radiographic Features

Atrial septal defect is relatively uncommon in dogs and cats. Its principal radiographic feature is right-sided enlargement, assuming that the defect is large enough to allow sufficient left to right shunting of blood across the defective atrial septum to produce right ventricular volume overload. Only in the advanced stages of this disease does pulmonary oligemia develop to the extent that it becomes radiographically recognizable. Small defects do not alter the heart sufficiently to allow radiographic detection, and moderately sized defects result in only slight cardiomegaly.

Sonographic Features

Sonographically, an atrial septal defect may be associated with an enlarged right heart, de-

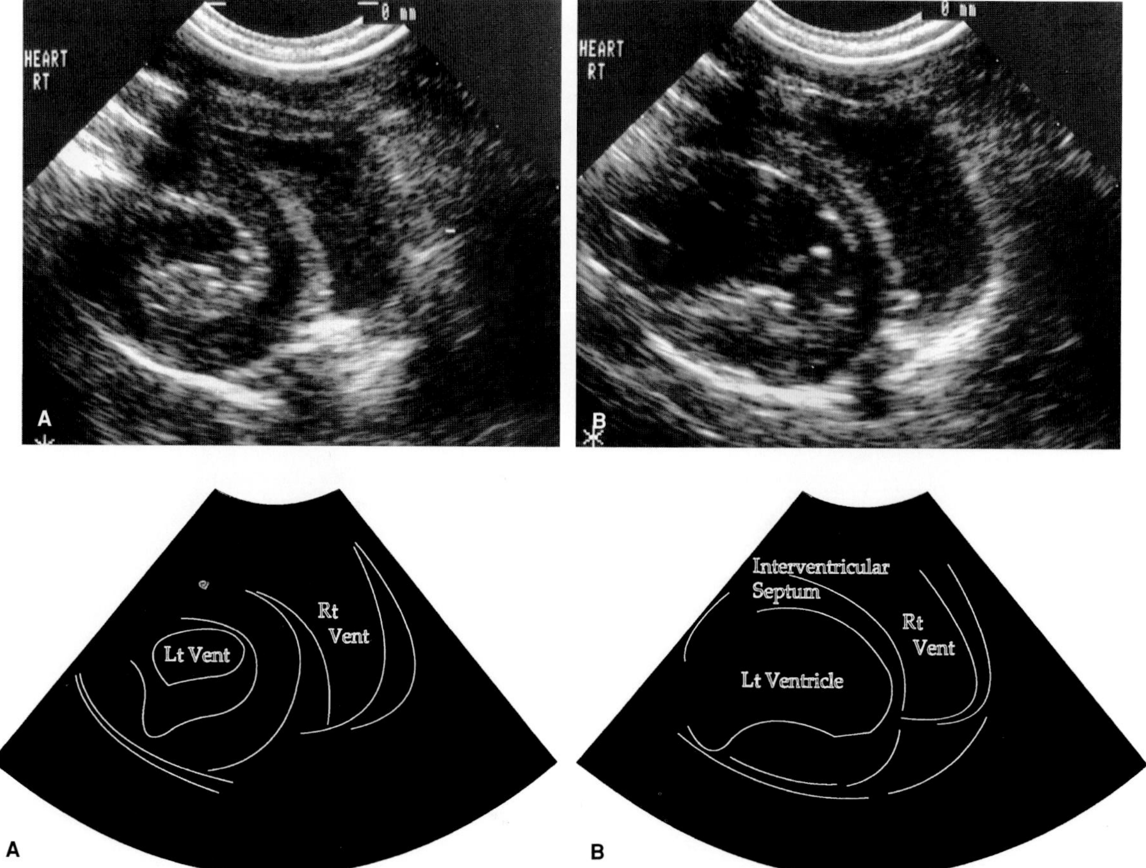

Figure 4-6. Normal cat. (**A**) Cross-sectional image and diagram of the left inflow and midlumen of the left ventricle (during systole). (**B**) Cross-sectional image and diagram of the left inflow and midlumen of the left ventricle (during diastole).

pending on its size and duration. Direct sonographic confirmation requires identification of septal discontinuity, with success largely predicated on the size of the defect, the quality of the scanning equipment, and the skill and experience of the examiner. If the defect is located in the ventral aspect of the septum near the atrioventricular valve, it is called an ostium primum type defect. A lesion in the central part of the atrial septum is classified as an ostium secundum defect, and a lesion located at the junction of the interatrial septum and caudal vena cava is designated a sinus venosus defect.

Care should be taken not to mistake the foramen ovale for a central (secondum) defect.[7]

Mitral and Tricuspid Dysplasia

Radiographic Features

Radiographically, atrioventricular valvular dysplasias are characterized by atrial enlargement causing the heart to appear taller and wider at the base in the lateral projection.

Sonographic Features

Sonographically, atrioventricular valvular dysplasia may be characterized by an abnormal right or left heart, depending on which valve is involved (Fig. 4-17). Using mitral dysplasia as

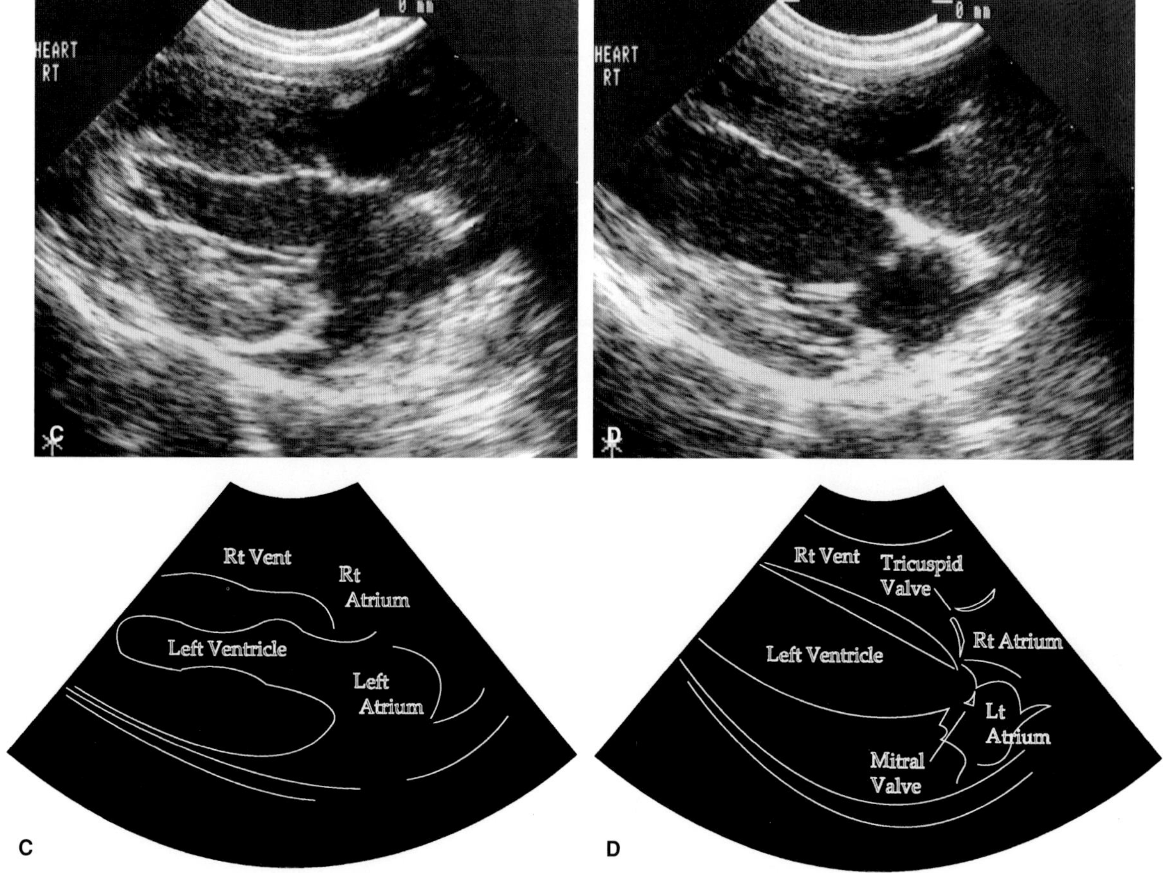

Figure 4-6. *(Continued)* (**C**) Long-sectional image and diagram of the left inflow (during systole). (**D**) Long-sectional image and diagram of the left inflow (during diastole). *(continued)*

an example, the left inflow tract shows dilation of left atrium and its incoming pulmonary veins, and the mitral valve is typically enlarged, deformed, and often moves abnormally.

Valvular dysplasia may also be diagnosed presumptively, on the basis of regurgitation demonstrated with Doppler (Fig. 4-18).

Ebstein's Anomaly

Radiographic Features

Radiographically, Ebstein's anomaly is a downward displacement of the tricuspid valves, resulting in the proximal part of the involved ventricle functioning as an atrial reservoir, and it is characterized by cardiomegaly with right-sided emphasis.

Sonographic Features

Sonographically, Ebstein's anomaly alters the right ventricular inflow tract in a characteristic manner (Fig. 4-19): extension of the tricuspid valves deeply into the right ventricle, right atrial dilation, and an abnormally shaped left ventricle.

Tetralogy of Fallot

Radiographic Features

Radiographically, tetralogy of Fallot is a complex cardiac anomaly composed of pulmonic stenosis, right ventricular hypertrophy, a large ventricular septal defect, and an abnormally small aorta. It characterized by right-sided en-

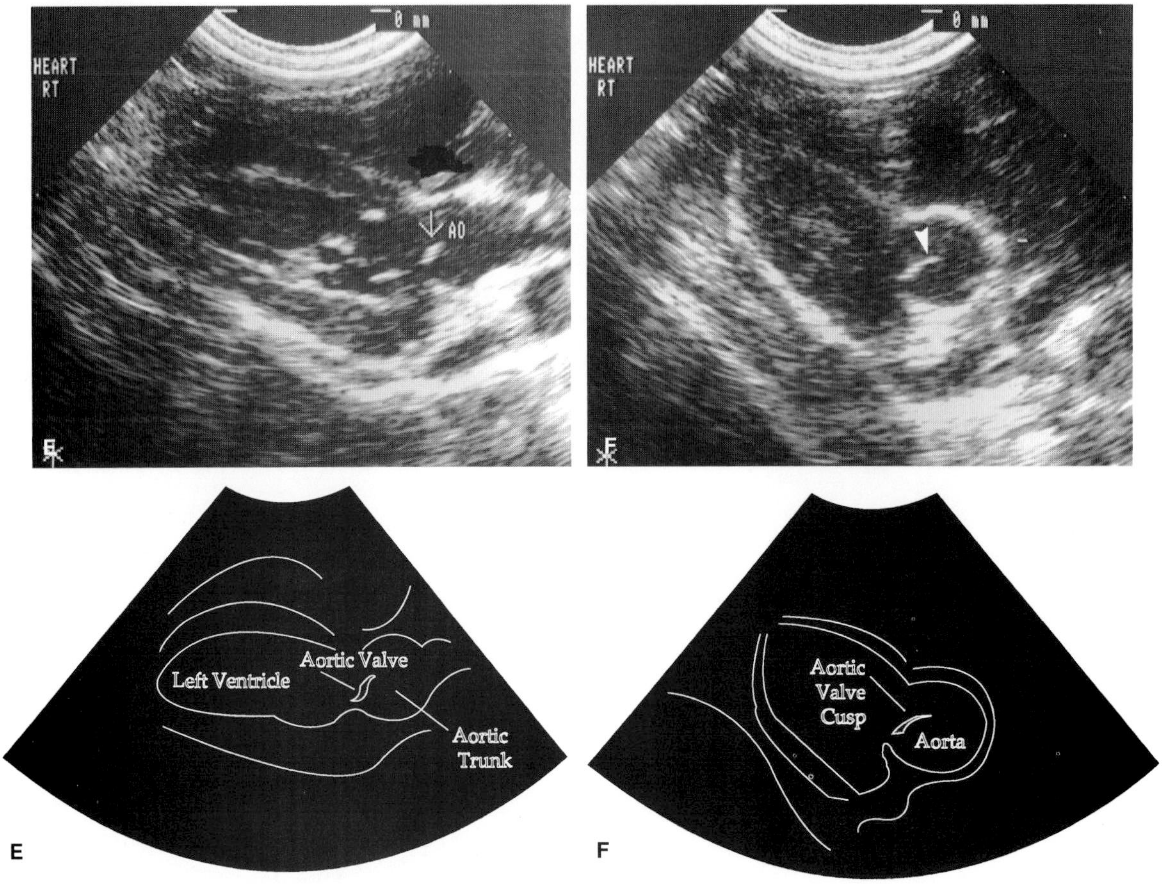

E

F

Figure 4-6. *(Continued)* (**E**) Long-sectional close-up image and diagram of the aortic valve region; the arrow marks the valve cusp. (**F**) Cross-sectional close-up image and diagram of the aortic valve region; the arrowhead marks the valve cusp.

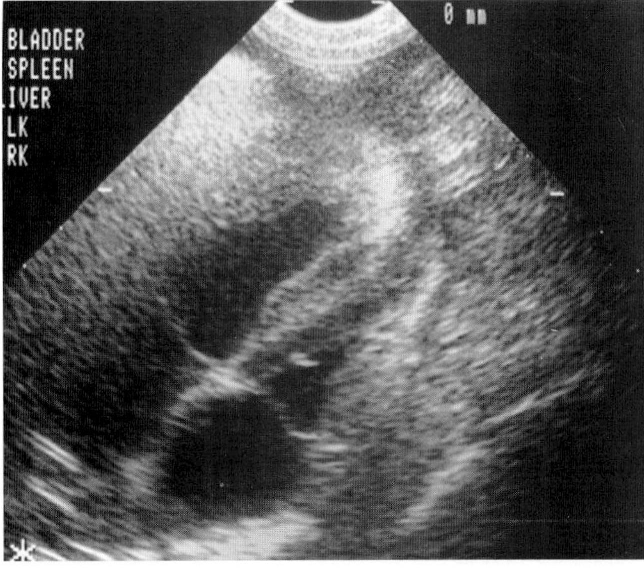

Figure 4-7. Four-chamber image of heart scanned transhepatically from the cranioventral aspect of the abdomen.

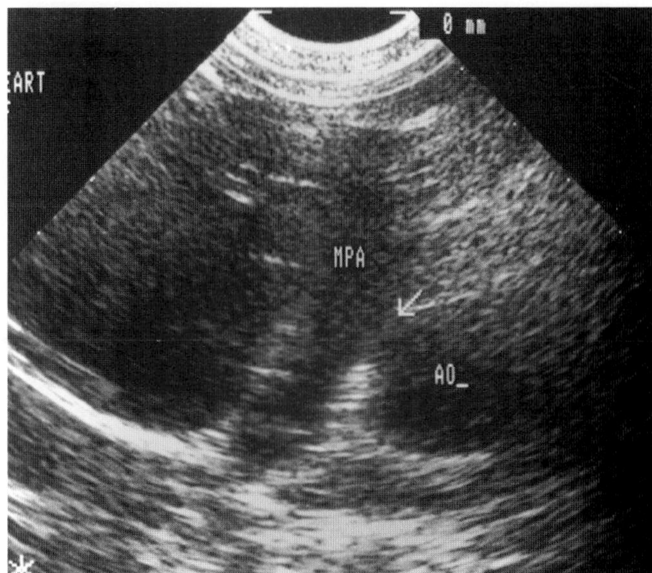

Figure 4-8. Cross-sectional image of the aorta and main pulmonary artery shows mural discontinuity representing the junction of patent ductus arteriosus (*arrow*).

largement, abnormal positioning or size of the aorta and main pulmonary artery, and pulmonary oligemia.

The combined anatomic abnormalities of pulmonic stenosis, right ventricular hypertrophy, and small ventricular septal defect (with a normally sized and positioned aorta) should not be mistaken for a tetralogy of Fallot and are more accurately called multiple congenital cardiac anomalies.

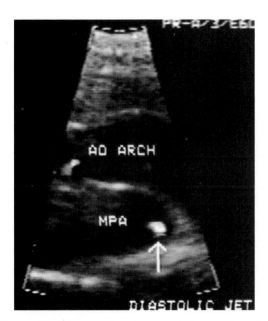

Figure 4-9. Long-sectional gray scale image of a color Doppler exam of the aortic and pulmonary trunks shows a diastolic jet (*arrow*) resulting from transarterial blood flow through a patent ductus arteriosus.

Sonographic Features

Sonographically, tetralogy of Fallot is characterized by an abnormal right heart. The right inflow shows a dilated right atrium and ventricle. The right ventricle wall is typically thickened. The right outflow tract is narrowed, and the pulmonic valve cusps are thickened and hyperechoic. Tissue bands, shelves, and strands may appear proximal or distal to the valve. The left outflow typically shows a large septal defect, above which a smaller than normal aorta is usually positioned.

COMMON ACQUIRED HEART DISEASES

Endocardiosis

Radiographic Features

Radiographically, endocardiosis results in cardiomegaly, which is right, left, or general-

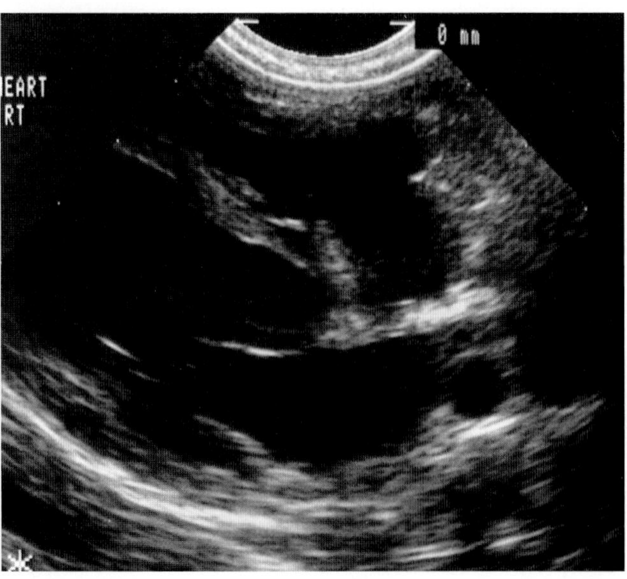

Figure 4-10. Long-sectional view of the left cardiac inflow shows mild to moderate dilation of the left ventricle compatible with, but not necessarily indicative of, a patent ductus arteriosus.

ized, depending on whether one or both atrioventricular valves are affected. The most common variation is mitral endocardiosis, which causes cardiomegaly with left-sided emphasis.

Sonographic Features

One or both inflows appear abnormal, depending on which atrioventricular valve is affected. If the mitral valve is endocardiotic, the left inflow is abnormal; if the tricuspid valve is endocardiotic, the right inflow is abnormal.

Mitral endocardiosis is characterized by several features (Fig. 4-20): dilation of the right inflow; various degrees of mitral deformity, including thickening, lumpiness, and discrete valvular masses (most often located at or near the extremity of the involved leaflet); valvular hyperechogenicity; and abnormal valvular motion.

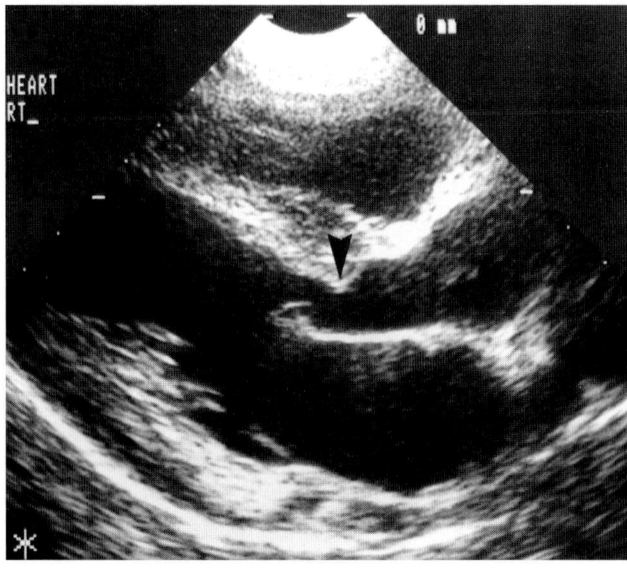

Figure 4-11. Long-sectional image of left cardic outflow shows a thickened, conical ventricular septum (*arrowhead*) extending into the left ventricular outflow tract proximal to the aortic valve (not shown).

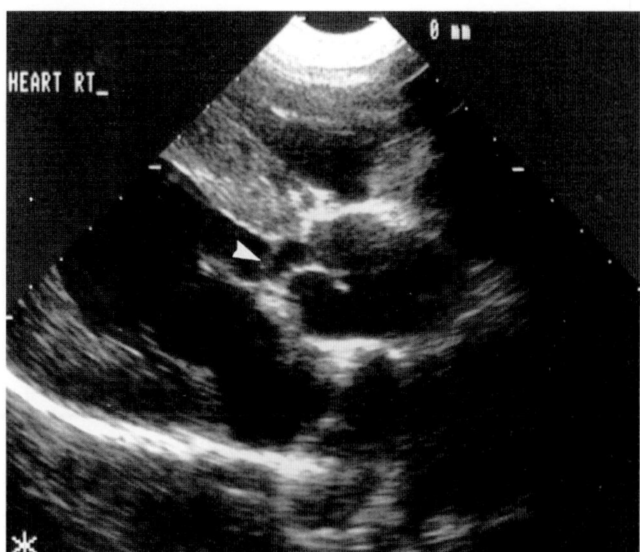

Figure 4-12. Long-sectional image of left cardiac outflow shows septal thickening proximally and an adjacent thin subaortic membrane (*arrowhead*).

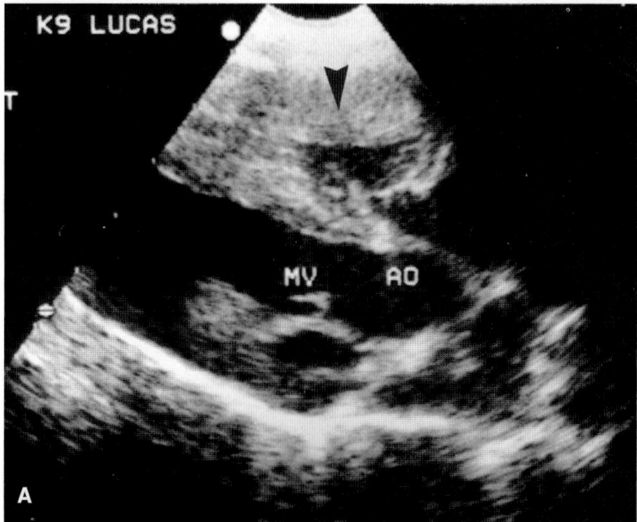

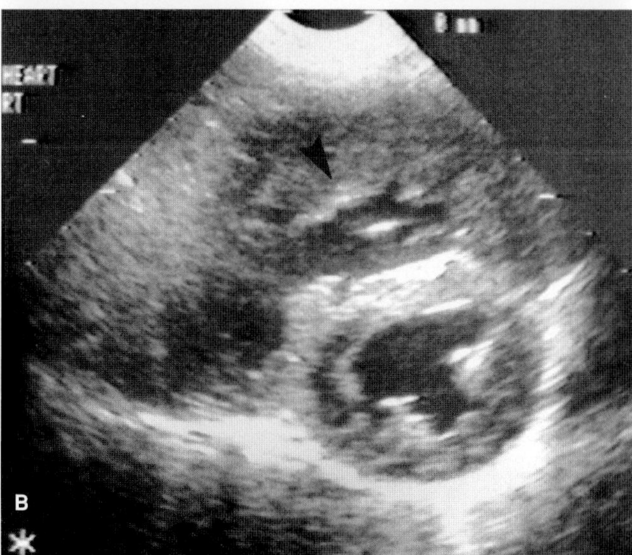

Figure 4-13. (**A**) Long- and (**B**) cross-sectional images (two different dogs) of the right cardiac inflow show severe ventricular thickening (*arrowheads*), including the septum, secondary to pulmonic stenosis.

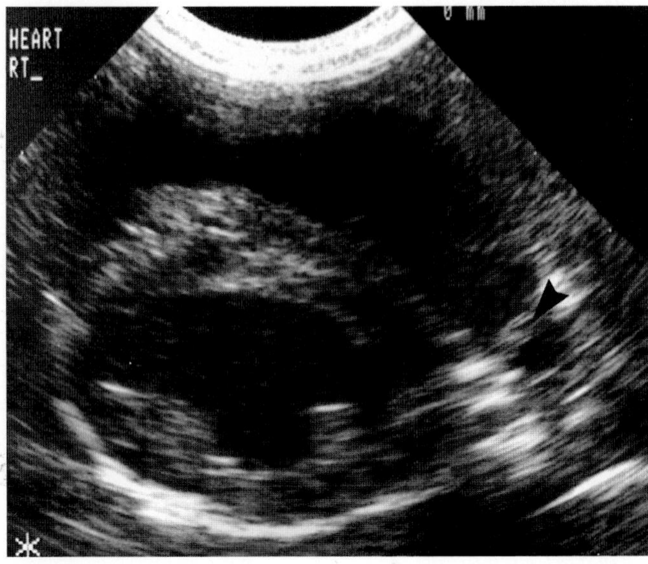

Figure 4-14. Cross-sectional image of the right cardiac outflow shows a greatly thickened pulmonic valve (*arrowhead*).

Valvular insufficiency causing a regurgitant jet (the most important direct consequence of endocardiosis), can only be evaluated using Doppler ultrasound. The ultrasound examiner does not observe insufficiency during cross-sectional cardiac imaging, although it may be inferred based on the indirect evidence described.

Endocarditis

Radiographic Features

Endocarditis is typically associated with a normal radiograph, especially in the early stages of the disease. Later, various types of car-

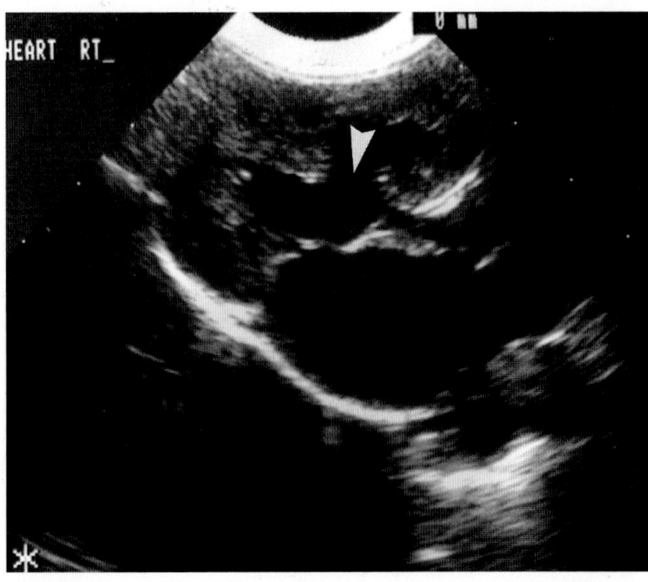

Figure 4-15. Long-sectional image of the left cardiac outflow shows a large ventricular septal defect (*arrowhead*).

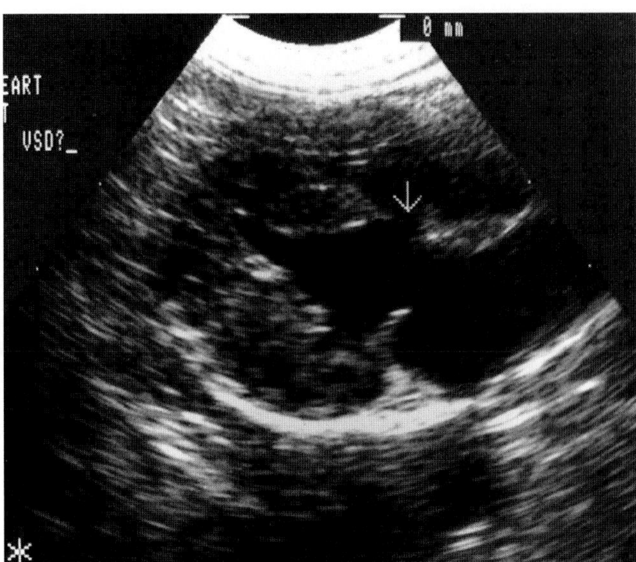

Figure 4-16. Long-sectional image of the left cardiac outflow shows a medium ventricular septal defect (*arrow*).

diomegaly may develop, depending on which valve or valves are affected.

Sonographic Features

Sonographically, endocarditis is most often characterized by abnormal aortic valves (Figs. 4-21 through 4-23). Occasionally, growths may develop on the cords, papillary muscles, or ventricular endocardium.

Affected valve leaflets typically appear thickened and hyperechoic. The valve may be uniformly affected or contain small or medium-sized clusters of granulation tissue and bacteria, called vegetations or vegetative lesions. Valvular motion is often mechanically altered as a result of endocarditic lesions.

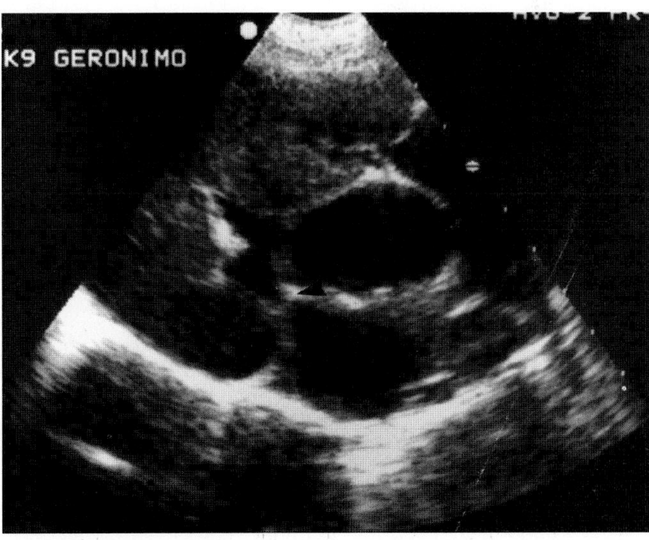

Figure 4-17. Long-sectional image of the left cardiac inflow shows enlarged, deformed, hyperechoic mitral leaflet (*arrowhead*), the result of dysplasia.

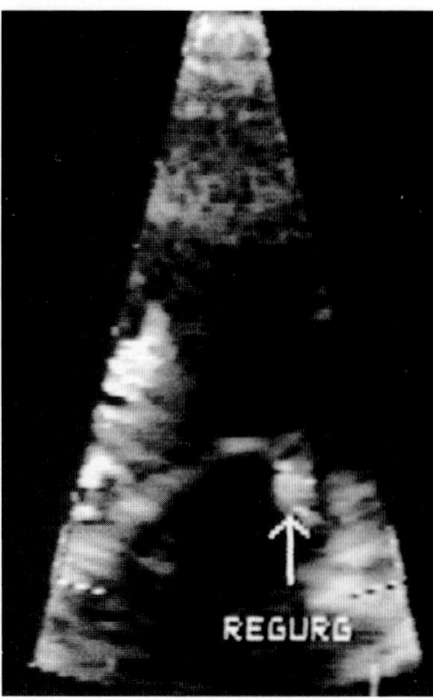

Figure 4-18. A close-up view of the tricuspid valve during systole using color-flow Doppler (gray-scale mode) shows a regurgitant jet on the atrial side of the valve (*arrow*), indicative of tricuspid insufficiency. Small jets of this magnitude are seen in some normal dogs.

Feline Hypertrophic Cardiomyopathy

Radiographic Features

Advanced hypertrophic cardiomyopathy of cats, thyroid-induced cardiomyopathy, and other forms are characterized by several radiographic features: cardiomegaly with left-sided emphasis; a distinctive bilobed appearance to the heart, with the upper lobe formed by an enlarged left atrium; and pulmonary overcirculation.

Milder forms of cardiomyopathy produce lesser amounts of cardiac enlargement, but in most instances, the heart gradually changes from its normal symmetric oval shape, to an asymmetric oval having a relatively broad base and narrow apex. Increased pulmonary vasculature tends to reflect increasing venous hypertension.

Sonographic Features

Sonographically, the hypertrophic heart is typically characterized by an abnormal left in-

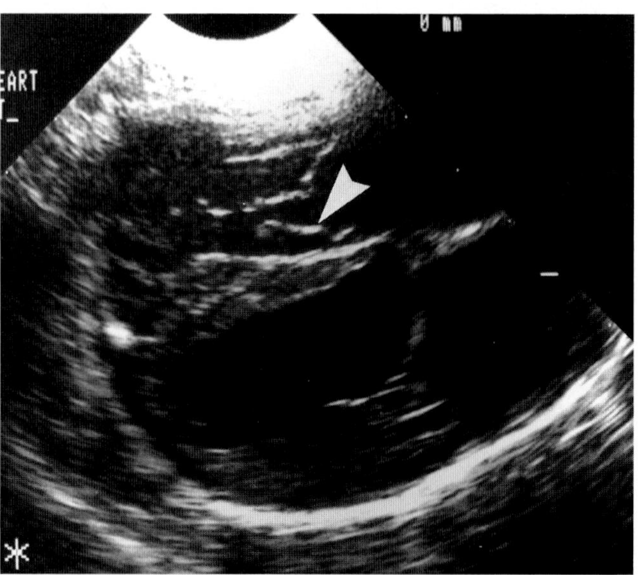

Figure 4-19. Long-sectional image of the right cardiac inflow shows tricuspid valves extending abnormally deep into the right ventricle (*arrowhead*), functionally creating a larger than normal right atrium and smaller than normal right ventricle.

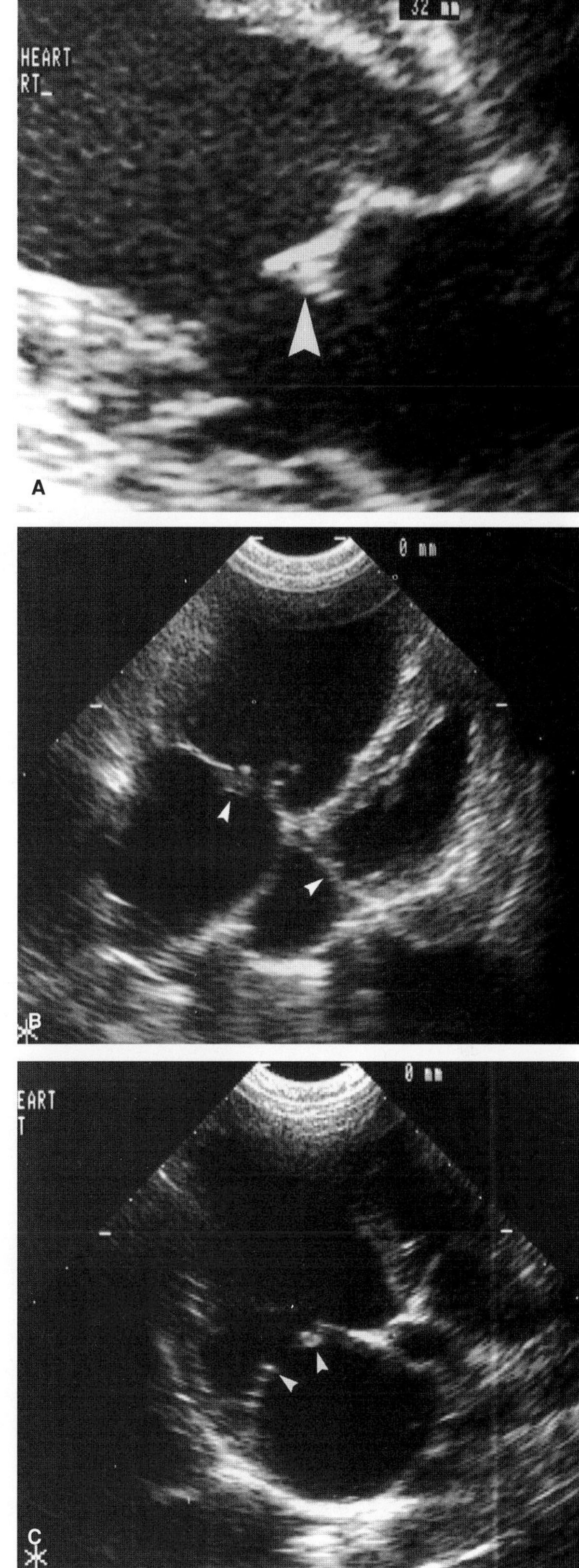

Figure 4-20. (**A**) Close-up, long-sectional view of the left cardiac inflow shows an endocardiotic mitral valve (*arrowhead*). (**B**) Long-sectional, four-chamber image of the heart shows dilation the right side and endocardiotic atrioventricular valves bilaterally (*arrowheads*). (**C**) Long-sectional, four-chamber image of the heart shows dilation the left side and endocardiotic mitral valves (*arrowheads*).

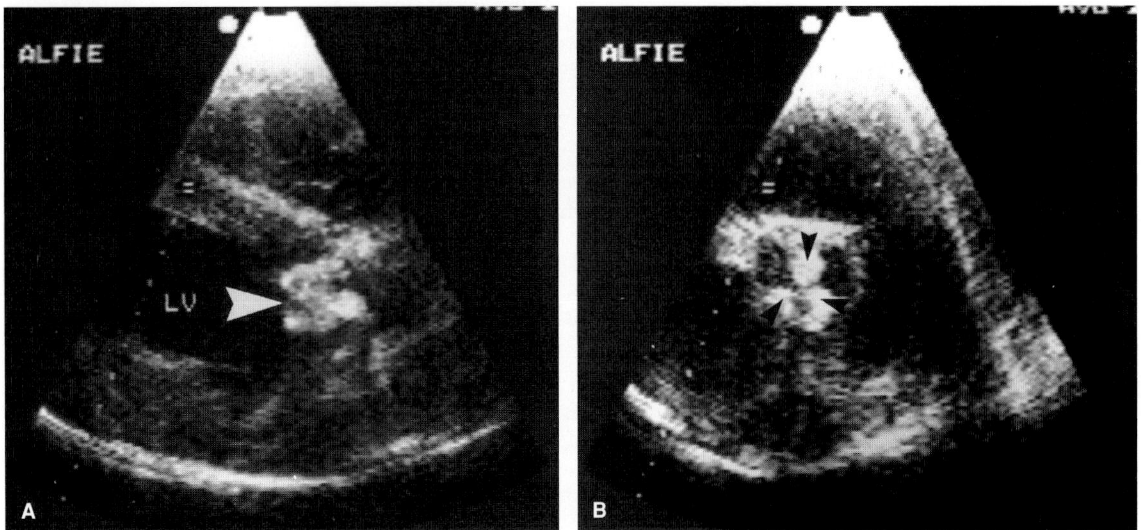

Figure 4-21. (**A**) Long- and (**B**) cross-sectional images of the left cardiac outflow show a greatly enlarged, hyperechoic aortic valve (*arrowhead*), the result of endocarditis.

flow (Figs. 4-24 through 4-26). Abnormal features may include left atrial dilation, reduced left ventricular chamber size, increased left ventricular wall thickness, and increased septal thickness (symmetric or asymmetric).

Canine Hypertrophic Cardiomyopathy

Radiographic Features

Radiographically, advanced hypertrophic

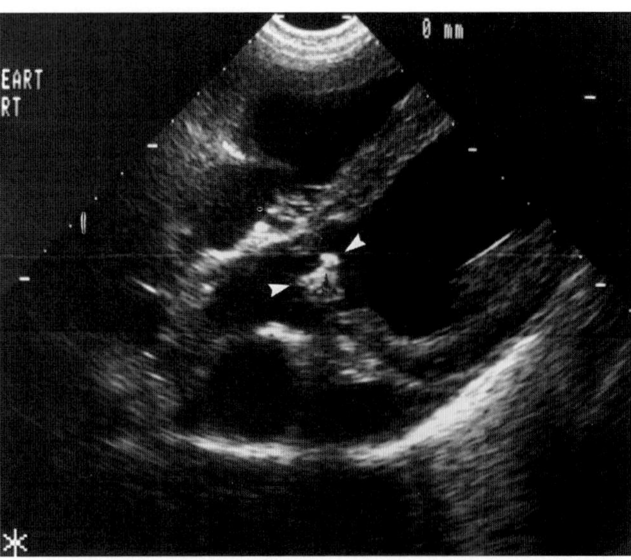

Figure 4-22. Long-sectional image of the left cardiac outflow shows a thickened, roughly marginated, hyperechoic aortic valve (*arrowhead*) indicative of endocarditis.

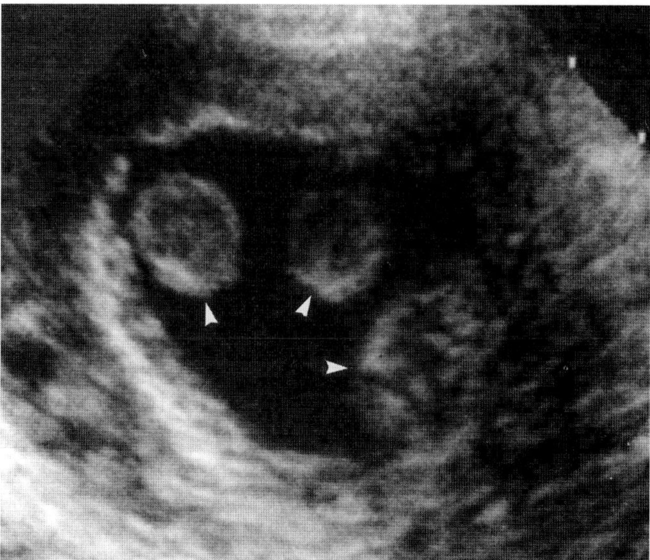

Figure 4-23. Cross-sectional image of the left ventricle (from the left side of the thorax) shows three circular objects resembling papillary muscles (*arrows*). The diagnosis was mural endocarditis.

cardiomyopathy in the dog is characterized by generalized cardiomegaly or cardiomegaly with left-sided emphasis.

Sonographic Features

Like the cat, hypertrophic cardiomyopathy in the dog is characterized by an abnormal left inflow (Fig. 4-27). Specific features may include a thickened ventricle wall, thickened ventricular septum, decreased ventricular volume, and an enlarged atrium.

Feline and Canine Dilated Cardiomyopathy

Radiographic Features

Radiographically, cardiomyopathy is characterized by generalized cardiomegaly.

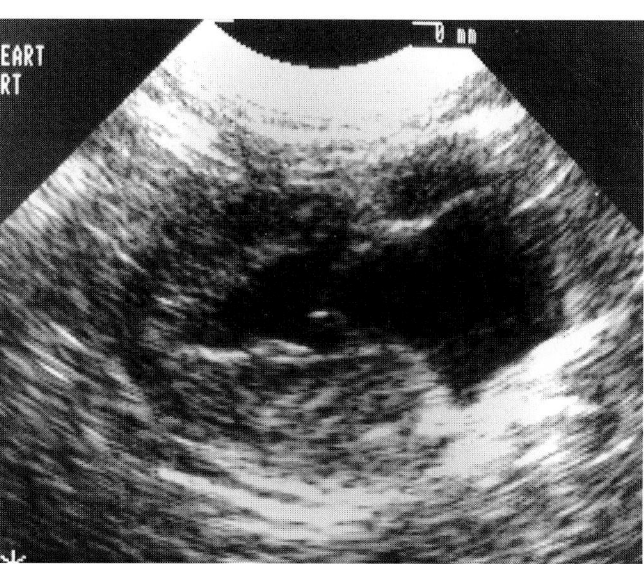

Figure 4-24. Long-sectional image of the left cardiac inflow shows a moderate to severe left ventricular thickening but only mild to moderate left atrial enlargement. The diagnosis was hypertrophic cardiomyopathy.

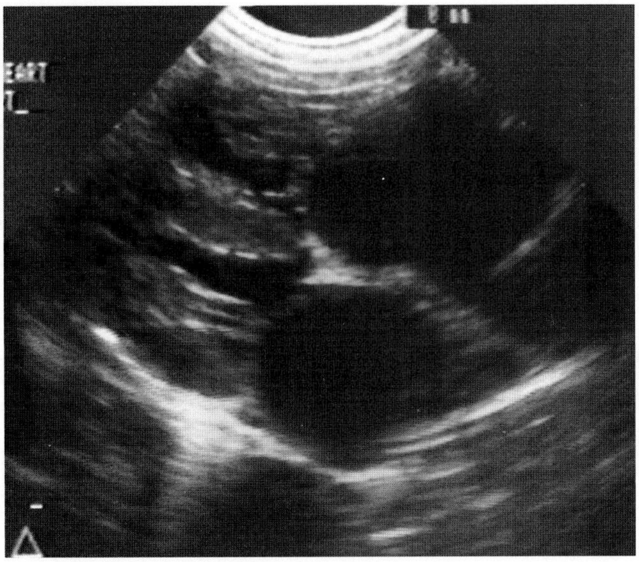

Figure 4-25. Long-sectional image of the left cardiac inflow shows moderate left and right ventricular and septal thickening and massive bilateral atrial enlargement. The latter finding indicates advanced pulmonary venous hypertension. The diagnosis was hypertrophic cardiomyopathy.

Sonographic Features

Sonographically, dilated cardiomyopathy is characterized by chamber enlargement and weak contraction (Figs. 4-28 and 4-29).

Pericardial Fluid

Radiographic Features

Large volumes of pericardial fluid cause the heart to assume a spherical shape rather than its normal oval configuration. Medium amounts of fluid usually alter the heart shape, but not as characteristically as large volumes do. Small quantities of fluid usually cannot be differentiated from cardiomegaly and usually go undetected. Large amounts of pericardial fluid are usually associated with diminished pulmonary blood flow, causing the lung to appear oligemic.

Sonographic Features

Sonographically, large and medium pericardial fluid accumulations affect the entire heart and result in characteristic features (Figs. 4-30

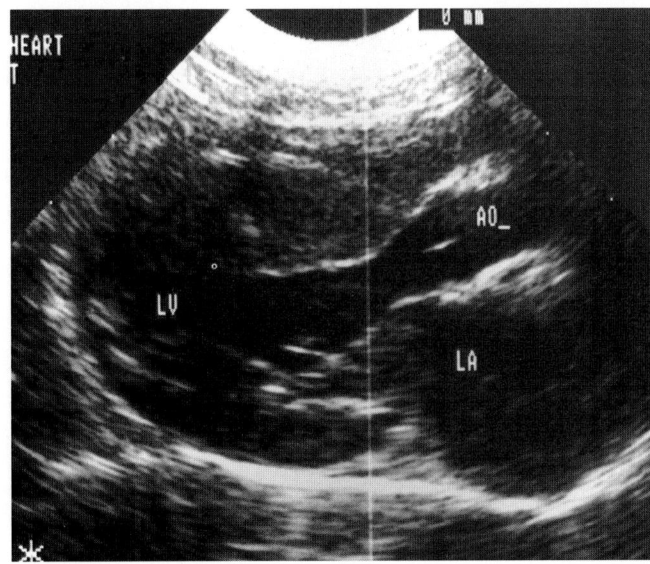

Figure 4-26. Long-sectional image of the left cardiac outflow shows moderate left ventricular thickening and severe septal thickening. The left atrium is also enlarged. The diagnosis was hypertrophic cardiomyopathy.

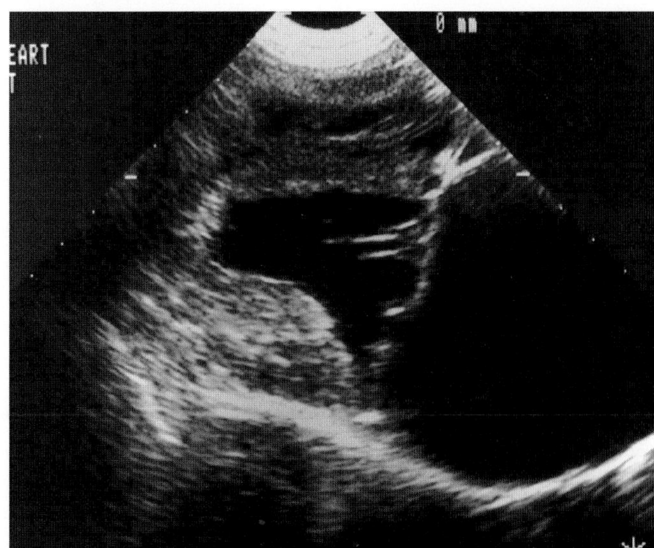

Figure 4-27. Long-sectional image of the left cardiac inflow shows a thickened left ventricle and massive left atrial dilation. The diagnosis was hypertrophic cardiomyopathy.

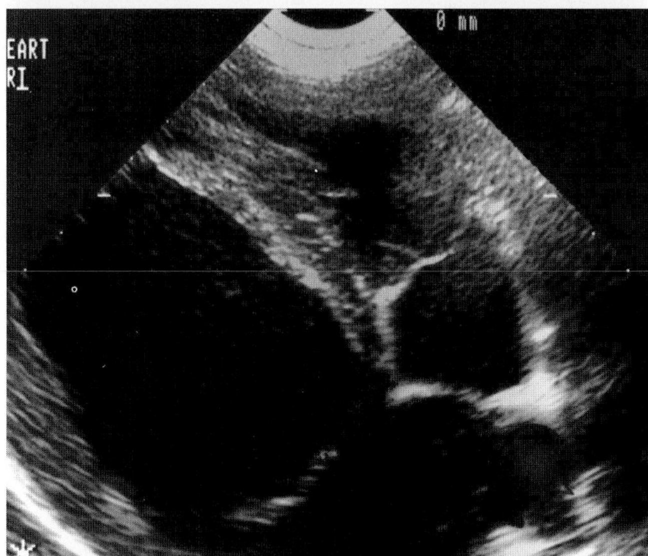

Figure 4-28. Long-sectional image of the left cardiac inflow shows moderate enlargement of the left ventricle and atrium, with normal wall thickness.

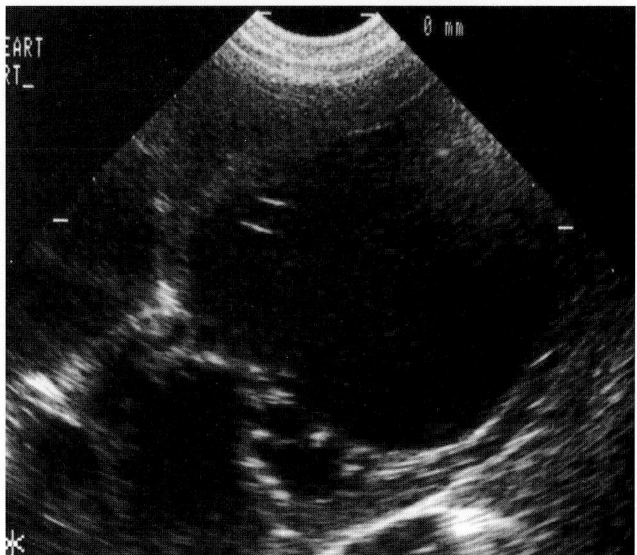

Figure 4-29. Long-sectional image of the left cardiac inflow shows severe dilation of all chambers, with marked thinning of ventricular wall.

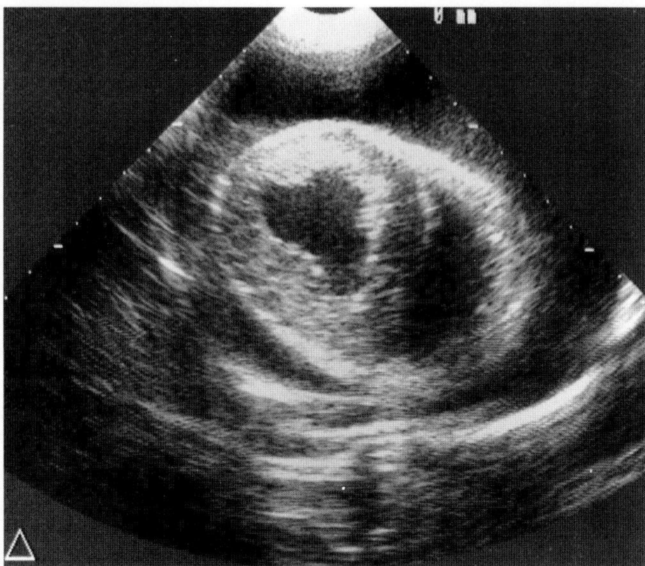

Figure 4-30. Cross-sectional image of ventricles (through the midchamber) shows a large volume of pericardial fluid bounded by pericardium. Notice the unusually bright or hyperechoic appearance of the myocardium, epicardium, and pericardium. The diagnosis was idiopathic pericardial fluid.

and 4-31). The myocardium appears unusually "bright" or hyperechoic. The cardiac perimeter is much more distinct than normal. The heart is surrounded by a thick anechoic zone, which is surrounded by a hyperechoic rim of variable thickness. Usually, the heart chambers appear smaller than normal. The margins of the right inflow frequently undulate as the heart contracts and expands within the surrounding pericardial fluid.

UNCOMMON ACQUIRED HEART DISEASES

Pericardial Mass and Mass Effect

Radiographic Features

A large pericardial mass such as a tumor or mass effect such as a blood clot or liver lobe (eg, pericardial-peritoneal communication), typi-

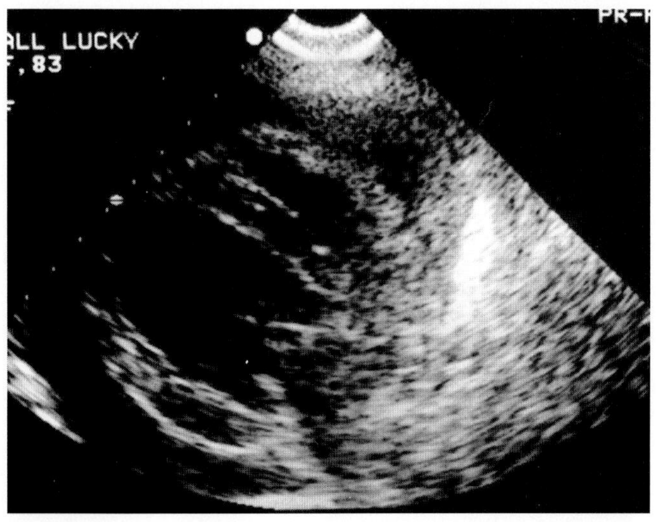

Figure 4-31. Long-sectional image of a heart shows a large volume of pericardial fluid, causing characteristically bright tissue-fluid interfaces. The diagnosis was idiopathic pericardial fluid.

cally alters the apparent size and shape of the cardiac silhouette to the extent that it may be mistaken for heart disease.

Sonographic Features

Some pericardial masses are associated with pericardial fluid. If fluid is present, the mass and the pericardium are often well marginated and readily identified (Fig. 4-32). It is more difficult to asses if large and medium-sized masses without surrounding fluid are intrapericardial or extrapericardial (Fig. 4-33).

Atrial Clot

Radiographic Features

There are no characteristic features of an atrial clot. Larger clots may obstruct venous return to the heart and cause the lung to appear oligemic.

Sonographic Features

Sonographically, most atrial clots move but are tethered to the inner surface of the atrium or valve. Clot echogenicity depends on size and duration (Fig. 4-34).

Hypertrophy Secondary to Systemic Hypertension

Radiographic Features

In my limited experience with this disorder, there appears to be no distinguishing radiographic feature to indicate the presence of hypertension or to differentiate it from other sources of hypertrophy such as cardiomyopathy.

Sonographic Features

Generalized ventricular hypertrophy combined with systemic hypertension and chronic renal disease suggests a cause-effect association (Fig. 4-35).

Traumatic Pericardial Rupture, Cardiac Herniation, and Entrapment

Radiographic Features

In this rare form of injury, the heart is partially ejected through a tear in the pericardium as a result of a severe blow to the chest. Subsequently, the heart may become entrapped

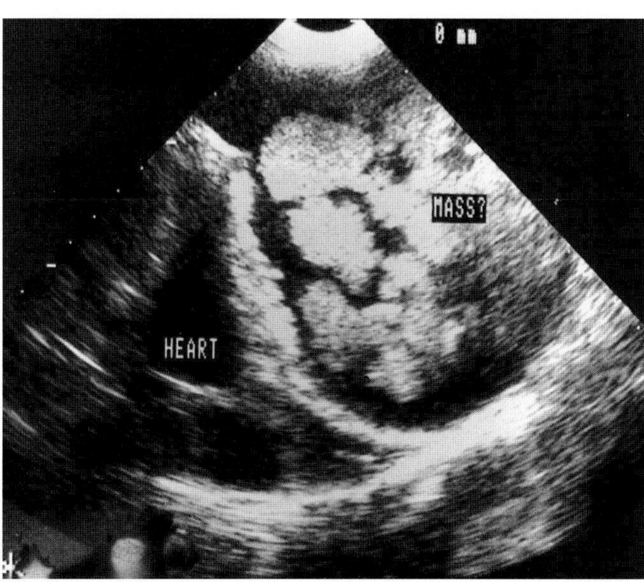

Figure 4-32. Oblique-sectional image of a heart shows a large, lobulated pericardial mass surrounded by fluid. The diagnosis was pericardial hematoma.

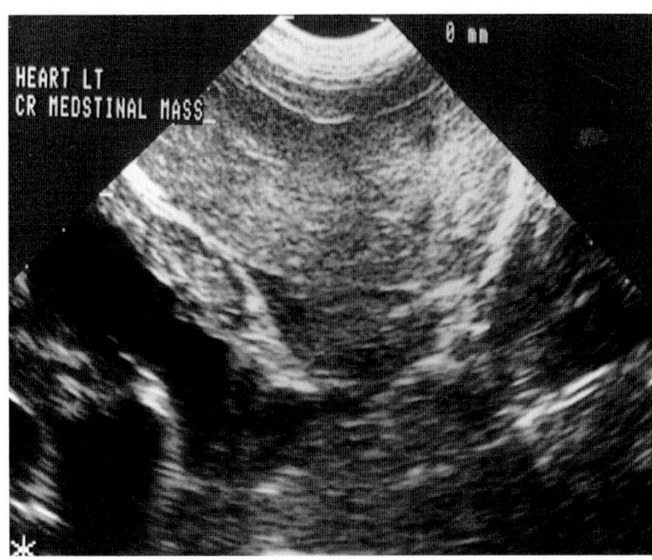

Figure 4-33. Oblique-sectional image of a heart shows a large, solid, extrapericardial mass. The diagnosis was lymphoma.

within the rent in the pericardium. This entrapment may lead to myocardial strangulation, ischemia, and infarct.

Sonographic Features

The key sonographic feature of this disorder is reduced or absent contractility of the extrapericardial component of the heart. When the heart has been completely exsheathed, it may be possible to identify the "rolled-up" pericardium at the heart base, which appears as an ill-defined mass. Under such conditions, the heart motion may appear excessive.

Acknowledgment
I gratefully acknowledge my medical imaging colleagues, Drs. John Pharr and Rachel Saint Vincent, who diagnosed many of the disorders presented in

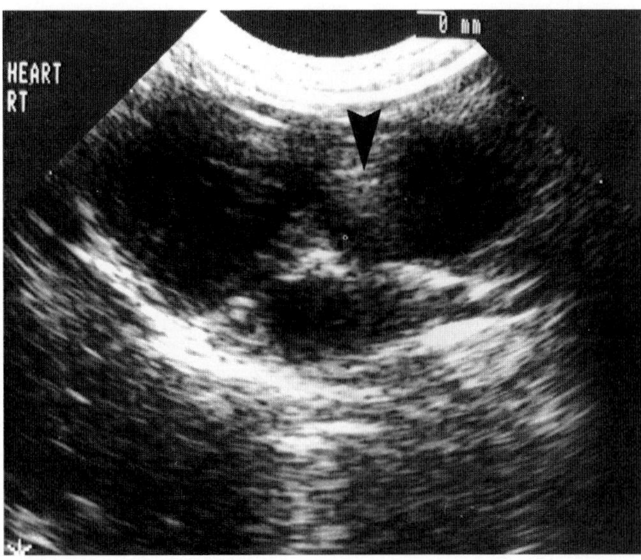

Figure 4-34. Oblique-sectional image of a heart shows a medium-sized right atrial mass (*arrowhead*). The presumptive diagnosis was a right atrial blood clot.

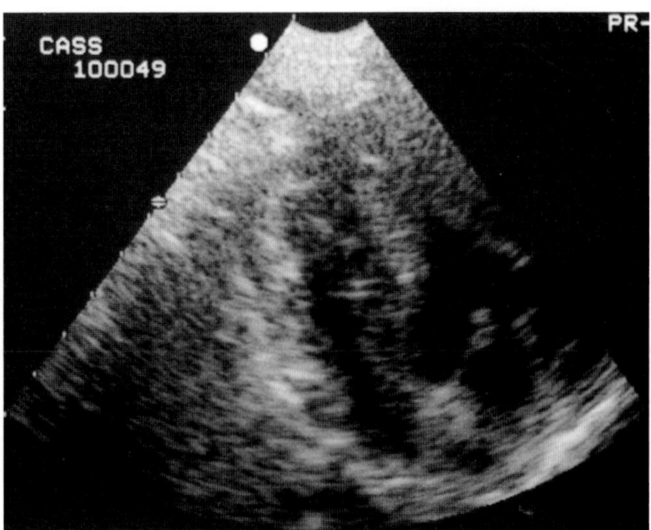

Figure 4-35. Four-chamber image of the heart shows thickening of both ventricles. The diagnosis was hypertrophic cardiomyopathy secondary to systemic hypertension.

this chapter. Like most of what we do, sonology is a collaborative endeavor.

REFERENCES

1. Sheiman RG. Traumatic Aorta Tear: Screening with chest CT. Radiology 1992;182:667.
2. Weyman AE. Principles and practice of echocardiography. 2nd ed. Philadelphia: Lea & Febiger, 1994:516.
3. Gaber CG. Doppler echocardiography. Vet Clin North Am 1991;3:479.
4. DeMaria A. Cardiac Doppler: the basics. Andover: Hewlett-Packard Medical Products Group, 1984.
5. Ruckerbusch Y, Phaneuf L-P, Dunlop R. The heart pump. In: Ruckerbusch Y, Phaneuf L-P, Dunlop R, eds. Physiology of small and large animals. Philadelphia: BC Decker, 1988:115.
6. Thomas WP, Gaber CE, Jacobs GJ, et al. Recommendations for standards in transthoracic two-dimensional echocardiography in the dog and the cat. Vet Radiol 1994;35:173.
7. Kaplan PM. Congenital heart disease. Vet Clin North Am 1991;21:479.

BIBLIOGRAPHY

Veterinary Cardiac Anatomy and Physiology

Feeny DA, Fletcher TF, Hardy RM. Thorax. In: Feeny DA, Fletcher TF, Hardy RM, eds. Atlas of correlative imaging anatomy of the normal dog. Philadelphia: WB Saunders, 1991:153.

Ruckerbusch Y, Phaneuf L-P, Dunlop R, eds. Physiology of small and large animals. Philadelphia: BC Decker, 1988:115.

Human Cardiac Anatomy and Physiology

Seely RR, Stephens TD, Tate P. Cardiovascular system: the heart. In: Seely RR, Stephens TD, Tate P, eds. Anatomy and physiology. 2nd ed. St. Louis, Mosby Year Book, 1992.

Veterinary General Cardiology

Bonagura JD, Darke PGG. Congenital heart disease. In: Ettinger SJ, Feldman EC, eds. Textbook of internal medicine. 3rd ed. Philadelphia: WB Saunders, 1995:892.

Fox PR. Canine and feline cardiology. New York: Churchill Livingstone, 1988.

O'Grady MR. Acquired valvular heart disease. In: Ettinger SJ, Feldman EC, eds. Textbook of internal medicine. 3rd ed. Philadelphia: WB Saunders, 1995:944.

Human General Cardiology

Hurst JW, Alpert JS. Diagnostic atlas of the heart. New York: Raven Press, 1994.

Netter FH. The CIBA collection of medical illustrations, vol 5: heart. Summit, NJ: CIBA Pharmaceutical, 1969.

Veterinary Cardiac Radiology

Bahr RJ, Root CR. The heart and great vessels. In: Thrall DE, ed. Textbook of veterinary diagnostic radiology. 2nd ed. Philadelphia: WB Saunders, 1994:304.

Farrow CS. The thorax. In: Farrow CS, ed. Radiology of the cat. St. Louis, Mosby Year Book, 1994:88.

Suter PF. Cardiac diseases. In: Thoracic radiology. Wettswil, Switzerland: Self-published (PF Suter), 1984:351.

Suter PF, Ettinger SJ. Canine cardiology. Philadelphia: WB Saunders, 1970.

Toombs JP, Widmar WR, Ogburn PN. Evaluating canine cardiovascular silhouettes: radiographic methods and normal radiographic anatomy. In: Moon M, ed. Radiology in practice. Trenton, NJ: Veterinary Learning Systems, 1994.

Human Cardiac Radiology

Elliott LP, Schiebler GL. The x-ray diagnosis of congenital heart disease in infants, children, and adults. 2nd ed. Springfield, IL: Charles C Thomas, 1979.

Shelton DK. Cardiac imaging in acquired disease. Baltimore: Williams & Wilkins, 1994.

Veterinary Echocardiography

Bonagura JD, Herring DS. Echocardiography: congenital heart disease. Vet Clin North Am 1985;15:1177.

Human Echocardiography

Nanda NC. Doppler echocardiography. 2nd ed. Philadelphia: Lea & Febiger, 1994.

Weyman AE. Principles and practice of echocardiography. 2nd ed. Philadelphia: Lea & Febiger, 1994.

Small Animal Ultrasound, edited by Ronald W. Green.
Lippincott-Raven Publishers, Philadelphia © 1996.

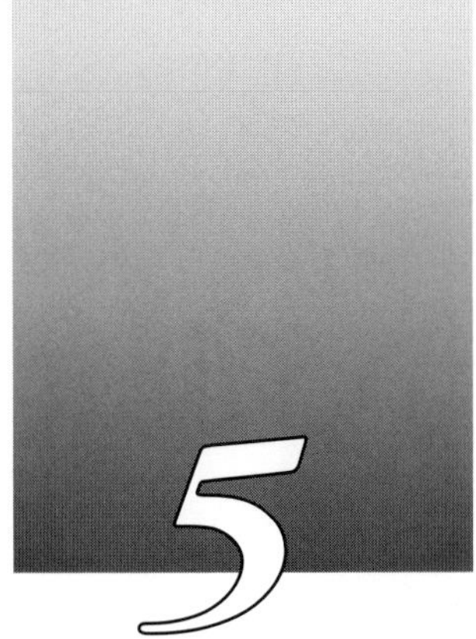

THORAX

Robert J. Bahr

Thoracic ultrasonography was initially directed at cardiac and pericardial disease, but the indications have expanded to include the pleural space, mediastinum, diaphragm, and lung.[1,2] These structures can be easily imaged if a suitable acoustic window is available. Thoracic sonography often provides diagnostic information unobtainable by routine radiography.[3] Pleural and mediastinal masses obscured by fluid on a conventional radiograph can be identified and measured, and the internal architecture can be examined with ultrasound. Diaphragmatic hernias can be easily diagnosed, and the actual rent in the diaphragm can sometimes be seen. Ultrasound can be used to examine consolidated lung and many pulmonary masses and to localize, measure, and characterize pleural effusion.

SCANNING TECHNIQUES FOR THORACIC ULTRASOUND

Tranquilization is seldom required for thoracic ultrasound. The positioning of the patient is often dictated by the clinical signs and the availability of an acoustic window. Pleural effusion makes a good acoustic window. A patient with a pleural effusion should be positioned to take advantage of this property. Because free fluids in the pleural space gravitate, the use of a cardiac table (see Chaps. 3 and 4) can help in scanning the lateral thorax. When positioning a patient with a large-volume pleural effusion, care must be taken not to compromise the vital signs of the patient. Scanning is most commonly done through an intercostal space.[2] Scanning of the caudal thorax may be performed by using a subcostal (ie, transhepatic) approach. The thoracic inlet can be used to scan the cranial portion of the mediastinum. Clipping of the hair, copious amounts of coupling gel, and a small footprint transducer are important in maximizing the image quality.

ULTRASOUND ANATOMY OF THE THORAX

The thorax is composed of the heart, lungs, mediastinum, trachea, esophagus, pleura, diaphragm, and thoracic wall. The heart is discussed in Chapter 4. Most of the normal thorax is air-filled lung, which makes it difficult or impossible to image (Fig. 5-1). An acoustic window is provided by free fluid, a fluid-filled cyst, an abscess, a solid mass, or a soft tissue organ such as the liver or heart. Because an acoustic window is necessary to image structures in the thorax, imaging of the thorax, other than the heart, is possible only when disease conditions exist.[4]

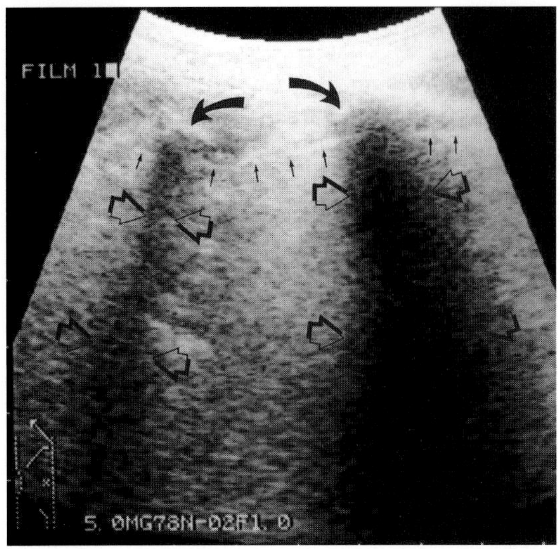

Figure 5-1. Short-axis ultrasound scan (dorsal is right) made at the right eighth intercostal space. Notice the bright, curvilinear echoes depicting the near side of two normal ribs (*curved arrows*) and the resultant anechoic acoustic shadowing (*open arrows*) distal to each rib. Between the ribs is a speckled, diffuse reverberation artifact caused by ultrasound striking the normal air-filled lung. Notice the thin, sharply defined, hyperechoic line (*small, straight arrows*) following the contour of the chest wall and caused by the combined echoes of the parietal and visceral pleural membranes.

Thoracic Wall

Ultrasound can generate an accurate picture of the size, shape, location, and internal echotexture of thoracic wall masses. Ultrasound can also detect extension of disease into adjacent ribs or the pleural space (Fig. 5-2).[5] Thoracic wall masses include osteosarcomas, chondrosarcomas, fibrosarcomas, mammary tumors, abscesses, granulomas, embedded foreign bodies, and hematomas. A standoff pad may be needed in the examination of small, superficial lesions. High-frequency transducers (7.5 or 10 MHz) are best for imaging thoracic wall masses.

Diaphragm

From the subcostal approach, the highly echogenic lung surface blends with echoes from the adjacent diaphragm and results in a broad hyperechoic band (Fig. 5-3).[2] This band of combined echoes is commonly referred to as the *diaphragm*. The actual diaphragm can be seen as a thin echogenic line when the lung is separated from the diaphragm by fluid or a mass (Fig. 5-4).[2,3,6]

(text continues on p. 93)

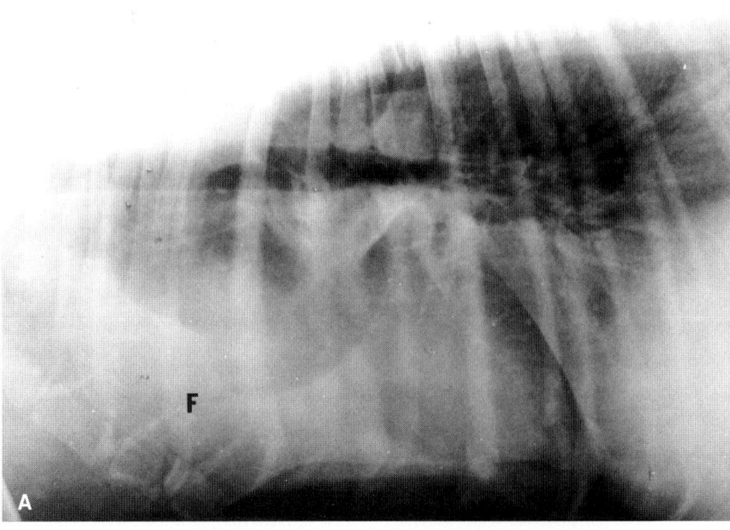

Figure 5-2. (**A**) Left lateral thoracic radiograph of a 7-year-old, spayed, female mixed-breed dog with moderate pleural effusion (*F*) and dorsal displacement of the cranial lung lobes.

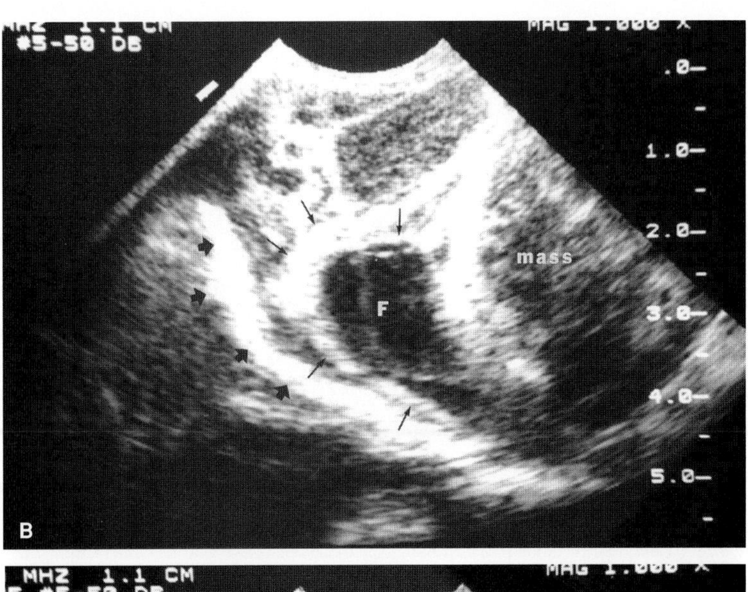

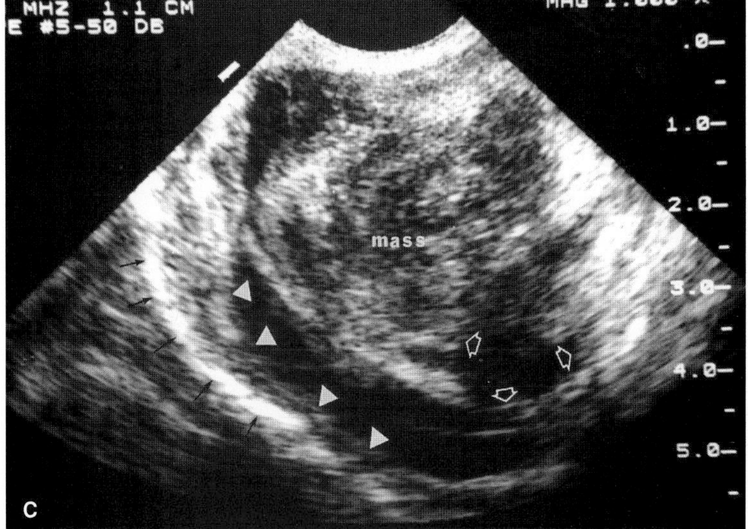

Figure 5-2. *(Continued)* (**B**) A long-axis sonogram of the cranial mediastinum from the left third intercostal space (ICS) shows multiple compartments of hypoechoic and anechoic mediastinal fluid (*F*); thickened, hyperechoic membranes (*small arrows*); a thickened, hyperechoic parietal pleura (*thick, short arrows*); and a large, hypoechoic mass (*mass*) in the cranial mediastinum. (**C**) A long-axis sonogram of the cranial mediastinum from the left fifth ICS shows this same mass but viewed from a more caudal acoustic window. The mass contains a cavitary space filled with anechoic fluid (*open arrows*) and is surrounded by anechoic fluid in this location. The floor of the mediastinum is lined by a poorly marginated, hypoechoic solid echoes (*white arrowheads*) that has firmly adhered to the thickened, hyperechoic parietal pleura (*small, black arrows*). The diagnosis was a poorly differentiated invasive chondrosarcoma arising from the sternum. (Courtesy of Ontario Veterinary College, University of Guelph, Guelph, Ontario.)

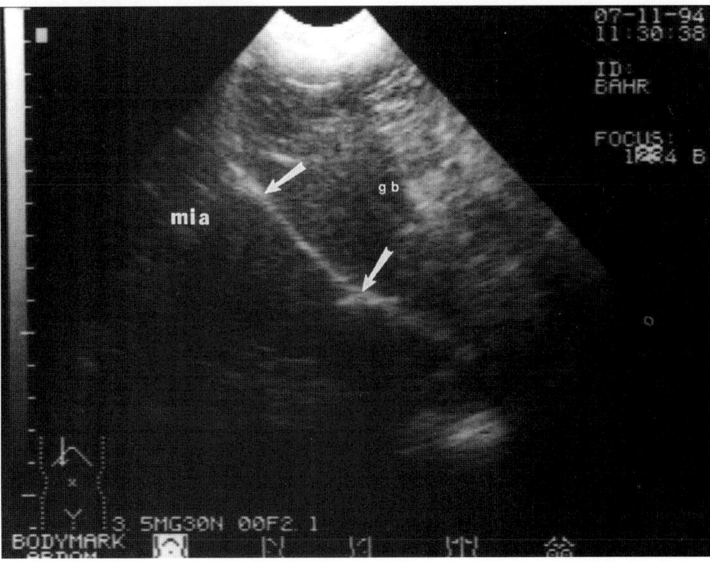

Figure 5-3. Long-axis sonogram of the liver just to the right of the midline in a normal dog shows the normal diaphragmatic echo (*arrows*) and a mirror-image artifact (*mia*) deep to the diaphragm, giving the erroneous impression of a liver on the thoracic side of the diaphragm. The gallbladder neck (*gb*) is partially visible.

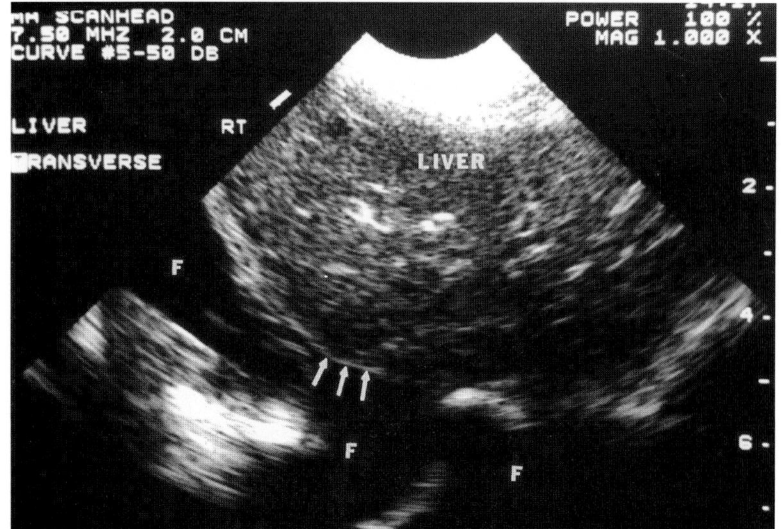

Figure 5-4. Transverse midline ultrasound scan using the subcostal approach with the liver as an acoustic window in a dog with right heart failure due to dilatory cardiomyopathy. Anechoic pleural fluid (*F*) is seen lying against the thin, hyperechoic diaphragm (*arrows*), and there is a loss of the usual mirror-image artifact. (Courtesy of Ontario Veterinary College, University of Guelph, Guelph, Ontario.)

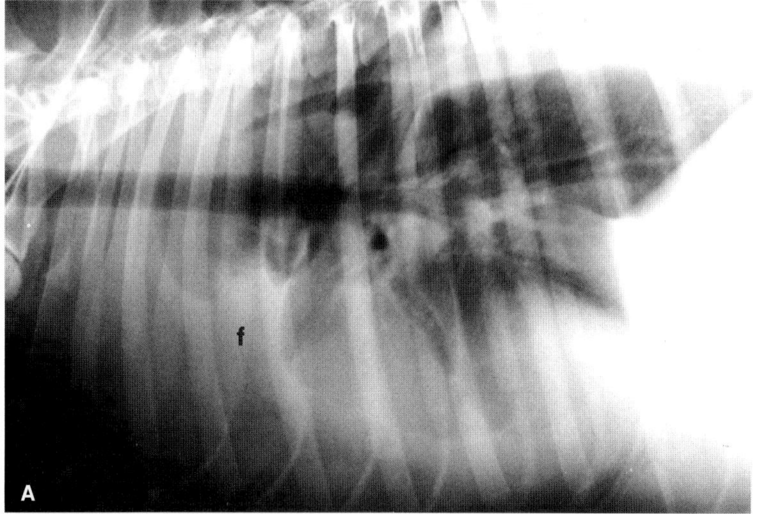

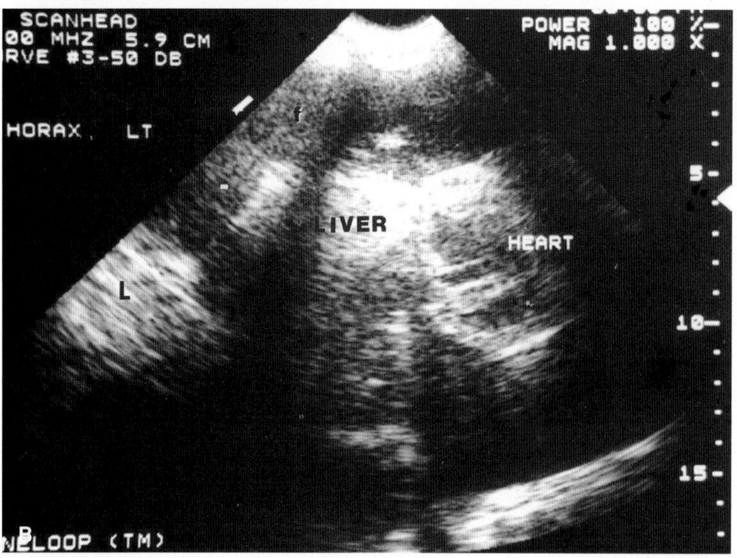

Figure 5-5. (**A**) Left lateral thoracic radiographs of a 3-year-old dog with severe pleural effusion (*f*). (**B**) The transverse sonogram made through the left eighth intercostal space (left side of image is dorsal) shows hypoechoic pleural fluid (*f*), an atelectatic left caudal lung lobe (*L*), and the liver lying adjacent to the left side of the heart without an interposed diaphragmatic echo. The diagnosis was a diaphragmatic hernia with the liver adhered to the pericardium. (Courtesy of Ontario Veterinary College, University of Guelph, Guelph, Ontario.)

In examining the diaphragm, a systematic approach should be used. The esophagus (esophageal hiatus), the aorta (aortic hiatus), and the vena cava (postcaval foramen) penetrate the diaphragm. Mirror-image artifacts are common when examining the diaphragm from thesubcostal approach. These artifacts must not be mistaken for a ruptured diaphragm with the liver in the thorax.

Ultrasound examination may be beneficial in diagnosing a diaphragmatic rupture, especially in patients with a small rupture and minimal displacement of viscera or if there is a large-volume pleural effusion (Fig. 5-5).[7–9] Visualization of a portion of the liver, without an adjacent diaphragmatic line, lateral to or in contact with the heart is indicative of a diaphragmatic rupture (see Fig. 5-5). Other abdominal viscera, such as omentum, stomach, spleen, and intestine, may also be visible in the pleural space, especially if surrounded by anechoic pleural fluid.[2,10] An additional sonographic sign of liver herniation from diaphragmatic rupture is paradoxical movement of the liver through the diaphragmatic defect. The herniated liver moves craniad, and the diaphragm moves caudad with each inspiratory effort.[11]

If two gallbladders are seen, one in the thorax and one in the abdomen, the error is caused by a mirror-image artifact (see Fig. 5-3) and not a diaphragmatic rupture. However, one gallbladder seen in the thorax is a result of a diaphragmatic rupture. A hiatal hernia (Fig. 5-6) or old, healed, subclinical diaphragmatic hernia (Fig. 5-7) may also be detected and characterized by ultrasound.[4,11]

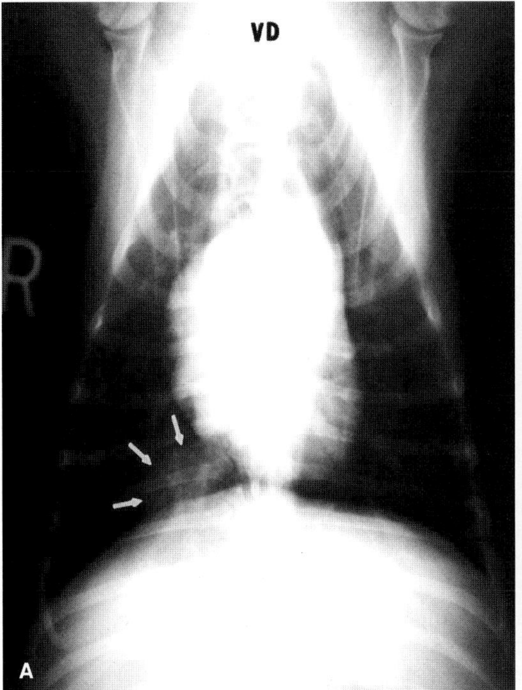

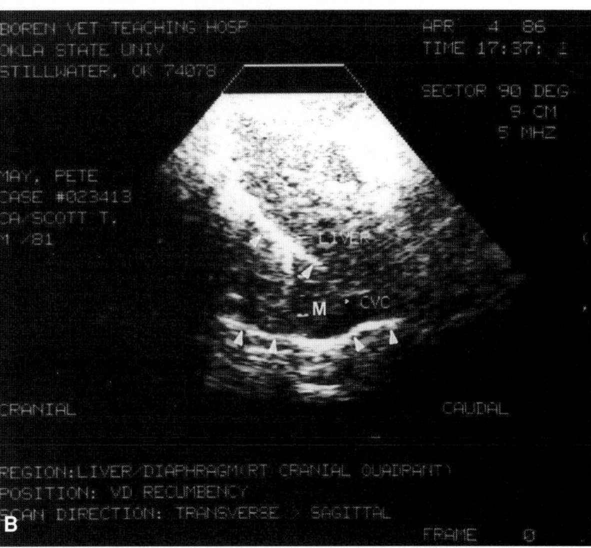

Figure 5-6. (**A**) Ventrodorsal thoracic radiograph of a 3-year-old male Scottish terrier with an incidental finding of an unusual opacity adjacent to the caudal vena cava (*arrows*), creating an irregular bulge on the diaphragmatic shadow. (**B**) Long-axis sonogram made at the right ninth intercostal space (using the liver as an acoustic window) shows compression of the caudal vena cava (*CVC*) by a hypoechoic, ill-defined mass (*M*) with the same echotexture as the liver. The mass protrudes through the caval hiatus of the diaphragm, which appears as an incomplete, hyperechoic line (*arrowheads*). The diagnosis was a diaphragmatic hernia with the liver herniated through the caval foramen.

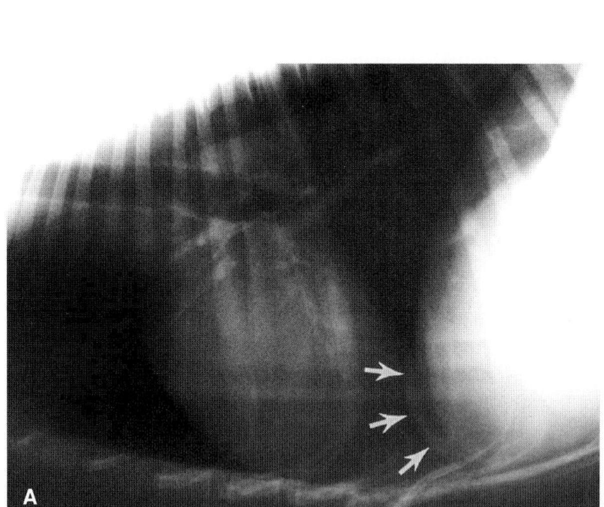

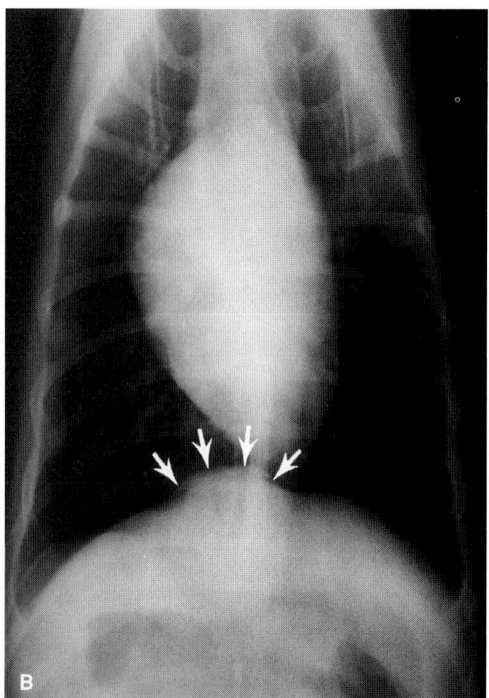

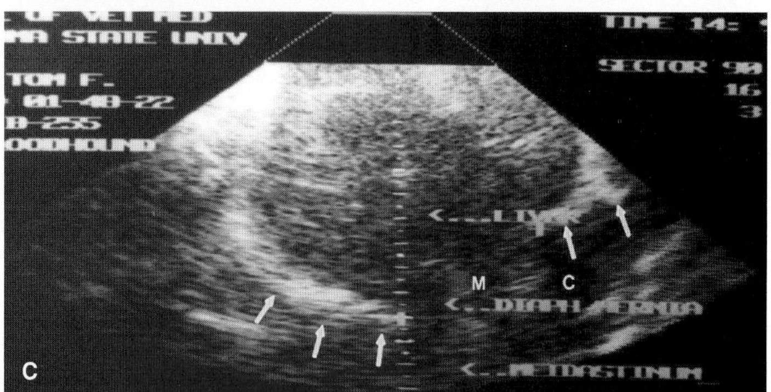

Figure 5-7. (**A**) Left lateral and (**B**) ventrodorsal thoracic radiographs of a 3.5-year-old male bloodhound with a history of intermittent fever spikes and inspiratory dyspnea, with harsh lung sounds on auscultation. The radiographs show an abnormal contour and opacity of the cupula of the diaphragm at the midline, with confluent water tissue opacity (*arrows*) between the diaphragm and apex of the heart. (**C**) Short-axis sonogram (subcostal approach) of the liver and diaphragm at the midline (left side of image is right side of dog) shows discontinuity of the cupula of the diaphragm with echogenic material (*M*) interspersed with hypoechoic, cavitary (*C*) spaces within this diaphragmatic defect. Two valvelike, linear, hyperechoic structures (*arrows*) lie parallel to each other and form the boundaries of this defect. These fluctuate like valves with each heart beat in the real-time image and are compatible with the edges of the torn diaphragm. The diagnosis was an old, occult diaphragmatic hernia with partial herniation of a liver lobe without pleural effusion.

Pleura and Pleural Space

Ultrasound can detect fluid, estimate its volume, and evaluate its character or echotexture, and it can locate mass lesions of the parietal and visceral pleura.

Pleural fluid appears as a hypoechoic (Fig. 5-8) or anechoic (see Fig. 5-4) space between the thoracic wall or diaphragm and the lung. Transudates usually appear anechoic, and exudates appear hypoechoic.[2] Exudates (eg, pyothorax), hemorrhage (eg, hemothorax), and neoplasia may contain enough protein or cellular material to produce "sludge" or to organize and subdivide the pleural space into multiple compartments (see Fig. 5-2).[2,12–14] The sonographic appearance of gas bubbles in pleural fluid may be a result of an anaerobic bacterial infection.[15]

After ultrasonography, thoracocentesis is necessary for fluid analysis to characterize a pleural effusion. A highly viscous collection of pus or clotted blood may appear hypoechoic.[2,16,17] These fluids may require a large-bore needle to obtain an adequate sample. Effusion with a complex echo pattern and a high degree of septation is consistent with fibrinous fluid (most likely septic) and is less likely to be successfully drained.[2,12,18]

Lungs

Normal lungs are not imaged well with ultrasound (see Fig. 5-1).[2] Conventional radiography remains the imaging method of choice for the initial evaluation of pulmonary disease.[10] Ultrasound can add valuable diagnostic information that complements radiographic findings.[2,4] Pleural effusion favors visualization of atelectatic lung lobes (Fig. 5-9). These lobes usually appear hyperechoic and wedge shaped.[2] Pulmonary masses or lung consolidations can be imaged directly through the chest wall if there are no interposed ribs or air-filled structures (Fig. 5-10). The liver or heart can often be used as an acoustic window to image lung lesions.

Pulmonary tumors have various degrees of echogenicity (see Fig. 5-10) and often have irregular borders (Fig. 5-11). They displace normal, air-filled lung tissue and may be differentiated from pulmonary consolidation by the lack of visualization of bronchial and vascular structures (see Fig. 5-11).[2] Tumors often erode and replace normal pulmonary parenchyma with aberrant, disorganized neoplastic tissue.[2] Dystrophic calcification of the lungs may appear sonographically as a cluster of irregular, hyperechoic echoes in the center of a mass. Acoustic shadowing is often seen with dystrophic calcification (Fig. 5-12).[2]

Pulmonary abscesses are uncommon in dogs and cats. Sonographically, pulmonary abscesses have thick echogenic walls with irregular inner margins.[19] The lumen of the abscess may be anechoic or hypoechoic and can be septated. Abscesses may have hyperechoic sediment that layers. Gas–fluid interfaces have been seen in pulmonary abscesses.[2] Primary or metastatic

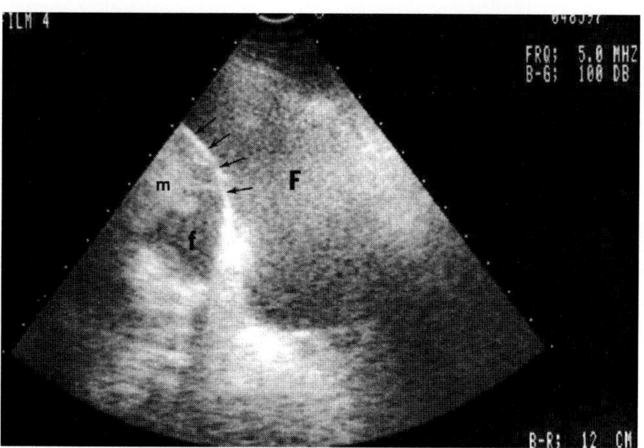

Figure 5-8. Transverse sonogram of a dog made through the right fourth intercostal space (left side of image is dorsal) shows a large amount of hypoechoic pleural effusion (*F*) surrounding the pericardium (*arrows*), which is distended by hypoechoic fluid (*f*) and which contains a mass lesion (*m*). The diagnosis was a pleural carcinomatosis secondary to primary right atrial appendage carcinoma.

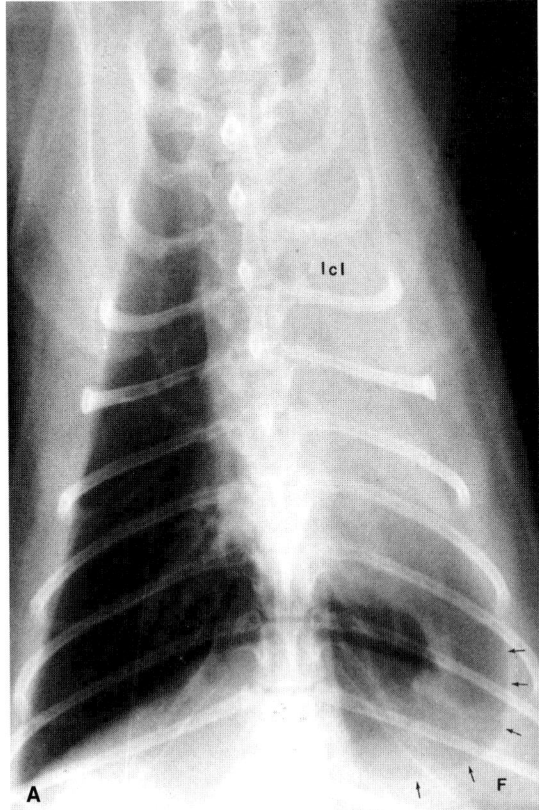

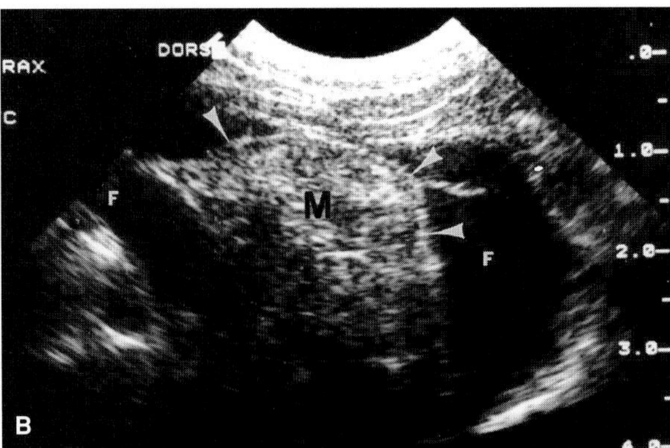

Figure 5-9. (**A**) Ventrodorsal thoracic radiograph of a 2-year-old, neutered male, domestic longhair cat with primarily left-sided pleural effusion (*F*). Notice the contracted, rounded, but aerating left caudal lung lobe with pleural thickening (*small arrows*) and the lack of an air-filled left cranial lobe (*lcl*). (**B**) Transverse sonogram made through the left fifth intercostal space (left side of image is dorsal) shows a somewhat rounded, hypoechoic mass (*M*) with a thin, hyperechoic margin (*white arrowheads*) surrounded by a large amount of hypoechoic pleural fluid (*F*). The mass is an atelectatic lung lobe that cannot inflate because of restrictive fibrosing pleuritis. The diagnosis was complete atelectasis of the left cranial lobe with thickened pleura. (Courtesy of Ontario Veterinary College, University of Guelph, Guelph, Ontario.)

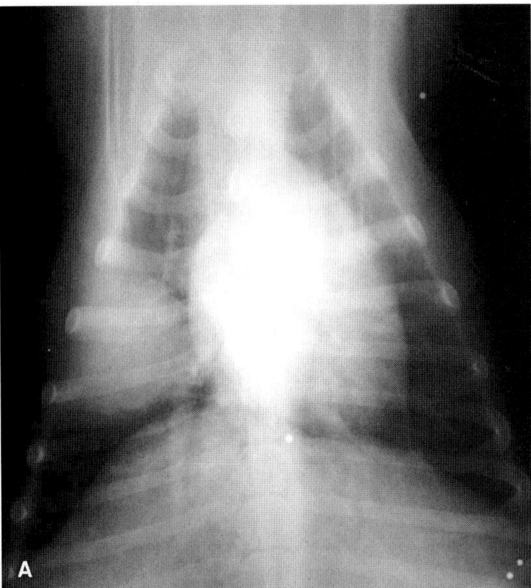

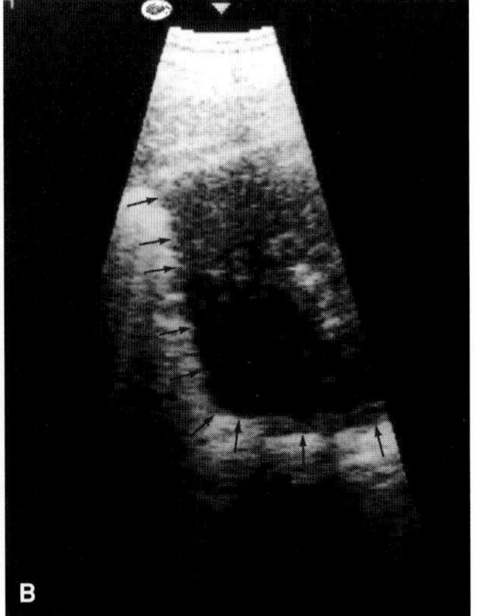

Figure 5-10. (**A**) Dorsoventral thoracic radiograph of a 9-year-old, male English pointer shows a large, well-circumscribed pulmonary mass in the right middle lobe touching the chest wall. (**B**) Transverse sonogram made at the right fifth intercostal space (dorsal is to the left side of the image), showing the dorsal margin of the pulmonary mass where it interfaces with the aerating lung (*arrows*) as demonstrated by the hyperechoic border. The diagnosis was pulmonary adenocarcinoma.

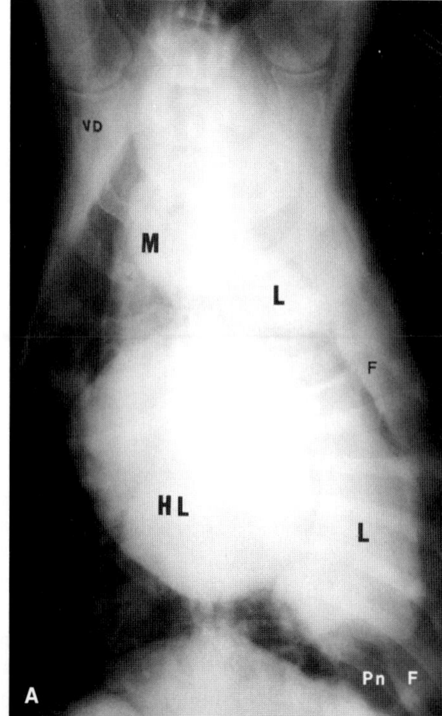

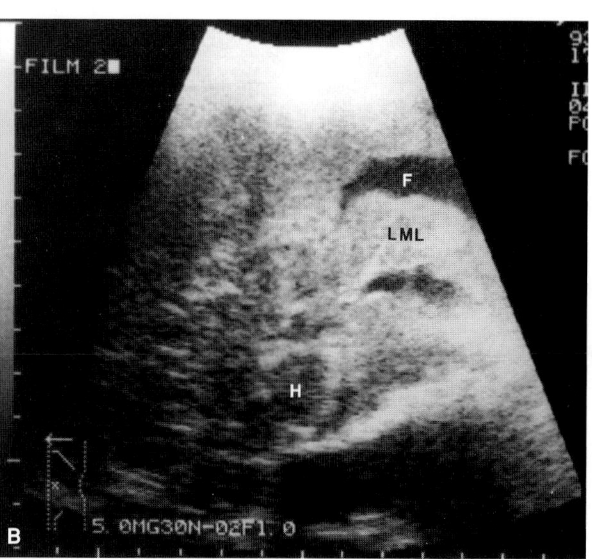

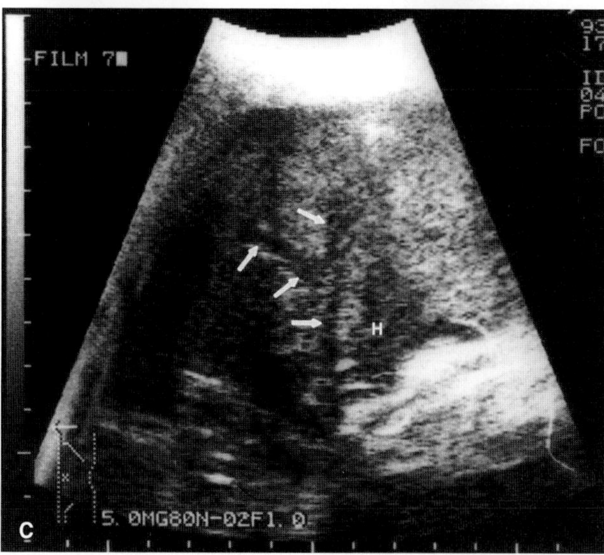

Figure 5-11. (**A**) Ventrodorsal thoracic radiograph of a 6-year-old female Doberman pinscher, showing apparent consolidation of most of the left lung (*L*) with associated left-sided pleural effusion (*F*), spontaneous pneumothorax (*Pn*), a huge cranial mediastinal mass (*M*), and hilar lymphadenopathy (*HL*). (**B**) Short-axis sonogram made at the left sixth intercostal space (left side of image is dorsal), scanning about midway between the sternum and spine. Notice the irregular border of the left middle lobe (*LML*), which has a hyperechoic echotexture superficially and a deeper, more complex echopattern with hypoechoic areas interspersed with darker hypoechoic (*H*) regions. Anechoic pleural fluid (*F*) with many low-level echoes is also seen. (**C**) Another short-axis sonogram made at the left seventh intercostal space over the left caudal lobe shows a solid, complex echoic mass with hypoechoic, irregularly shaped areas (*H*), some of which are linear and branching (*arrows*), caused by fluid-filled bronchi. The diagnosis was lymphomatoid granulomatosis.

tumors with necrotic centers and abscesses have similar sonographic findings (Fig. 5-13).

Lung consolidation, most commonly caused by bronchopneumonia, has a sonographic appearance similar to that of the liver.[20] Fluid-filled pulmonary vessels and bronchi may appear as anechoic, branching, tubular structures (Fig. 5-14), not unlike the portal veins seen in the liver. Small pockets of trapped air in consolidated lung may produce reverberation artifacts, which may aid in the differentiation of consolidated lung from herniated liver, pleural fibrin deposits, or neoplasia.[21]

In addition to scattered echogenic foci from residual pockets of air, consolidated lung parenchyma in human patients is defined by

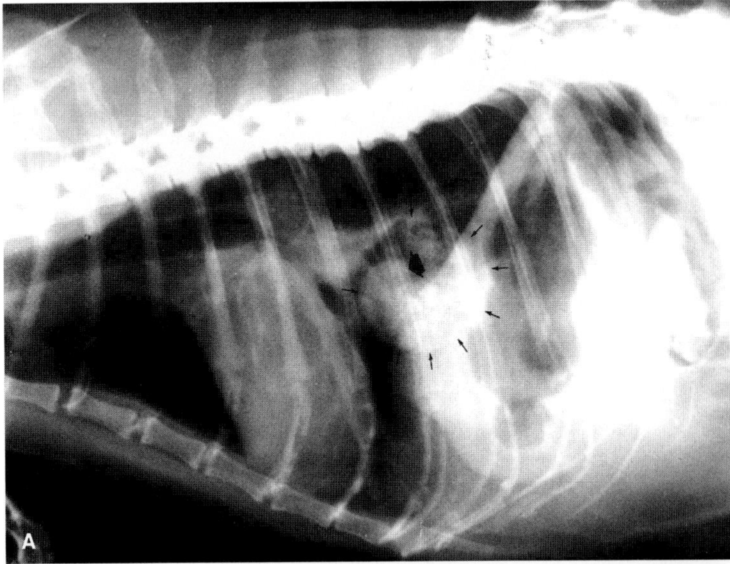

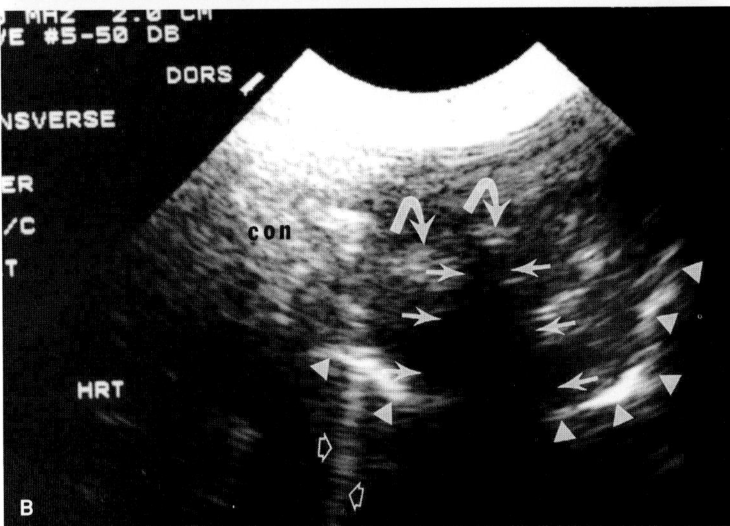

Figure 5-12. (**A**) Right lateral thoracic radiograph of a 12.5-year-old spayed female domestic shorthair cat, showing a pulmonary mass (*small arrows*) in the periphery of the left caudal lobe with internal dystrophic mineralization (*large, wide arrow*). (**B**) Transverse sonogram made at the left eighth intercostal space shows a hypoechoic mass with a hyperechoic margin (*white arrowheads*) and a fan-shaped, anechoic region (*white arrows*) caused by acoustic shadowing from the multiple areas of irregularly shaped dystrophic mineralizations (*curved arrows*) within the mass. A comet-tail artifact (*open arrows*) is also visible adjacent to the mass, and a consolidated lung with a liver-like echotexture (*con*) is seen dorsal to the mass. (Courtesy of Ontario Veterinary College, University of Guelph, Guelph, Ontario.)

"ultrasound fluid bronchograms" (ie, multiple, nonpulsatile, anechoic tubular structures consistent with fluid-filled bronchi) and "ultrasound air bronchograms" (ie, strong echogenic branching lines converging toward the hilus of the lung).[21] The scattered, echogenic, nonlinear foci seen in different scanning planes are considered to be caused by residual air pockets within consolidated lung (see Fig. 5-14).[2,21]

The direction in which visible pulmonary vessels and bronchi taper may also help differentiate consolidated lung from herniated liver.[10] Pulmonary vessels and bronchi taper toward the caudal direction, and portal vessels and bile ducts in a herniated lobe of liver probably taper in a cranial or lateral direction.

Mediastinum

Mediastinal structures may be imaged through a suitable acoustic window.[2,10,22] The imaging

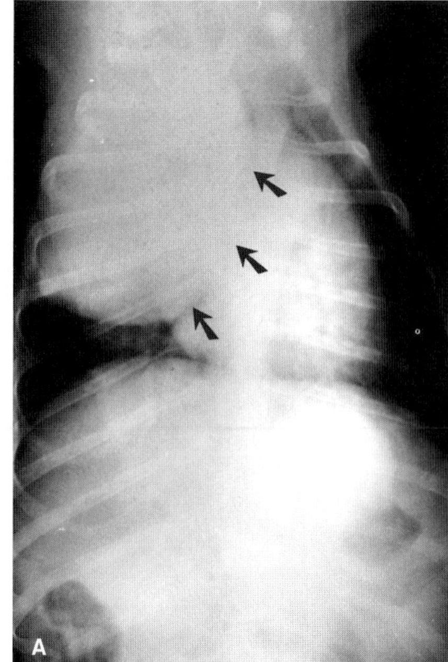

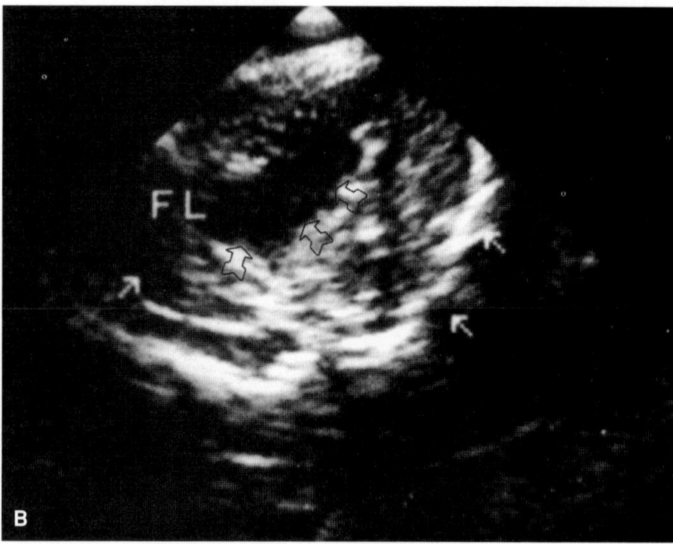

Figure 5-13. (**A**) Dorsoventral thoracic radiograph of a 12.5-year-old, spayed female, mixed-breed dog shows a large pulmonary mass in the right cranial lung lobe (*arrows*). (**B**) Transverse sonogram made at the right third intercostal space (dorsal is on left side of image) shows the hyperechoic margin (*white arrows*) of the hypoechoic mass, which also contains an anechoic, fluid-filled central cavity (*FL*). This mass was bordered by a thick, echogenic wall (*open arrows*). The diagnosis was a papillary adenocarcinoma with a well-encapsulated, sterile abscess of the right cranial lobe. (Courtesy of Ontario Veterinary College, University of Guelph, Guelph Ontario.)

portals are suprasternal (ie, between the sternum and spine), parasternal (ie, dorsal to the sternum), and substernal (ie, subcostal or transhepatic). Ultrasound is more sensitive than radiography in detecting mediastinal masses in dogs and cats.[22]

Ultrasound can be used to evaluate the echogenicity, number, size, relation to vascular

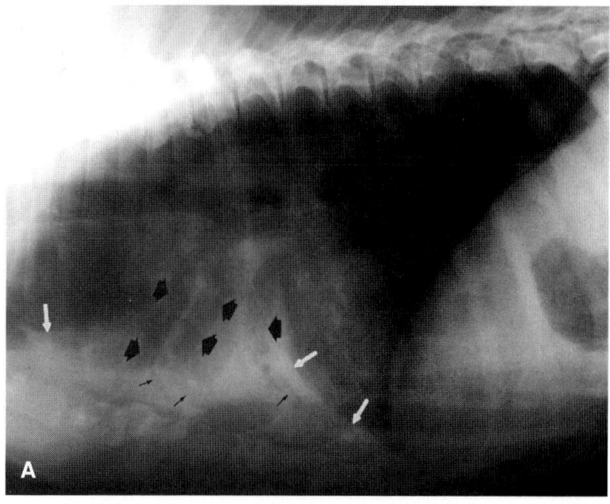

Figure 5-14. (**A**) Left lateral thoracic radiograph of an 11.5-year-old, spayed female Saint Bernard with chronic bronchopneumonia resulting in pulmonary consolidation of the ventral periphery of the right cranial and middle lobes (*small white arrows*), with numerous air bronchograms (*small black arrows*) and cylindrical bronchiectasis (*wide black arrows*). *(continued)*

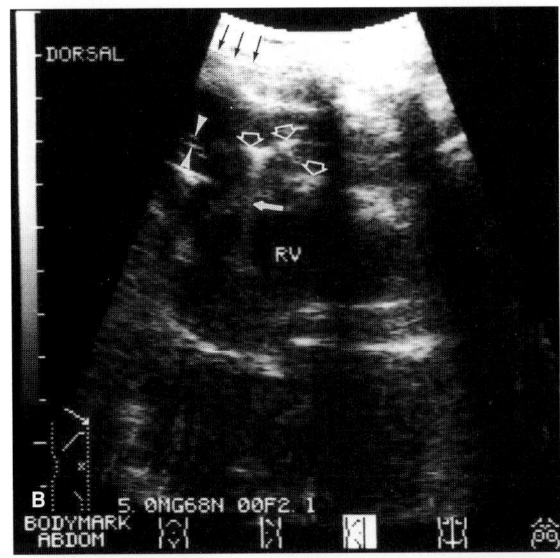

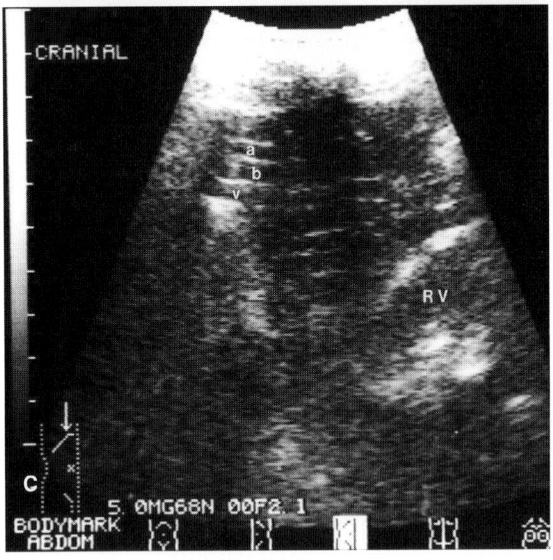

Figure 5-14. *(Continued)* (**B**) Transverse sonogram made at the right third intercostal space (left side of image is dorsal) shows the thin, hyperechoic line caused by the parietal pleura (*small black arrows*) immediately superficial to the hypoechoic, consolidated right cranial lobe, which extends over the heart (*RV*). An anechoic vessel with hyperechoic, parallel walls (*small white arrowheads*) is seen, and multiple, small hyperechoic foci (*open arrows*) with a reverberation artifact (*white arrow*) represent air. (**C**) A long-axis sonogram made at the right third intercostal space (cranial is to the left) shows a segment of consolidated right cranial lobe (hypoechoic) with a pulmonary artery (*a*), a fluid bronchogram (*b*), and a pulmonary vein (*v*) along with other probable fluid bronchograms cranial and superficial to the heart (*RV*). The diagnosis was purulent inflammation.

structures, and margination of mediastinal masses (Fig. 5-15). Mediastinal effusion can also be detected with ultrasound.

Malignant tumors such as lymphosarcoma often involve the mediastinum. Sonographically, mediastinal tumors may have a well-circumscribed hyperechoic rim with a hypoechoic center (Figs. 5-16 and 5-17).[22] As with most tumors, the sonographic appearance varies, and fine-needle aspirates or biopsies should be obtained.

Mediastinal lymphadenopathy is seen in infectious and neoplastic disease (see Chap. 17).

ULTRASOUND-GUIDED BIOPSIES

Ultrasound guidance enables accurate placement of biopsy needles while avoiding critical structures such as large blood vessels.[2] Chest wall tumors, mediastinal masses, and pleural

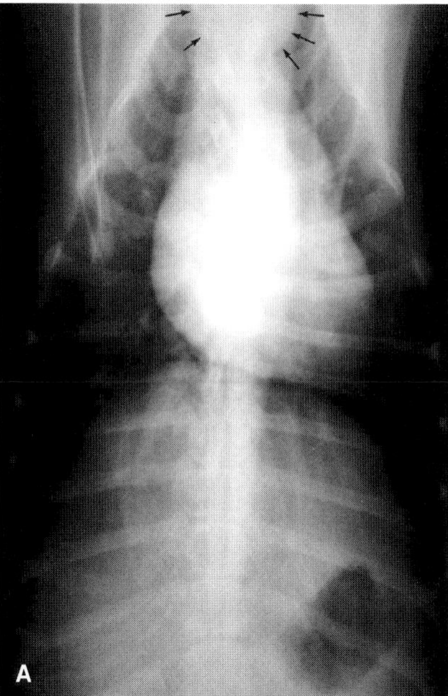

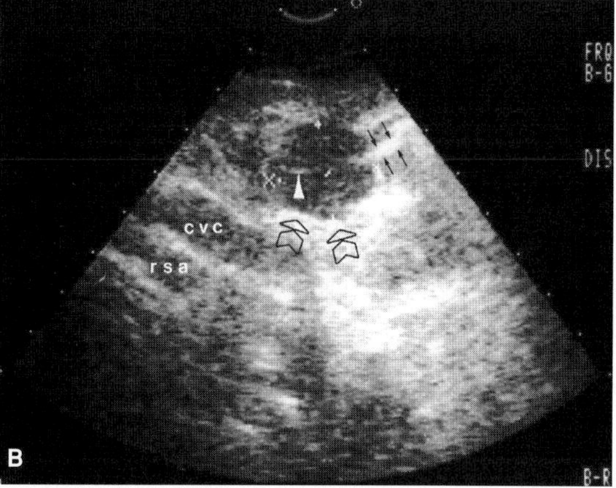

Figure 5-15. (**A**) Dorsoventral thoracic radiograph of a 7-year-old male boxer shows a relatively small mass (*arrows*) in the cranial mediastinum. (**B**) Long-axis sonogram made at the left first intercostal space using the parasternal acoustic window with the dog in dorsal recumbency and the sternum tipped slightly to the right side. The small, round, solid, hypoechoic mass (with calipers measuring size) appears encapsulated with a distant hyperechoic rim (*open arrows*) and has only a small remnant of the central echogenic hilum (*white arrowhead*) usually seen in normal lymph nodes. The cranial vena cava (*cvc*) and right subclavian artery (*rsa*) are seen just deep to the mass. A biopsy needle (*small black arrows*) is seen entering the caudoventral aspect of the mass. The diagnosis was thymic lymphosarcoma.

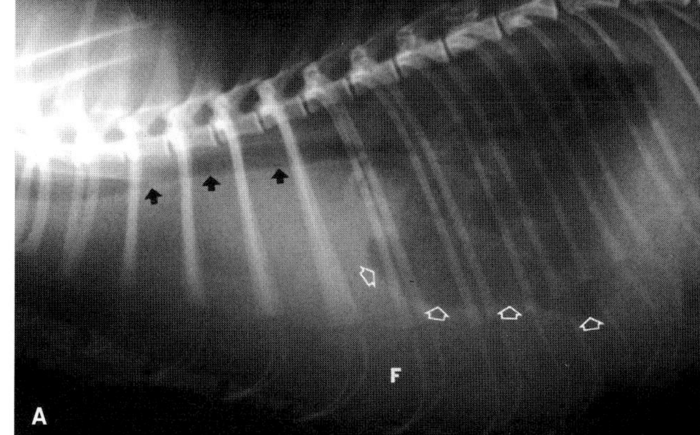

Figure 5-16. (**A**) Right lateral thoracic radiograph of a 3-year-old spayed female domestic shorthair cat shows severe, pleural effusion (*F*) with secondary pulmonary atelectasis (*open arrows*) and dorsal and rightward displacement (*solid arrows*) of the trachea, suggesting a cranial mediastinal mass. *(continued)*

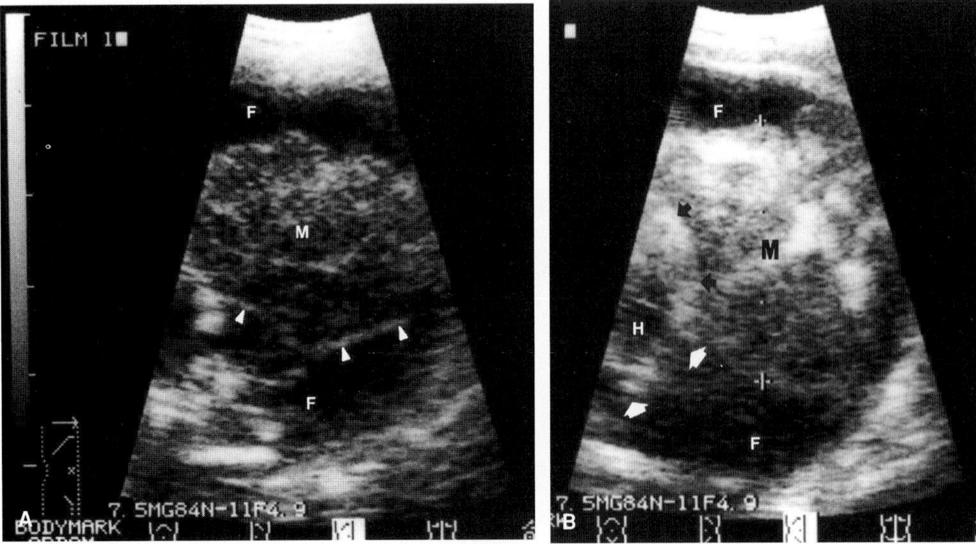

Figure 5-16. *(Continued)* (**B**) Transverse sonogram made with an upper surface approach to the right fourth intercostal space with the cat in left lateral recumbency (dorsal to the left of the image) shows a complex cranial mediastinal mass (*M*) with a hyperechoic rim (*arrowheads*) surrounded by anechoic pleural fluid (*F*). **(C)** Another transverse sonogram made with the same approach, but to the right fifth intercostal space (same orientation), shows the heterogeneous mass (*M*) in a slightly more ventral location, with the mass wrapping around the right ventrolateral border (*arrows*) of the heart (*H*). Anechoic pleural fluid (*F*) is still evident. The diagnosis was lymphosarcoma.

lesions and small pulmonary lesions adjacent to the chest wall or diaphragm are easily biopsied with the aid of ultrasound (see Chap. 3).[10,23]

Sonography is a valuable addition to radiography in the evaluation of the thorax. Sonography is especially valuable in cases of large fluid volumes or large masses. Many lesions require fine-needle aspirates or biopsies for definitive diagnosis, and ultrasound is ideal for localizing biopsy or aspiration sites.

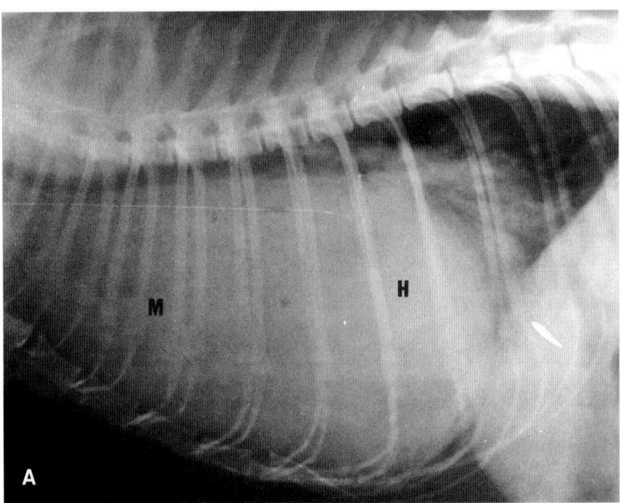

Figure 5-17. (**A**) Left lateral thoracic radiograph of a 9-year-old, neutered male domestic shorthair cat shows a large cranial mediastinal mass (*M*) that completely obscures the cranial border of the heart (*H*) and displaces the trachea.

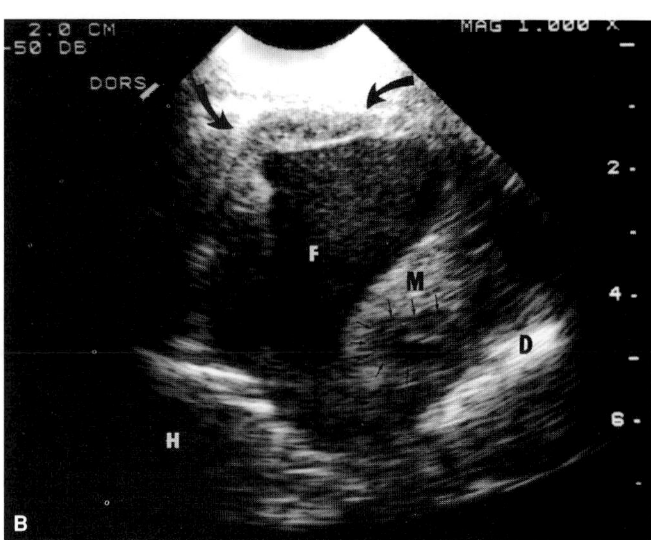

Figure 5-17. *(Continued)* (**B**) Transverse sonogram made at the left ninth intercostal space with the cat in dorsal recumbency (dorsal is to the left of image) shows a thick-walled, cavitary mass (*M*) containing hypoechoic fluid (*F*) with many homogeneous, low-level echoes typical of that associated with a high protein or cell count. The mass appears well-encapsulated (*curved arrows*) and highly vascularized, with a well-defined, curving vessel (*small arrows*). The mass is adjacent to the diaphragm (*D*) and is displacing the heart (*H*). The diagnosis was abscessed thymoma. (Courtesy of Ontario Veterinary College, University of Guelph, Guelph, Ontario.)

REFERENCES

1. Lamb CR, Stowater JL, Pipers FS. The first 21 years of veterinary diagnostic ultrasound. A bibliography. Vet Radiol 1988;29:37.
2. Stowater JL, Lamb CR. Ultrasonography of non-cardiac thoracic disease in small animals. J Am Vet Med Assoc 1989; 195:514.
3. Hashimoto A, Kudo T, Sawashima I. Diagnostic ultrasonography of non-cardiac intrathoracic disorders in small animals. Research Bulletin of the Faculty of Agriculture Gifu University 1990; 55:235.
4. Rosenberg HK. The complementary roles of ultrasound and plain film radiography in differentiating pediatric chest abnormalities. Radiographics 1986;6:427.
5. Targhetta R, Balmes P, Marty-Double C, et al. Ultrasonically guided aspiration biopsy in osteolytic bone lesions of the chest wall. Chest 1993;103:1403.
6. Cosgrove DO, Garbutt P, Hill CR. Echoes across the diaphragm. Ultrasound Med Biol 1978;3:385.
7. Ammann AM, Brewer WH, Maull KI, Walsh JW. Traumatic rupture of the diaphragm: real-time sonographic diagnosis. Am J Roentgenol 1983;140:915.
8. Middleton WD, Melson GL. Diaphragmatic discontinuity associated with perihepatic ascites: a sonographic refractive artifact. Am J Roentgenol 1988;151: 709.
9. Rao KG, Woodlief RM. Grey scale ultrasonic demonstration of ruptured right hemi-diaphragm. Br J Radiol 1980;53:812.
10. Tidwell AS. Diagnostic pulmonary imaging. Probl Vet Med 1992;4:239.
11. Merten DF, Bowie JD, Kirks DR, Grossman H. Anteromedial diaphragmatic defects in infancy: current approaches to diagnostic imaging. Radiology 1982; 142:361.
12. Hirsh JH, Rogers JV, Mack LA. Real-time sonography of pleural opacities. Am J Roentgenol 1981;136:297.
13. Goldenberg JN, Spitz HB, Mitchell SE. Gray scale ultrasonography of the chest. Semin Ultrasound 1982;3:263.
14. Simeone JF, Mueller PR, van Sonnenberg E. The uses of diagnostic ultrasound in the thorax. Clin Chest Med 1984;5:281.
15. Reimer JM, Reef VB, Spencer PA. Ultrasonography as a diagnostic aid in horses with anaerobic bacterial pleuropneumonia and/or pulmonary abscessation: 27 cases (1984–1986). J Am Vet Med Assoc 1989;194:278.

16. Cunningham JJ, Wooten W, Cunningham MA. Gray scale echography of soluble protein and protein aggregate fluid collections (in vitro study). J Clin Ultrasound 1976;4:417.
17. Laing FC, Filly RA. Problems in the application of ultrasonography for the evaluation of pleural opacities. Radiology 1978;126:211.
18. Marks WM, Filly RA, Callen PW. Real-time evaluation of pleural lesions: new observations regarding the probability of obtaining free fluid. Radiology 1982; 142:163.
19. Rantanen NW. Diseases of the thorax. In: Rantanen NW, ed. Veterinary clinics of North America. Equine practice. Philadelphia: WB Saunders, 1986;2:49.
20. Hirsch JH, Carter SJ, Chikos PM, Colacircio C. Ultrasonic evaluation of radiographic opacities of the chest. Am J Roentgenol 1978;130:1153.
21. Acunas B, Celik L, Acunas A. Chest sonography—differentiation of pulmonary consolidation from pleural disease. Acta Radiol 1989;30:273.
22. Konde LJ, Spaulding K. Sonographic evaluation of the cranial mediastinum in small animals. Vet Radiol 1991;32:178.
23. Ikezoe J, Sone S, Higashihara T, et al. Sonographically guided needle biopsy for diagnosis of thoracic lesions. Am J Roentgenol 1984;143:229.

Small Animal Ultrasound, edited by Ronald W. Green.
Lippincott-Raven Publishers, Philadelphia © 1996.

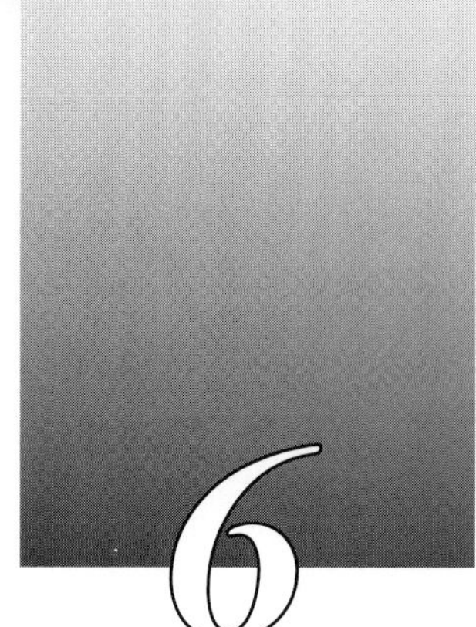

LIVER

Beth Paugh Partington and David S. Biller

Ultrasonography is an ideal complementary diagnostic tool to abdominal radiology, physical examination, and laboratory data in the evaluation of the liver. Hepatic ultrasound can noninvasively examine the internal architecture of the hepatic parenchyma, biliary system, perihepatic structures, and portal and hepatic vascular supply. Hepatic ultrasound findings are rarely pathognomonic and therefore require the results of hepatic sampling by means of biopsy or fine-needle aspiration for a specific diagnosis.

SCANNING TECHNIQUES FOR HEPATIC ULTRASOUND

The patient is positioned in dorsal recumbency on a padded table for hepatic ultrasonography. A V-trough surgical table with a vinyl-covered foam pad is ideal for maintaining the animal comfortably in dorsal recumbency. Gentle manual restraint usually is sufficient to prevent excess motion by the patient. Few patients require tranquilization for abdominal ultrasound.

Hair should be clipped on the cranioventral abdomen from the umbilicus to the tenth intercostal space. The sides of the patient should be clipped up to the center of the ribs. If possible, the patient should be fasted for 24 hours before the procedure. This preparation helps to limit the sonographic barriers of excessive gas in the stomach and intestine. In busy practices, fasting may be somewhat impractical and reserved for cases for which an immediate examination is unnecessary or if gastrointestinal gas has been proven to compromise the examination. In these cases, the examination should be repeated in 24 hours, after the appropriate patient preparation. Increasing the volume of gastric fluid may sometimes provide a sonographic window to parts of the liver. This can be accomplished by placing a moderate volume of water in the stomach through an orogastric tube. Force-feeding water using a dose syringe or allowing the animal to drink voluntarily may increase the volume of gastric fluid, but it may also increase the volume of gas, compromising the examination.

The cranioventral abdomen and caudoventral thorax are covered with coupling gel. To scan the liver in the transverse and longitudinal planes, place the transducer just distal to the xiphoid and angle the transducer beam cranially. Pass the transducer from the left to right over the entire ventral abdomen, just distal to the last costal cartilages. Right and left lateral longitudinal and transverse scans are performed by placing the transducer in the last three intercostal spaces on the right and left.[1–3]

In cats and small dogs (≤15 lb), the entire liver can be imaged subcostally. For the larger dog and especially for the deep-chested breeds, the examiner needs to place the transducer intercostally in the last three to four rib spaces to image the entire liver. In some very-deep-chested dogs with small livers, the operator may not be able to image the entire liver because of overlying lung tissue. If the V-trough table can tilt, some increased access may be gained by evaluating the cranial portion of the patient, allowing the liver to drop slightly caudally with gravity. If bile duct obstruction is suspected, tilting the animal slightly to the right may increase the fluid in the pylorus and duodenum and allow greater sonographic access to the distal portion of the bile duct.

A 7.5-MHz transducer is used for cats and dogs weighing less than 20 pounds. A 5.0-MHz transducer is used for larger dogs.[4] Depending on the penetration capabilities of the equipment, a 3.0-MHz transducer may be necessary to image the entire dorsal liver in some very-deep-chested giant breeds. A sector scanner with a small footprint or contact zone is preferred for hepatic imaging. Mechanical or electronic sector scanners, phased-array, and annular-array transducers are acceptable for liver ultrasound. Linear-array transrectal large-footprint transducers are insufficient for hepatic imaging because of their inability to image intercostally and subcostally.

ULTRASOUND ANATOMY OF THE LIVER

Approaches and Normal Landmarks

The liver is bounded cranially by the concave echogenic structure of the diaphragm-lung interface. It is bordered caudally by the fundus and body of the stomach, the spleen to the far left, and the pylorus and right kidney to the right. In obese animals, a large volume of falciform fat may increase the separation of the liver from the ventral body wall. Falciform fat may appear similar to the liver to the novice ultrasonographer, but fat has a slightly coarser echotexture and is more echogenic than normal liver. The liver has a relatively homogenous echogenicity and should be less echogenic than the spleen and falciform fat, approximately isoechoic to slightly hyperechoic compared to the renal cortex and should have sharp smooth margins.

The hepatic ultrasonographer should attempt to obtain images of the liver adjacent to the spleen in the left cranial portion of the abdomen (Fig. 6-1) and the liver touching the right renal cortex in the right cranial portion of the abdomen (Fig. 6-2). The first image (ie, spleen and

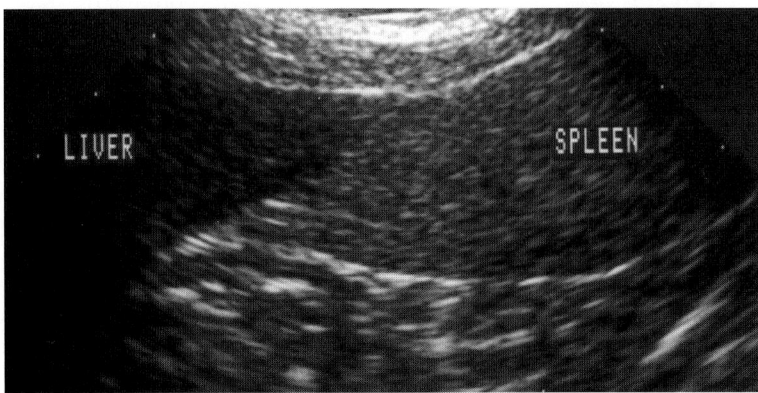

Figure 6-1. Longitudinal scan of the left lateral liver lobe touching the head of the spleen in the left cranial portion of the abdomen. The normal liver is less echogenic than the spleen and has a coarser, less uniform echoic texture. (From Biller DS, Kantrowitz B, Miyabayashi T. Ultrasonography of Diffuse Liver Disease. J Vet Intern Med 1992;6:71.)

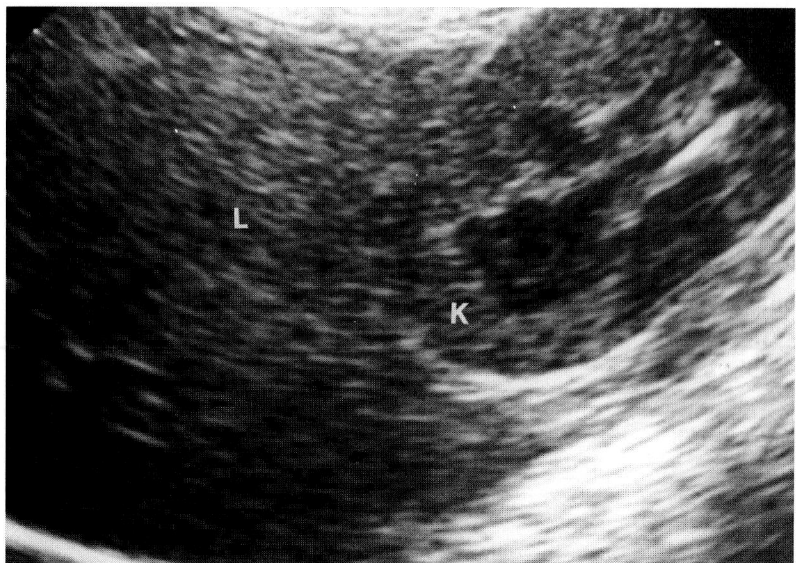

Figure 6-2. Longitudinal scan of the right kidney (*K*) in the renal fossa of the caudate liver (*L*) lobe in the right cranial portion of the abdomen. The liver and renal cortex normally have the same echogenicity. (From Biller DS, Kantrowitz B, Miyabayashi T. Ultrasonography of Diffuse Liver Disease. J Vet Intern Med 1992; 6:71.)

liver) may be somewhat difficult in the normal animal, but the second image (ie, liver and kidney) should be obtainable in every patient, because the right kidney lies in the renal fossa of the caudate lobe of the liver. These two images allow comparison of the relative hepatic echogenicity at the same depth and control settings when diffuse hepatic disease is suspected. If the liver and right renal cortex are isoechoic, the finding rules out improper control settings as a cause of altered hepatic echogenicity, although this depends on having a normal right kidney.

The hepatic parenchyma contains numerous circular and tubular anechoic structures of various sizes that represent the hepatic and portal veins (Fig. 6-3). Portal veins have an apparent echogenic wall because of the fat and fibrous tissue surrounding the vessel. Portal veins are largest at the junction of the main portal vein at the porta hepatis and taper as they progress into the hepatic parenchyma. Hepatic veins do not have an echogenic margin, except where they are very large near the junction of the caudal vena cava in the craniodorsal liver.[5] However, even at the junction to the caudal vena cava, the echogenicity of hepatic vein margins is less than a portal vein of similar size. Hepatic arteries and intrahepatic bile ducts are not routinely identified with ultrasound.

It is important to know the ultrasound anatomy of the major abdominal vasculature as it enters or passes the liver at the porta hepatis. If the ultrasonographer can clearly identify the perihepatic vessels, locating the bile duct, pancreas, adrenals, and vascular anomalies is much easier. The aorta is identified as the most dorsal, midline, large, pulsatile vascular structure that appears to pass over the echogenic diaphragm. Just ventral and slightly to the patient's right is the caudal vena cava. Deep abdominal compression with the transducer may narrow the caudal vena cava lumen, but it rarely significantly alters the lumen of the aorta. Just ventral and slightly to the left of the caudal vena cava is the prehepatic portal vein (Fig. 6-4). The bile duct lies ventral, slightly to the patient's right and parallel to the portal vein. Transverse imaging through the right caudal intercostal spaces may be the best way to identify the major vascular orientation (Fig. 6-5).[6]

The biliary system consists of the gallbladder, the cystic duct, and the intrahepatic and extrahepatic bile ducts. Bile flows from the bile canaliculi into the interlobar ducts, into the lobar ducts, and on into the hepatic ducts, which empty into the bile duct. The cystic duct carries bile to and from the gallbladder and connects to the bile duct proximal to the hepatic ducts. The

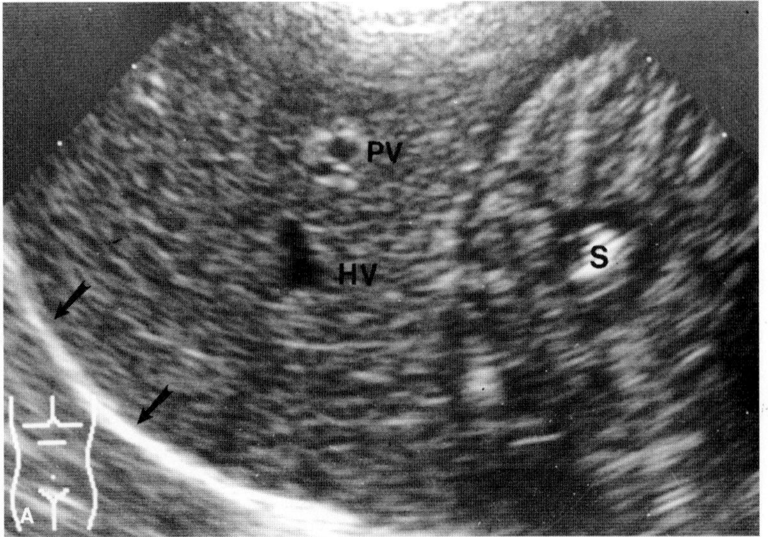

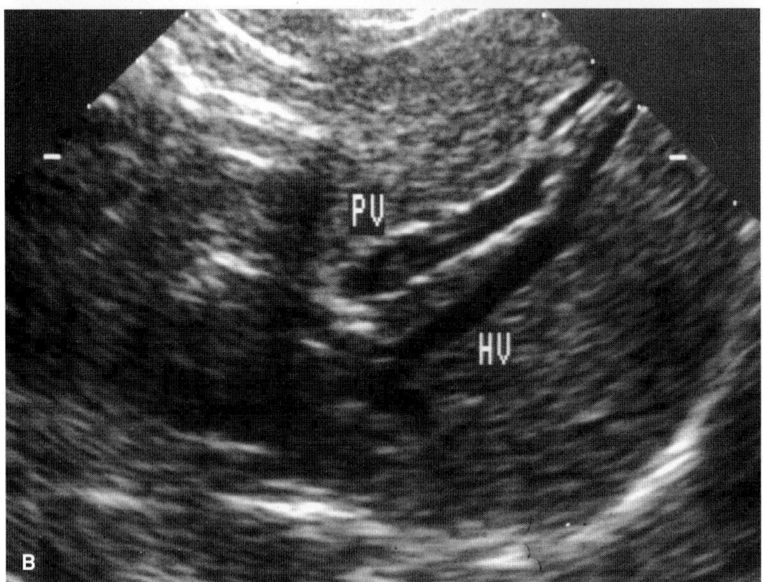

Figure 6-3. (**A**) Longitudinal scan of the left liver with a cross section of a portal vein and hepatic vein. The arrows identify the echogenic line of the diaphragm–lung interface. The center of the fundus of the stomach (*S*) is also identified. (**B**) Transverse scan of the liver shows a longitudinal image of an echogenic-walled portal vein (*PV*) and hypoechoic hepatic vein (*HV*). (From Biller DS, Kantrowitz B, Miyabayashi T. Ultrasonography of Diffuse Liver Disease. J Vet Intern Med 1992;6:71.)

hepatic, lobar, and interlobar bile ducts are not appreciated in a normal hepatic ultrasound. In the normal patient, the gallbladder, cystic duct, and bile duct should be visible ultrasonographically. The gallbladder is found to the right of midline and should be anechoic and have a very thin wall. It is an oval to pear-shaped structure in the dog and cat (Fig. 6-6). The cystic duct is identified as a continuation of the gallbladder neck, which tapers until it enters the common bile duct. Exact determination of where the cystic duct ends and the bile duct begins is difficult and unnecessary in the normal patient. The bile duct continues out of the liver and is identified as a 1- to 3-mm, tubular, anechoic structure just ventral to the portal vein.[6,7] Bile ducts as long as 4 mm have been recorded in normal cats. The bile duct continues its course through the pancreas and enters the duodenum at the major papilla.

The gallbladder is a good place to look for two common ultrasound artifacts: acoustic

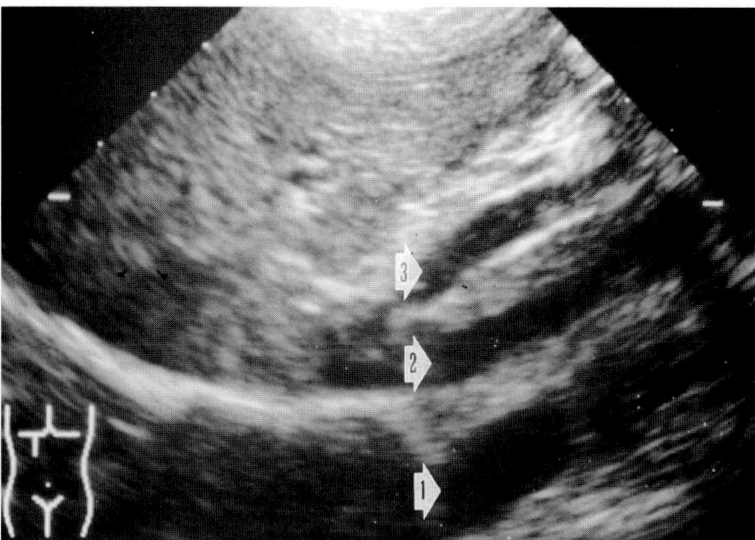

Figure 6-4. Longitudinal scan in the cranial portion of the right central abdomen shows the aorta (*arrow 1*) dorsal to the caudal vena cava (*arrow 2*), which is dorsal to the prehepatic portal vein (*arrow 3*). The common bile duct (not visualized on this scan) lies just ventral (closer to the transducer) to the portal vein.

enhancement (ie, through transmission) and mirror-image artifacts. Through transmission is identified as a diverging area of increased echogenicity distal to the gallbladder (Fig. 6-7). It is created because the sound beam is less attenuated as it crosses the fluid-filled gallbladder than the adjacent liver.[4,8] Acoustic enhancement at the gallbladder is of little importance, but recognition of this artifact in other areas can aid the ultrasonographer in interpretation.

A mirror-image artifact is created when the sound beam produces a single reverberation between the walls of the gallbladder and the gallbladder and diaphragm.[4,8] It is identified as a mirror or reversed duplication of the gallbladder and the diaphragm image distal to the actual gallbladder and diaphragm (Fig. 6-8). The single reverberation delays the echoes' return to the transducer. Because depth placement of the image is based on the round-trip time of the pulse and echo, the computer places the tardy echo deep to the original structure. The gallbladder mirror-image artifact is of little significance except when searching for a diaphrag-

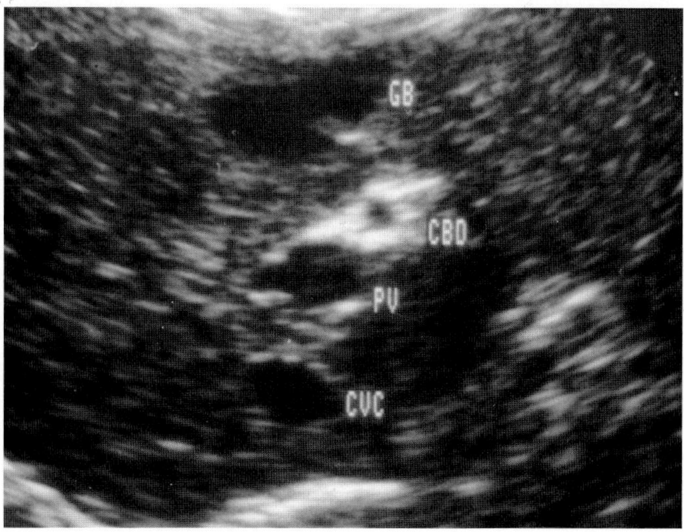

Figure 6-5. Transverse scan through the caudal intercostal spaces in the cranial portion of the right central abdomen shows the caudal vena cava (*CVC*), intrahepatic portal vein (*PV*), common bile duct (*CBD*) and neck of the gallbladder (*GB*).

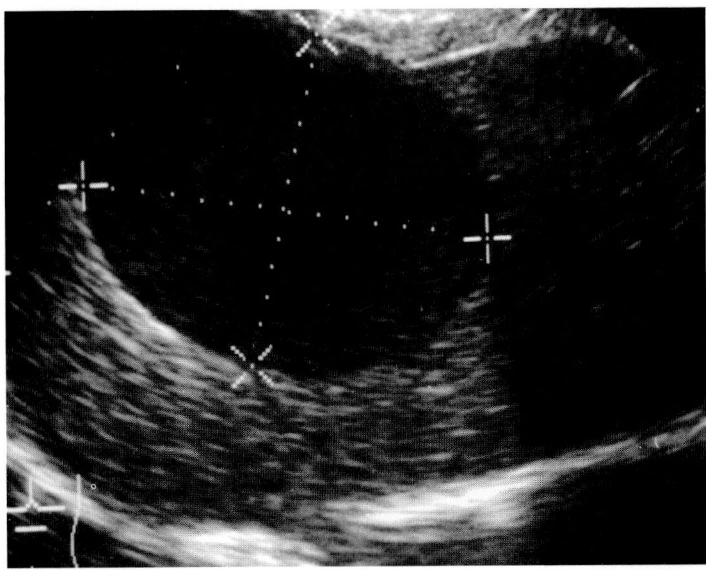

Figure 6-6. Transverse liver scan, with a normal gallbladder outlined by vertical and transverse cursors. The gallbladder is slightly right of the midline and has a very thin wall surrounding the anechoic bile.

matic hernia; then, the appearance of a gallbladder in front of the diaphragm can be confusing. However, the gallbladder in front of the diaphragm is accompanied by a normally positioned gallbladder behind the diaphragm, preventing misinterpretation of a diaphragmatic hernia. A bilobed gallbladder has been reported as a common anomaly in cats (Fig. 6-9).[9] This usually is an incidental finding and should not be confused with a mirror-image artifact.

Liver Size

Two studies dealing with the ultrasonographic measurement of liver size came to somewhat opposite conclusions.[10–12] Both used longitudinal and transverse measurements from the ventral liver tip to the craniodorsal diaphragm margin as an estimation of overall liver weight. One group of researchers concluded that real-time ultrasound measurements were of little value in

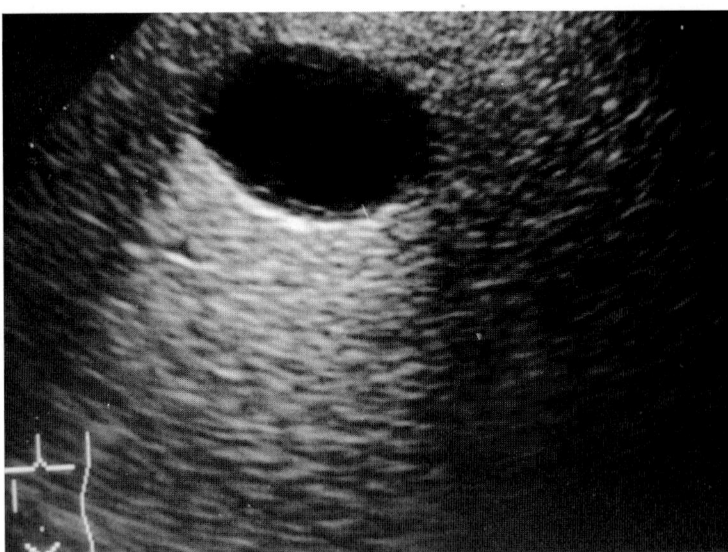

Figure 6-7. Acoustic enhancement or through transmission. Longitudinal scan of the right liver demonstrates the diverging echogenic wedge distal to the gallbladder. This area of increased echogenicity is caused by the lack of attenuation of the ultrasound beam as it passes through the fluid-filled gallbladder.

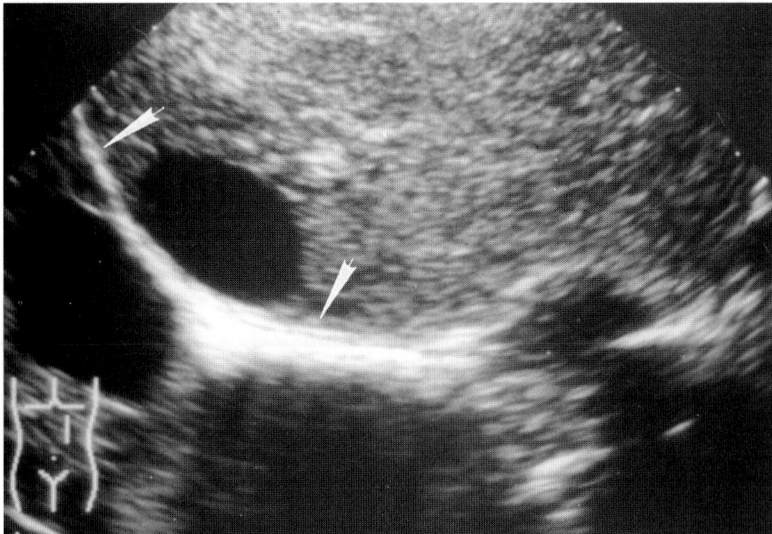

Figure 6-8. Mirror-image artifact in a longitudinal scan through a hepatic cyst adjacent to the diaphragm. Duplication of the hepatic cyst in front of the diaphragm occurs because of reverberation of the echoes between the cyst walls and diaphragm. Arrowheads identify the echogenic diaphragm-lung interface.

predicting liver weight.[12] Another researcher concluded that longitudinal or transverse measurements provided a useful estimation of liver mass.[10,11] We think that ultrasound is valuable in the subjective estimation of liver size. Large livers are easily imaged and provide a large separation between diaphragm and stomach. Large livers often have rounded margins, unlike the sharp edges of the normal liver. Small livers are narrow and difficult to image between the lung and stomach gas reverberations. We also refer to the standard lateral radiographic examination of the abdomen for correlation of the ultrasound estimation of the liver size.

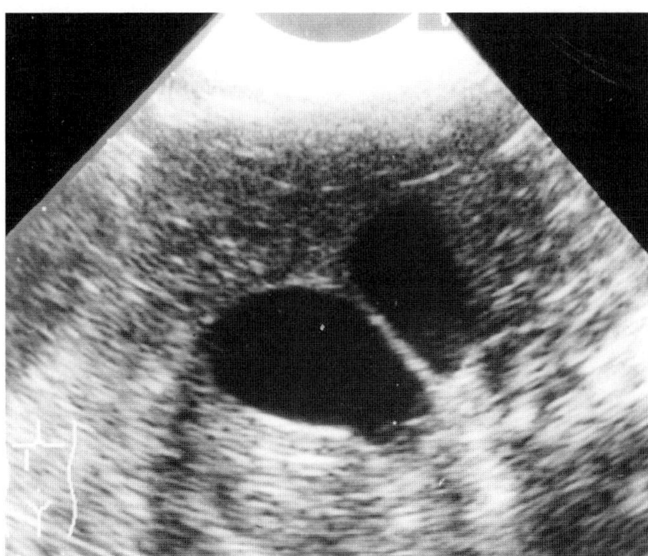

Figure 6-9. Duplication of the gallbladder in a normal Siamese cat. This is an incidental finding and can be differentiated from a mirror-image artifact because there is no diaphragm between the two gallbladders. A similar appearance may occur with a dilated gallbladder that partially folds on itself.

ULTRASOUND APPEARANCE OF ABNORMALITIES AND DISEASE STATES

Diffuse Hepatic Disease

The hepatic ultrasound parameters that are routinely evaluated include size, margination, echogenicity, vascularity, beam penetration, biliary mensuration, and perihepatic abnormalities. Diffuse hepatic disease may affect any or all of these parameters. One problem with diffuse hepatic disease is that the most common ultrasonographic findings is a normal-appearing liver. For identification of a specific disease process in the liver, the examiner must have a sample of hepatic tissue from a fine-needle aspirate or preferably a biopsy for culture and histopathology. Ultrasound findings may allow a more narrow, prioritized differential diagnosis, but the final diagnosis usually requires a tissue sample.

Diffuse hepatic disease may cause a change in the echogenicity of the hepatic parenchyma. The liver should be less echogenic than the spleen and isoechoic or slightly hyperechoic compared with the renal cortex. Increased echogenicity is identified as hepatic echogenicity greater than the renal cortex and similar to the spleen. The echogenic portal vein margins may also appear less distinct with diffuse hyperechoic liver disease. Increased beam attenuation with decreased visualization of deeper structures is also characteristic of a hyperechoic liver.[13] Diseases that commonly cause an increase in hepatic echogenicity include cirrhosis, hepatic lipidosis, and steroid hepatopathy (Table 6-1). Other disease that may cause an increase in liver echogenicity are diabetes mellitus, lymphosarcoma, chronic cholangeohepatitis, and some toxic hepatopathies. Hepatic lipidosis, diabetes mellitus, steroid hepatopathy, lymphosarcoma, and toxic hepatopathies are more commonly present in a normal-sized to enlarged liver (Fig. 6-10). Cirrhosis and chronic cholangeohepatitis are generally present in a small, irregularly marginated liver.

Besides an increase in liver echogenicity and a decrease in liver size, cirrhosis may appear as multiple hepatic nodules from macronodular regeneration (Fig. 6-11). Perihepatic changes such as ascites, portal and splenic vein dilation, and splenomegaly may occur with cirrhosis because of portal hypertension. Unilateral adrenal enlargement with a functional adrenal mass or bilateral adrenal enlargement with pituitary-dependent hyperadrenalcorticalism may be present with endogenous steroid hepatopathy. Hepatic lipidosis usually appears as an enlarged liver that is isoechoic to hyperechoic compared with the falciform fat (Fig. 6-12).[14,15]

Diffuse hepatic disease may result in liver hypoechogenicity. A hypoechoic liver has more prominent portal vein walls compared with the hepatic parenchyma and is less echogenic than the renal cortex. Hypoechoic liver diseases in-

TABLE 6-1
Hyperechoic Liver Disease

	Size	Beam Penetration	Vascularity	Ancillary Abnormalities
Fatty Liver	Increased	Normal–decreased	Normal	
Steroid Hepatopathy	Increased	Normal–decreased	Normal	Adrenomegaly*
Cirrhosis	Increased	Normal–decreased	Decreased PV flow & velocity†	Ascites, splenomegaly

*Endogenous steroid hepatopathy—bilateral enlargement with pituitary dependent and unilateral enlargement with adrenal tumors. Exogenous steroid hepatopathy will result in small adrenals bilaterally.

†Portal veins may appear smaller and will demonstrate decreased flow and velocity on duplex Doppler.

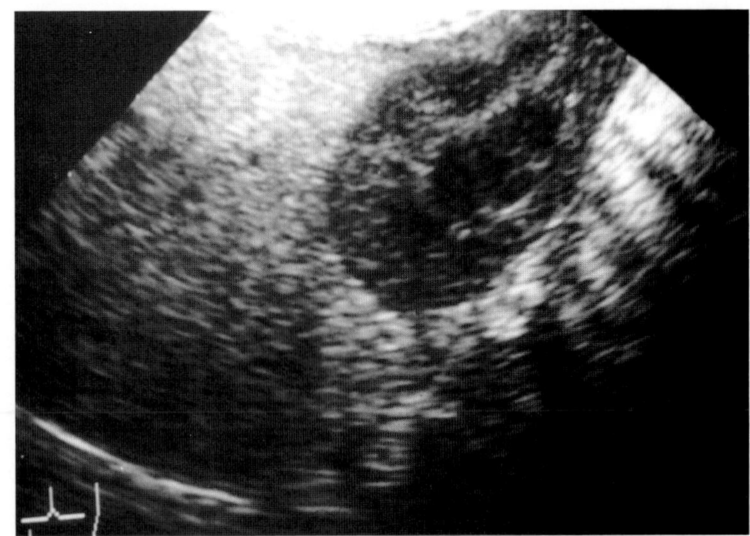

Figure 6-10. Diffuse hyperechoic liver disease.The longitudinal image of the right kidney in the renal fossa of the caudate liver lobe demonstrates diffuse liver hyperechogenicity compared with the normal renal cortex. Notice the increased attenuation of the ultrasound beam in the deeper liver structures, which is not present deep to the kidney. The biopsy diagnosis was hepatic fibrosis due to bile stasis secondary to biliary carcinoma.

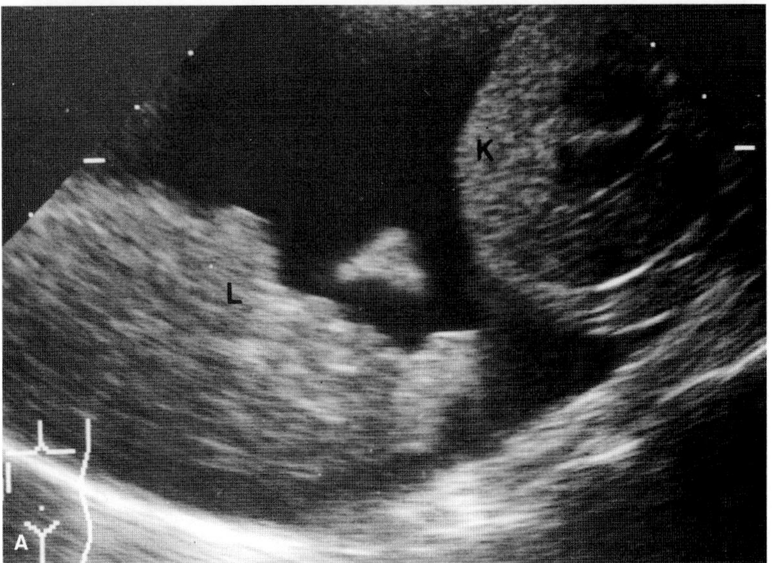

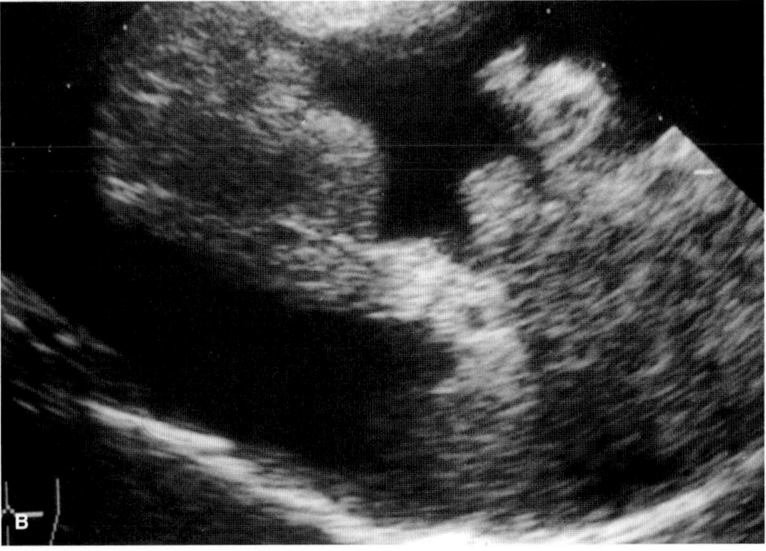

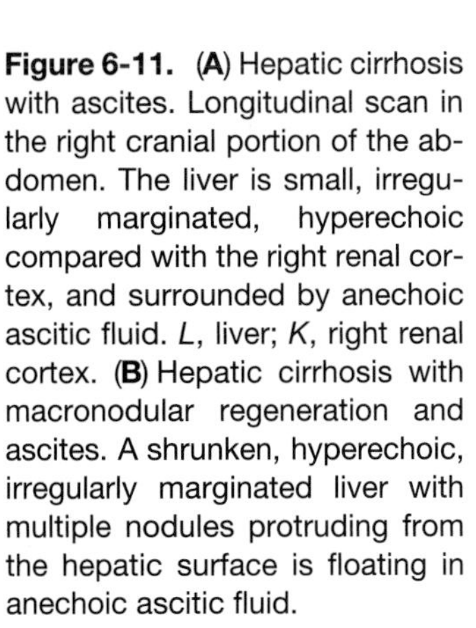

Figure 6-11. (**A**) Hepatic cirrhosis with ascites. Longitudinal scan in the right cranial portion of the abdomen. The liver is small, irregularly marginated, hyperechoic compared with the right renal cortex, and surrounded by anechoic ascitic fluid. *L*, liver; *K*, right renal cortex. (**B**) Hepatic cirrhosis with macronodular regeneration and ascites. A shrunken, hyperechoic, irregularly marginated liver with multiple nodules protruding from the hepatic surface is floating in anechoic ascitic fluid.

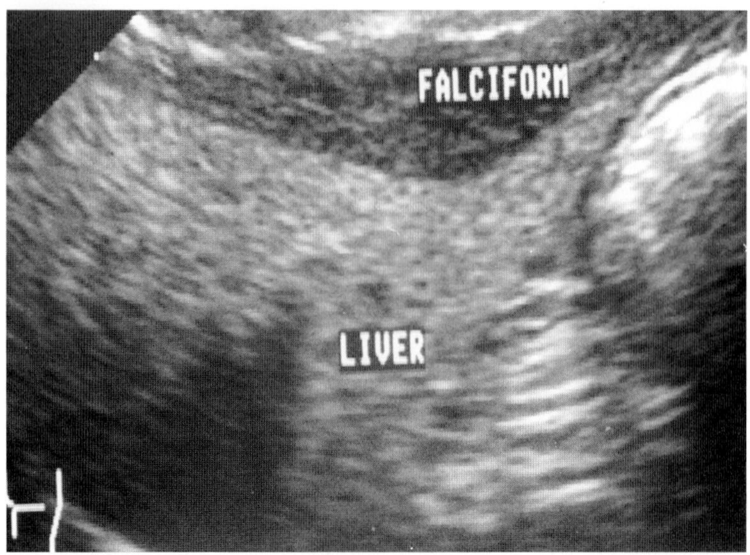

Figure 6-12. Hepatic lipidosis in a Persian cat. The liver is enlarged and hyperechoic compared with the falciform fat.

clude inflammatory hepatitis (eg, suppurative), lymphosarcoma, leukemia, and chronic passive congestion (Table 6-2).[1–3,13] The hypoechogenicity results because the uniform cellular infiltrates or increased liver blood volume is less attenuating than normal liver parenchyma. Suppurative hepatitis may cause a dramatic decrease in liver echogenicity with minimal other changes (Fig. 6-13). Chronic passive congestion, most commonly from right heart disease, can cause hepatomegaly, decreased echogenicity, splenomegaly, and dilation of the hepatic veins and caudal vena cava.

Hepatic lymphosarcoma has a varied ultrasonographic appearance.[16–18] It may present as a diffuse decreased or increased echogenicity in a normal to enlarged liver (Fig. 6-14). It may also present as focal or multifocal poorly circumscribed hypoechoic areas or well-circumscribed hyperechoic nodules surrounded by areas of decreased echogenicity (Fig. 6-15). Hepatic lymphosarcoma may represent only a portion of the abdominal lymphosarcoma tumor burden. Careful ultrasound evaluation should be performed to detect abdominal lymphadenopathy and splenic involvement (Fig. 6-16). Hepatic

TABLE 6-2
Hypoechoic Liver Disease

	Size	Beam Penetration	Vascularity	Ancillary Abnormalities
Suppurative Hepatitis	Increased	Normal–increased	Normal	Abscesses, lymphadenopathy
Hepatic Congestion	Increased	Normal–increased	Increased CVC and hepatic vein	Ascites, splenomegaly
Lymphoma	Increased	Normal–increased	Normal	Lymphadenopathy, hepatic and splenic masses, splenomegaly

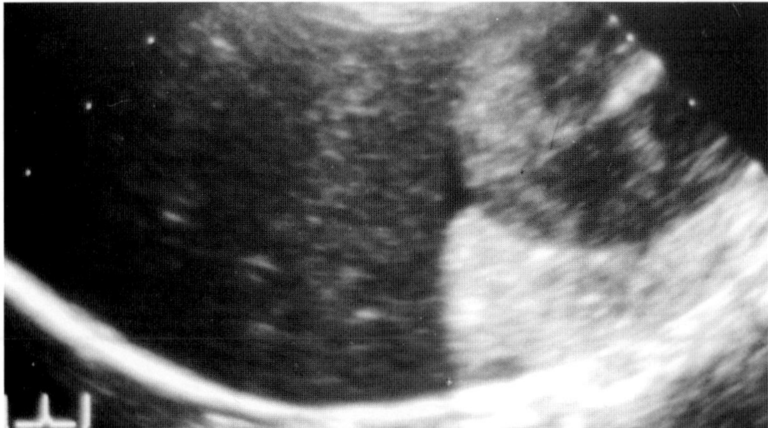

Figure 6-13. Diffuse hypoechoic liver disease. This longitudinal image of the liver and right kidney shows the liver to be much less echogenic than the adjacent renal cortex. The needle aspirate diagnosis was suppurative hepatitis due to *Escherichia coli.*

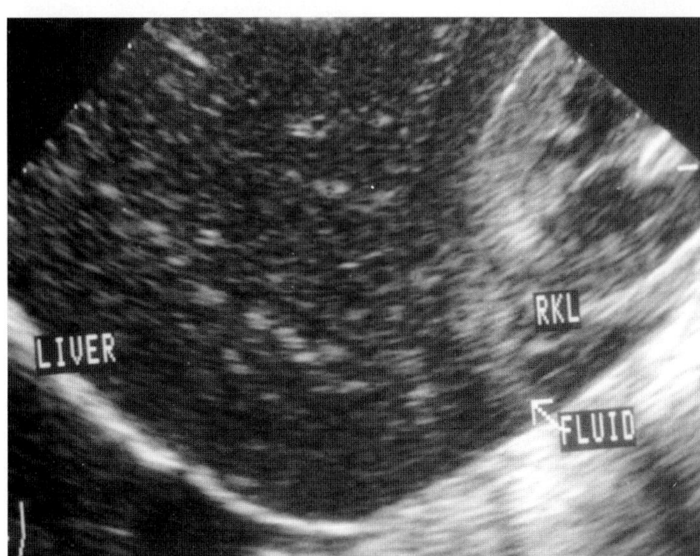

Figure 6-14. Diffuse hypoechoic liver disease due to lymphosarcoma. The liver is hypoechoic compared with the renal cortex, and the hyperechoic walls of the portal veins stand out more prominently throughout the hepatic parenchyma.

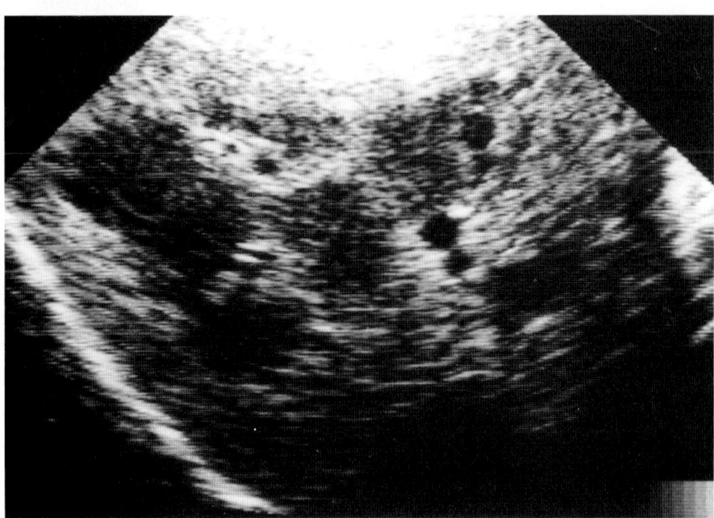

Figure 6-15. Hepatic lymphosarcoma. The longitudinal scan shows multifocal hypoechoic nodules scattered throughout the hepatic parenchyma.

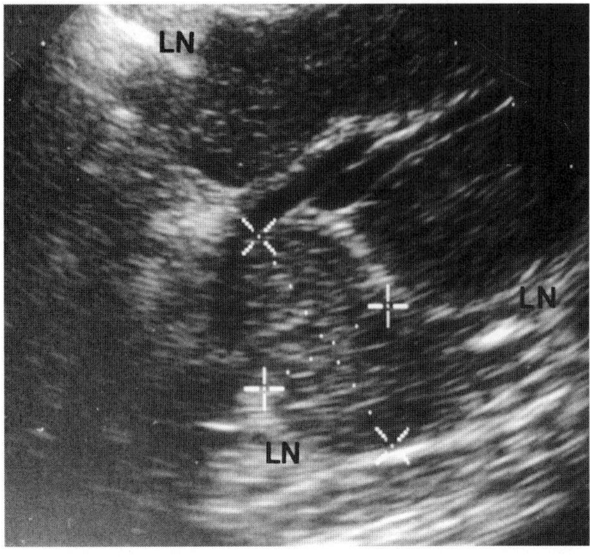

Figure 6-16. Central abdominal lymphadenopathy in a cocker spaniel with generalized abdominal lymphosarcoma. The lymph nodes (*LN*) are well-circumscribed hypoechoic masses that are oval to round. The linear anechoic tubular structures between the nodes are the abdominal aorta and caudal vena cava. Cross-hatch cursors measure the most ventral lymph node.

lymphosarcoma and other diffuse hepatic disease may produce completely normal hepatic ultrasound scans.[13,17]

A normal liver ultrasound examination does not rule out the possibility of diffuse hepatic disease. If hepatic disease is suspected from the clinical examination and laboratory results, the presence of a normal liver ultrasound should not deter the clinician from obtaining a liver aspirate or biopsy.

Focal Hepatic Disease

Focal hepatic disease is more easily recognized ultrasonographically because focal lesions have an altered architecture or echogenicity and are surrounded by normal liver.[19] Focal hepatic disease includes cysts, hematomas, abscesses, granulomas, regenerative nodules, primary and metastatic neoplasms, and less commonly, bilomas and infarcts. As with diffuse hepatic disease, there are few focal lesions that can be diagnosed merely by their ultrasonographic characteristics. Each focal lesion has a spectrum of appearances that depends on the cause and duration of disease. Definitive diagnosis usually requires fine-needle aspiration or biopsy.

Hepatic cysts may be the most characteristic focal lesion (Fig. 6-17). Hepatic cysts may be congenital or caused by prior trauma. They typically are round, have a smooth and distinct wall, are anechoic, and demonstrate through transmission or acoustic enhancement. Hepatic cysts may be single or multiple and may be septated or contain internal echoes from cellular debris or hemorrhage.

Bilomas (ie, biliary pseudocyst) are uncommon thin-walled, circular, anechoic structures found in the liver (Fig. 6-18). Bilomas form secondary to trauma as an encapsulated collection of bile outside the biliary tract.[20] Bilomas and hepatic cysts can be differentiated by fine-needle aspiration of the fluid. Hepatic cysts and bilomas usually do not cause clinical signs unless they are very large, causing focal compression of adjacent structures.

The ultrasound appearance of hematomas depends on the degree of clot formation. Hematomas usually are hyperechoic initially during active blood loss and become hypoechoic to mixed as they mature.[1,2] A very large, old hematoma may appear as a well-demarcated, mixed hyperechoic mass.

The ultrasound appearances of hepatic abscesses and granulomas depend on their cellular composition and duration.[21] Abscesses typically are hyperechoic early and may or may not have a defined margin. As the abscess matures, it may become hypoechoic or anechoic, with or with-

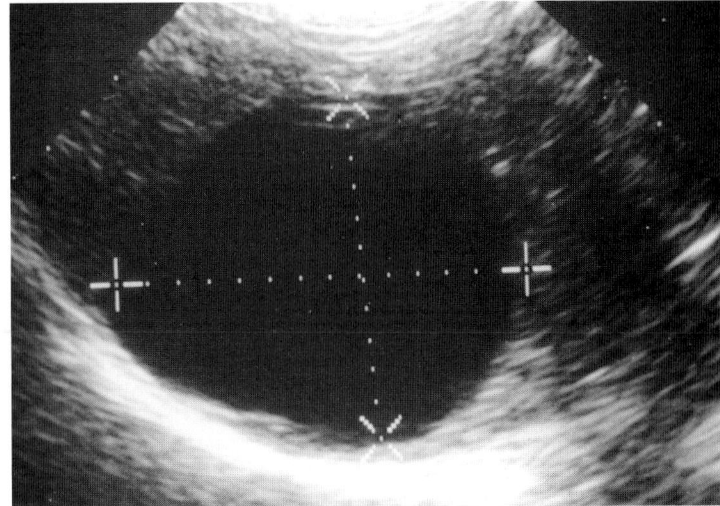

Figure 6-17. Hepatic cyst. The crosshatch cursors measure a large, single hepatic cyst that is adjacent to the diaphragm. Hepatic cysts are round, thin-walled, and anechoic, and they demonstrate through transmission. They can be differentiated from the gallbladder by their location, lack of contraction after feeding a meal containing fat, and the lack of a gallbladder neck or cystic duct.

out gravity-dependent hyperechoic cellular debris. Abscesses may also appear as mixed echogenic lesions. The most common appearance is an irregularly marginated hypoechoic mass without a well-defined wall or through transmission (Fig. 6-19). Abscesses may contain microbubbles of gas that appear as a highly reflective interface that may reverberate at the proximal margin or shadow distally. Some chronic abscesses may have so low a cellularity as to demonstrate through transmission, appearing cyst-like.

Hyperplastic hepatic nodules are benign reorganized masses of hepatic tissue that contain lipid, blood-filled sinusoids, lymphocytes, and areas of atrophied or necrotic hepatocytes. They have a variable appearance and can be hypoechoic, isoechoic, mixed, or hyperechoic.[22] In our experience, the nodules are most commonly hypoechoic. The nodules can be multiple and variably sized and may cause the margin of the liver to be lumpy or irregular. They are commonly mistaken for neoplasia and require a fine-needle aspirate or biopsy sample for confirmation. Var-

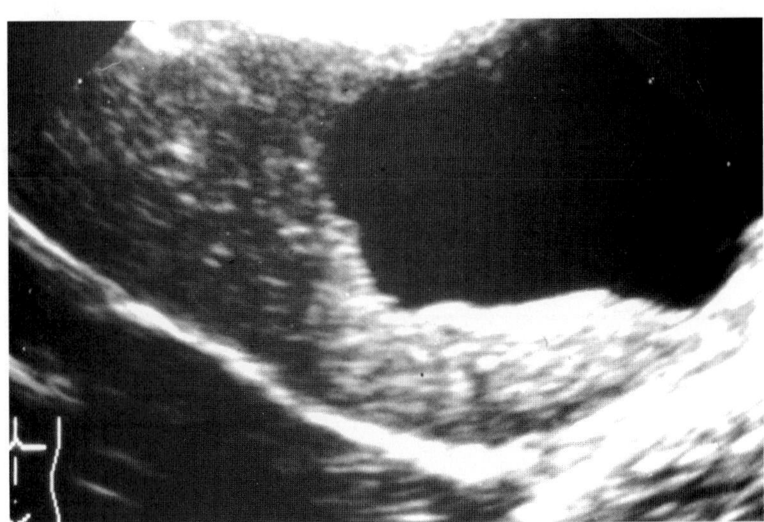

Figure 6-18. Biloma or hepatic pseudocyst. Bilomas may be irregularly circumscribed, as in this example, or very thin walled and round.

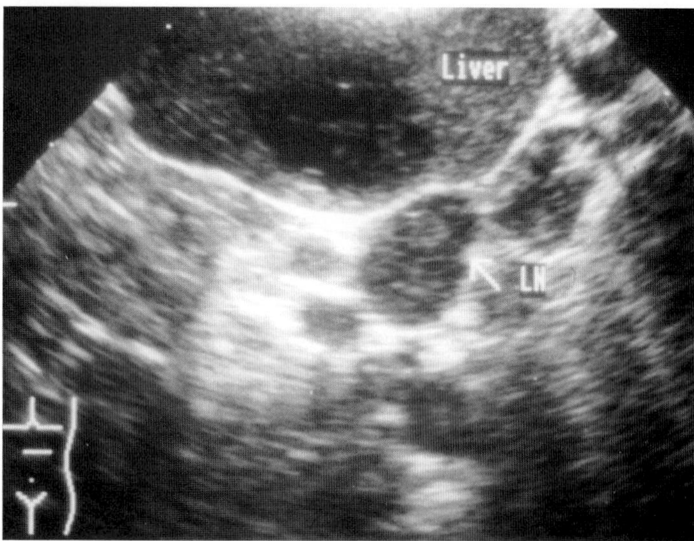

Figure 6-19. Hepatic abscess with perihepatic lymphadenopathy. The abscess appears as a poorly circumscribed hypoechoic liver mass. The well-circumscribed hypoechoic nodules surrounding the margin of the liver are enlarged hepatic lymph nodes.

ious sizes of hypoechoic nodules may also represent islands of extramedullary hematopoiesis in patients with chronic blood loss.

The ultrasound appearance of primary hepatic neoplasia varies greatly.[23] It may appear as a very large, moderately circumscribed, infiltrating mass that bulges beyond the normal liver margins with an echogenicity slightly more mixed than normal liver. It can also be a diffuse inhomogeneity with areas of mixed echogenicity (Fig. 6-20). Solitary or multiple focal lesions of altered echogenicity can also be seen. The ultrasonographic appearance of liver neoplasia is not characteristic for the histopathologic cell type because of the presence of edema, necrosis, fibrosis, neovascularization, hemorrhage, and inflammatory response elements (Fig. 6-21).

Metastatic neoplasia usually appears as solitary or multiple, circumscribed masses scattered throughout the hepatic parenchyma.[1–3,16,23] These nodules may be homogeneously hypoechoic or hyperechoic, or the lesion may appear as a target lesion with a hyperechoic center and hypoechoic outer rim (Fig. 6-22). When the nod-

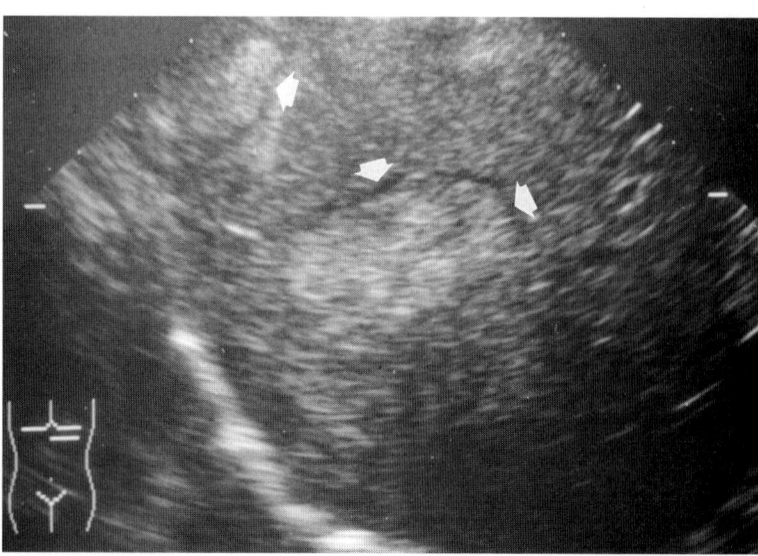

Figure 6-20. Primary hepatic neoplasia. The neoplasm appears as multifocal, poorly circumscribed areas of mixed echogenicity slightly more echogenic than the surrounding normal liver (*arrowheads*). The biopsy diagnosis was hepatocellular carcinoma.

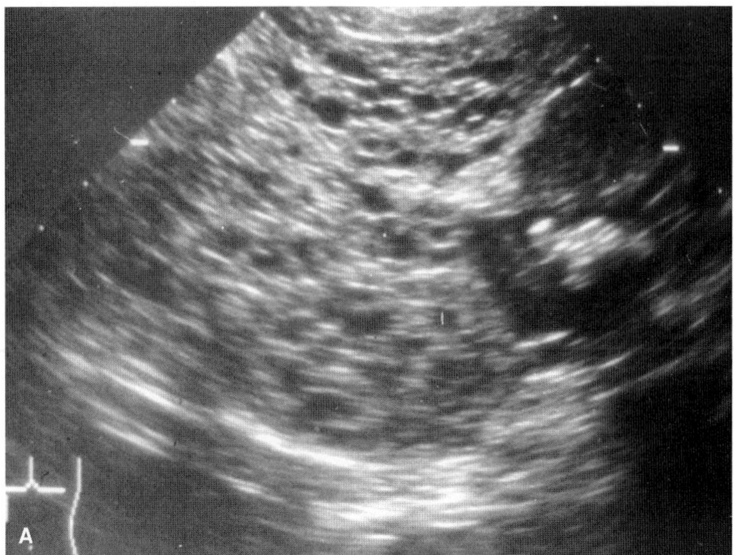

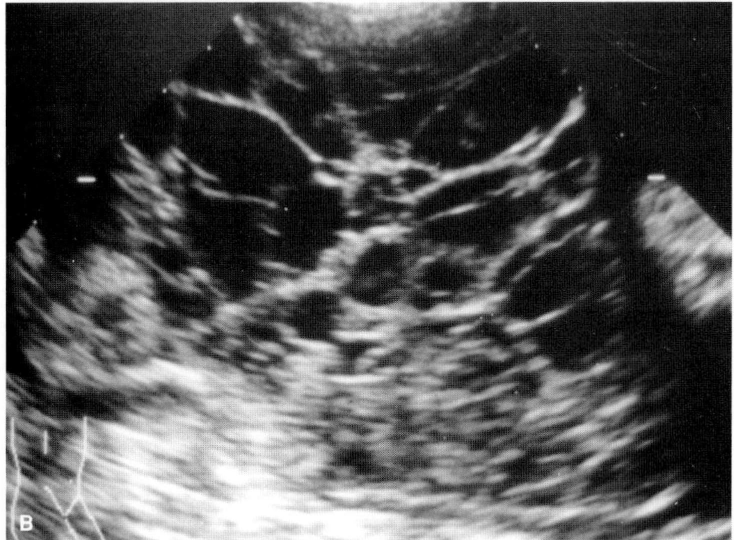

Figure 6-21. (**A**) Hepatic hemangiosarcoma. Multifocal anechoic masses throughout the hepatic parenchyma give the liver a moth-eaten appearance. (**B**) Hepatic hemangiosarcoma. Multiple anechoic cavitations throughout the liver represent various amounts of tumor, hematoma, and blood-filled cavitations.

ules are fairly isoechoic, they may be difficult to detect without careful examination with a high-frequency transducer. Diffuse secondary neoplastic infiltration may also cause an extensive inhomogeneity or mottled appearance to the liver. The ultrasonographic appearance is not characteristic of cell type, and fine-needle aspiration or biopsy is required for definitive diagnosis. However, a high index of suspicion because of the presence of a known primary neoplasm or diffuse abdominal neoplasia may decrease the clinical relevance of a biopsy.

Disease of the Gallbladder and Biliary Tract

Gallbladder disease is uncommon in dogs and cats.[24] The gallbladder appear distended or large in almost all patients that are ill enough to be anorexic. Gallbladder sludge or partial inspissation of bile is a common ultrasonographic finding. Sludge appears as a gravity-dependent, mobile layer of echogenic bile, which may indicate a mild degree of biliary stasis, but the patient usually is not symptomatic (Fig. 6-23).

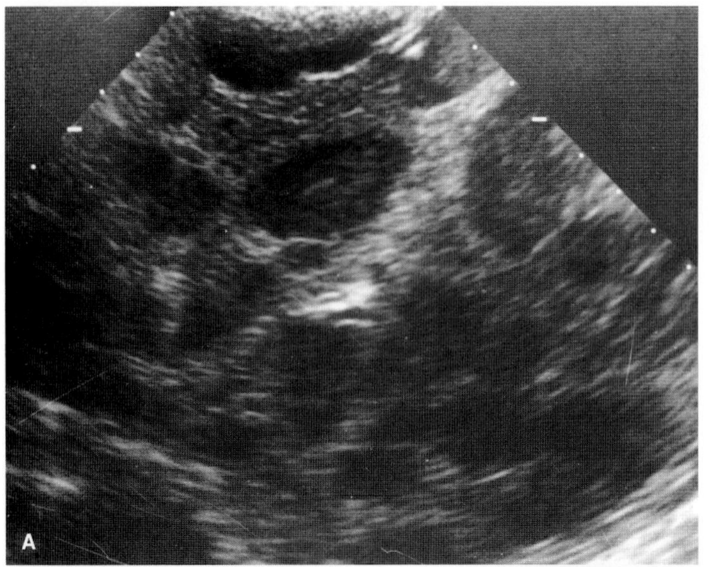

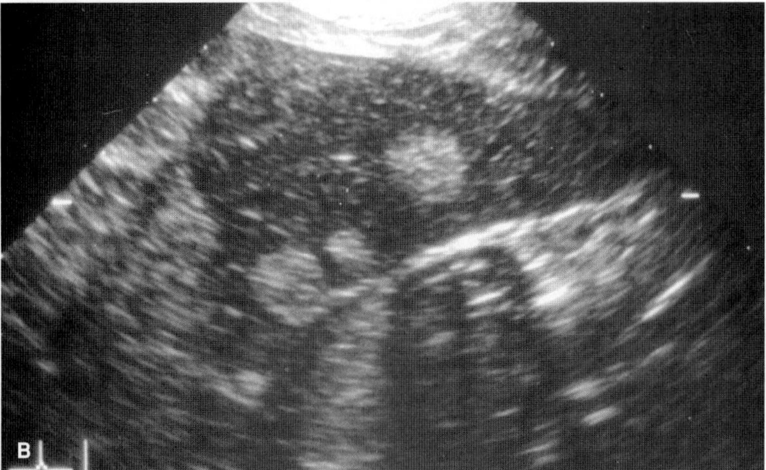

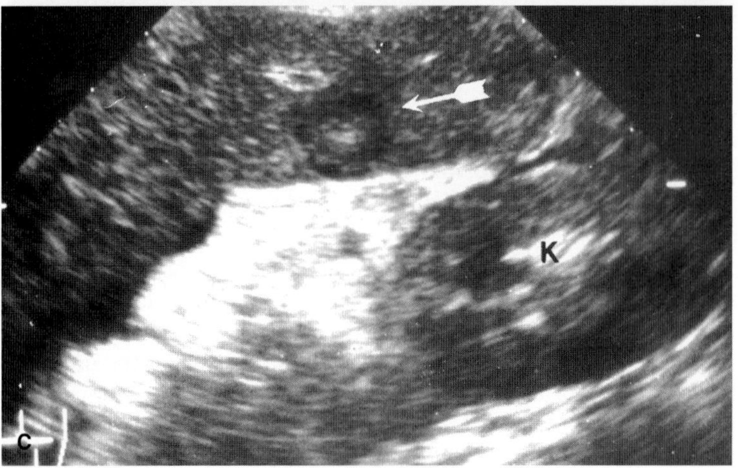

Figure 6-22. (**A**) Metastatic neoplasia in the liver. Metastatic nodules may appear as solitary or multifocal hypoechoic nodules, as in this poodle with metastatic fibrosarcoma. (**B**) Metastatic neoplasia in the liver. Metastatic nodules may appear as solitary or multifocal hyperechoic nodules, as in this Laborador retriever with metastatic renal cell carcinoma. (**C**) Metastatic neoplasia in the liver. Metastatic nodules may also appear as target (*white arrow*) lesions. Areas of hyperechogenicity may be surrounded by areas of hypoechogenicity, as in this Cairn terrier with metastatic pancreatic adenocarcinoma. *K*, kidney.

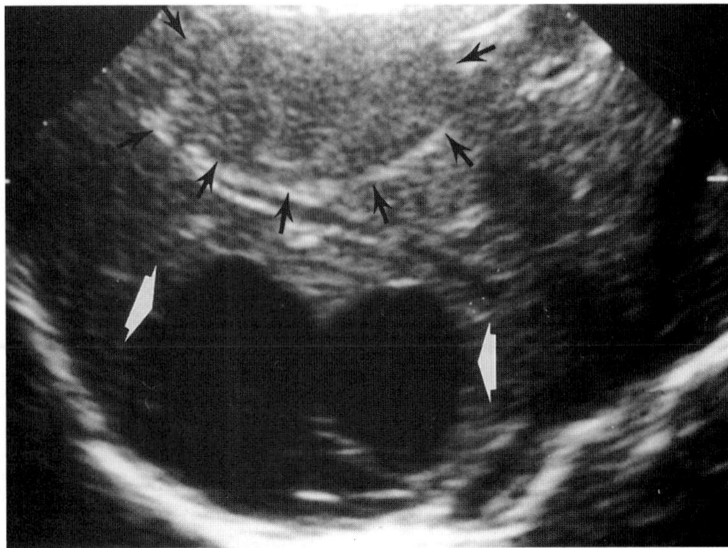

Figure 6-23. Hepatic cysts (*white arrowheads*) and a sludge-filled gallbladder (*black arrows*). The gallbladder is completely filled with echogenic sludge, which makes it appear as a hyperechoic pseudomass. The bilobed anechoic hepatic cysts could be mistaken for the gallbladder without careful sonographic examination.

The gallbladder wall is normally unseen or appears as a very thin border between the anechoic bile and the normal hepatic parenchyma. Generalized gallbladder wall thickening can be seen with cholecystitis, any form of peritoneal fluid, hypoproteinemia, hepatitis, and cholangiohepatitis (Fig. 6-24).[1–3] The thickened gallbladder wall may take on a layered appearance because of the visualization of the inner and outer wall with abdominal fluid or a peripheral margin of edema with inflammatory conditions (Fig. 6-25). Focal gallbladder wall thickening can be seen in cases of benign cystic hyperplasia or the mucus-producing glands and less commonly with adenomas or adenocarcinomas (Fig. 6-26).[1–3]

Cholelithiasis and choledocholithiasis are uncommon. Choleliths have not been associated with consistent clinical signs, and their significance is under investigation.[25] They appear as a

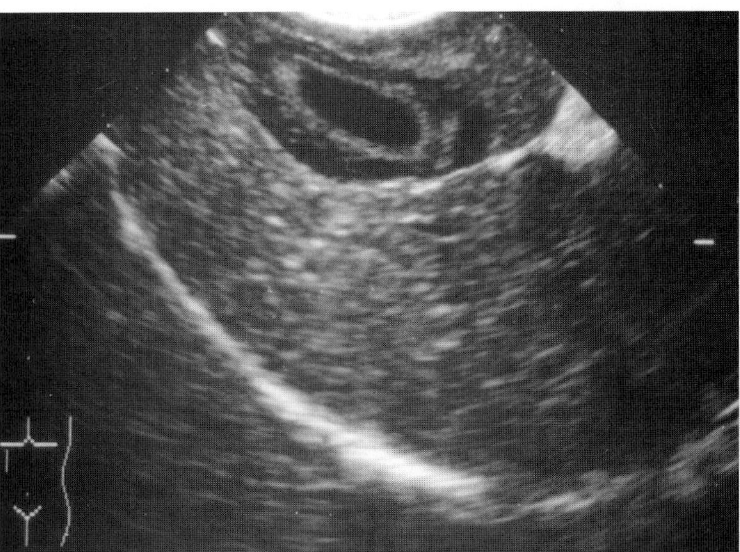

Figure 6-24. Acute cholecystitis. The gallbladder is contracted and has a thickened hyperechoic wall surrounded by a hypoechoic rim of edema.

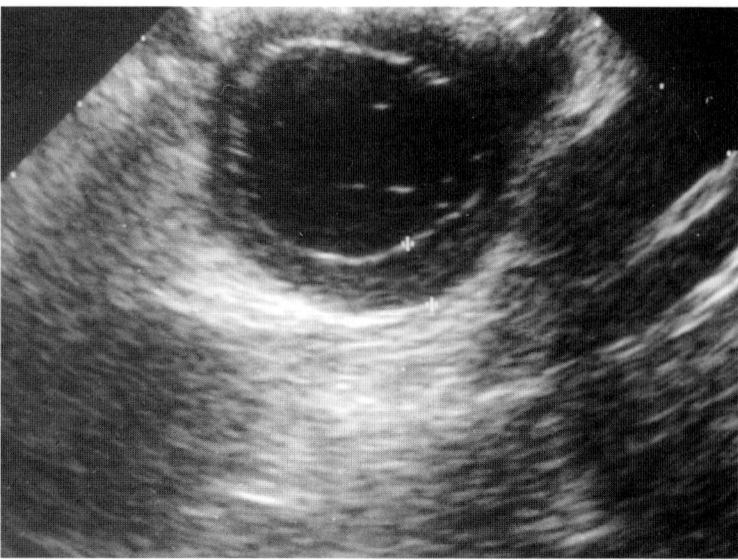

Figure 6-25. Pseudocholecystitis. The gallbladder is normal sized and has a thin hyperechoic wall surrounded by a thick hypoechoic rim of fluid or edema in this patient with ascites.

focal gravity-dependent hyperechoic foci within the gallbladder that produce posterior shadowing (Fig. 6-27). The amount of shadowing depends on the degree of mineralization, size of the calculus, and the transducer frequency. Placing the calculus within a high-frequency transducer focal zone increases the acoustic shadowing. Biliary sludge that contains no mineral or cholesterol choleliths usually does not cause acoustic shadowing. Choledocholithiasis (ie, biliary duct calculi) is more commonly associated with the clinical signs of obstruction or cholangitis.[24] They are hyperechoic foci within the bile ducts that may be difficult to see because of overlying bowel gas. Choledocholithiasis is more easily identified when they are surrounded by anechoic bile in a dilated obstructed duct.

Primary biliary tract disease generally falls into three categories: neoplasia, inflammation, and obstruction. Cholangiocellular carcinomas cannot be differentiated from other hepatic neoplasms.[16,23] They may appear as solitary or multiple hypoechoic masses scattered throughout the hepatic parenchyma (Fig. 6-28). Cholangitis

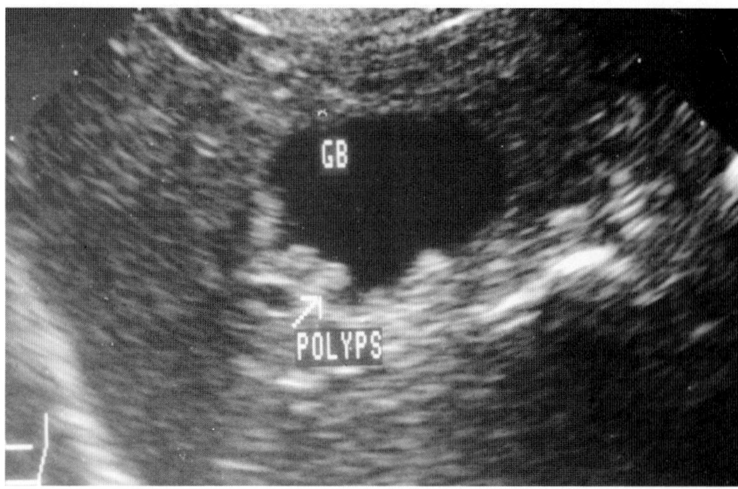

Figure 6-26. Benign cystic hyperplasia of the mucus-producing glands of the gallbladder. The benign hyperechoic polyps are an incidental finding in older patients but are impossible to differentiate from early gallbladder malignancy by ultrasound alone.

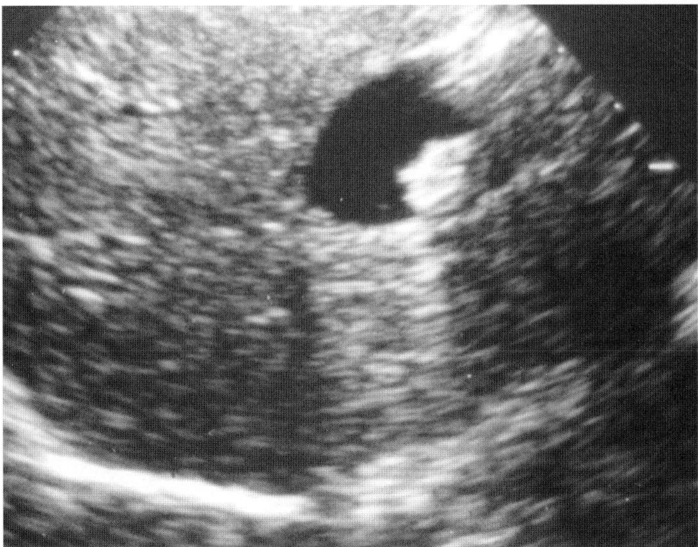

Figure 6-27. Large solitary hyperechoic cholelith within the gravity-dependent portion of a small, contracted gallbladder. Notice the lack of acoustic enhancement beneath the cholelith. This cholelith causes little shadowing distally.

or cholangiohepatitis has a variable appearance, including diffuse decreased hepatic echogenicity and diffuse inhomogeneity of hepatic echogenicity.

Ultrasound is the ideal imaging modality for differentiating hepatocellular disease from biliary obstruction in the icteric patient. Ultrasound-guided biopsy or fine-needle aspiration of the liver can diagnose hepatocellular disease. Samples are taken from any area of the liver with an altered sonographic appearance, or random samples are removed from a normal-appearing liver. A normal liver sonogram does not rule out diffuse liver disease.

Biliary obstruction in small animals may result from pancreatitis, cholelithiasis, lymphadenopathy, inflammation, neoplasia, granulomas, or abscesses of the pancreas, duodenum, liver, and adjacent areas. Extrahepatic biliary obstruction first appears as a distention of the gallbladder and a loss of the tapering of the gallbladder neck or cystic duct. This occurs experi-

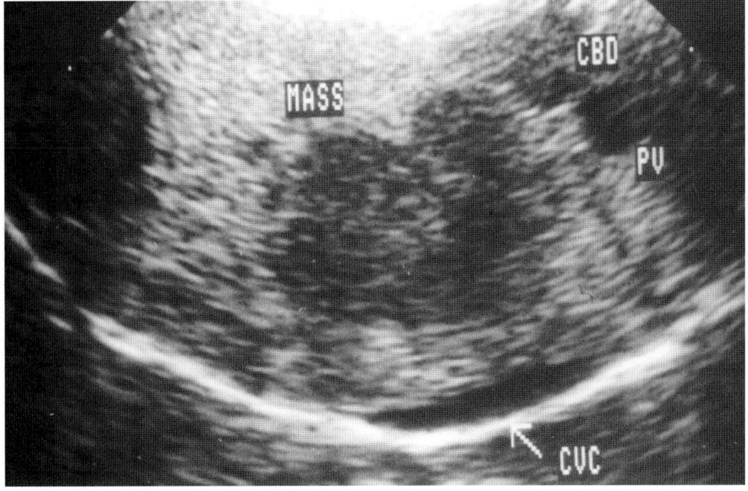

Figure 6-28. Cholangiocellular carcinoma in a Boston terrier. The liver is hyperechoic as a result of bile stasis and fibrosis. The tumor appears an irregularly circumscribed, hypoechoic mass within the hepatic parenchyma. Primary hepatic and biliary neoplasms cannot be differentiated based on the ultrasound appearance alone.

mentally in the dog 24 hours after ligation of the bile duct.[6,7] If the obstruction continues, there is rapid retrograde dilation of the biliary system, with enlargement of the duct at 48 hours, dilation of the extrahepatic ducts at 72 hours, and dilation of the intrahepatic ducts at 1 week (Fig. 6-29).[6] The dilated bile duct is a tubular, anechoic structure with acoustic enhancement just ventral to the portal vein (Fig. 6-30). Dilated extrahepatic bile ducts appear as numerous, tortuous, anechoic, tubular structures in the area of the porta hepatis between the gallbladder and the pancreas. Dilated intrahepatic ducts appear as tortuous, irregularly branching, anechoic, tubular structures with echogenic walls throughout the liver.[6]

After the biliary system has been dilated, it may remain enlarged despite the absence of continued obstruction. A study suggested the need to evaluate gallbladder dynamics to differentiate a dilated nonobstructed system from true obstruction.[26] This is done by measuring the gallbladder volume, slowly injecting intravenously 0.04 μg/kg of a synthetic cholecystokinin (Kinevac, E.R. Squibb and Sons, Inc., Princeton, NJ), and measuring the gallbladder volume 1 hour later.[26] In a nonobstructed patient, the gallbladder volume should decrease by approximately 40%. In dogs with biliary obstruction, the gallbladder emptied less than 20% 1 hour after injection.

Another technique that aids in the diagnosis of biliary obstruction is the transhepatic cholecystogram.[27] This is performed with ionic or nonionic iodinated contrast, the same contrast the veterinarian would use intravenously for excretory urography. A 22-gauge 3.5-in (9-cm) spinal needle is placed with ultrasound guidance through the liver into the gallbladder (Fig. 6-31). Approximately 25% of the bile in the gallbladder is withdrawn and replaced with an equal volume of contrast medium. Radiographs of the cranial portion of the abdomen are taken at 5 minutes, 45 minutes, and 2 hours after injection. The normal cholecystogram outlines the gallbladder, cystic duct, and bile duct, and on later films, contrast is seen in the duodenum or jejunum. With complete extrahepatic biliary obstruction, contrast cannot enter the small intestine, and the site of biliary obstruction usually is identifiable (Fig. 6-32).

Abnormalities of the Hepatic Vasculature

Four categories of hepatic vasculature disease are described for small animal patients: hepatic venous congestion, portal hypertension, portosystemic shunts, and arteriovenous malformations. Central hepatic venous congestion is recognized as an enlarged hypoechoic liver with

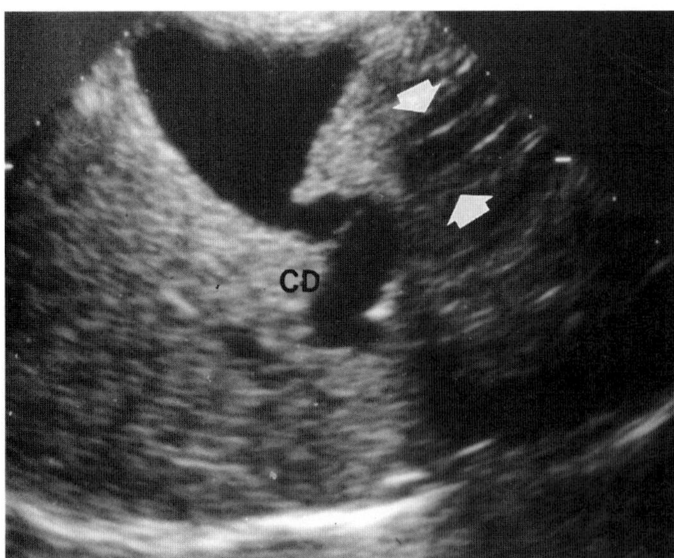

Figure 6-29. Dilated cystic duct (*CD*) and intrahepatic bile ducts (*white arrowheads*) in a terrier mix. The bile duct was partially obstructed at the level of the duodenal papilla by fibrosis from chronic recurrent pancreatitis.

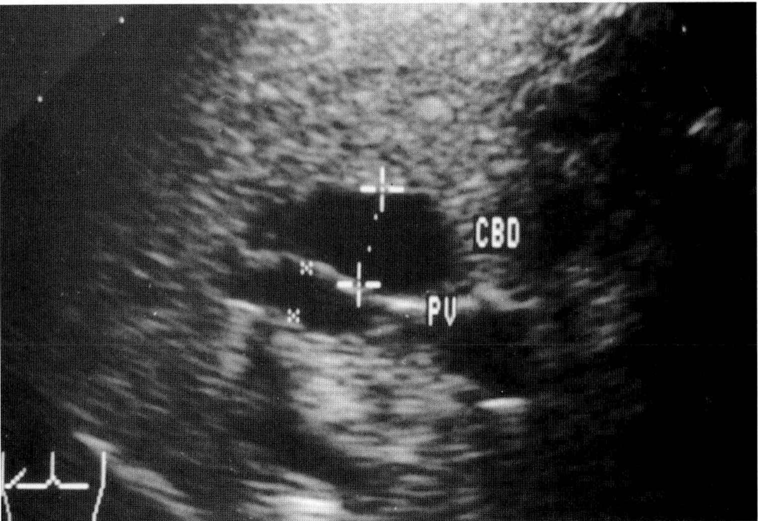

Figure 6-30. Longitudinal view of a dilated bile duct (*CBD*) just ventral (closer to the transducer) to the portal vein (*PV*) in a patient with extrahepatic biliary obstruction causing jaundice. This area may be easiest to image from the caudal right intercostal approach.

enlarged hepatic veins joining the caudal vena cava at the level of the diaphragm.[1–3,28,29] This is most easily seen with the transducer placed subcostally on the midventral abdomen in a transverse plane (Fig. 6-33). Hepatic venous congestion is most commonly caused by right heart failure, but it is seen with any obstruction to caudal vena cava flow or increased central venous pressure.

Portal hypertension is difficult to diagnose with standard ultrasonographic imaging. The main portal and extrahepatic portal veins may have an enlarged diameter, but this is not a consistent finding. The presence of multiple portosystemic collateral vessels, ascites, splenomegaly, and an abnormal liver ultrasound is highly suggestive of portal hypertension. Portal hypertension is best diagnosed with duplex Doppler ultrasound.[30,31] Doppler ultrasound can measure portal blood flow volume and velocities. Portal hypertensive patients generally have reduced velocity and flow.[30] Newer ultrasound machines have Doppler capabilities, but the cost may be prohibitive except in very large practices.

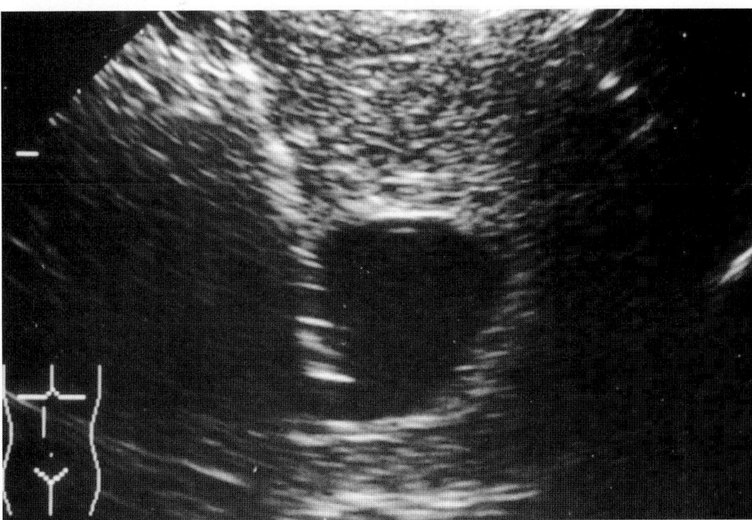

Figure 6-31. Needle passing into the gallbladder using ultrasound guidance for a transhepatic cholecystogram. Approximately 25% of the gallbladder volume is removed and replaced with an equal volume of iodinated contrast medium.

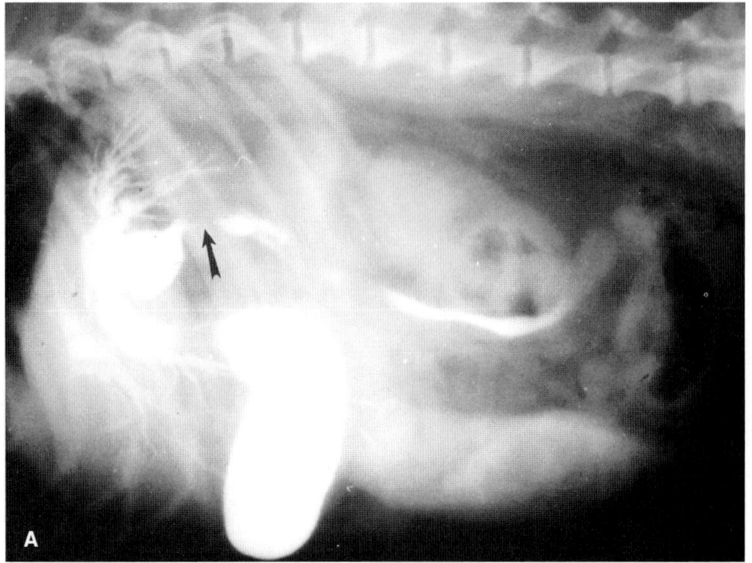

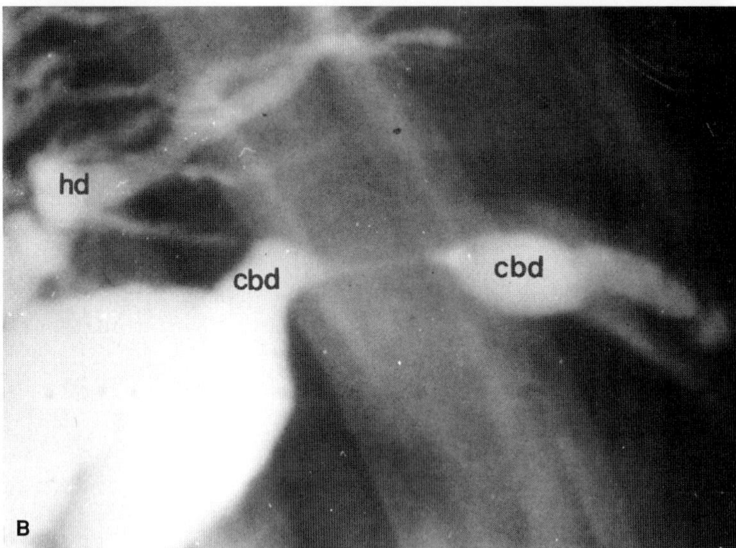

Figure 6-32. (**A**) Transhepatic cholecystogram of a dog with partial extrahepatic biliary obstruction secondary to fibrosis around the common bile duct from chronic recurrent pancreatitis. Notice the dilated gallbladder, contrast medium filling the dilated intrahepatic bile ducts, and the stricture (*black arrow*) of the bile duct just proximal to its entrance into the duodenum, which also contains a small volume of contrast. (**B**) Close-up of the stricture of the same bile duct. *CBD*, dilated bile duct; *HD*, dilated intrahepatic bile ducts. The hepatic ultrasound of this patient is shown in Figure 6-29.

Portosystemic shunts may be intrahepatic or extrahepatic, congenital or acquired, and single or multiple.[32,33] A gross clinical simplification is that young, small-breed dogs most commonly have congenital, single, extrahepatic shunts; young large-breed dogs have congenital, single, intrahepatic shunts; and adult dogs more likely have multiple, acquired, extrahepatic shunts. The ultrasonographic findings associated with portosystemic shunting include a small liver, decreased size and number of vascular structures within the liver, and an abnormal connection between the portal vein and the systemic venous circulation.[13,29,34–36] Other findings may include an increased diameter of the caudal vena cava, a decreased diameter of the portal vein, and splenomegaly.

Portosystemic shunts may be identified ultrasonographically in about 40% of affected patients.[36] Intrahepatic shunts are best identified by scanning transversely from the right intercostal space. The caudal vena cava and portal vein should be imaged from the midabdomen through the porta hepatis to the diaphragm. In-

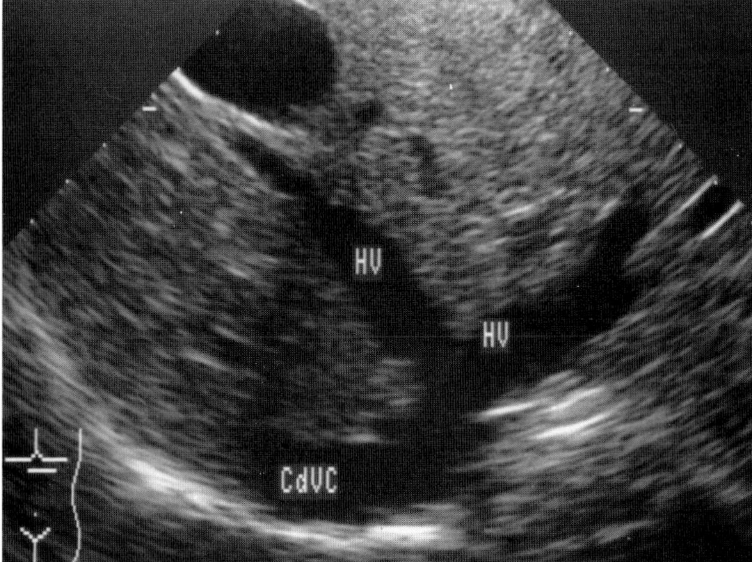

Figure 6-33. Hepatic venous congestion secondary to right heart failure. The liver is hypoechoic, and the hepatic veins (*HV*) are dilated as they enter a dilated caudal vena cava (*CdVC*). (From Biller DS, Kantrowitz B, Miyabayashi T. Ultrasonography of diffuse liver disease. J Vet Intern Med 1992;6:71.)

trahepatic shunt vessels often appear as large, mildly tortuous, anechoic, tubular structures connecting the portal vein to a large hepatic vein or the caudal vena cava (Fig. 6-34).[36,37] These vessels often run dorsally from the portal vein within the hepatic parenchyma. The connection may be difficult to identify distinctly because of its tortuosity, and because of the cranial displacement of the small liver under the lungs. General anesthesia and positive-pressure ventilation may assist identification of intrahepatic shunts by pushing the diaphragm caudally and increasing the central venous pressure.[36,37]

Extrahepatic shunts are more difficult to confirm with ultrasound because of the various locations of the vascular connections and overlying bowel gas. Extrahepatic shunts may appear as an abnormal, large branch off the portal vein connecting most commonly to the colic vein, splenic vein, caudal vena cava, renal vein, or azygous vein (Fig. 6-35). The cranial extension of the portal vein generally decreases in di-

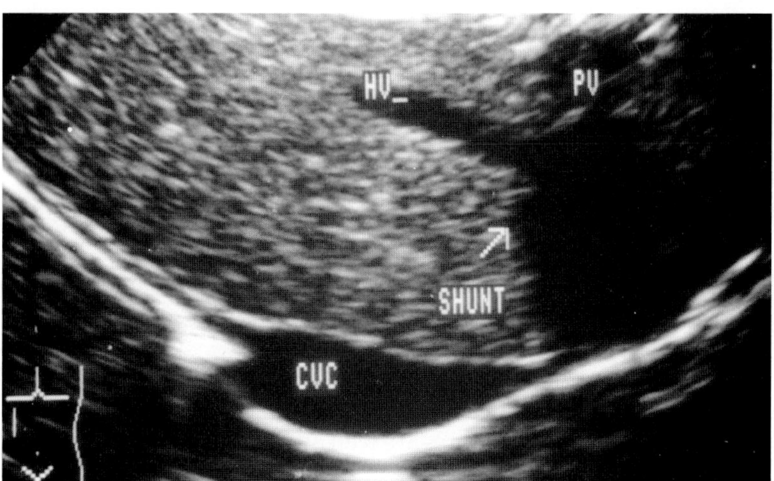

Figure 6-34. Intrahepatic portocaval shunt. The shunt is a large, anechoic, tubular structure connecting an intrahepatic portal vein to the caudal vena cava.

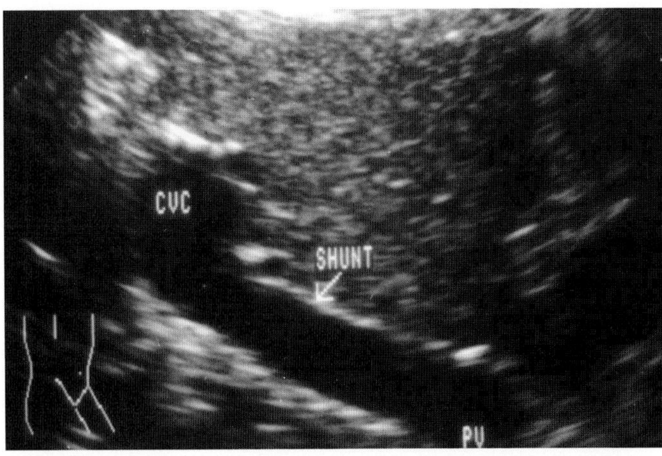

Figure 6-35. Extrahepatic portocaval shunt. The shunt is located just caudal to the liver and is visualized as a large anechoic vessel connecting the prehepatic portal vein (*PV*) to the caudal vena cava (*CVC*).

ameter, and the caudal vena cava may increase in size after the shunt vessel anastomosis. Multiple extrahepatic shunts often appear as a collection of tortuous vessels in the vicinity of the kidney or spleen. If a portosystemic shunt is suspected clinically and not identified ultrasonographically, a splenoportogram, cranial mesenteric arteriogram, or operative mesenteric portogram should be performed for diagnosis.

Hepatic arteriovenous malformations appear as tortuous, tubular, anechoic structures within or closely adjacent to the liver.[38] Specular reflections associated with flowing blood can often be seen within the dilated veins of the malformation. Ascites is often concurrently present, unlike cases of portosystemic shunts, which rarely have ascites. Arteriovenous malformations can be differentiated from dilated biliary structures because of the visualized flow, absence of acoustic enhancement, and the fact that they are often restricted to only one lobe of the liver.[38] Duplex Doppler can be used to confirm direction and velocity of flow within the abnormal vessels. Confirmation before surgical removal of the liver lobe may require a celiac arteriogram.

LIVER BIOPSY

Sampling of tissue with fine-needle aspiration or biopsy is the single most important diagnostic tool for liver disease. Standard ultrasound-guided or -directed procedures are well adapted to liver sampling.[39–41] Assessment of the packed cell volume and an activated clotting time, bleeding time, or prothrombin time and partial thromboplastin time are performed before biopsy. Core biopsies are performed with a 16- or 18-gauge Tru-Cut–type needle and are generally sufficient for diagnosis. The surgeon should take an additional core for culture if inflammatory disease is suspected. Fine-needle aspiration with a 22-gauge needle for cytology may also be diagnostic if someone in the practice or area has hepatic cytology experience.

In cases of diffuse liver disease, the left lateral liver lobe is most commonly biopsied. The needle is inserted subcostally in the cranial portion of the left abdomen and directed dorsally, cranially, and laterally. The biopsy path is chosen to avoid the fundus of the stomach and major liver vessels. If the stomach is grossly distended, the right lateral liver lobe can be sampled in a similar manner using ultrasound to avoid the gallbladder and major vasculature. Very small livers may require a lateral intercostal approach. Care should be taken to place the needle during expiration to avoid the pleural space.

In focal liver disease, ultrasound guidance for tissue sampling is unsurpassed. The lesion is approached by whatever angle is necessary to avoid critical structures. The needle is then observed to pass directly into the area of abnormality, preventing misdiagnosis from faulty sampling. Lesions as small as 2 to 3 mm can be sampled, depending on the machine's resolution. Complications from ultrasound liver biopsies are few.[42] Repeating ultrasound examinations 1 and 4 hours after the biopsy usually identifies any significant hemorrhage that may require clinical intervention.

REFERENCES

1. Nyland TG, Hager DA. Sonography of the liver, gallbladder and spleen. Vet Clin North Am 1985;15:1123.
2. Nyland TG, Hager DA, Herring DS. Sonography of the liver, gallbladder, and spleen. Semin Vet Med Surg 1989; 4:13.
3. Nyland TG, Park RD. Hepatic ultrasonography in the dog. Vet Radiology, 1983;24:74.
4. Herring DS. Physics, facts and artifacts of diagnostic ultrasound. Vet Clin North Am 1985;15:1107.
5. Carlisle CH, Wu JX, Heath TORE. The ultrasonic anatomy of the hepatic and portal veins of the canine liver. Vet Radiol 1991;32:170.
6. Nyland TG, Tore NA. Sonographic evaluation of experimental bile duct ligation in the dog. Vet Radiol 1982;23:252.
7. Zeman RK, Taylor KJW, Rosenfield AT, et al. Acute experimental biliary obstruction in the dog: sonographic findings and clinical implications. Am J Roentgenol 1981;136:965.
8. Park RD, Nyland TG, Lattimer JC, et al. B-mode gray-scale ultrasound: imaging artifacts and interpretation principles. Vet Radiol 1981;22:204.
9. Moentk J, Biller DS. Bilobed gallbladder in a cat; ultrasonographic appearance. Vet Radiol 1993:34:354.
10. Barr F. Normal hepatic measurements in the mature dog. J Small Anim Pract 1992; 33:367.
11. Barr F. Ultrasonographic assessment of the liver size in the dog. J Small Anim Pract 1992;33:359.
12. Godshalk CP, Badertscher RR, Rippy MK, Ghent AW. Quantitative ultrasonic assessment of liver size in the dog. Vet Radiol 1988;29:162.
13. Biller DS. Kantrowitz B, Miyabayashi T. Ultrasonography of diffuse liver disease: A review. J Vet Intern Med 1992;6:71.
14. Yeager AE, Mohammed H. Accuracy of ultrasonography in the detection of severe hepatic lipidosis in cats. Am J Vet Res 1992;53:597.
15. Center BA. Hepatic lipidosis. In: August J, ed. Consultations in feline internal medicine. Philadelphia: WB Saunders, 1991:451.
16. Feeney DA, Johnston GR, Hardy RM. Two-dimensional, gray-scale ultrasonography for assessment of hepatic and splenic neoplasia in the dog and cat. J Am Vet Med Assoc 1984;184:68.
17. Lamb CR, Hartzband LE, Tidwell AS, Pearson SH. Ultrasonographic findings in hepatic and splenic lymphosarcoma in dogs and cats. Vet Radiol 1991; 32:117.
18. Nyland TG. Ultrasonic patterns of canine hepatic lymphosarcoma. Vet Radiol 1984; 25:167.
19. Cartee RE. Diagnostic real time ultrasonography of the liver and the dog and cat. J Am Anim Hosp Assoc 1981;17: 731.
20. Berry CR, Ackerman N, Charach M, Lawrence D. Iatrogenic biloma (biliary pseudocyst) in a cat with hepatic lipidosis. Vet Radiol 1992;33:145.
21. Konde LJ, Lebel JL, Park RD. Sonographic application in the diagnosis of intra-abdominal abscesses in the dog. Vet Radiol 1986;27:151.
22. Stowater CR, Lamb CH, Schelling SH. Ultrasonographic features of canine nodular hyperplasia. Vet Radiol 1990; 32:268.
23. Whiteley MB, Feeney DA, Whiteley LO. Ultrasonographic appearance of primary and metastatic canine hepatic tumors: a review of 48 cases. J Ultrasound Med 1989;8:621.
24. Hagar DA. Diseases of the gallbladder and extrahepatic biliary system. In: Ettinger SJ, ed. Textbook of veterinary internal medicine, 3rd ed. Philadelphia: WB Saunders, 1989:1555.

25. Schall WD, Chapman WL, Finco DR, et al. Cholelithiasis in dogs. J Am Vet Med Assoc 1973;163:469.
26. Finn ST, Park RD, Twedt DC, Curtis CR. Ultrasonographic assessment of sincalide-induced canine gallbladder emptying; an aid to the diagnosis of biliary obstruction. Vet Radiol 1991;32:269.
27. Wrigley RH. Radiographic and ultrasonographic diagnosis of liver disease in dogs and cats. Vet Clin North Am 1985; 15:21.
28. Lamb CR. Abdominal ultrasonography in small animals: examination of the liver, spleen and pancreas. J Small Anim Pract 1990;31:5.
29. Lamb CR. Ultrasonography of the liver and biliary tract. Probl Vet Med 1991; 3:555.
30. Kantrowitz BM, Nyland TG, Fisher R. Estimation of portal blood flow using duplex real-time and pulsed doppler ultrasound imaging in the dog. Vet Radiol 1989;30:222.
31. Nyland TG, Fisher PE. Evaluation of experimentally induced canine hepatic cirrhosis using duplex doppler ultrasound. Vet Radiol 1990;31:189.
32. Vulgamott JC. Portosystemic shunts. Vet Clin North Am 1985;15:229.
33. Johnson CA, Armstrong PJ, Hauptman JG. Congenital portosystemic shunts in dogs: 46 cases (1979–1986). J Am Vet Med Assoc 1987;191:1478.
34. Moon ML. Diagnostic imaging of portosystemic shunts. Semin Vet Med Surg (Small Anim) 1990;5:120.
35. Saunders HM, Pugh CR, Rhodes RM. Expanding applications of abdominal ultrasonography. J Am Anim Hosp Assoc 1992;28:369.
36. Wrigley RH, Knode LJ, Park RD, Lebel JL. Ultrasonographic diagnosis of portocaval shunts in young dogs. J Am Vet Assoc 1987;191:421.
37. Wrigley RH, Macy DW, Wykes PM. Ligation of a ductus venous in a dog using ultrasonographic guidance. J Am Vet Med Assoc 1983;183:1461.
38. Bailey MQ, WIllard MD, McLoughlin MA, et al. Ultrasonographic findings associated with congenital hepatic arteriovenous fistula in three dogs. J Am Vet Med Assoc 1988;192:1009.
39. Hager DA, Nyland TG, Fisher R. Ultrasound-guided biopsy of the canine liver, kidney and prostate. Vet Radiol 1984; 26:82.
40. Hoppe FE, Hager DA, Poulos PW, et al. A comparison of manual and automatic ultrasound guided biopsy techniques. Vet Radiol 1986;27:99.
41. Selcer B, Cornelius LM. Percutaneous liver biopsy using the ultrasound guided biopsy instrument. Vet Med Rep 1989; 1:412.
42. Leveille R, Partington BP, Biller DS, Miyabayashi T. Complications after ultrasound guided biopsy of abdominal structures in dogs and cats (246 cases). J Am Vet Med Assoc 1988;203:413.

Small Animal Ultrasound, edited by Ronald W. Green.
Lippincott-Raven Publishers, Philadelphia © 1996.

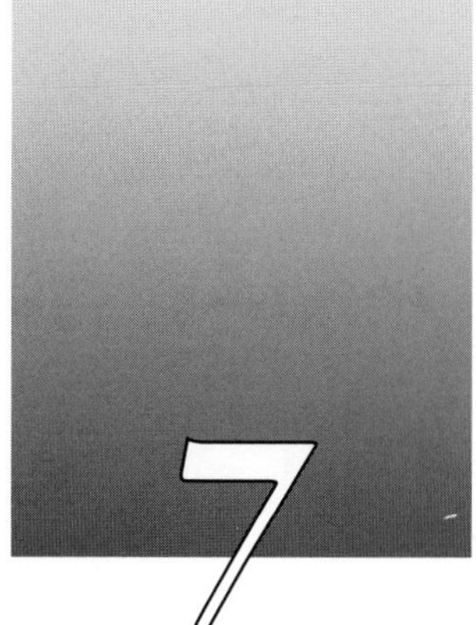

SPLEEN

Beth Paugh Partington and David S. Biller

The spleen should be scanned thoroughly during every abdominal ultrasound examination. Specific indicators for splenic examination include any abdominal mass, splenomegaly, hemoperitoneum, abdominal trauma, anemia, hypotension, and suspected metastasis. Regardless of the clinical indication for abdominal ultrasound, the entire abdomen always should be evaluated.

SCANNING TECHNIQUES FOR SPLENIC ULTRASOUND

The hair on the abdomen should be carefully clipped ventrally and along the left side, from the costal arch to the pubis. In large, deep-chested breeds, the spleen may lie beneath the ribs, which extends the area to be clipped to include the last few intercostal spaces on the left. The animal is scanned in dorsal recumbency or right lateral recumbency on a padded table or a padded V-trough table, which may be more comfortable. The patient is restrained manually as for other abdominal ultrasound examinations. Tranquilization is rarely required for abdominal ultrasound and is discouraged for splenic ultrasound, because acetylpromazine and barbiturates relax the splenic smooth muscle, resulting in red pulp congestion and splenomegaly.[1]

Coupling gel is applied to displace air, which may act as an ultrasonographic barrier. The spleen is examined in longitudinal and transverse planes by passing the transducer over the ventral abdomen from the left cranial portion of the abdomen to the pubis and along the left lateral aspect of the abdomen.

The transducer is angled dorsally and to the left from the ventral approach and toward the center of the abdomen from the left lateral approach.

The head of the spleen is attached to the greater curvature of the stomach by the gastrosplenic ligament. The body and tail of the spleen are mobile and may be found along the left lateral abdomen, left ventral abdomen, or central ventral abdomen, or the body of the spleen may cross the central abdomen, with the tail found in the right ventral abdomen. If the animal is imaged in right lateral recumbency, the spleen may pass dorsoventrally across the left abdominal wall from the last two intercostal spaces to an area just caudal to the rib cage.[2] The spleen usually lies superficial to the fundus of the stomach cranially, the small intestine centrally, and the left kidney caudally. Its superficial location enables complete ultrasound examination without the sonographic barrier of bowel gas.

Because of its proximity to the body wall, it is important to adjust the near-gain and scanning depth for maximum near-field visualization.[3,4]

A 7.5-MHz transducer is used in cats and dogs weighing less than 20 pounds. A 5.0-MHz transducer is preferred for larger dogs.[5,6] In-line sector scanners with a small footprint are ideal, but linear-array transducers can image the spleen in patients heavier than 20 pounds. The near-field bright band artifact that occurs at the transducer-skin interface with mechanical sector scanners may preclude visualization of the superficial portion of the spleen. In the cat, this is especially important, because the feline spleen is very thin. Using an ultrasound standoff pad or angling the transducer almost horizontally from the central abdomen to the left ventral abdominal wall may increase the superficial image quality.

ULTRASOUND ANATOMY OF THE SPLEEN

Approaches and Anatomic Landmarks

The spleen is attached to the greater omentum along the concave visceral surface or hilus. When the animal is in dorsal recumbency, the visceral surface of the spleen usually faces the midline. The parietal surface is smooth and convex and typically faces the left lateral body wall. The splenic artery and vein join the spleen along the hilar border at the proximal third of its length. The splenic artery arises from a branch of the celiac artery and forms a variable vascular ramus along the hilar margin. The splenic arteries usually are not seen, but when visualized, they have a small diameter and an echogenic wall.[2] Splenic veins do not have an echogenic wall, are of larger diameter than splenic arteries, and are commonly recognized as a Y-shaped vascular confluence at the splenic hilus (Fig. 7-1). Larger splenic veins can be identified as tubular, anechoic structures imaged within the splenic parenchyma.[2] The splenic vein empties the splenic venous return into the liver through the portal vein.

The splenic parenchyma has a uniformly mottled echogenicity, with a finer, more dense echotexture than falciform fat or liver (Fig. 7-2). The spleen should be more echogenic than the renal cortex or liver, but it is less echogenic than the fat in the renal sinus. The examiner should be able to image the left kidney and part of the spleen at the same time (Fig. 7-3). This maneuver allows comparison of splenic and renal cortical echogenicities at the same control settings. In some patients, the left lateral liver lobe and spleen can be imaged in the same scan. This allows comparison of the splenic and hepatic echogenicities at the same depth and control settings (see Fig. 6-1). When the splenic echogenicity is similar to the liver or the renal cortex, the spleen can be considered hypoechoic; this assumption is based on a known normal liver and kidney.

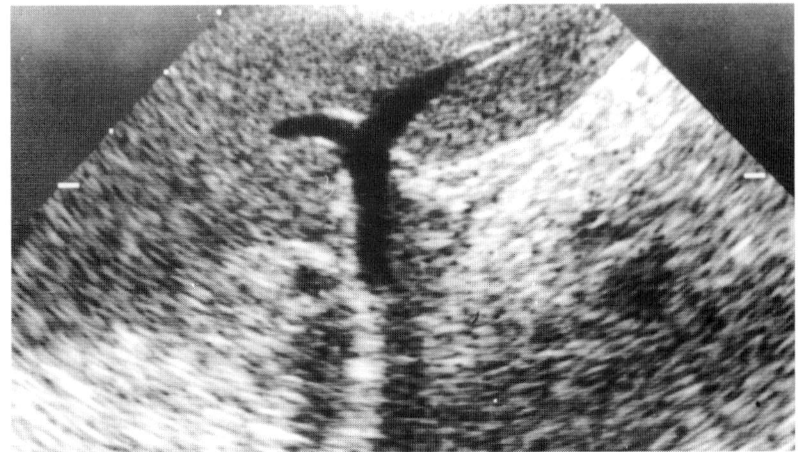

Figure 7-1. Y-shaped splenic venous hilus along the visceral surface of a normal canine spleen. The parallel echogenic lines extending beyond the caudal vein branch are echogenic artery walls on the edge of the ultrasound beam slice.

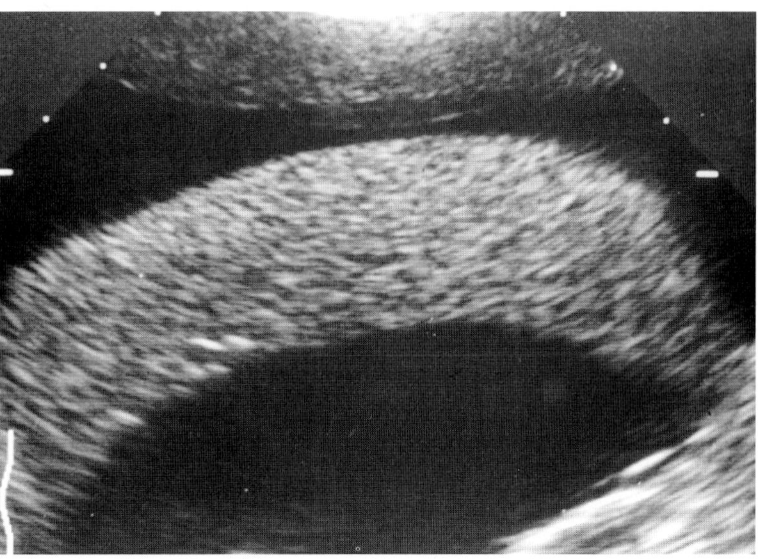

Figure 7-2. Normal canine spleen floating in ascitic fluid. Notice the fine splenic echotexture devoid of frequent large vascular markings, as is seen in the normal liver.

The splenic capsule is identified as the thin, well-defined echogenic margin surrounding the organ. A focal hyperechoic region surrounding the splenic vessels as they enter the body of the spleen may be present in some patients. This is a normal variant and should not be misinterpreted as pathology. This hyperechoic perivascular region is caused by capsular invagination of fibrous connective tissue and fat from the hilus (Fig. 7-4). The tail of the spleen may fold inward on itself, mimicking a mass or nodular enlargement. Careful ultrasound examination in two planes can identify the splenic capsule surrounding the folded spleen (Fig. 7-5).

Splenic Size

Ultrasound assessment of splenic size remains largely subjective.[4,7] Small, contracted spleens may exist in patients with acute blood loss or hypotension. Small spleens are very thin and difficult to identify because they often lie within the near-field artifact. Use of a standoff pad and

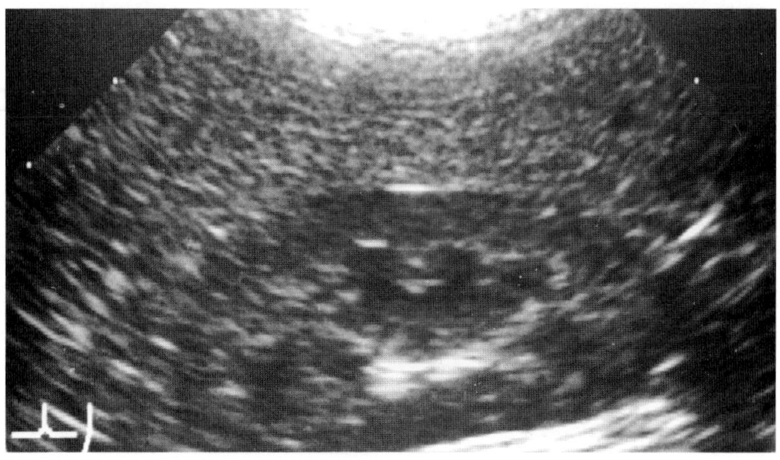

Figure 7-3. Longitudinal view of the left kidney completely shrouded by a normal canine spleen. The normal splenic echogenicity is greater than the normal renal cortex. The outer parietal surface of the spleen is within the near-field artifact.

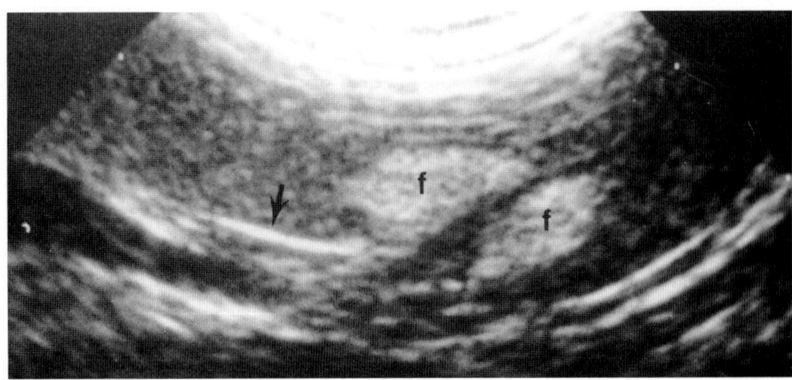

Figure 7-4. Thin normal spleen with echogenic perivascular capsular invaginations (*f*) surrounding an anechoic splenic hilar vessel. The splenic capsule (*arrow*) is seen as the thin hyperechoic band surrounding the spleen.

maximizing the near-field resolution may help in imaging small organs. As the spleen enlarges, it becomes thicker, wider, longer, and easier to image. As it thickens, it occupies the near and middle field of the ultrasound image and pushes the left kidney farther into the dorsal midabdomen. Very large spleens may fold on themselves, extend into the pelvic inlet, and appear to cover the entire ventral abdomen.[7]

Ultrasound assessment of splenic size should be carefully correlated with abdominal radiographs and abdominal palpation. The spleen is a dynamic, mobile organ, and its size and position may change fairly rapidly.

The Abnormal Spleen

The spleen is the largest component of the reticuloendothelial system in the body of the dog and cat.[1,8] The white pulp traps bacteria and other blood-borne antigens, which results in immunologic recognition and subsequent antibody production. The red pulp acts as a filter to clear damaged or aged erythrocytes, and in the dog, it is responsible for the removal of erythrocyte inclusions such as Heinz and Howell-Jolly bodies. The spleen also functions as a storage site for as much as 10% of the red cell volume and contains pluripotential stem cells for extramedullary hematopoiesis.[1,8] Because of its multiple func-

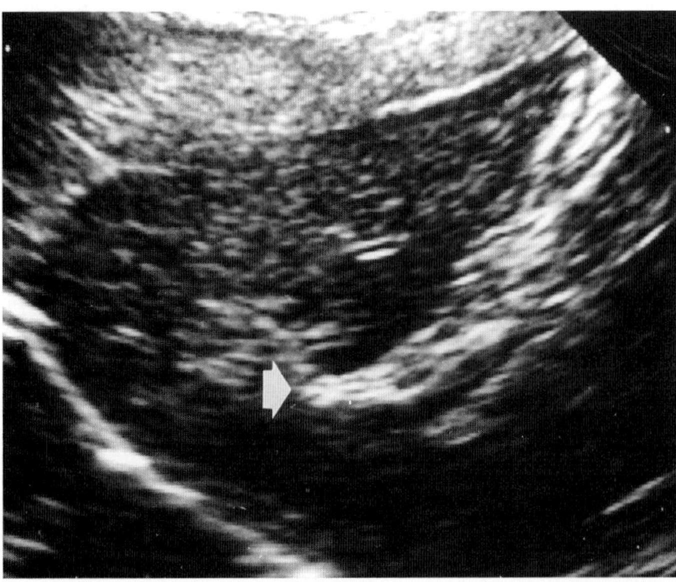

Figure 7-5. Splenomegaly due to acetylpromazine tranquilization. Notice that the enlarged hypoechoic spleen is folded on itself. The splenic capsule appears twice as thick at the folded junction (*arrowhead*).

tions, the spleen may be involved in a variety of vascular, infectious, neoplastic, and immunologic processes.[7] Ultrasound is the ideal method for imaging the abnormal spleen.[9,10]

ULTRASOUND APPEARANCE OF ABNORMALITIES AND DISEASE STATES

Diffuse Splenic Disease

Diffuse splenic disease characteristically presents as a uniformly enlarged spleen with normal or decreased echogenicity and a normal or inhomogeneous echotexture. The degree of splenomegaly varies with the disease condition. Diffuse splenic disease can be categorized as infiltrative splenomegaly, congestive splenomegaly, hyperplasia of the reticuloendothelial system, and secondary to infectious or inflammatory conditions.[8] Fine-needle aspiration of the spleen for cytologic analysis and biopsy for histopathologic examination are the most important tests for the diagnosis of diffuse splenic disease.[11–13]

Infiltrative Splenic Disease

Infiltrative splenomegaly includes acute and chronic myeloid and lymphoid leukemias, extramedullary hematopoiesis, amyloidosis, multiple myeloma, systemic mast cell disease, malignant histiocytosis, lymphosarcoma, and other metastatic neoplasms.[8] Although these diseases are presented as diffuse conditions, focal nodules can also be present with most infiltrative disease processes.

Splenic lymphosarcoma has three common ultrasound presentations. The first is an enlarged, slightly irregularly marginated spleen with a hypoechoic, moth-eaten, inhomogeneous echo pattern (Fig. 7-6).[14–17] The second appearance is of multiple, poorly marginated, hypoechoic to anechoic nodules (Fig. 7-7). The third, less common presentation is an enlarged spleen with a small number of large, complexly echogenic, cavitated, or hypoechoic masses.[17] These larger masses may sometimes represent hematomas or regenerative nodules forming within a diffusely infiltrated spleen. Splenic lymphosarcoma is often just a portion of the cancer burden of the patient with multicentric lymphosarcoma (Fig. 7-8). It is important to examine the abdomen carefully for lymphadenopathy and hepatic or gastrointestinal involvement (see Figs. 6-14 through 6-16).[18]

Leukemias, multiple myeloma, and systemic mast cell disease may cause an enlarged normoechoic to hypoechoic spleen or multiple hypoechoic nodules of various sizes. Abdominal ultrasound rarely assists in the diagnosis of these conditions, except for splenic fine-needle aspiration in systemic mast cell disease. Systemic mastocytosis in the cat usually causes diffuse splenic enlargement (Fig. 7-9).[1] Malignant histiocytosis may appear as a diffusely hypoechoic spleen, but it can also exist as multiple, large, complexly echogenic splenic masses. A portion of these larger masses may represent hematoma formation due to disruption of the splenic vasculature by the malignant infiltration (Fig. 7-10).

When the demand for blood cells is high, the pluripotential stem cells in the spleen may differentiate and form islands of extramedullary hematopoiesis. This process may result in diffuse, mildly hypoechoic splenomegaly. Splenic extramedullary hematopoiesis occurs most commonly with chronic hemolytic or hypoplastic anemias, pancytopenias due to myelofibrosis, and chronic inflammatory disorders such as pyometra and brucellosis.[8]

Congestive Splenic Disease

Congestive splenomegaly can be seen in animals with portal hypertension, right heart failure, pericardial effusion, vena cava syndrome of heartworm disease, splenic torsion, and thrombosis of the splenic, hepatic, or portal veins.[1,3,4,8,19] The spleen usually is mildly enlarged and hypoechoic, with portal hypertension and increased caudal vena cava pressures (eg, right heart failure, pericardial effusion, heartworm disease). With portal hypertension, the splenic veins may be enlarged, and the liver may have an abnormal ultrasonographic appearance. Congestive splenomegaly due to increased caudal vena cava pressure can generally

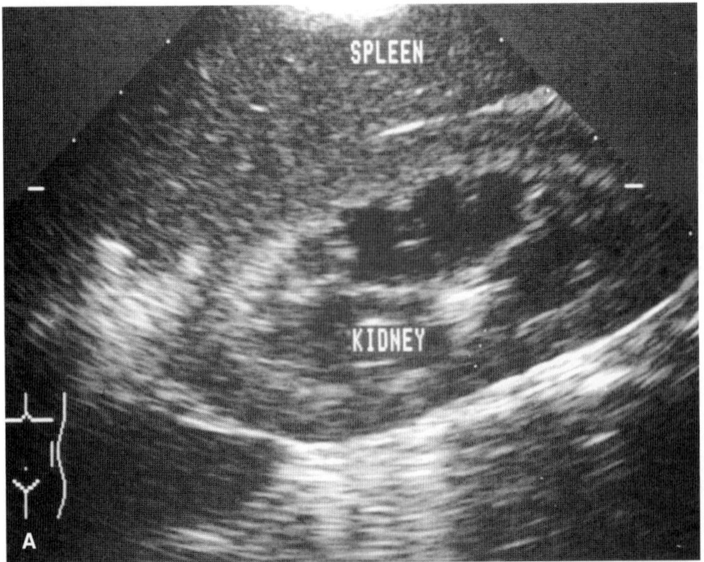

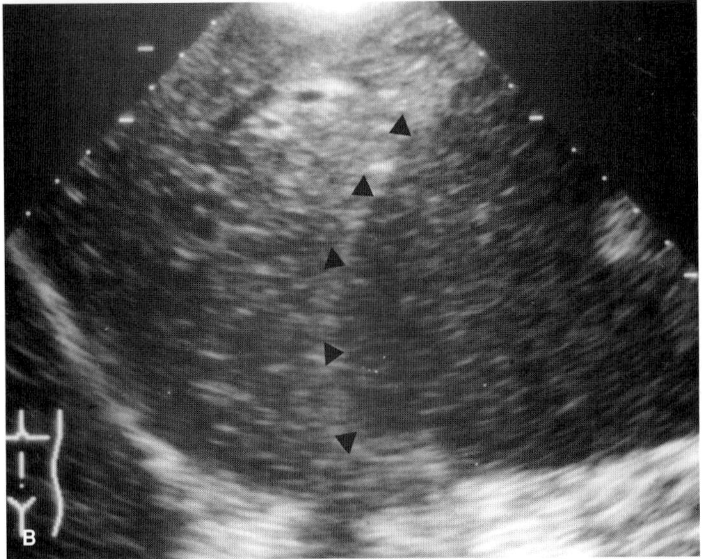

Figure 7-6. (**A**) Splenic lymphosarcoma. The spleen is enlarged and hypoechoic, with approximately the same echogenicity as the adjacent left kidney. (**B**) Splenic lymphosarcoma. The spleen is very large, folded on itself, and in close contact with the liver. The spleen is hypoechoic and has a slightly moth-eaten, inhomogeneous echotexture. The black triangles identify the liver-spleen junction, with the liver to the left and the spleen to the right. The spleen is less echogenic than the liver.

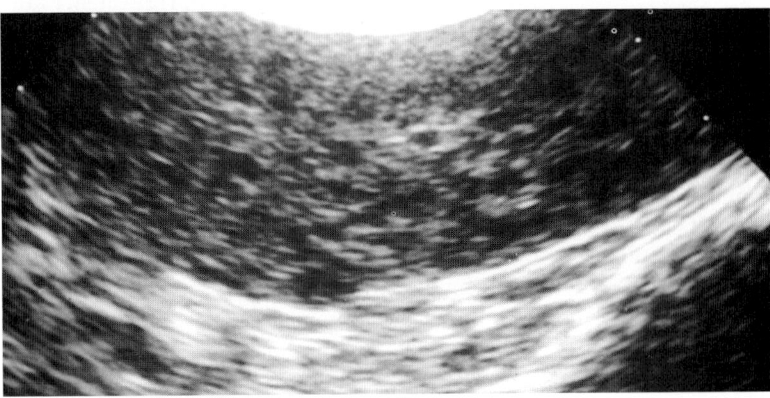

Figure 7-7. Splenic lymphosarcoma. The spleen is large, hypoechoic, and contains numerous poorly circumscribed hypoechoic to anechoic nodules.

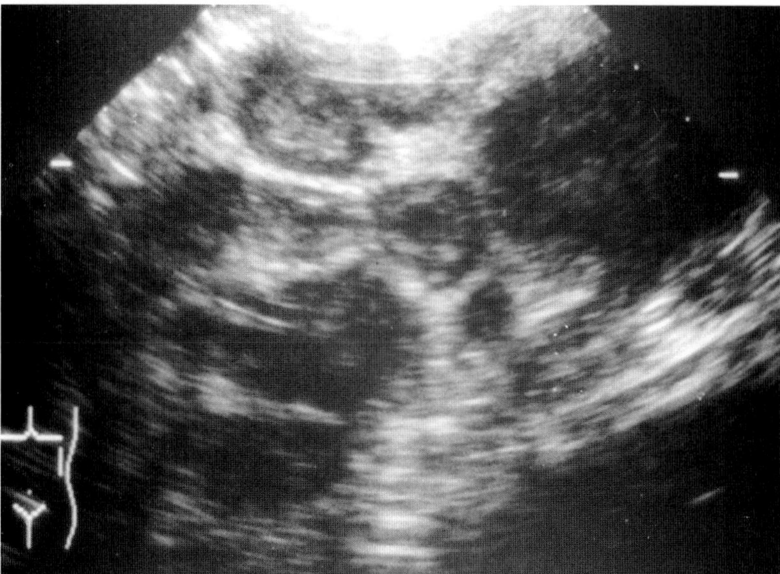

Figure 7-8. Splenic lymphosarcoma. The spleen is large and contains numerous hypoechoic, target, and complexly echogenic masses.

be differentiated because of the enlargement of the caudal vena cava, hepatic veins, and splenic veins (Fig. 7-11). The source of the increased caval pressure can often be identified with echocardiography.

Congestive splenomegaly due to thrombosis and suppurative infarction can be focal, regional, or involve the entire spleen.[3,4,7,19] Predisposing conditions include septicemia, neoplasia, cardiomyopathy, and valvular endocarditis. Infarcted areas may appear as a focal hypoechoic or isoechoic nodule deforming the splenic margin.[19] An infarct may also appear as a wedge-shaped hypoechoic area of the splenic margin, which later becomes hyperechoic. Diffuse infarction or necrosis of the spleen is characterized by a heterogeneous, hypoechoic, coarse, lacy parenchymal pattern (Fig. 7-12).[19] Splenic ischemia associated with gas-forming anaerobic bacteria may result in gangrenous or

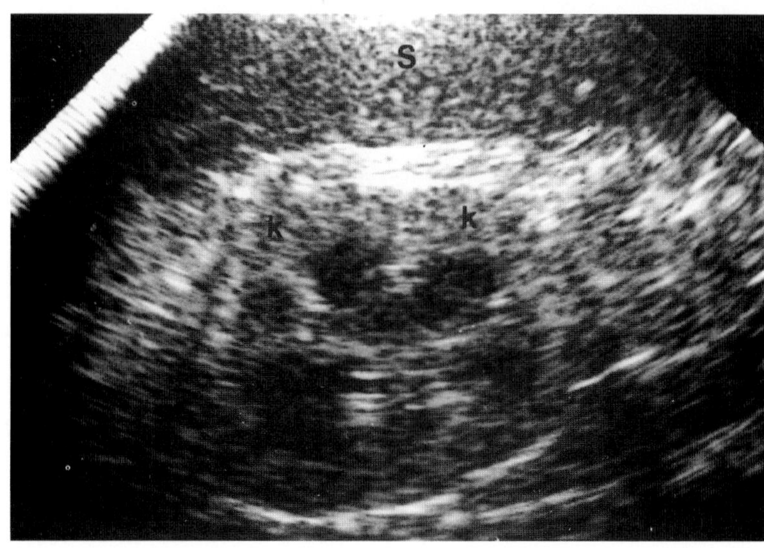

Figure 7-9. Splenic mastocytosis in a cat. The spleen (*s*) is large and hypoechoic compared with the left renal cortex (*k*).

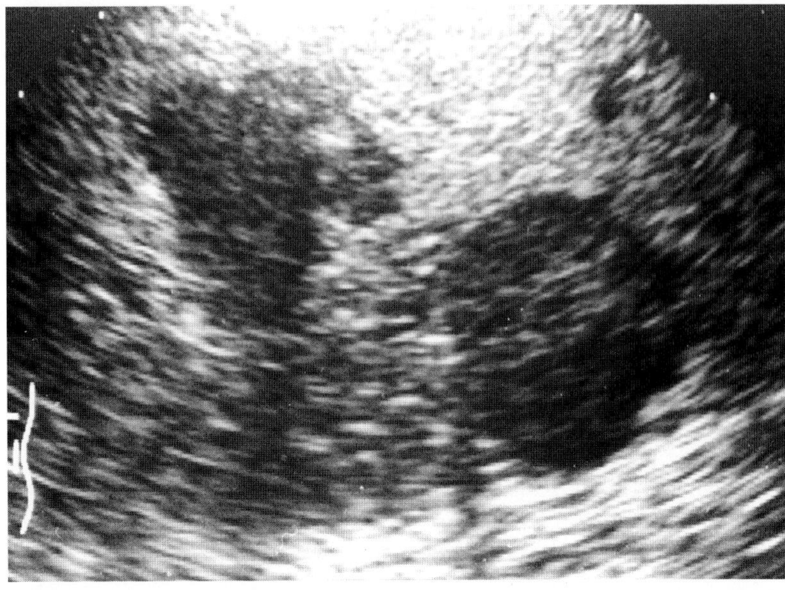

Figure 7-10. Malignant histiocytosis in a rottweiler. The spleen is large and contains numerous very large, irregularly circumscribed hypoechoic masses.

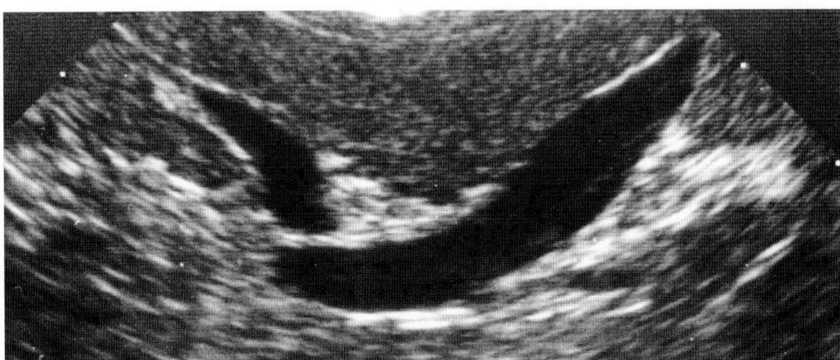

Figure 7-11. Congestive splenomegaly in a Doberman pinscher with hepatic cirrhosis. The spleen is enlarged and hypoechoic, with very large central hilar splenic veins.

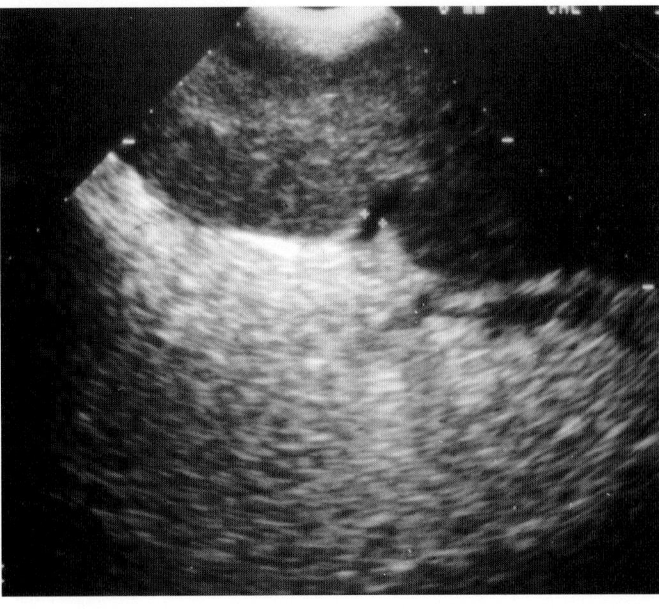

Figure 7-12. Diffuse splenic infarction. The spleen in large, hypoechoic, and irregularly marginated, with a coarse lacy echotexture. The cursors (+) outline the splenic hilar vessels.

emphysematous splenitis. Gas pockets within the spleen appear as intensely hyperechoic focal areas with distal reverberation artifacts (Fig. 7-13).[19] The radiolucent gas pockets may be visible on abdominal radiographs (Fig. 7-14).

Torsion of the spleen is a rare, life-threatening emergency that is seen primarily in large- or giant-breed dogs.[19–21] Splenic torsion patients typically present with anorexia, weight loss, lethargy, vomiting, depression, and palpable splenomegaly.[22,23] Clinical findings include mild anemia, leukocytosis, hemoglobinemia, and hemoglobinuria.[23] The sonographic appearance of splenic torsion is a grossly enlarged spleen with diffuse anechoic areas separated by parallel linear echoes (Fig. 7-15).[19,21] The proximal splenic vessels may be enlarged, and the hilar pedicle torsion may appear as a complexly echogenic mass deep to the spleen. Partial splenic torsion or congestion due to venous occlusion often accompanies gastric dilation with volvulus.

Splenic Hyperplasia

Hyperplasia of the reticuloendothelial system occurs in small animal patients with immune-mediated hemolytic anemias, drug-induced hemolytic anemias, immune-mediated thrombocytopenias, and blood parasites.[8] The damaged erythrocytes and inclusion bodies that occur with these diseases are removed by the spleen. Splenic hyperplasia causes smooth, generalized splenomegaly with a normal to hypoechoic echogenicity and normal echotexture.

Infectious and Inflammatory Splenomegaly

Generalized splenomegaly may occur in a variety of inflammatory and infectious conditions. The spleen enlarges because of a combination of extramedullary hematopoiesis, reticuloendothelial system (RES) hyperplasia, and lymphocytic-plasmacytic splenitis. The degree of involvement of these three mechanisms in the generation of the splenomegaly varies with the etiologic agent and duration of disease. Conditions that may stimulate this response include systemic mycosis such as histoplasmosis, coccidioidomycosis, and blastomycosis; viral disease such as canine distemper and infections canine hepatitis; blood parasites and organisms such as *Hemobartonella, Salmonella, Brucella, Clostridia, Babesia, Ehrlichia,* and *Toxoplasma.*[8] The ultrasonographic appearance has not been documented for all these diseases, but the physiology suggests that the spleen should be large and smooth, with a normal to hypoechoic

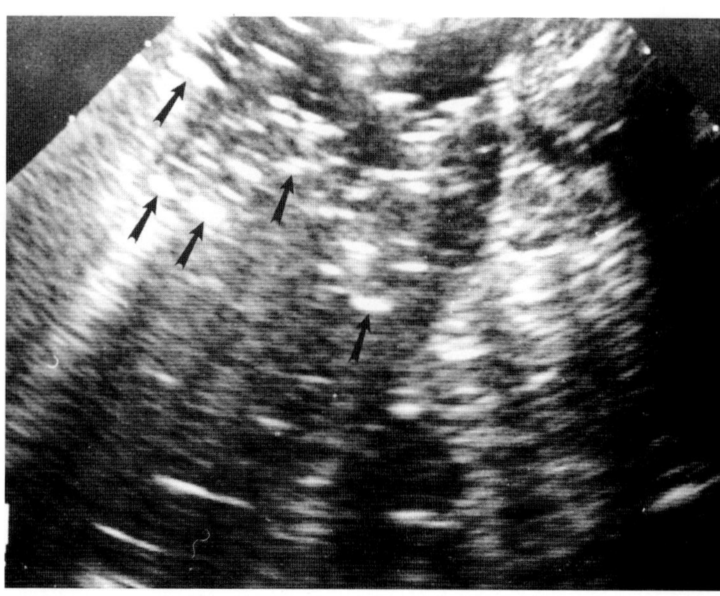

Figure 7-13. Emphysematous splenitis. The spleen is enlarged, hypoechoic, and contains numerous intensely hyperechoic foci of gas (*arrows*) that reverberate distally.

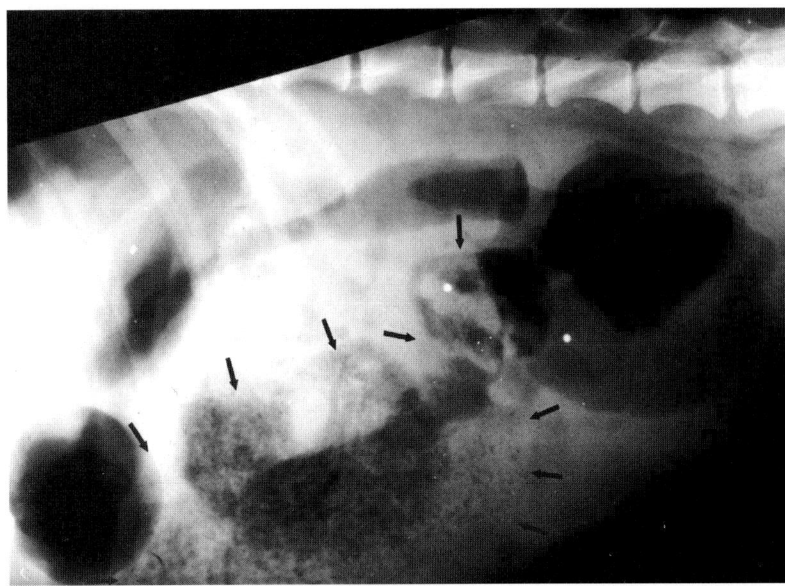

Figure 7-14. Radiograph of gangrenous splenitis. The spleen is enlarged and contains various sizes of particulate and linear gas collections throughout the parenchyma. The arrows outline the splenic margin. (Courtesy of Dr. Robert D. Pechman, Louisiana State University, Baton Rouge, LA.)

echogenicity and normal echotexture. This is a nonspecific change that can be seen with many disease entities.

Focal Splenic Disease

Focal splenic disease is more easily recognized ultrasonographically than diffuse disease because the lesions are surrounded by normal splenic parenchyma or bulge from the splenic surface. Focal splenic disease is characterized by size, shape, margination, echogenicity, presence of gas or mineralization, and beam attenuation properties. As with diffuse conditions, the sonographic appearance of focal disease is rarely pathognomonic and usually requires a fine-needle aspirate or biopsy for diagnosis.[11,14] Focal

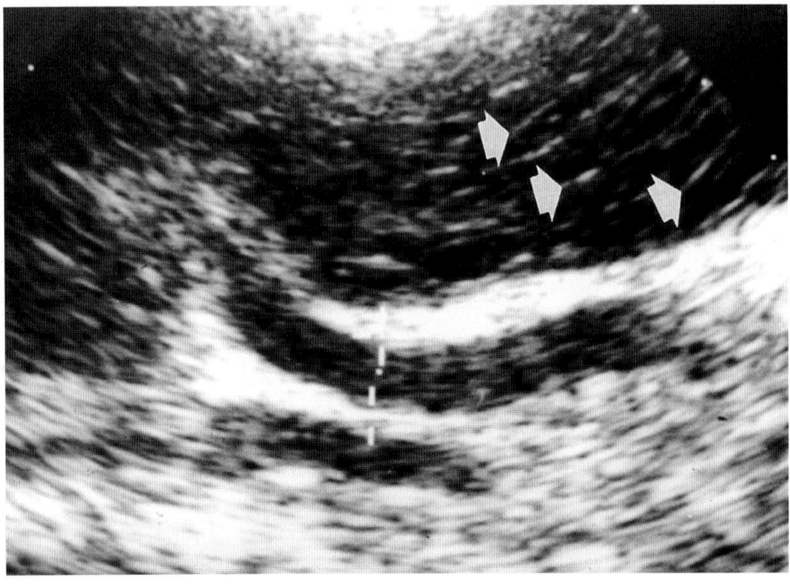

Figure 7-15. Splenic torsion. The spleen is grossly enlarged and hypoechoic and contains anechoic areas separated by parallel linear echoes (*arrowheads*). One of the enlarged proximal splenic vessels is outlined by cursors (+).

splenic diseases include neoplasms, infarcts, hematomas, regenerative nodules, cysts, abscesses, and granulomas.

Focal Splenic Neoplasia

The most common canine splenic neoplasm is hemangiosarcoma. Hemangiosarcoma is a malignant tumor composed of immature endothelial cells lining blood-filled cavitations. Hemangiosarcoma is more common in older male dogs, with a predilection for the German shepherd breed. Patients are weak, depressed, and anemic, with elevated pulse and respiratory rates and weight loss at presentation.[24–26] These tumors often cause periodic splenic hemorrhage that results in splenic hematoma formation and abdominal distention due to bloody peritoneal effusion. Radiography may reveal solitary or multiple splenic masses, but because of the large number of patients that present with abdominal effusion, ultrasonography is the most accurate diagnostic tool.[14,27]

Ultrasonographically, hemangiosarcoma has a variable but somewhat characteristic appearance. The spleen is enlarged and contains multiple masses, which range from 1 cm to greater than 10 cm in diameter. These masses often protrude from the splenic surface or may appear adjacent to or near the spleen. The masses have a mixed appearance; some are largely hypoechoic because of very large cavitations, and others are complexly echogenic, with an equal mix of anechoic cavitations and heterogeneous hyperechogenicity. Other masses are predominantly heterogeneously hyperechoic and have few cavitations.[27] This variability probably reflects a combination of different volumes of tumor mass, hematomas, and posthemorrhagic cyst formation (Fig. 7-16). The tumors are often well-defined lesions but lack a capsular margin. The anechoic cavitations may demonstrate acoustic enhancement. Fifty percent of patients have some volume of hypoechoic peritoneal effusion.[27] The effusion is generally more echogenic than normal urine in the bladder because of the high erythrocyte content (Fig. 7-17).

Splenic hemangiosarcoma is a highly metastatic tumor that characteristically spreads to the liver and diffusely spreads throughout the peritoneal cavity. Liver metastases are often irregularly circumscribed anechoic to hypoechoic nodules that vary in size from just visible to several centimeters in diameter (see Fig. 6-21). Chest radiographs and an echocardiogram are an important part of the clinical workup because of the high prevalence of pulmonary metastasis and right atrial hemangiosarcoma with pericardial hemorrhage.[28]

Besides its diffusely affected appearance, splenic lymphosarcoma may appear focally as multiple, poorly marginated, hypoechoic to anechoic nodules or as an enlarged spleen with a small number of large, complexly echogenic, cavitated or hypoechoic masses.[15]

Other focal malignant neoplasms commonly found in the spleen include leiomyosarcomas, fibrosarcomas, anaplastic sarcomas, plasma cell tumors, and mast cell tumors.[26] Leiomyosarcoma, plasma cell tumors, and mast cell tumors are frequently more homogeneously hypoechoic than fibrosarcomas and anaplastic sarcomas, but the ultrasonographic appearance of primary and metastatic splenic tumors is not specific for cell type (Fig. 7-18).[14,18] Because these tumors often disrupt splenic vasculature, hematoma formation within and around the tumor mass may complicate the sonographic appearance. Ultrasound-guided fine-needle aspiration or biopsy is an ideal method for obtaining samples of focal splenic disease for diagnosis.

Nonmalignant Focal Splenic Disease

The most common focal splenic mass detected with ultrasound is nodular hyperplasia.[29] Hyperplastic nodules are often mistaken for neoplastic disease. These nodules can be single or multiple and typically are homogeneously hypoechoic to isoechoic compared with the spleen. Regenerative nodules usually have a well-defined border without a capsule. These nodules may bulge from the splenic surface and vary in size from 1 cm to more than 5 cm in diameter. Hyperplastic nodules may have a slightly mottled echotexture, but small to moderate sized nodules usually do not contain the anechoic cavitations frequently found in hemangiosarcoma and hematomas (Fig. 7-19).

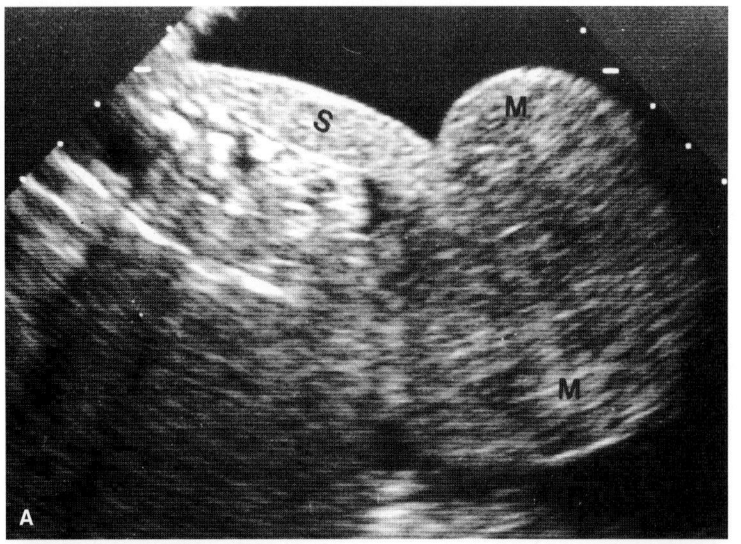

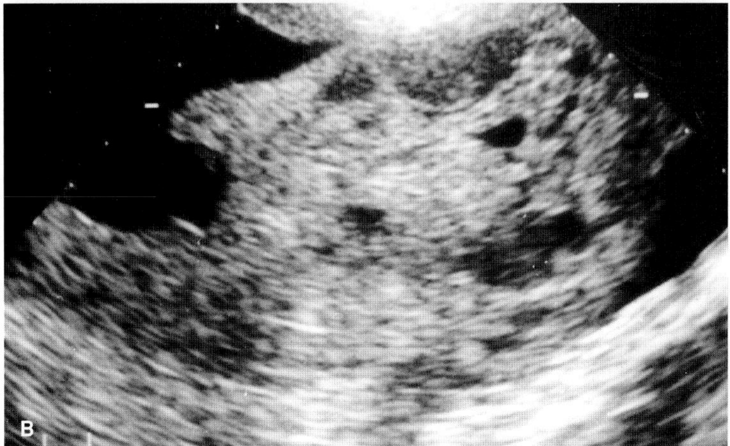

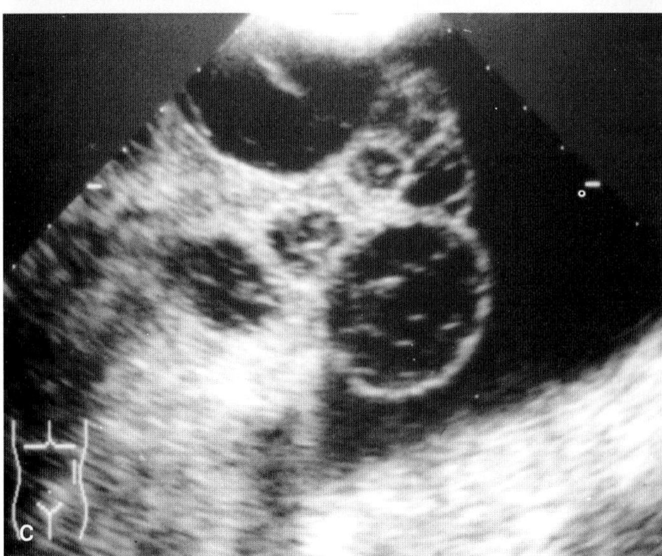

Figure 7-16. (**A**) Splenic hemangiosarcoma. A large, complexly echogenic solid mass (*M*) protrudes from the tail of the spleen (*S*). The spleen is surrounded by hypoechoic abdominal hemorrhage. (**B**) Splenic hemangiosarcoma. A large, complexly echogenic mass contains numerous hypoechoic and anechoic cavitations. The mass is surrounded by hypoechoic abdominal hemorrhage. (**C**) Splenic hemangiosarcoma. Numerous bubble-like, anechoic blood-filled cavitations are scattered throughout the spleen. The spleen is surrounded by hypoechoic abdominal hemorrhage.

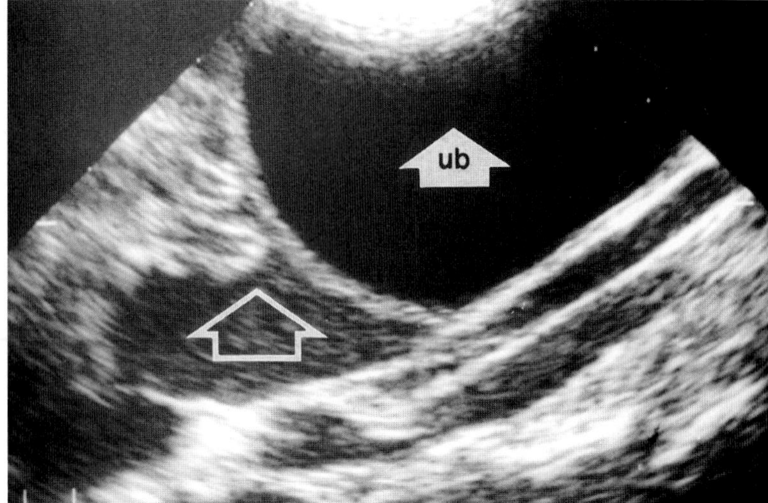

Figure 7-17. Abdominal hemorrhage secondary to hemangiosarcoma. This longitudinal view of the urinary bladder (*white arrows, ub*) shows a fluid collection dorsal to the bladder margin (*open arrow*). The echogenicity of the abdominal fluid is much greater than the urine in the bladder. This indicates a protein or cellular composition (erythrocytes in this case) much higher than urine.

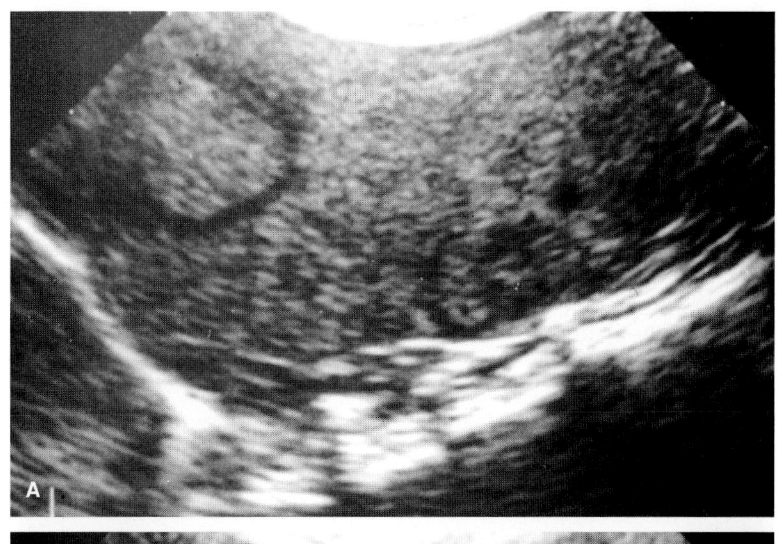

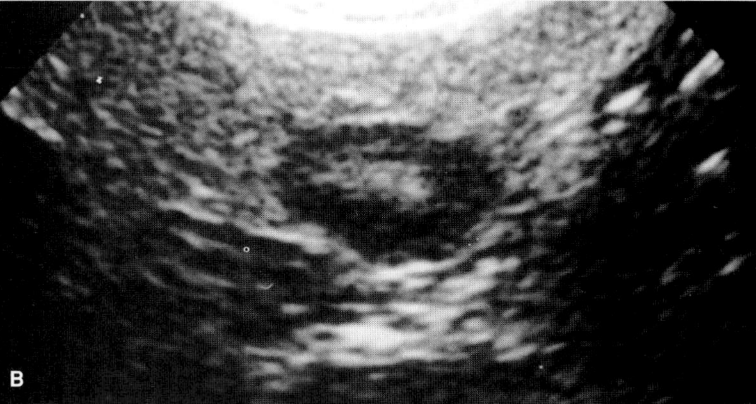

Figure 7-18. (**A**) Multiple, irregularly circumscribed target masses within the spleen. The biopsy showed anaplastic carcinoma. (**B**) Solitary, fairly well-circumscribed target mass within the spleen. The biopsy revealed a mast cell tumor.

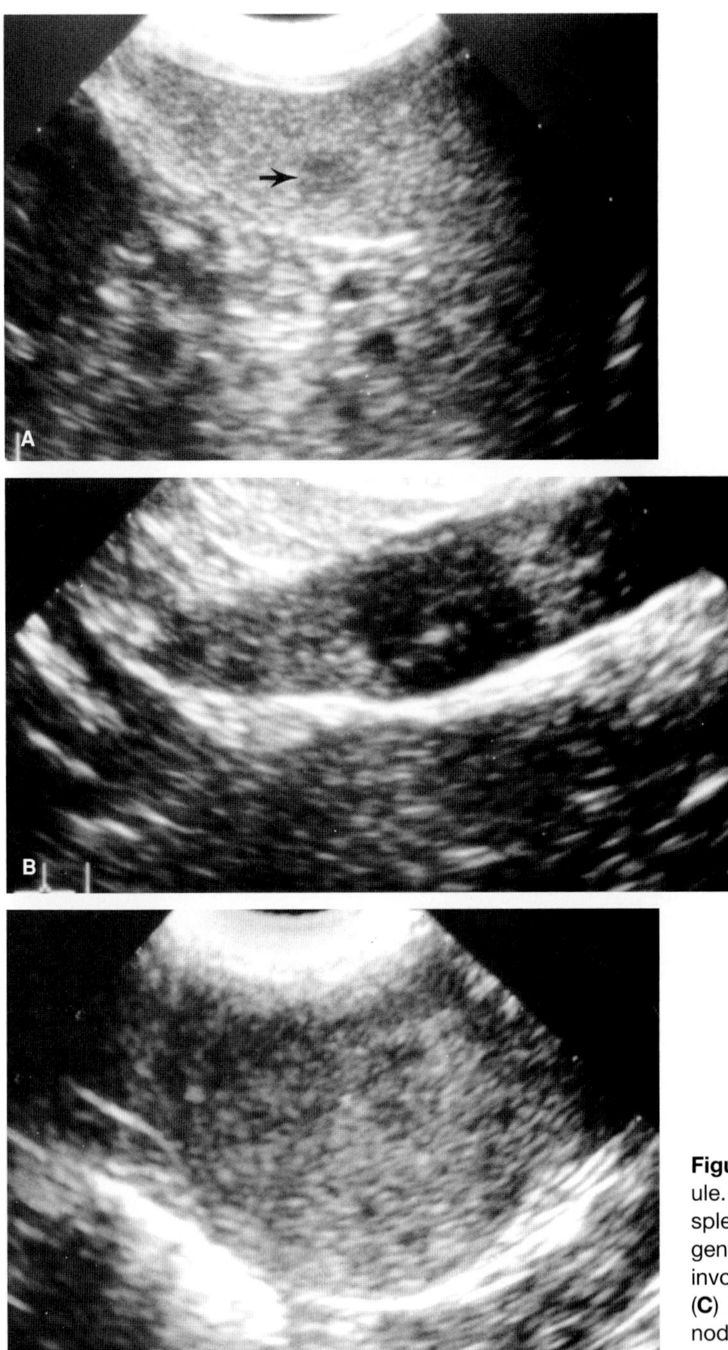

Figure 7-19. (**A**) Splenic regenerative nodule. A small, hypoechoic mass within the splenic parenchyma (*arrow*). (**B**) Splenic regenerative nodule. A large, hypoechoic mass involves almost the entire width of the spleen. (**C**) Splenic regenerative nodule. This 5-cm nodule bulges from the surface of the spleen and has a slightly mottled echotexture, with normal splenic echogenicity.

Splenic hematomas commonly are detected by abdominal ultrasound. Hematomas may form spontaneously, secondary to trauma, and secondary to neoplastic infiltration. The patients often present with various combinations of vague signs such as anorexia, abdominal pain, depression, nausea, weight loss, and lethargy.[30] Most patients are older, and splenic masses are readily detected on the abdominal radiographs. Splenic hematomas can be single or multiple, and they vary from small (1 to 2 cm) to very large (>22 cm). The masses may be present within the splenic parenchyma or protrude from the capsular surface. The smaller hematomas tend to be more hypoechoic, but the larger ones are complexly hyperechoic, with areas of hypoechogenicity and septation. Hematomas are usually well-defined lesions and may encapsulate (Fig. 7-20).[31] When the masses are very large, there is an incorrect tendency to suspect malignancy. This may lead to a failure to perform a splenectomy because of a poor preoperative prognosis.[32] Unlike patients with hemangiosarcoma, chronic splenic hematoma patients do not present in hypovolemic shock and generally do not have detectable peritoneal hemorrhage. Because 20% of the splenic hematoma patients in one study had underlying splenic lymphosarcoma, it is important to obtain histopathology examination of the mass and splenic body.[30]

Splenic abscesses are uncommon.[3,4,7] The typical sonographic appearance is an irregularly circumscribed, hypoechoic mass with little or no through transmission (Fig. 7-21).[31] Splenic cysts (ie, pseudocysts) are also uncommon.[3,4] Cysts may form secondary to trauma and hematoma resorption. Sonographically, cysts are round, anechoic, thin-walled, fluid-filled nodules that

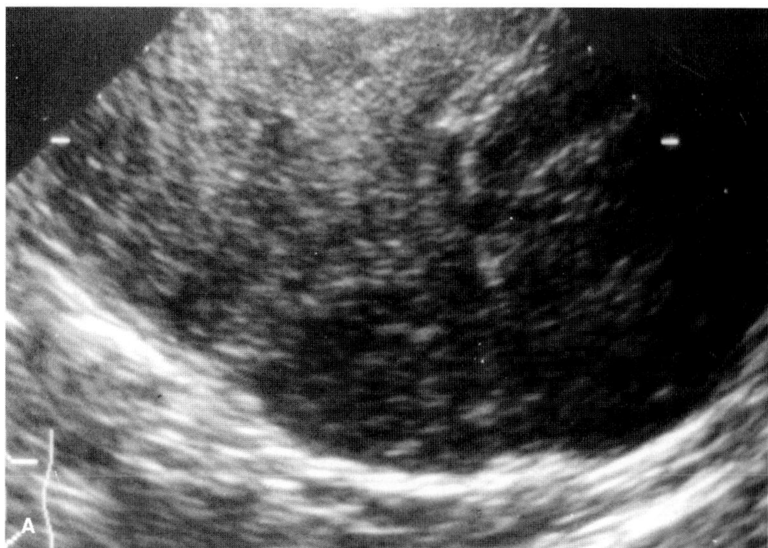

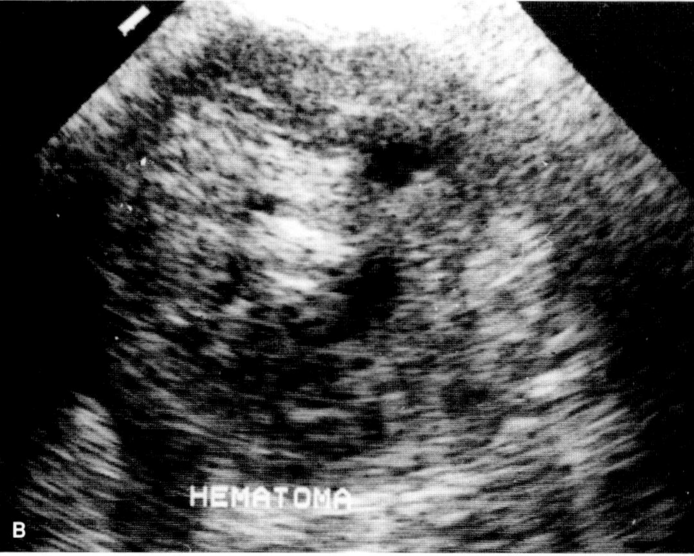

Figure 7-20. (**A**) Splenic hematoma. This mass was larger than 10 cm in diameter and encompassed more than one half of the spleen. It is fairly homogeneously hypoechoic, solid, and contains a well-defined capsule. (**B**) Splenic hematoma. This mass was 6 cm in diameter, complexly echogenic, and contained several cavitations.

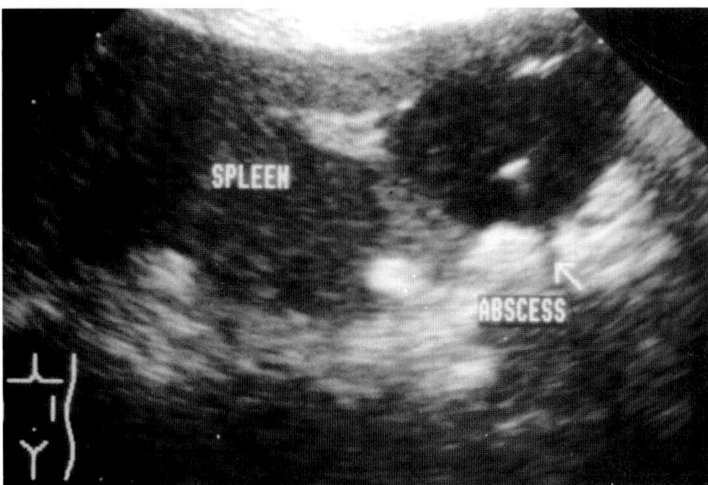

Figure 7-21. Splenic abscess. The abscess is hypoechoic, irregularly circumscribed, and contains two focal bright echoes, which represent small gas collections.

show acoustic enhancement (Fig. 7-22). Definitive diagnosis of these lesions is easily obtained with ultrasound-guided fine-needle aspiration.

Splenic Trauma

The spleen may be fractured by any form of abdominal trauma, but it is uncommonly a source of life-threatening hemorrhage after trauma. The most common form of trauma in small animals is being hit by a car. Only 3 of 600 dogs examined in one study had splenic rupture after being hit by a car.[33] Acute, serious splenic trauma patients present with tachycardia, abdominal pain, increased respiratory rate, slow capillary refill, and other clinical signs of hypovolemic shock. The abdomen may be distended, and abdominal radiographic detail is poor. Abdominal ultrasound reveals a moderately echogenic peritoneal fluid. The echogenicity is caused by the high cell count in acute hemorrhage. Fresh free blood in the peritoneal cavity is more echogenic than normal urine in the bladder. The spleen may have an irregular surface, with disruption of the smooth capsular margin.

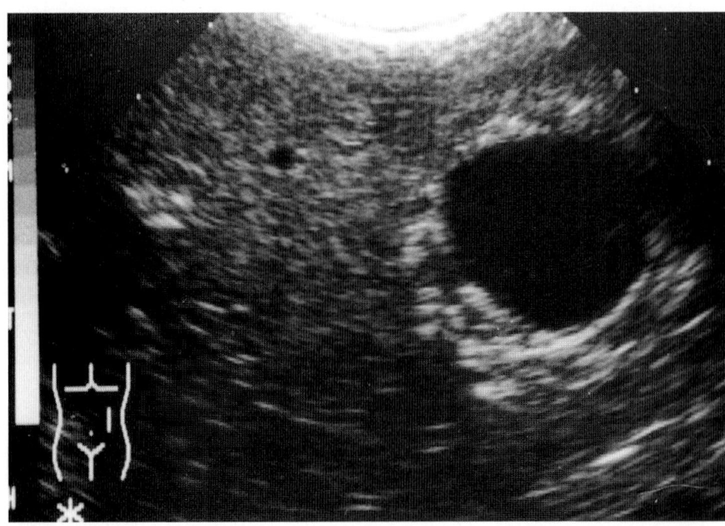

Figure 7-22. Splenic cyst. The cyst is round, anechoic, and demonstrates through transmission.

The spleen is often difficult to image because of splenic contraction and early hematoma formation surrounding the trauma site. If serious abdominal hemorrhage occurs after minimal trauma, a splenic tumor or coagulopathy should be suspected.

FINE-NEEDLE ASPIRATION AND BIOPSY OF THE SPLEEN

Fine-needle aspiration for cytologic samples of focal or diffuse splenic disease is performed similarly to other organs. The area to be sampled is identified on ultrasound, and a needle path that does not cross vital structures is chosen. The needle can be placed through an ultrasound biopsy guide or free-hand directed into the site using ultrasound visualization. A 22- to 25-gauge 1- to 1.5-in needle is attached to a 12- to 20-mL syringe. The needle is gently but quickly passed into the lesion, and full suction is applied two or three times without moving the needle. The suction is released, and the needle is withdrawn. Splenic samples appear as a small volume of blood-tinged material in the hub of the syringe. The sample is placed one drop at a time on glass slides and smeared as a peripheral blood smear. Because samples clot quickly, the smears should be made rapidly.[11–13]

Diffuse, noncavitated and focal, solid splenic lesions can be aspirated without hesitation in a patient with normal coagulation. Large, complexly echogenic focal masses with numerous cavitations and peritoneal fluid may be hemangiosarcoma and should not be sampled. These masses are prone to hemorrhage, and needle penetration can cause peritoneal seeding of the tumor.[12] These patients should undergo splenectomy after careful sonographic evaluation of the liver and radiographic evaluation of the lungs for metastasis.

If the cytologic sample is insufficient for diagnosis, a needle-core biopsy of the splenic lesion can be taken. Automatic 18-gauge needle-core biopsy needles (Biopty, Monopty, Temno) are preferred, because they yield higher sample quality with less tissue trauma.[34–36] Only generalized or focal solid splenic lesions are recommended for biopsy. Abdominal ultrasound can be used to monitor for hemorrhage after the biopsy procedure.

REFERENCES

1. Lipowitz AJ, Blue J, Perman V. The spleen. In: Slatter DH, ed. Textbook of small animal surgery. Philadelphia: WB Saunders, 1985;1204.
2. Wood AKW, McCarthy PH, Angles JM. Ultrasonographic-anatomic correlation and imaging protocol for the spleen in anesthetized dogs. J Am Vet Med Assoc 1990;51:1433.
3. Myland TG, Hagar DA. Sonography of the liver, gallbladder and spleen. Vet Clin North Am 1985;15:1123.
4. Myland TG, Hager DA, Derring DS. Sonography of the liver, gallbladder, and spleen. Semin Vet Med Surg 1989;4:13.
5. Herring DS. Physics, facts and artifacts of diagnostic ultrasound. Vet Clin North Am 1985;15:1107.
6. Park RD, Myland TG, Lattimer JC, et al. B-mode gray-scale ultrasound: imaging artifacts and interpretation principles. Vet Radiol 1981;22:204.
7. Lamb DR. Abdominal ultrasonography in small animals: examination of the liver, spleen and pancreas. J Small Anim Pract 1990;31:5.
8. Couto CG. Splenomegaly. In: American Animal Hospital Association scientific proceedings, Orlando, March 23–29, 1985. Mishawaka, IN: American Animal Hospital Association, 1985; 342.
9. Foss RR, Wrigley RH, Park RD, et al. A new frontier—veterinary ultrasound: the spleen. Med Ultrasound 1983;7:152.
10. Saunders HM, Pugh CR, Rhodes RM. Expanding applications of abdominal ultrasonography. J Am Anim Hosp Assoc 1192;28:369.
11. O'Keefe DA, Couto CG. Fine needle aspiration of the spleen as an aid in the diagnosis of splenomegaly. J Vet Intern Med 1987;1:102.

12. Osborne CA, Perman V, Stevens JB. Needle biopsy of the spleen. Vet Clin North Am 1974;4:311.
13. Swischer SN, Dale WA. Splenic aspiration biopsy in the dog. Blood 1955;10:812.
14. Feeney DA, Johnston GR, Hardy RM. Two-dimensional, gray-scale ultrasonography for assessment of hepatic and splenic neoplasia in the dog and cat. J Am Vet Med Assoc 1984;184:68.
15. Lamb CR, Hartzband LE, Tidwell AS, Pearson SH. Ultrasonographic findings in hepatic and splenic lymphosarcoma in dogs and cats. Vet Radiol 1991;32:117.
16. Whiteley MB, Feeney DA, Whiteley LO. Ultrasonographic appearance of primary and metastatic canine hepatic tumors; a review of 48 cases. J Ultrasound Med 1989;8:621.
17. Wrigley RH, Konde LJ, Park RD, Lebel JL. Ultrasonographic features of splenic lymphosarcoma in dogs: 12 cases (1980–1986). J Am Vet Med Assoc 1988;193: 1565.
18. Nyland TG, Kantrowitz BM. Ultrasound in diagnosis and staging of abdominal neoplasia. In: Gorman N, ed. Oncology—contemporary issues in small animal medicine. New York: Churchill Livingstone, 1986:1.
19. Schelling CG, Wortman JA, Saunders M. Ultrasonographic detection of splenic necrosis in the dog. Vet Radiol 1988; 29:227.
20. Konde LJ, Wrigley RH, Lebel JL, et al. Sonographic and radiographic changes associated with splenic torsion in the dog. Vet Radiol 1989;1:41.
21. Wrigley RH. Ultrasonography of the spleen—life threatening splenic disorders. Probl Vet Med 1991;3:574.
22. Stead AC, Frankland AL, Borthwich R. Splenic torsion in dogs. J Small Anim Pract 1983;24:549.
23. Stevenson C, Chew DJ, Kociba GJ. Torsion of the splenic pedicle in the dog: a review. J Am Anim Hosp Assoc 1981; 17:239.
24. Brown NO, Parnaik AK, MacEwen EG. Canine Hemangiosarcoma. J Am Vet Med Assoc 1985;186:56.
25. Fees DL, Withrow SJ. Canine Hemangiosarcoma. Compend Contin Educ Pract Vet 1981;3:1047.
26. Frey AJ, Betts CW. A retrospective study of splenectomy in the dog. J Am Anim Hosp Assoc 1877;13:730.
27. Wrigley RH, Park RD, Konde LJ, Lebel JL. Ultrasonographic features of splenic hemangiosarcoma in dogs: 18 cases (1980 to 1986). J Am Vet Med Assoc 1988;192: 1113.
28. Kaplan PM, Murtaugh RJ, Ross JN. Ultrasound in emergency veterinary medicine. Semin Vet Med Surg 1988;3:245.
29. Ishmael J, McHowell J. Neoplasia of the spleen of the dog with a note on nodular hyperplasia. J Comp Pathol 1968;78:59.
30. Wrigley R H, Konde LJ, Park RD, Lebel JL. Clinical features and diagnosis of splenic hematomas in dogs; 10 cases (1980 to 1987). J Am Anim Hosp Assoc 1989;25:371.
31. Konde LJ, Lebel JL, Park RD. Sonographic application in the diagnosis of intra-abdominal abscesses in the dog. Vet Radiol 1986;27:151.
32. Bartels P. Indications for splenectomy and post-operative survival rate. J Small Anim Pract 1970;10:781.
33. Kolata RJ, Johnson DE. Motor vehicle accidents in urban dogs: a study of 600 cases. J Am Vet Med Assoc 1975;167:938.
34. Hager DA, Nyland TG, Fisher R. Ultrasound-guided biopsy of the canine liver, kidney and prostate. Vet Radiol 1985; 26:82.
35. Hoppe FE, Hager DA, Poulos PW, et al. A comparison of manual and automatic ultrasound guided biopsy techniques. Vet Radiol 1986;27:99.
36. Partington BP, Leveille R, Bradley G. Ultrasound biopsy of the canine spleen. Presented in the American College of Veterinary Radiology annual proceedings, November 1990. Chicago, IL, 1990.

Small Animal Ultrasound, edited by Ronald W. Green.
Lippincott-Raven Publishers, Philadelphia © 1996.

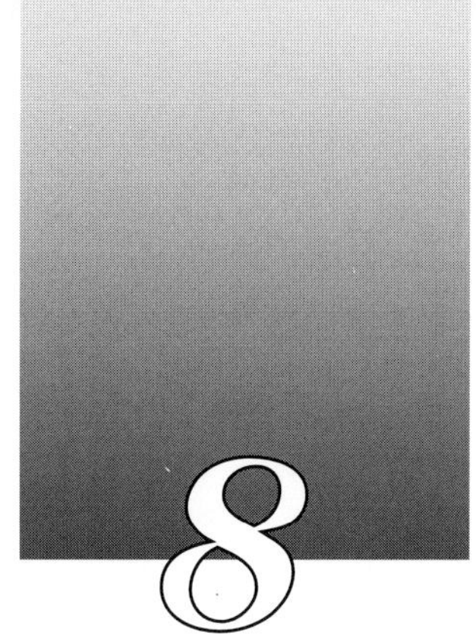

GASTROINTESTINAL TRACT

Linda D. Homco

Ultrasonography of the gastrointestinal (GI) tract presents problems and challenges for the sonographer. Sonography of the GI viscera was once thought to be impossible because of artifacts created by gas within the lumen.[1] Organs such as the small intestine and colon were considered "no man's land," with GI ultrasound scanning considered "rarely of any value."[2] Sonographically, ingesta and feces can produce highly reflective pseudomasses that create acoustic shadowing and add to the diagnostic difficulty.[1] Because the intestines move within the peritoneal cavity, localization of a lesion can be difficult. However, technical advancements have made GI sonography a valuable tool in diagnosing GI diseases. The image quality has improved enough to identify the layers of the bowel wall by transabdominal sonography, and even greater detail of the mucosa can be obtained with endoscopic sonography.[3] Peristalsis, which is often diminished in diseased bowel, can be assessed with real-time ultrasound.[1]

NORMAL ANATOMY AND LOCATION

The GI organs vary normally in size and position. The *stomach* varies more than the small and large intestines in its capacity to change size and shape. The major regions of the stomach are the cardia, fundus, body, and the pylorus, which consists of the pyloric antrum and the pyloric canal.[4] In the dog, the stomach lies in a transverse plane within the cranial abdomen, with the pylorus to the right of midline and much of the stomach to the left of midline.[4] In the cat, the stomach is more acutely angled, with the pyloric portion located at or near midline.[5]

The *duodenum* is the most fixed part of the *small intestine*.[6] It begins at the pylorus and runs caudally along the visceral surface of the liver and the right lateral abdomen to the level of the tuber coxae, where it turns medially and passes cranially to join the jejunum at the root of the mesentery.[6] The *jejunum* and *ileum* make up the largest portion of the small intestine and are the most mobile segments of the GI.[4] The jejunum, with no gross changes to differentiate it from the ileum, is the longest segment.

The *large intestine* is only slightly larger in diameter than the small intestine and is divided into the cecum, colon, and rectum.[4] The wall of the canine and feline large intestine, because of the absence of the sacculations or bands seen in other species, is similar in appearance to the small intestine.[4,6] The *cecum* in the dog and the cat does not communicate with the ileum and therefore acts as a diverticulum of the proximal colon.[6] The cecum is large and spiral or corkscrew shaped in the dog, and it is small and comma shaped in the cat.[6]

The colon is divided into the ascending, transverse, and descending portions, each named for the position it occupies and for the direction ingesta moves within the abdominal cavity rather than for any distinctive appearance. The short *ascending colon* passes along the medial surface of the duodenum and right lobe of the pancreas to the pylorus of the stomach, where it turns and crosses medially to form the *transverse colon*. The transverse colon is caudoventral to the stomach and the left limb of the pancreas. The transverse colon turns to the left of the root of the mesentery near the splenic hilum and forms the *descending colon*, which runs caudally in the left abdomen ventral to the left kidney and dorsal to the urinary bladder to the pelvic inlet. The *rectum* begins at the pelvic inlet and ends at the anal canal.[4]

SCANNING TECHNIQUES

Because of variability in the locations of portions of the GI viscera, it is difficult to evaluate specific areas of the tract. The stomach, although somewhat fixed in position, varies in size and shape depending on its contents, and the presence of gas prevents evaluation of many of its regions. The GI tract cannot be "run" from one end to the other as in surgery. Interference from gas and the normal peristalsis make it difficult to follow any segment for more than a few centimeters.

Because the normal GI tract contains a variety of materials, such as fluid, gas, mucus, ingesta, and feces, preparation of the animal for GI ultrasonography is recommended. The animal should be fasted for at least 12 hours before scanning, and restricting the water intake also decreases the amount of swallowed gas. To allow gas introduced during an enema to be eliminated, cleansing enemas are recommended at least 2 hours before scanning of the large bowel. In GI emergencies, such as intussusception or linear foreign body, abdominal preparation is usually not done.

To avoid interference from intraluminal gas, the sonographer should make use of the effects of gravity on the luminal contents when scanning the GI tract. When the pyloric outflow tract is to be evaluated, scanning with the patient in right lateral recumbency fills this area with fluid, and gas "floats" to the body and fundus. Tipping the dog's sternum toward the right with the animal in dorsal recumbency also fills the pylorus with any fluid present.[7] If a wall lesion of the greater curvature is to be assessed, left lateral recumbency creates a similar imaging window effect.

Scanning of the entire GI tract is done with the patient in dorsal recumbency. Although gas "rises" toward the ventral midline with the animal in this position, gentle pressure with the transducer during scanning easily displaces the gas-filled loops from the area of interest, a method called the graded compression technique.[8] The use of imaging windows, such as provided by the spleen or a full urinary bladder in assessing the small intestines and the descending colon, respectively, is also helpful.

Imaging of the stomach is best performed with a 7.5-MHz transducer. A 5.0-MHz transducer can be used to assess peristalsis or identify masses, but with lower frequencies, resolution of the layers in the wall is not possible. Small-footprint transducers are the best choice because of the limitations the ribs pose in accessing this area of the abdomen.

In the dog, sagittal scanning relative to the patient's long axis provides transverse images of the pylorus and body, and scanning in a transverse plane relative to the body yields long-axis views of these areas of the stomach. Sagittal and transverse imaging of a cat's stomach is accomplished in oblique imaging planes because of its orientation in the cranial portion of the abdomen.

To improve imaging of the stomach, the empty stomach can be filled with water.[1,9,10] Removal of air from the stomach before the introduction of water reduces the artifacts created by bubbles.[11] If some gas remains within the stomach, changing the patient's position displaces the water into the dependent portions of the stomach to provide an acoustic window.[9]

No special technique is needed to evaluate the small intestine. The graded compression technique displaces gas-filled loops away from the field of view of the transducer. To aid in imaging of the large bowel, a water enema can be used.[9]

After colonic preparation, a Foley-type catheter is inserted into the rectum, and the colon is gently distended with water. Tranquilization or a very light plane of anesthesia is recommended, because the increased pressure within the rectum may cause some patient discomfort.

Transrectal ultrasound, which has been used to evaluate adjacent organs such as the prostate gland, can also be used to evaluate the wall of the rectum and the descending colon. Flexible and rigid probes designed for endocavity use are available in the veterinary market. Endoscopic ultrasonography, which combines endoscopy and sonography, is one of the newest technologic advances in human medicine.[12]

Barium sulfate can interfere with scanning the GI tract.[13,14] In one study, settling of barium, allowing visualization of structures posterior to the intestinal wall, occurred within 4 hours.[14] If possible, ultrasound scanning is recommended before barium contrast studies. Iodinated GI contrast media do not cause a problem.[13]

NORMAL SONOGRAPHIC APPEARANCE

Stomach

The entire stomach is usually not visualized during routine sonography. Portions of the body and fundus along the greater curvature are seen in the near field, because these areas are typically the most ventral (Fig. 8-1). In sagittal scanning of the right cranial quadrant of the canine abdomen, the pyloric antrum is easily recognized as a small target sign just caudal to the liver (Fig. 8-2). The abdominal portion of the esophagus can occasionally be recognized between the esophageal hiatus of the diaphragm and the cardia. The empty contracted body and fundus of the stomach may appear as a large rosette in the left cranial abdomen (Fig. 8-3). However, most of the stomach is not usually visualized without fluid distention (Fig. 8-4).[9]

With higher-frequency transducers and with minimal gas in the stomach, five distinct layers of the stomach wall can be recognized (Fig. 8-5).[15] These layers are similar to those of the intestines and are discussed in the next section. The normal thickness of the stomach wall, depending on the degree of distention, is 3 to 5 mm when measured between rugal folds.[11] After distention, rugal folds are no longer detectable.[16]

Peristalsis can be assessed during real-time imaging. The mean number of contractions is four to five per minute, with a slight increase seen when the stomachs of fasted dogs are filled with water.[11]

Small Intestines

The normal sagittally scanned small intestine appears as alternating echodense and hypoechoic layers. These layers in cross section pro-

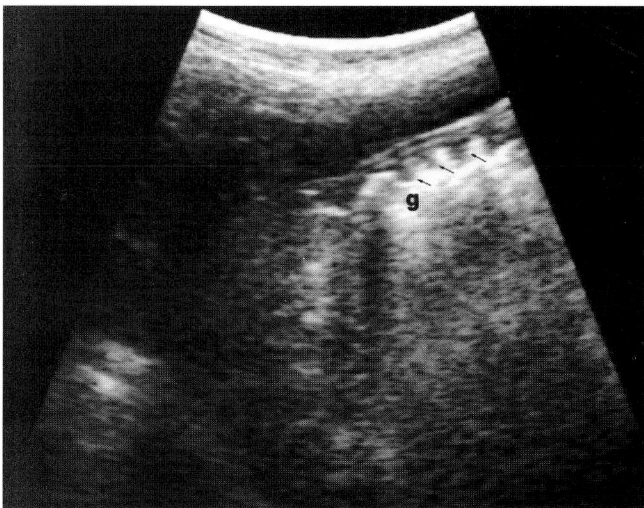

Figure 8-1. Sagittal sonogram of the normal stomach in a dog. Only the near-field wall with normal layers and rugal folds (*arrows*) is seen because of a gas artifact (*g*).

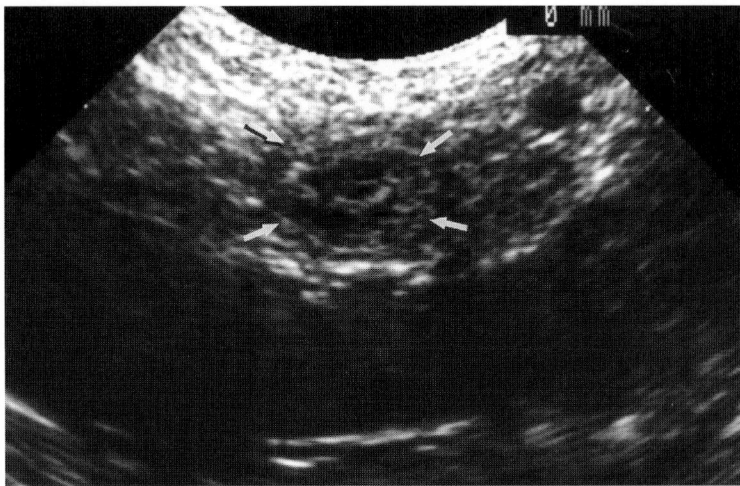

Figure 8-2. The sonogram of a transverse view of the pylorus (*arrows*) of a dog's stomach shows the normal target or bull's eye configuration.

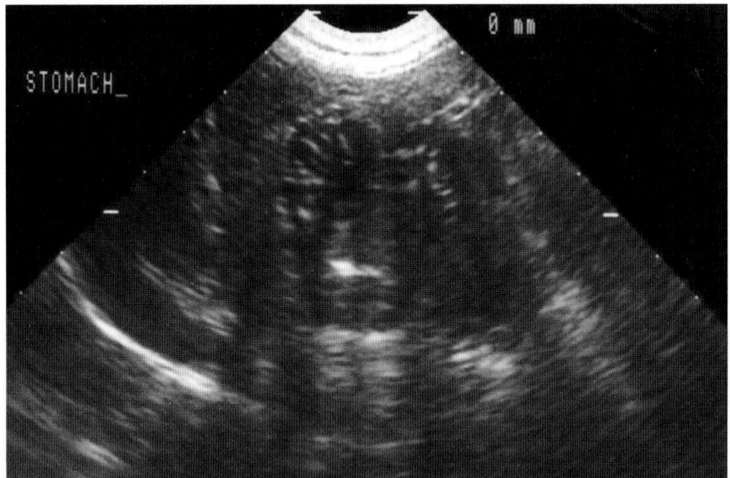

Figure 8-3. The sonogram of the fundus and body of an empty stomach in a dog shows the rugal folds and the normal layers of the stomach wall. The small shadows are caused by refraction artifacts from the rugal folds.

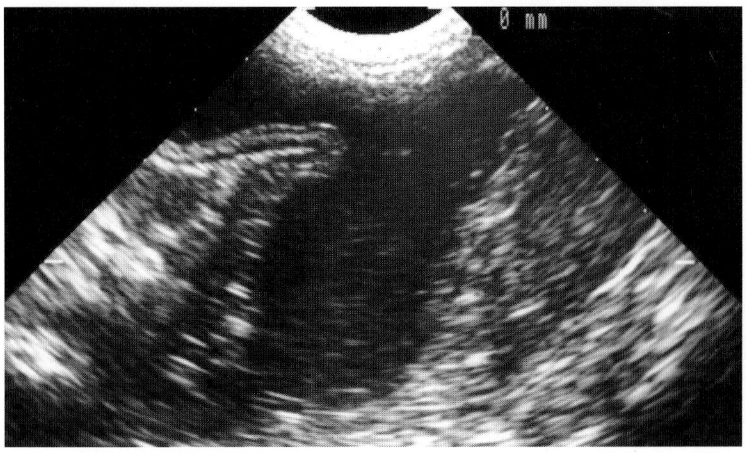

Figure 8-4. The sonogram of a normal fluid-filled stomach shows distention of the wall and a lack of rugal folds.

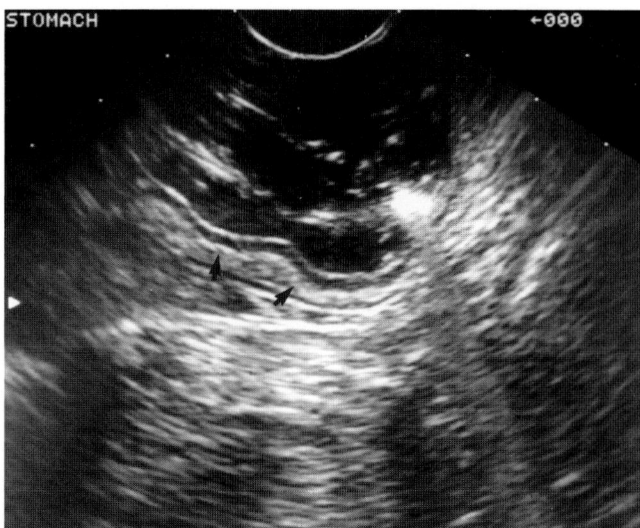

Figure 8-5. Endoscopic ultrasound image of the normal stomach wall (*arrows*). Gas and particles of food within the lumen create numerous artifacts.

duce a target sign or bull's-eye appearance (Fig. 8-6). Histologic correlations of these ultrasonographically recognizable layers have been well documented in the literature.[17] The five layers of the small intestine and the stomach, moving from the lumen outward, are:

- A thin, bright white echodense line that represents the interface of the adjacent mucosal surfaces in the empty bowel or the interface of the mucosa with gas or intestinal content
- A broad, hypoechoic to almost anechoic band that represents the mucosa
- A thin, echodense line that represents the submucosa
- A thin, hypoechoic band that represents the muscularis propria layer
- A thin, bright echodense line that is composed of the subserosa and serosa and the interface of the serosa with the mesentery (Fig. 8-7).[17]

Sonographic patterns that arise from the normal small bowel may be placed into three major categories.[3,18] A *mucous pattern* appears when echogenic material is seen within the bowel but does not have any associated artifacts such as reverberation or acoustic shadowing (Fig. 8-8). A *fluid pattern* arises from the presence of anechoic intraluminal material (Fig. 8-9). A *gas pattern* is seen when highly reflective gas within the

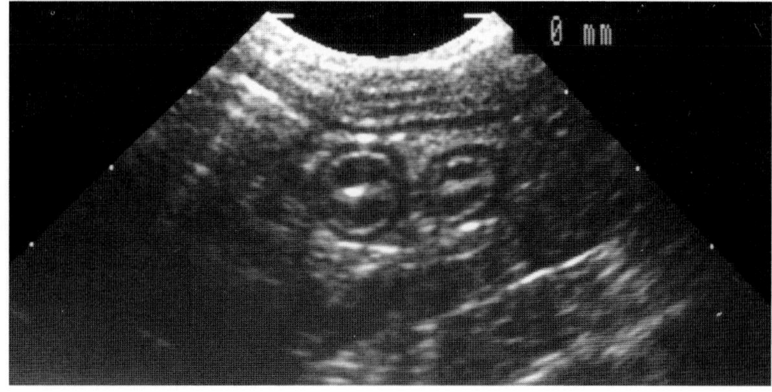

Figure 8-6. The transverse sonogram of the normal small intestine in a dog shows the alternating layers and the characteristic bull's-eye pattern. The mucosal interface appears as a white line rather than a dot, because the empty small intestine is a collapsed tube.

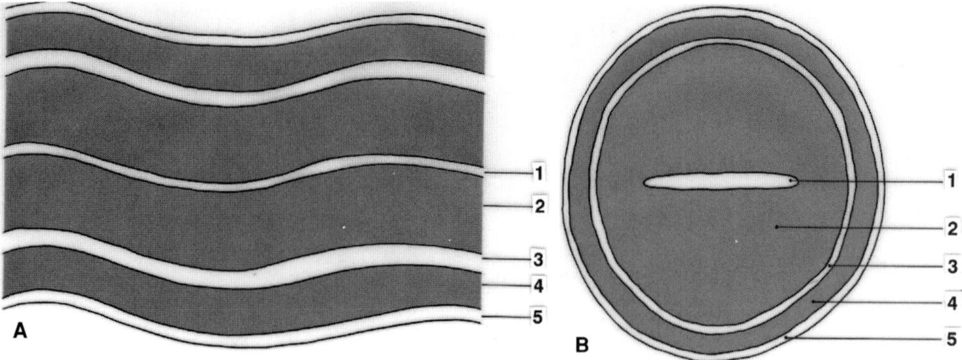

Figure 8-7. Line drawings illustrate (**A**) sagittal and (**B**) transverse views of the sonographic appearance of the normal small intestine. *1*, mucosal interface; *2*, mucosa; *3*, submucosa; *4*, muscularis propria; *5*, subserosa, serosa, and its interface with the mesentery.

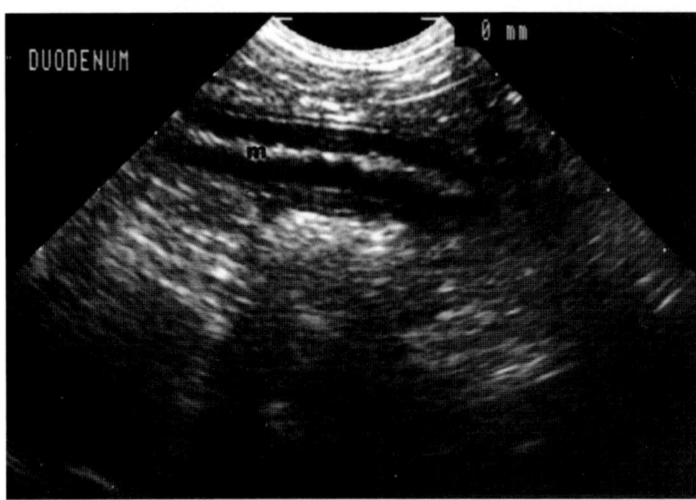

Figure 8-8. The sagittal sonogram of a normal small intestine demonstrates a mucous pattern. Echodense material in the lumen (*m*) interfaces with the mucosa without causing artifacts such as reverberation or shadowing.

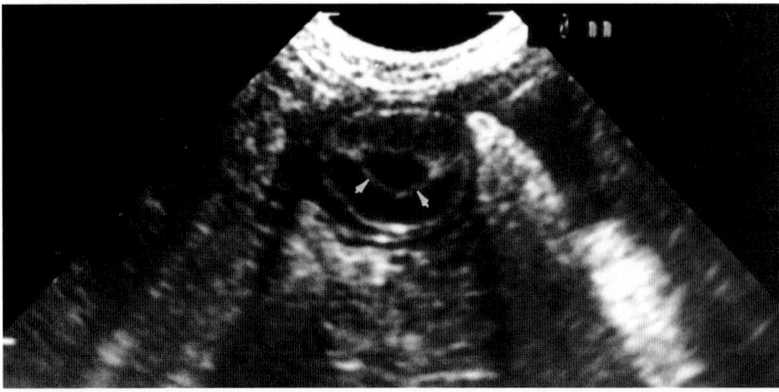

Figure 8-9. The transverse sonogram of a normal small intestine demonstrates a fluid pattern. Anechoic fluid is present within the lumen, and the mucosal interface (*arrows*) is a distinct bright line.

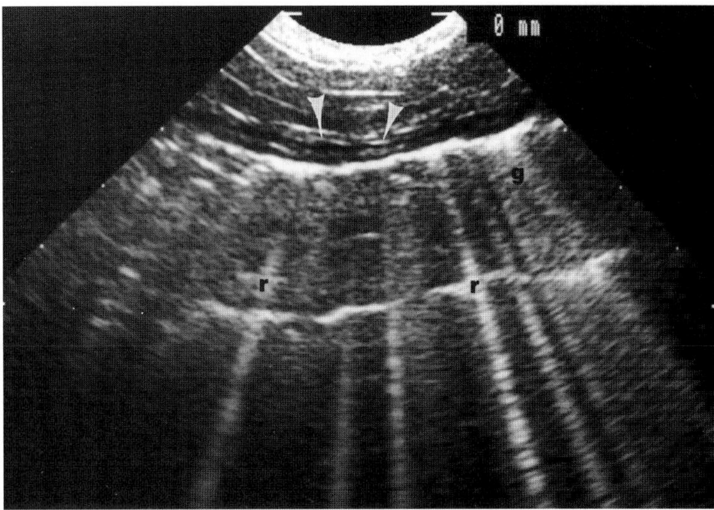

Figure 8-10. The sagittal sonogram of a normal small intestine shows a gas pattern. "Dirty" white acoustic shadows (*g*) and reverberation (*r*) artifacts prevent imaging of the entire circumference of the intestine. Only the layers of the near-field wall are seen (*arrows*).

bowel causes reverberations or a "dirty" or incomplete acoustic shadow (Fig. 8-10).[18,19]

The normal wall thickness of the canine small intestines has been reported as 2 to 3 mm.[11] Others, using high-resolution endoluminal transducers, have reported the normal range as 3.0 to 4.2 mm.[20] In my experience, the normal duodenal wall can be as thick as 5 mm. The thickness of the bowel should be measured only on images obtained in transverse sections, because oblique images may overestimate the wall thickness (Fig. 8-11).[21]

Normal proximal duodenal peristalsis is 4 to 5 contractions per minute, while small bowel contractions in the midabdominal region average 1 to 3 per minute.[11]

No distinction can be made among the different divisions of the small intestine with ultrasound. However, areas such as the duodenum may be identified by the location within the abdomen. The duodenum can be identified and followed by scanning it in a transverse plane as it exits the stomach.

Large Intestines

The large intestine or colon is nonsacculated in dogs and cats, and the cecum is not recognized as a separate entity. When the fluid-filled colon is imaged with high-resolution or transrectal transducers, five distinct layers with alternating echogenicity will be resolved (Fig. 8-12).[9] These layers are the same as those described for the small intestine and the stomach. However, resolution of all five layers during real-time imaging

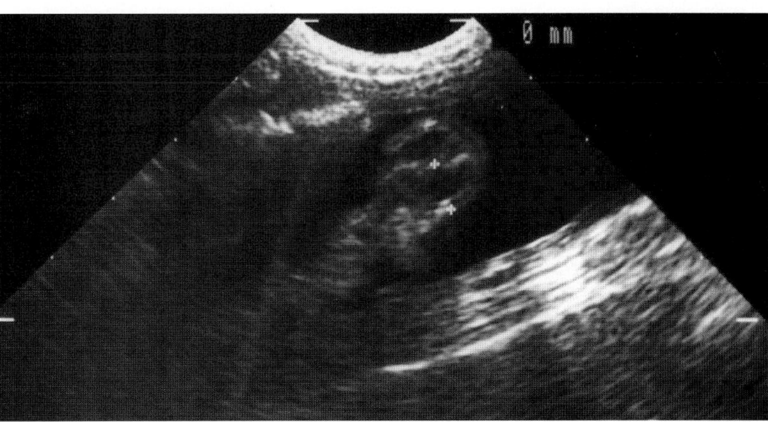

Figure 8-11. Calipers (+) demonstrate measurement of the normal small intestine in a dog with ascites.

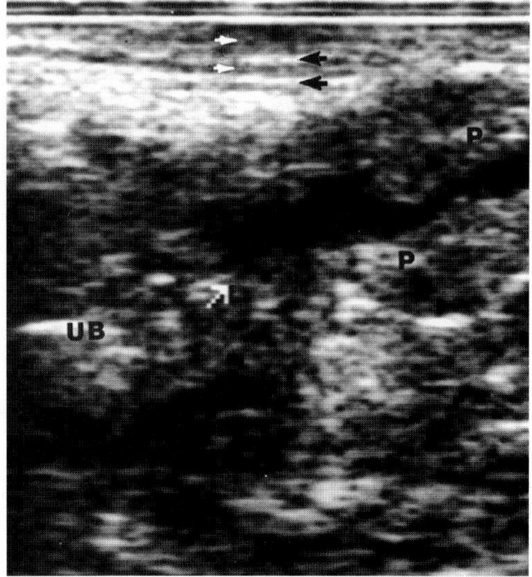

Figure 8-12. The transrectal ultrasound image of a mass in the urinary bladder neck (*UB*), urethra (*cursor arrow*), and prostate gland (*P*) in a dog shows the normal colonic wall in the near field. The mucosal interface is not seen because of transducer contact, but all other layers can be recognized (*alternating black and white arrows*).

is uncommon. The resolution is hampered by the presence of gas-containing feces within the lumen, which often appear as a mass that creates a dirty acoustic shadow or reverberation artifact, degrading the resolution of the wall layers (Fig. 8-13).

The normal thickness of the large intestinal wall is the same as for the small intestinal wall.[11] Peristalsis is not often observed when imaging the colon in real time.[11]

Colonic fluid with suspended echogenic material and large fecal masses may produce a highly reflective pseudomass with distant acoustic shadowing.[1,3] These artifacts create diagnostic dilemmas when imaging the pancreas and the urinary bladder (Fig. 8-14).

DISEASES OF THE GASTROINTESTINAL TRACT

Abnormalities of the GI tract are usually recognized by an alteration in the normal mucous or target pattern previously described.[1] Thickening of the wall gives rise to a target, pseudokidney, bull's-eye, cockade, or ring sign.[3,22–24] These changes are nonspecific for any one disease process; the term pseudokidney has been used to describe the wall thickening seen with neoplasia, inflammatory disease of the gut, or intussusception.[1]

Gastric Abnormalities

Hypertrophic Pyloric Stenosis

Hypertrophic pyloric stenosis occurs most often in small middle-aged or older purebred dogs. The disease is characterized by chronic, intermittent vomiting that occurs a few hours after eating.[25] Radiographically, the stomach may be distended and fluid filled.

Sonographically, the pylorus is circumferentially thickened, measuring 9 mm or greater in

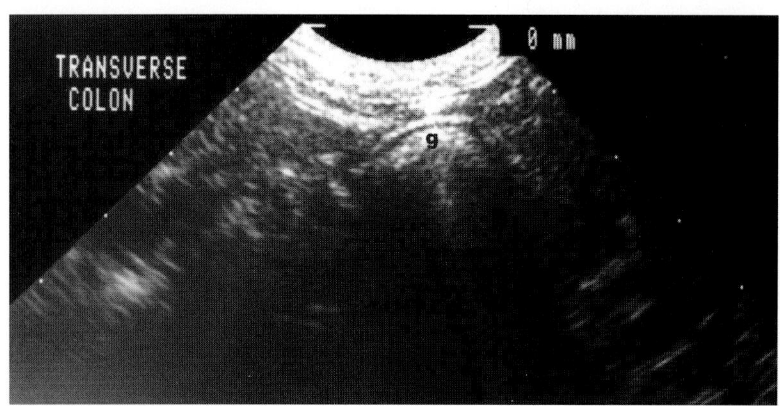

Figure 8-13. The transverse sonogram of a portion of the normal transverse colon in a dog shows a "dirty" acoustic shadow (*g*) resulting from the presence of gas and feces within the lumen.

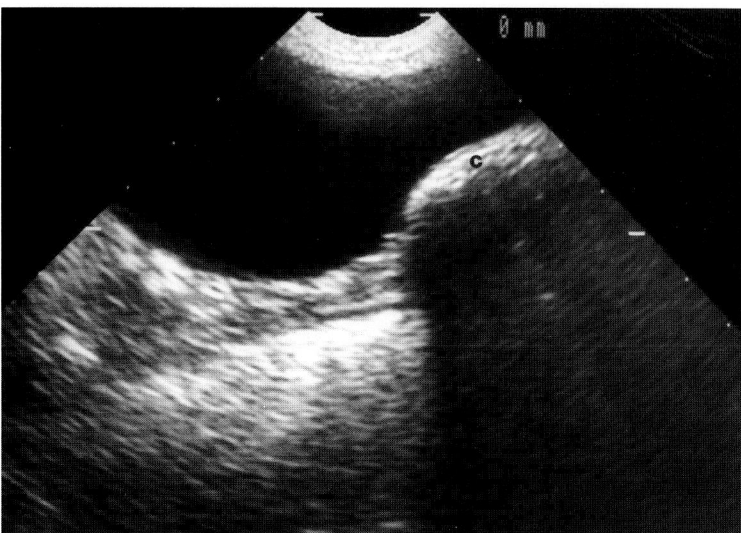

Figure 8-14. The sagittal sonogram of the urinary bladder demonstrates the pseudomass (*c*) created by the feces-filled descending colon. This type of artifact is often mistaken for cystic calculi because of its acoustic shadow.

diameter.[7,16] The muscularis layer remains hypoechoic and is 4 mm thick or larger.[7,26] On transverse imaging of the pylorus, this thickened muscular wall appears as a hypoechoic ring (Fig. 8-15*A*).[7,27] The stomach usually is distended with fluid or food, and peristalsis may be exaggerated (Fig. 8-15*B*). Little or no filling of the duodenum is evident during real-time imaging.

Gastric Foreign Bodies

The ultrasonographic appearance of ingested foreign objects depends on the nature of the foreign material and its ability to transmit or attenuate the ultrasound beam.[19] Many solid foreign bodies, whether radiopaque or radiolucent on routine abdominal radiographs, cast an acoustic shadow (Fig. 8-16*A*). The surface of many foreign objects acts as a strong reflector that creates a bright echogenic border and an acoustic shadow.[19] Gastric dilatation and hyperperistalsis may be evident in patients with gastric foreign bodies within the pyloric outflow tract (Fig. 8-16*B*). In addition to ingested foreign objects such as rubber balls and rocks, other gastric foreign objects such as trichobezoars may be detected with ultrasound.[28] Distention of the stomach with water and positional imaging of the animal may help to define free-moving echogenic foreign objects.

Gastritis

Gastritis most often appears as a diffusely thickened stomach wall. The layers are maintained, with thickening of the mucosa evident (Fig. 8-17).[29] Preliminary work in dogs suggests that pathologic thickening should be suspected when the stomach wall is more than 6 to 7 mm thick.[11] Acute and severe inflammation causes a uniform thickening of the wall (Fig. 8-18), and chronic gastritis may result in localized or diffuse thickening.[9] Localized thickening, which is often associated with ulcers, cannot be differentiated from neoplasia by ultrasound alone (Fig. 8-19).[9]

Gastric Ulcers

With gastric ulcers, a focal area of thickening of the stomach wall often contains a central echogenic focus (Fig. 8-20).[1,29] The ulcer crater may not be evident, and the thickness of the wall at the level of the ulcer may actually be reduced.[9] Because a large portion of the stomach is often inaccessible, sonography is not routinely used to evaluate ulcer disease.[9]

Uremic Gastropathy

In animals with renal dysfunction and uremia, several GI complications are observed. Those that can be recognized sonographically

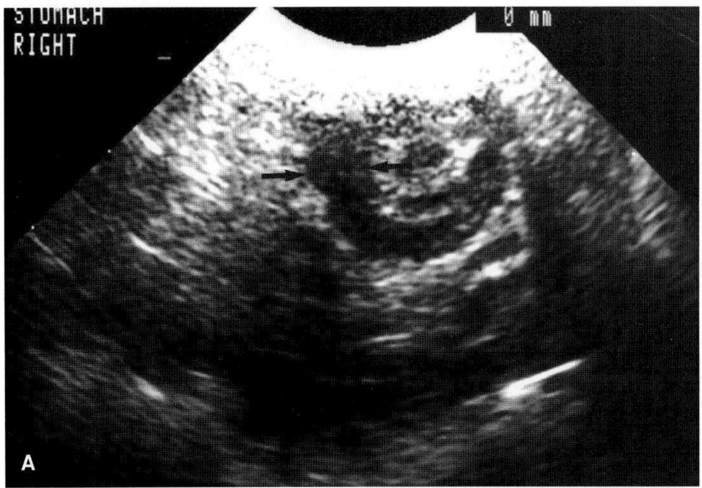

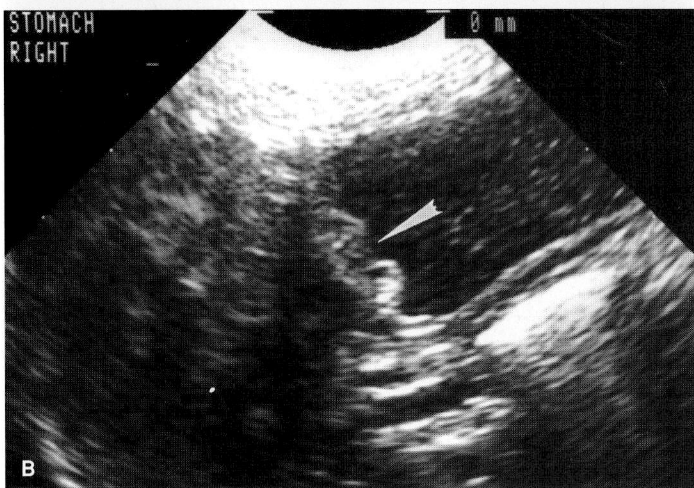

Figure 8-15. Hypertrophic pyloric stenosis. (**A**) Transverse sonogram of the pylorus of the stomach in a dog with hypertrophic pyloric stenosis. The muscular layer (*arrows*) is 5 mm thick. (**B**) Sagittal sonogram of the pyloric antrum of the stomach of the dog in **A**, showing the entrance to the pyloric canal (*arrowhead*). The stomach was fluid-filled, and increased peristalsis was evident on real-time imaging.

include hypertrophy of the gastric wall and its rugal folds and mineralization of the gastric mucosa and submucosal vasculature.[30,31] The thickness of the gastric wall often exceeds 9 mm, and the rugal folds will also appear thickened.[31] Mineralization of the gastric mucosa is indicated by an echogenic line of variable thickness within the superficial portion of the mucosa. The location differentiates mucosal mineralization from gas, which appears as a thin echogenic line on the mucosal surface (Fig. 8-21). Poor definition of the normal layers of the gastric wall may also be evident, which is probably associated with edema, hemorrhage, and inflammatory infiltrates, which are common histologic findings for dogs with severe uremia.[31]

Gastric Neoplasia

Gastric tumors have been reported in dogs and cats, but the incidence is relatively low. These include benign tumors, such as leiomyomas and adenomatous polyps, and malignant neoplasms, such as adenocarcinoma, lymphosarcoma, and leiomyosarcoma.[25] Metastatic neoplasia to the stomach is rare.

Small benign *polyps* are usually only seen with a fluid-filled stomach. Polyps have variable echogenicity and protrude into the gastric lumen (Fig. 8-22). *Leiomyomas* often appear as a circular hypoechoic mass continuous with the muscular layer of the stomach (Fig. 8-23).[9,10,16] *Adenocarcinoma* is the most common malignant

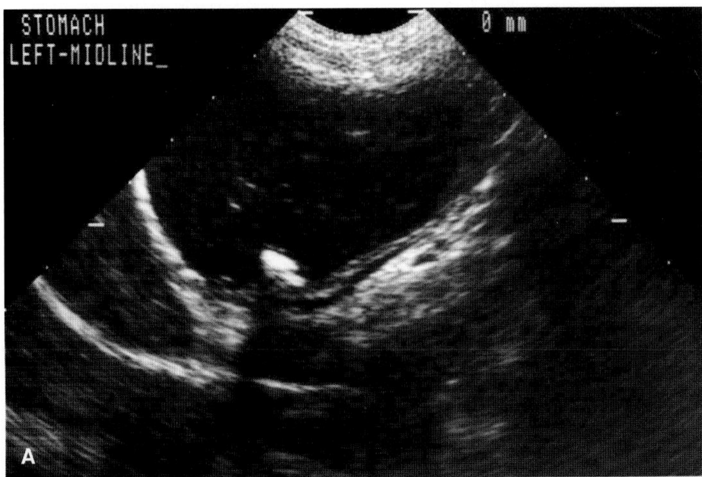

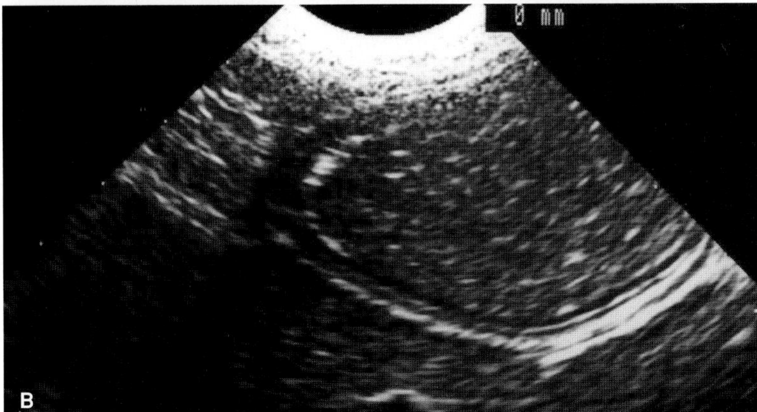

Figure 8-16. Gastric foreign bodies. (**A**) A small, irregular gastric foreign body (piece of rubber dog toy) casts an acoustic shadow in the stomach of the dog in Figure 8-15. This foreign body was freely movable in the fluid-filled stomach but too large to pass through the stenotic pyloric canal. (**B**) Gastric dilatation is a common finding with gastric foreign bodies that obstruct the pyloric outflow tract. Even though the fluid is moderately echoic, the normal wall layers can still be seen.

neoplasm in the canine stomach.[25] Sonographic identification depends on the location and extent of the tumor. Because a large part of the stomach is often not visualized, the water distention technique may be beneficial. Localized or diffuse wall thickening may be seen. Carcinomas may appear hypoechoic or moderately echoic, with irregular margins and disruption of the mucosa and muscularis due to infiltration (Fig. 8-24).[9,32] The stomach wall with a neoplasm is rigid and is unlikely to show peristalsis during real-time imaging.[10] When the neoplasm

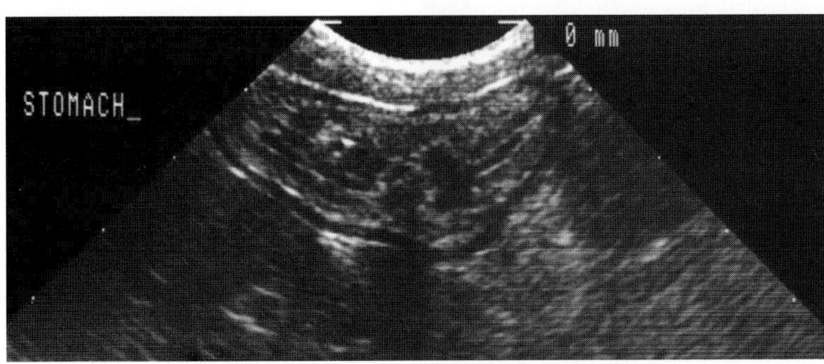

Figure 8-17. Sonogram of the stomach in a dog with diffuse mild gastric wall thickening (7 mm) associated with severe pancreatitis. The mucosa is thick and hyperechoic, and the wall layers are preserved.

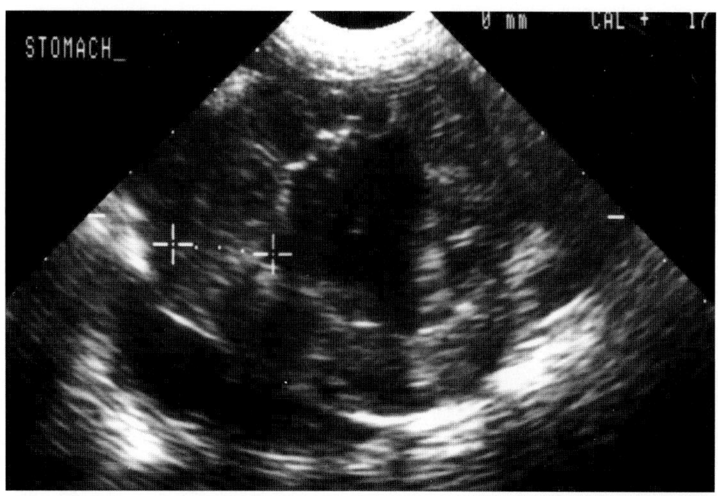

Figure 8-18. The sonogram of the stomach in a dog with acute severe gastritis shows diffuse wall thickening.

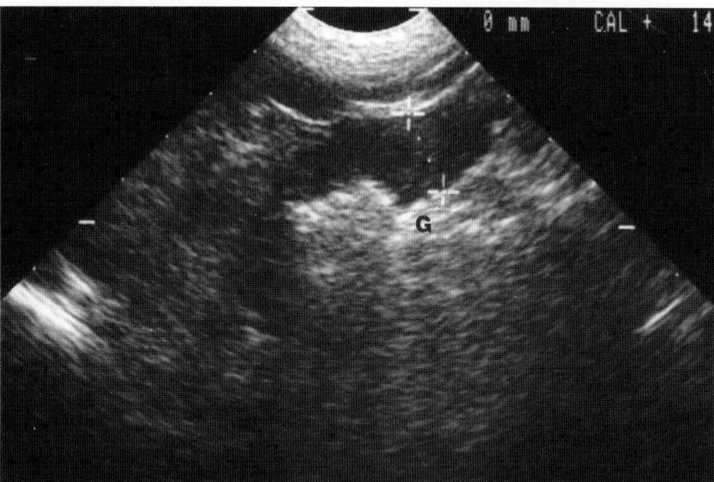

Figure 8-19. The sonogram of the stomach demonstrates localized gastric wall thickening in a dog with gastric ulcers. The layers are ill defined. The ulcer crater is not seen on this view. The lumen contains gas (*G*).

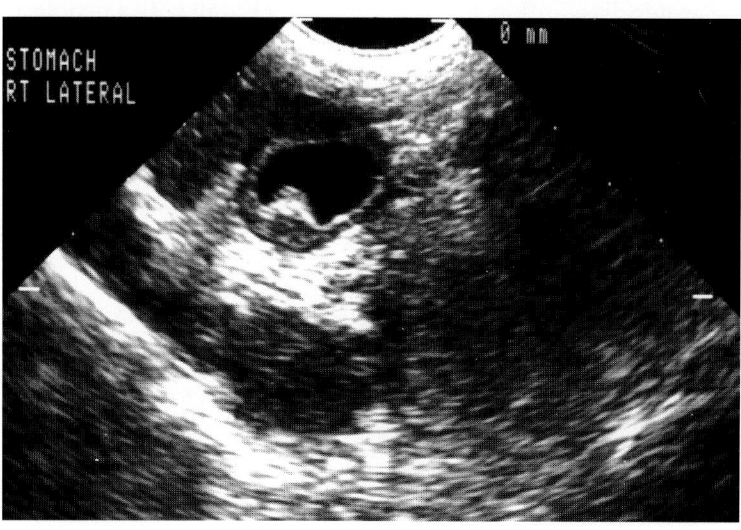

Figure 8-20. The sonogram of the stomach in a dog with an endoscopically confirmed large gastric ulcer near the pyloric antrum shows focal thickening involving the mucosa.

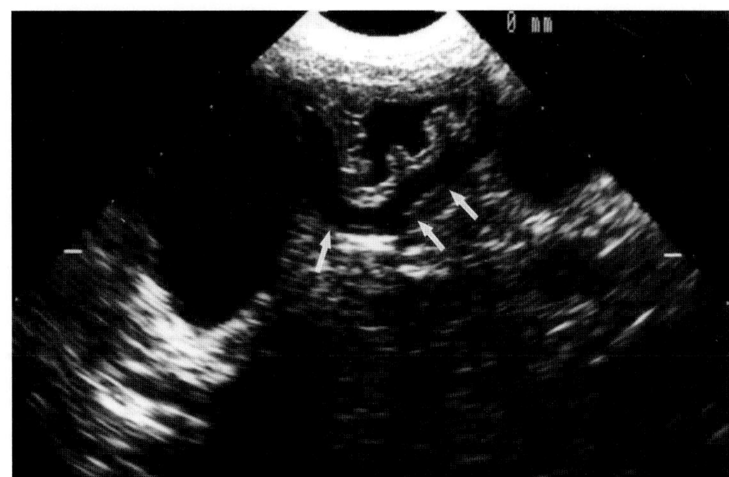

Figure 8-21. Transverse sonogram of the body of the stomach in a dog with uremic gastropathy. A thin, echodense line is evident within the superficial aspect of the mucosa, which is diffusely thickened. Small arrows indicate the serosal margin of the stomach.

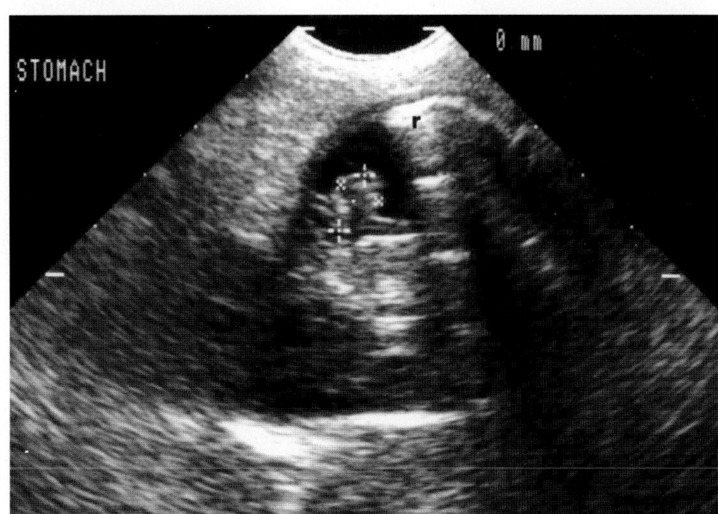

Figure 8-22. Sonogram of the stomach in a dog with a benign polyp. Notice the reverberation artifact (*r*) resulting from gas, which obliterates portions of the stomach wall.

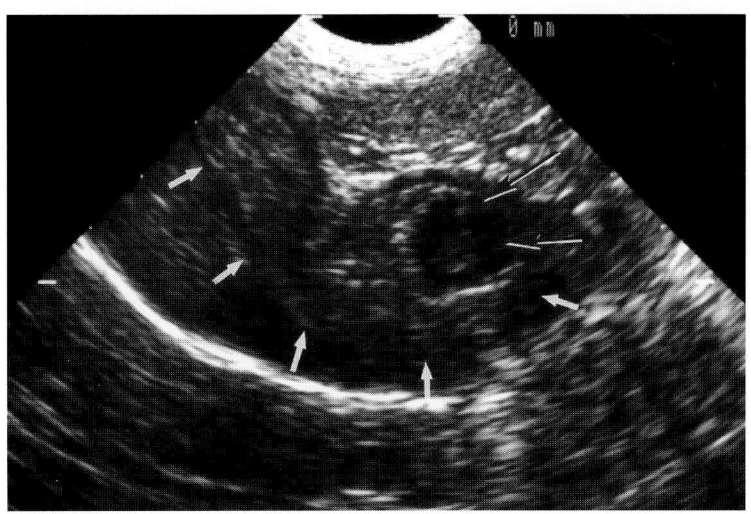

Figure 8-23. Sonogram of the empty stomach (*white arrows*) in a dog with a leiomyoma. The mass (*black arrows*) is circular and hypoechoic and most likely arises from the muscularis propria. Filling the stomach with fluid is necessary to determine which layers are involved.

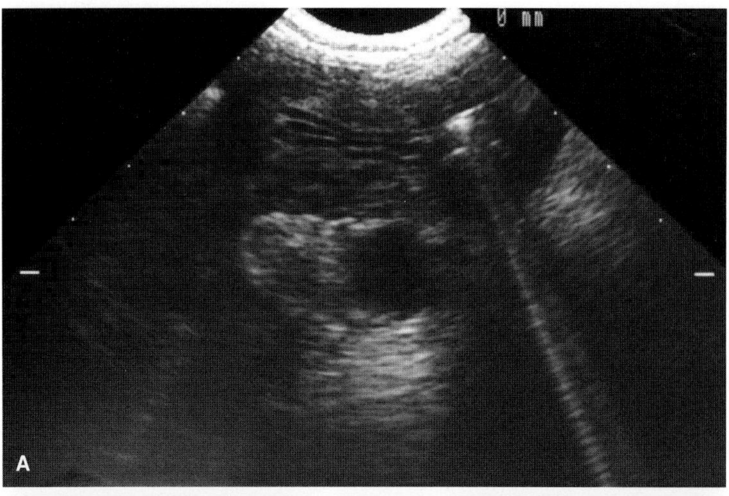

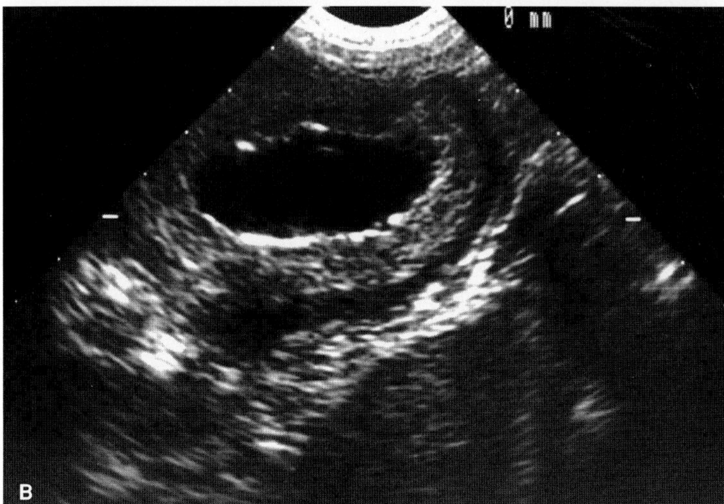

Figure 8-24. Gastric adenocarcinoma. (**A**) Localized wall thickening of a portion of the body of the stomach in a dog. The mucosa is thickened and moderately echoic. Decreased peristalsis was seen during real-time imaging. The remainder of the stomach wall was normal. (**B**) Diffuse gastric wall thickening in a dog, with moderately echoic uniform thickening of the mucosa throughout. No peristalsis was observed during real-time imaging. The diagnosis was made by ultrasound-guided fine-needle aspiration.

involves the pyloric antrum, gastric dilatation may be evident because of outflow obstruction.

Lymphosarcoma is the most common gastric neoplasm in the cat.[25] Typically, gastric lymphoma appears as thickened hypoechoic mucosa, which is caused by tumor infiltration (Fig. 8-25). The transverse view of the empty stomach affected with lymphosarcoma gives a classic pseudokidney appearance. However, other patterns have also been reported.[32,33]

Leiomyosarcomas are large solitary masses of intramural origin, usually found in the muscularis propria, although they can arise from the muscularis mucosa.[32] As it rapidly outgrows the blood supply, the center of the tumor often becomes echogenic. Large leiomyosarcomas can also appear to be extragastric. If gastric neoplasia is detected, it is important to examine the patient for regional lymphadenopathy and hepatic metastasis.

Small Intestine Abnormalities

Obstruction and Dilatation

Ileus, which is the failure of transit or passage of GI contents, may be caused by mechanical obstruction or an absence of peristalsis. In either case, the most significant sonographic feature is the intraluminal accumulation of fluid.[9]

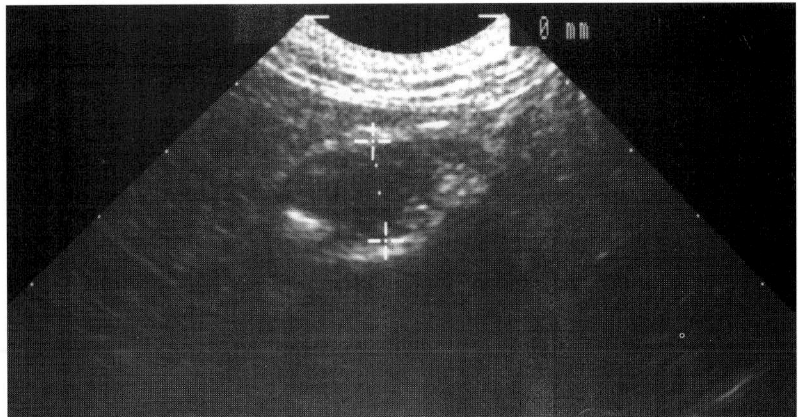

Figure 8-25. Sonogram of the stomach in a cat with lymphosarcoma. The wall is irregularly thickened and hypoechoic. Notice the similarity of this lesion to the focal gastritis lesion in Figure 8-19.

Small bowel *obstruction* often causes dilation of bowel loops proximal to the obstruction (Fig. 8-26). Because the small intestine cannot be "run" with ultrasound as in surgery, contrast radiography may be more helpful in identifying the area of obstruction. With small bowel obstruction, the dilated bowel loops are normal or have increased peristaltic activity, unless the obstruction has been longstanding.[34,35] The fluid-filled loops have normal wall thickness (2 to 3 mm) and appear anechoic centrally, with tubular (long-axis view) or round (cross-sectional view) shapes (Fig. 8-27).[9]

Paralytic ileus also causes fluid-filled loops of intestines. These loops of bowel lack peristalsis and are uniform in size (Fig. 8-28). Viral enteritis and other inflammatory diseases such as pancreatitis and peritonitis can cause paralytic ileus.[16,34]

Intestinal Foreign Bodies

Whenever small bowel dilatation is recognized sonographically, mechanical obstruction due to foreign objects must be considered. Ultrasound characteristics of small bowel obstruction include variable-sized intestinal loops, with large fluid-filled loops proximal to the foreign body, an abrupt change in bowel diameter at the obstruction (Fig. 8-29*A*), and a consistent intraluminal object that causes acoustic shadowing

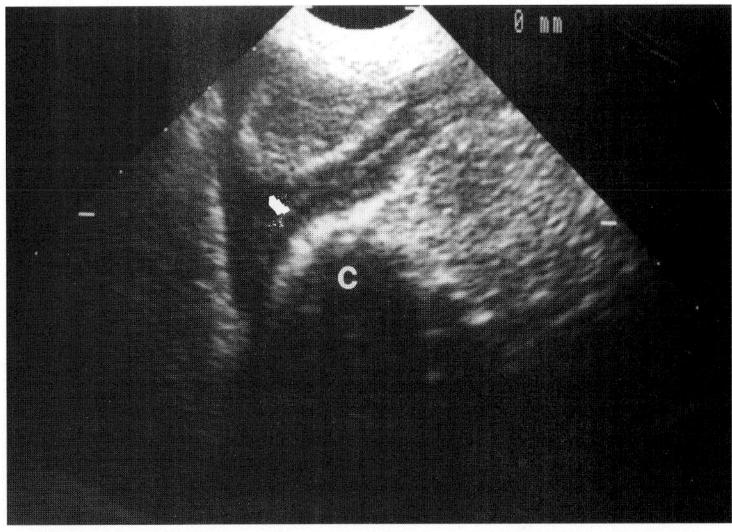

Figure 8-26. Sonogram of small bowel dilatation due to obstruction. The bowel loops are distended with echoic fluid, and peristalsis was increased on real-time imaging. The obstruction was a corncob foreign body (C).

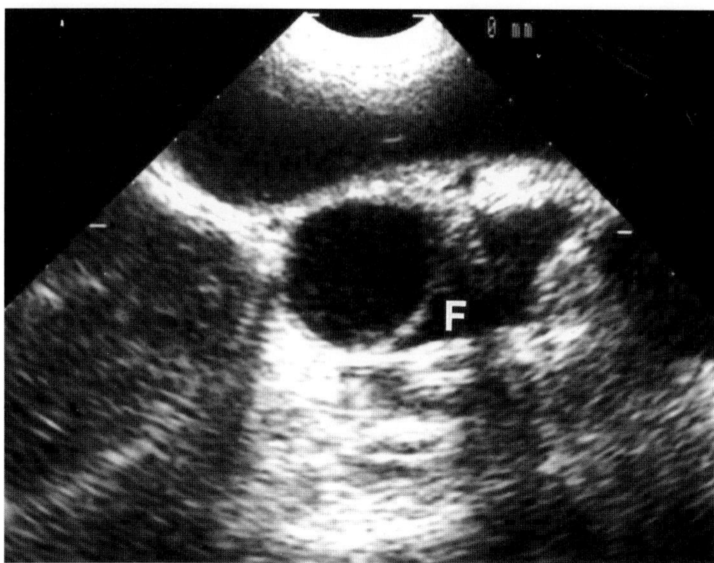

Figure 8-27. Sonogram of small bowel dilatation due to obstruction. The fluid-filled loops are seen in long- and short-axis views, and a small amount of ascites is evident (*F*). This long-standing obstruction resulted in decreased peristalsis on real-time imaging. The obstruction was caused by intussusception.

(Fig. 8-29*B*, *C*).[34] The bowel commonly is hypermotile proximal to the obstruction, unless the obstruction is chronic.

Many types of intestinal foreign bodies have been recognized sonographically.[19,36] Linear foreign bodies may not be visible, but plication or corrugation of the bowel is considered diagnostic (Fig. 8-29*D*).[19,37] If the GI obstruction results in excess gas, diagnosis with ultrasound becomes difficult or impossible.[34]

Intussusception

Most intussusceptions are ileocolic, although small intestinal intussusception and cecocolic intussusceptions occur. The sonographic appearance is a bull's-eye or target-like lesion with multiple concentric rings, which results from viewing the involved segment in cross section (Fig. 8-30*A*).[38,39] With low-frequency transducers, a thickened hypoechoic outer rim and an echogenic center are seen. These layers represent the edematous intussuscipiens surrounding the compressed mucosal and serosal surfaces of the intussusceptum (Fig. 8-30*B*).[38] With higher-frequency transducers, a multiple concentric ring appearance may be detected as the various layers of the bowel walls of the intussusceptum and the intussuscipiens are resolved (Fig. 8-30*C*).[9,16,40,41] The sonographic pattern

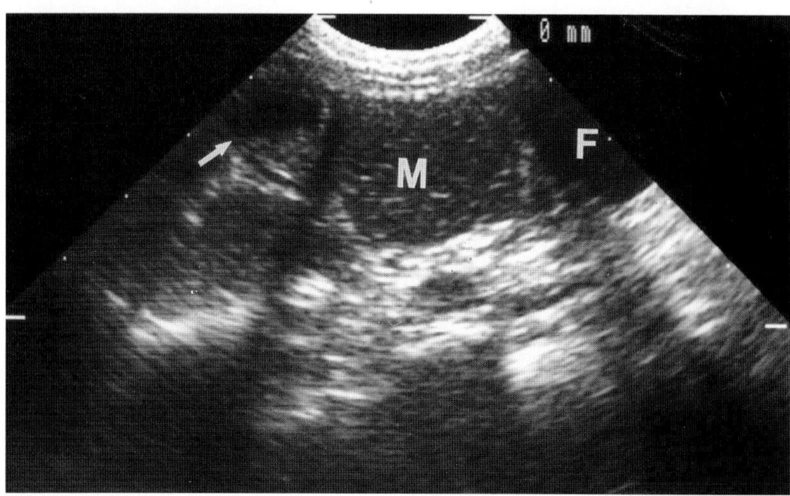

Figure 8-28. Sonogram of small bowel dilatation due to paralytic ileus. Three bowel loops are seen in cross section. One is filled with anechoic fluid (*F*); another is filled with echoic fluid, creating a pseudomass effect (*M*); and the third shows layering of echoic particles within the fluid (*arrow*). The latter is indicative of bowel stasis and poor mixing of intestinal contents. This dog had parvoviral enteritis.

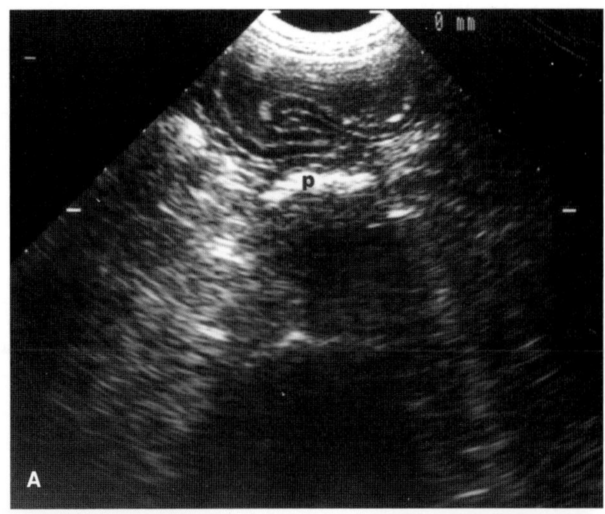

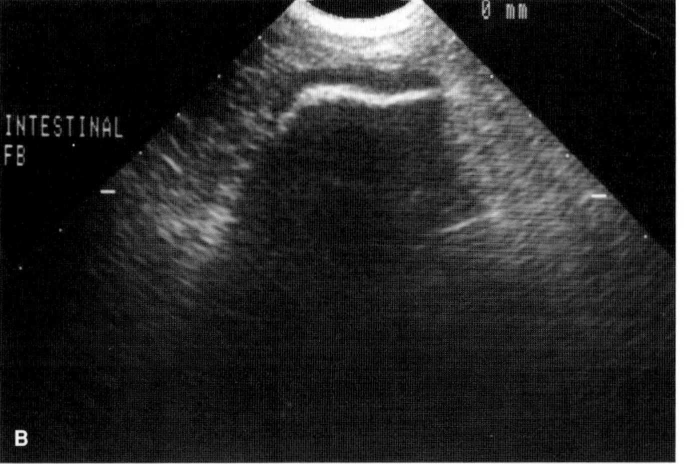

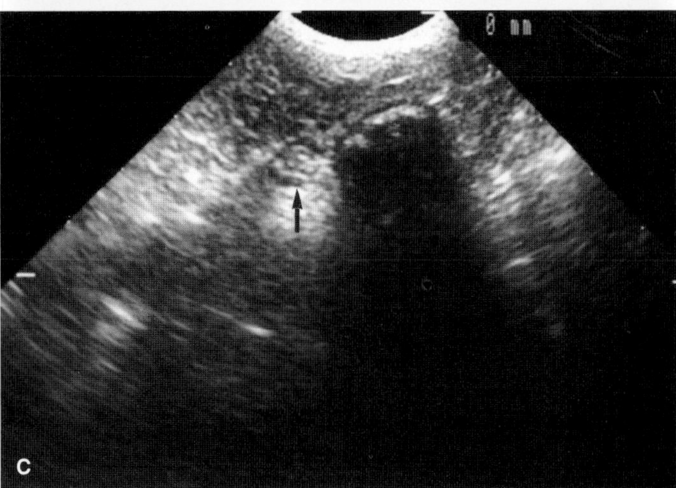

Figure 8-29. Small intestinal foreign bodies. (**A**) Sonogram of the intestine in a dog with a foreign body with portions of the pecan shell intact (*P*). Notice the abrupt change in bowel diameter near the foreign body. On real-time imaging, the proximal intestine was hypermotile. (**B**) Sonogram of the intestine in a dog with a bone foreign body. The acoustic shadow created by the foreign object was consistent in shape and location on real-time imaging. Notice the hypoechoic bowel wall due to inflammation. (**C**) Sonogram of the intestine in a cat with a cloth-covered plastic button foreign body. Compare the size with the cross section of normal empty small intestine (*arrow*). *(continued)*

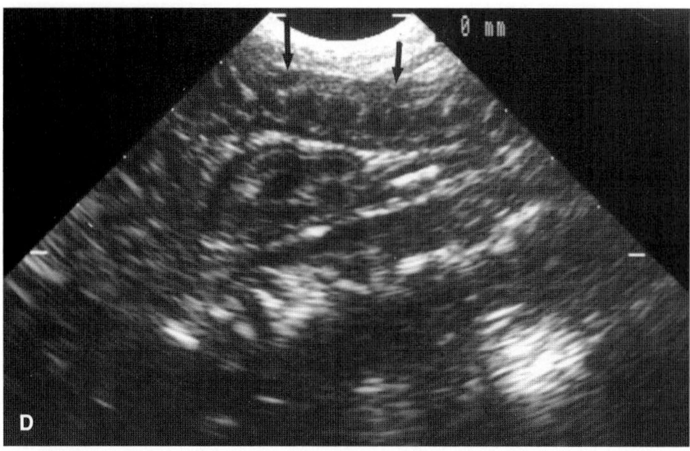

(**Figure 8-29.** *(Continued)* (**D**) Sonogram of the intestine in a puppy with a linear foreign body. Notice the corrugation of the intestine (*arrows*).

varies with the length of the segment of bowel involved and the orientation of the scanning plane relative to the long axis of the intussusception.[38] In a longitudinal view, a lumen within a lumen is often seen (Fig. 8-30*D*).[42] Scanning the affected area in long axis helps to make a definitive diagnosis of intussusception, because the target lesion itself is a nonspecific finding.[3,9]

Inflammatory Disease

Unless the inflammatory process produces thickening of the bowel wall, ultrasound is unlikely to demonstrate any abnormality.[3] Preliminary work suggests that pathologic thickening should be suspected when the bowel wall is more than 5 mm thick.[11,21] Although inflammatory bowel wall thickening varies in symmetry and degree, it usually involves a long segment of the bowel (Fig. 8-31*A*).[3] Typical ultrasound features of diffuse GI inflammatory and infiltrative diseases are dilatation with reduced peristalsis, diffusely thickened bowel wall (Fig 8-31*B–D*), and regional (mesenteric) lymphadenopathy. Parvoviral enteritis causes paralytic ileus with no change in the thickness of the GI wall.[16] Severe pancreatitis may cause thickening of the duodenal wall, with disruption of the normal layered appearance (Fig. 8-31*E*).[16] *(text continues on p. 170)*

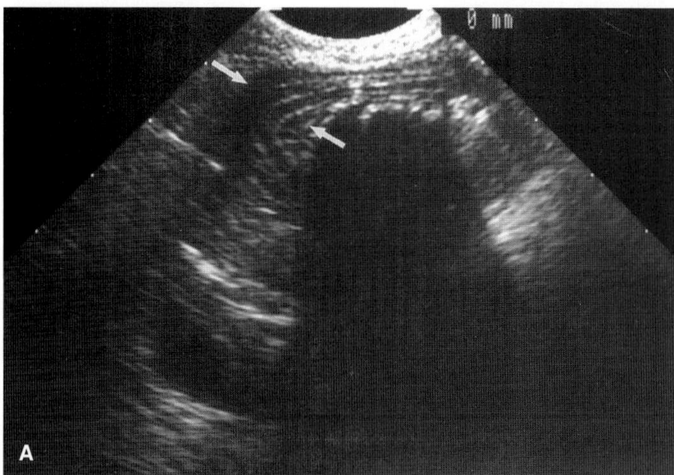

Figure 8-30. Intussusception. (**A**) Transverse sonogram of an intussusception in a dog, showing the multiple concentric rings from the bowel wall layers (*between arrows*). The central acoustic shadows were the result of small bone fragments trapped at this level.

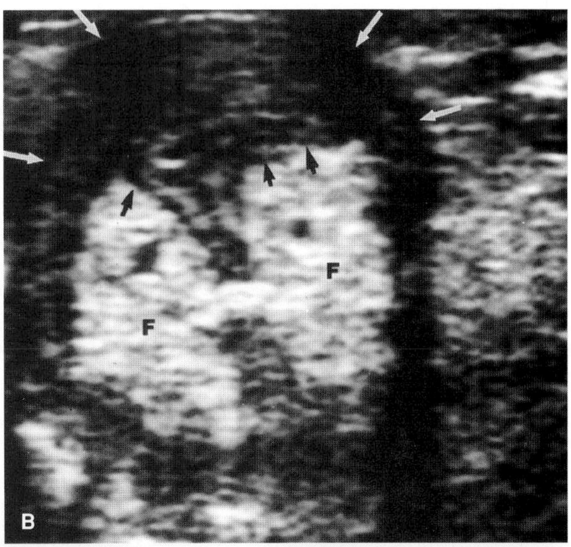

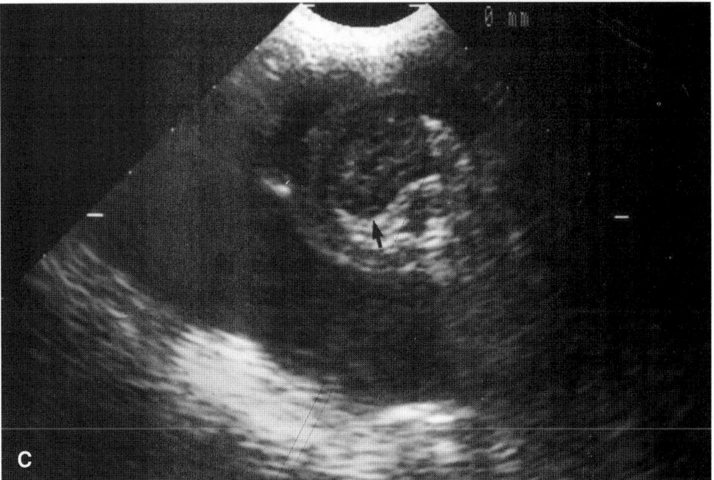

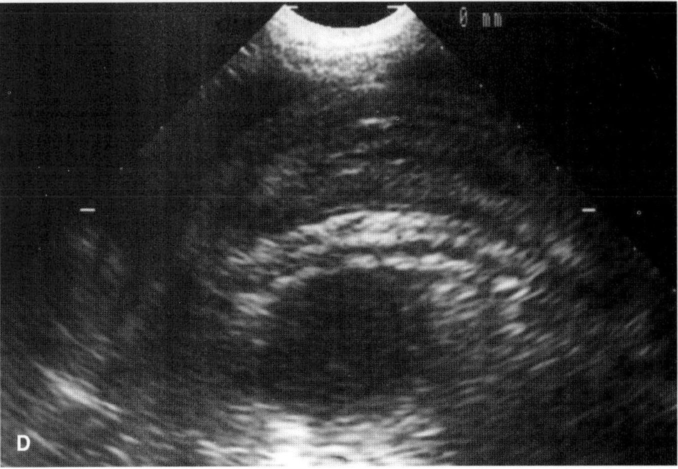

Figure 8-30. *(Continued)* (**B**) Transverse sonogram of an intussusception in a dog, showing the compressed bowel wall of the intussuscipiens (*black arrows*) within the intussusceptum (*white arrows*). The echodense area within the intussusceptum is entrapped mesenteric fat (*F*). (**C**) Transverse sonogram of an intussusception in a dog, showing the layers of the wall of the intussuscipiens (*arrow*). (**D**) Long-axis or sagittal sonogram of the intussusception seen in **C**, showing the lumen within a lumen.

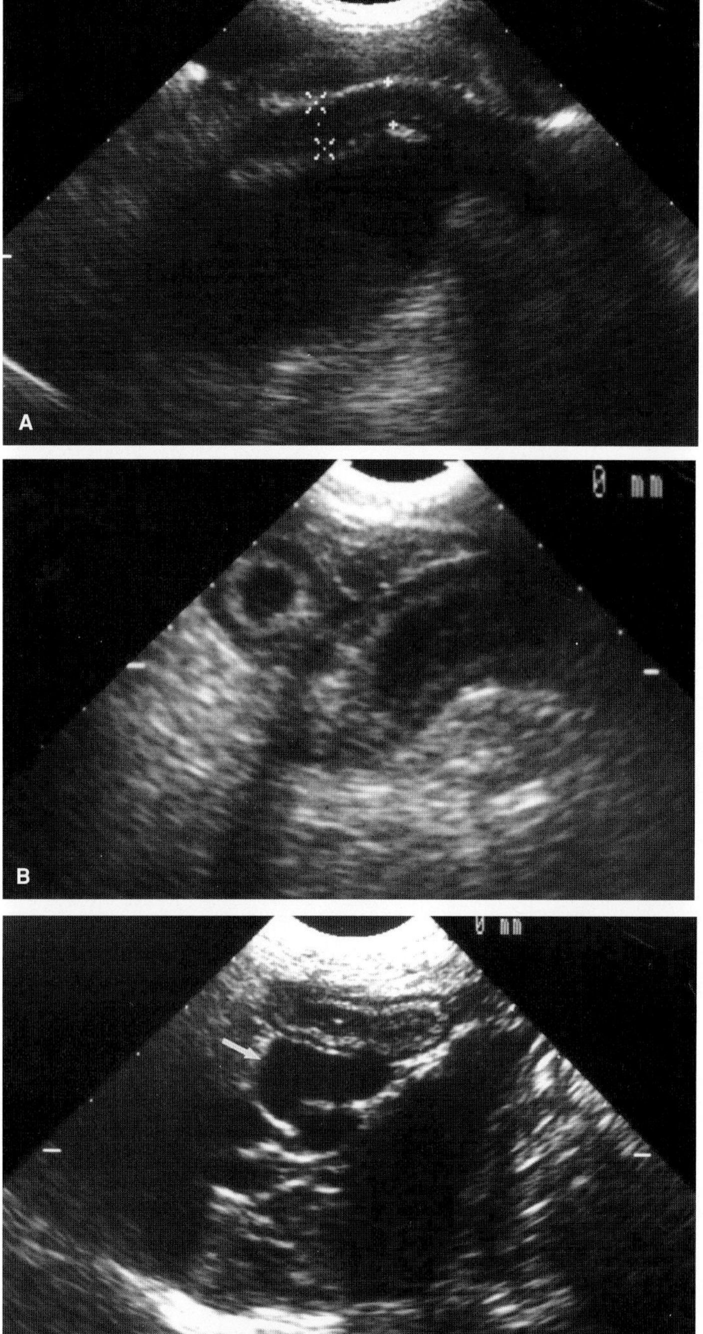

Figure 8-31. Inflammatory bowel disease. (**A**) Sagittal sonogram of the descending duodenum in a dog with lymphocytic, plasmacytic enteritis and lymphangiectasia with ascites. Notice the uniform involvement of the duodenum, which was 7 mm thick. (**B**) Sagittal and transverse views of diffusely thickened small intestine in a dog with extensive gastrointestinal wall hemorrhage secondary to disseminated intravascular coagulation. (**C**) Transverse sonogram of the proximal duodenum in a dog with severe necrotizing enteritis (cause undetermined). Although the bowel wall is not noticeably thickened, the mucosa and submucosa are prominent. The tortuous anechoic structure (*arrow*) deep to the intestine is the dilated bile duct.

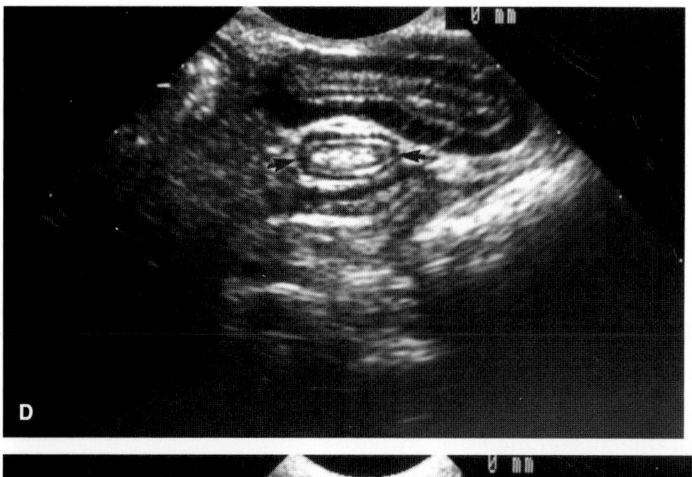

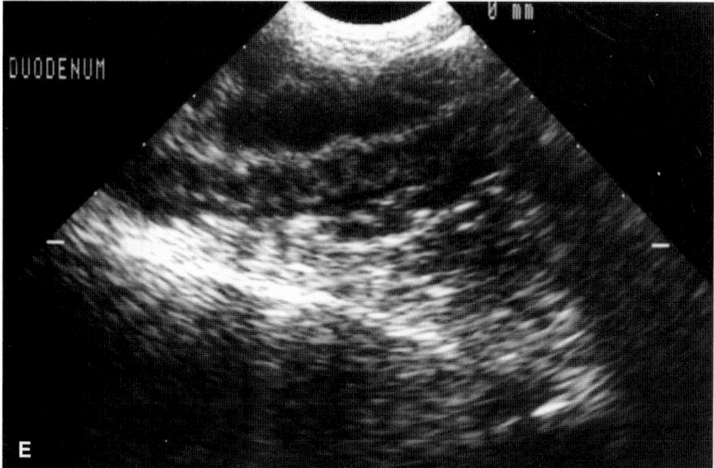

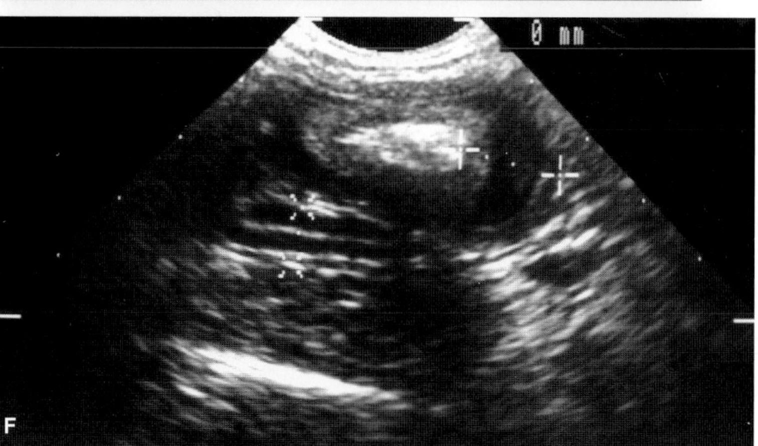

Figure 8-31 *(Continued)* (**D**) Sonogram of a uniformly thickened segment of small intestine in a cat with feline infectious peritonitis. Compare the wall thickness and appearance with the nearby small intestine (*arrows*). (**E**) Sagittal sonogram of the duodenum in a dog with severe pancretitis. The duodenum is distended with fluid. The pleated appearance of the bowel wall persisted during real-time imaging, implying spasticity or paralytic ileus. (**F**) Transverse sonogram of a segment of intestine in a dog with infiltration due to intestinal phycomycosis. The mucosa and submucosa are thickened, and the bowel wall is 14 mm thick.

Granulomatous or Infiltrative Disease

Some of the mycotic infections involve the GI tract, more commonly the small bowel, but they can also affect the stomach.[25,43] These organisms include *Histoplasma capsulatum*, *Pythium* spp., *Aspergillus* spp., and *Candida albicans*.[30] As these diseases infiltrate the mucosa or submucosa, they can cause focal, mass-like, or diffuse wall thickening (Fig. 8-31*F*). As a result of this infiltration, a reduction in peristalsis of the affected area of the GI tract may be noticed. This type of inflammation cannot be differentiated from neoplasia on the basis of wall thickening or the symmetry of this thickening.[9,16]

Small Intestinal Neoplasia

The distinction between inflammation and neoplasia cannot be made on the basis of wall symmetry or thickness. However, it seems that the morphology of the layers is more often preserved in inflammatory diseases, but not in tumors.[16]

Lymphosarcoma and adenocarcinoma are the most common small intestinal tumors in dogs and cats.[43] With the exclusion of lymphosarcoma, all other small intestinal neoplasms are sonographically characterized by a localized mass. Tumors such as adenocarcinoma and leiomyosarcoma disrupt the bowel wall layers, are often eccentric, and may be hypoechoic (Fig. 8-32).[24] Leiomyosarcomas in people frequently have solid and cystic areas as a result of necrosis (Fig. 8-33).[1,3] Lymphosarcoma may appear as a discrete mass or diffuse involvement.[43] Intestinal lymphosarcoma typically causes diffuse bowel wall thickening that appears as a single homogeneous, thick, hypoechoic layer between the hyperechoic mucosal and serosal interfaces (Fig. 8-34).[3,9] The lumen may be empty or dilated with fluid, and peristalsis is lacking (Fig. 8-35). The appearance may be indistinguishable from bowel wall thickening from other causes.[1,3] Identification of the wall layers involved may help to determine the primary tumor site.[16] As with neoplasms of the stomach, scanning for regional lymphadenopathy should be done.

Large Intestine Abnormalities

Disease of the large bowel can be detected transabdominally and also transrectally with the use of endorectal or transrectal ultrasound probes. The introduction of higher-frequency transducers has increased the potential for ultrasound diagnosis of intestinal diseases, because the transducer is in direct contact with the mucosal surface, avoiding gas-tissue interfaces. Detection of regional metastases may be less accurate with the ultrahigh-frequency probes because of their limited depth of penetration.

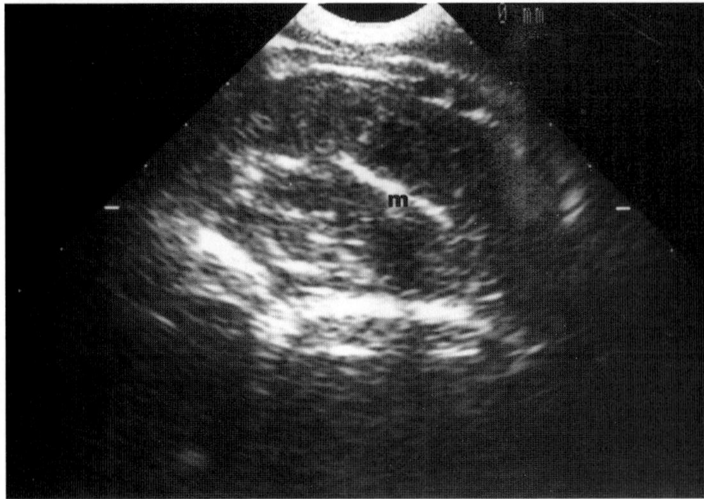

Figure 8-32. Sonogram of an annular adenocarcinoma of the small intestine in a dog. The mucosal interface is represented by a bright white central line (*m*). All other bowel wall layers are disrupted.

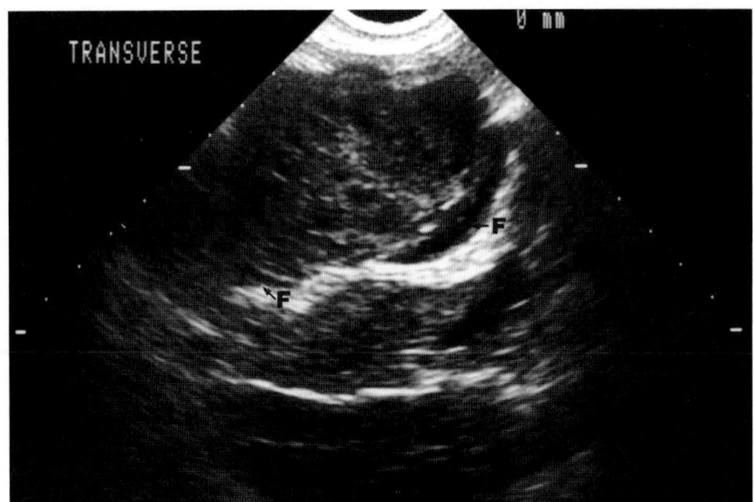

Figure 8-33. Sonogram of a leiomyosarcoma of the small intestine in a dog. The tumor has mixed echogenicity and is eccentric. The lumen contains a small amount of anechoic fluid (*F*).

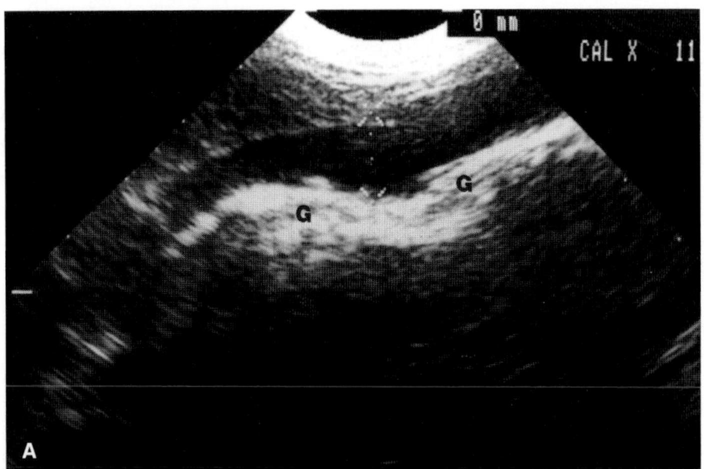

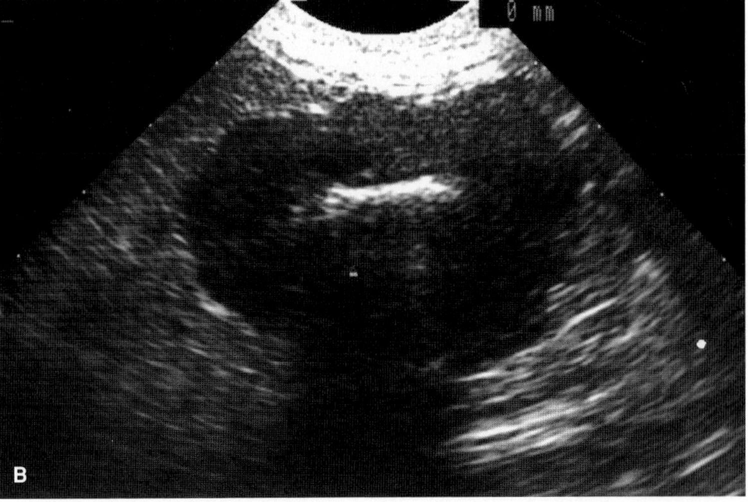

Figure 8-34. (**A**) Sagittal and (**B**) transverse sonograms of the small intestine in a cat with lymphosarcoma. Notice the thick hypoechoic bowel wall with only the mucosa and serosa evident. Only the near wall of the intestine is seen in the sagittal view because of the gas in the lumen (*G*).

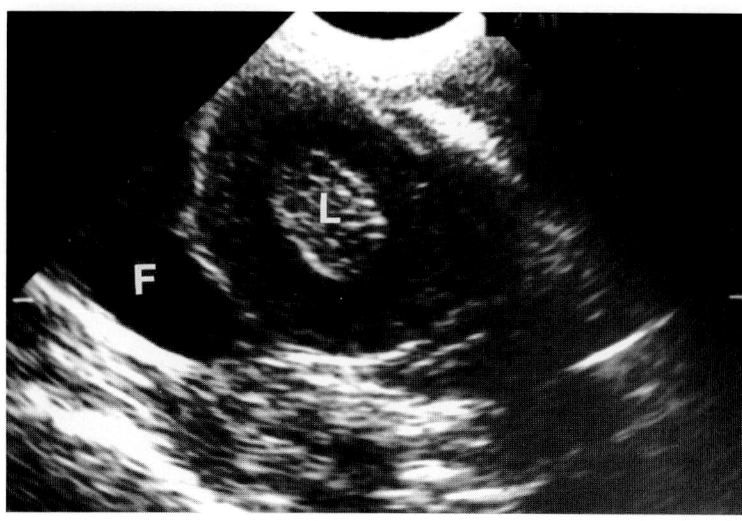

Figure 8-35. Transverse sonogram of intestinal lymphosarcoma in a cat. The lumen (*L*) is distended with echoic fluid. Ascites (*F*) is also present. Notice the classic target or bull's-eye pattern.

The sonographic findings for inflammatory diseases of the large bowel are similar to those for the small intestine.[24,44] The sonographic findings of intussusception have already been described.

The most common neoplasm in the canine large intestine is adenocarcinoma (Fig. 8-36), and lymphosarcoma is the most common neoplasm in the feline large intestine (Fig. 8-37).[45] Benign adenomatous polyps and leiomyomas occur as well.[45] Numerous reports from the human medical literature make use of endorectal sonography for diagnosis and staging of colorectal neoplasms.[1,9] Staging is possible with

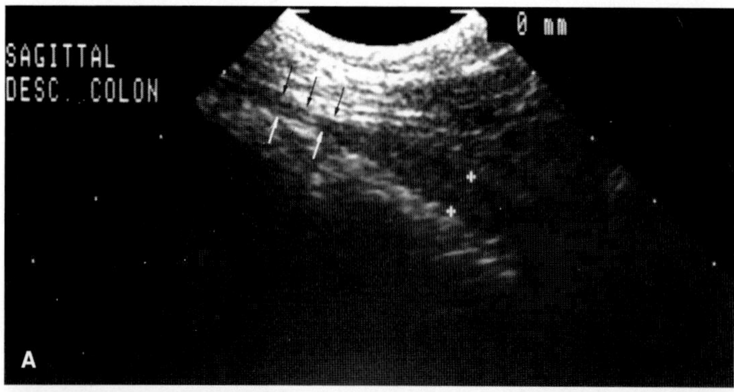

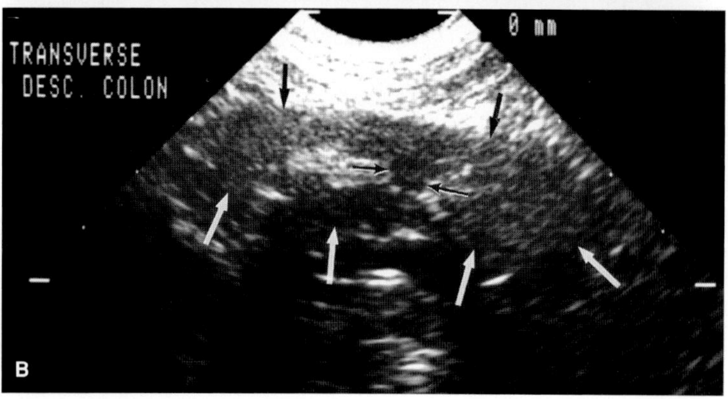

Figure 8-36. (**A**) Sagittal and (**B**) transverse sonograms of the descending colon in a dog with adenocarcinoma. (**A**) The ill-defined borders of this tumor are seen between the layered normal colon wall (*arrows*) and the infiltrative tumor (+ calipers). The far wall of the colon is not seen because of artifacts from gas and feces. (**B**) The transverse view shows the nonuniform bowel wall thickening and a polypoid extension of the tumor into the lumen (*small black arrows*). Large arrows delineate the serosal margins of the colon.

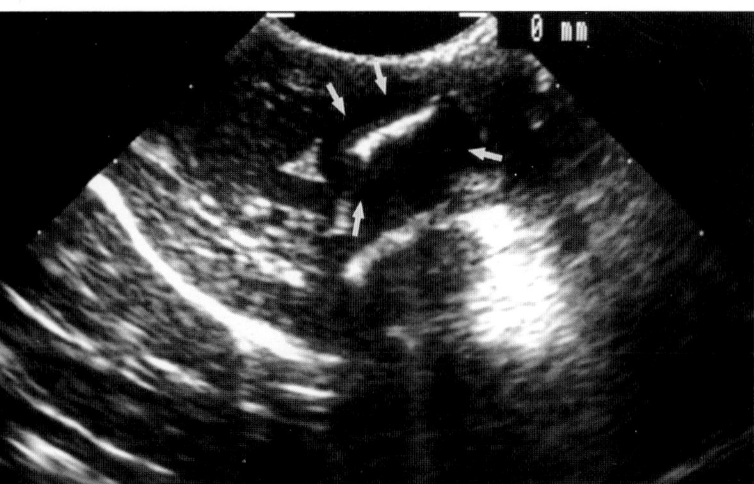

Figure 8-37. Sonogram of the hepatic flexure of the transverse colon in a cat with lymphosarcoma. The diffuse, infiltrative appearance of this tumor may be indistinguishable from bowel wall thickening due to other causes *(arrows)*.

high-frequency transducers, which can be used to identify the extent of involvement of the layers of the wall.[46,47]

BIOPSY TECHNIQUES

The techniques for performing ultrasound-guided biopsies or fine-needle aspirates of GI lesions have been reported in the veterinary literature.[48,49] Masses and infiltrative lesions usually result in less peristalsis, and motility of the segment to be sampled is usually not a problem. Although the normal thickness of the wall is less than 5 mm, focal masses or areas of infiltration may be large enough to be sampled with fine-needle aspiration. Ultrasound-guided tissue biopsies are reserved for larger masses.

Bowel wall thickness greatly influences the ability to achieve an accurate diagnosis.[49] Localization of the needle tip is important in sampling the bowel wall. Large lesions are easier to sample, and needle tip location is less critical.[48,49]

CONCLUSION

Improvements in technology and scanning techniques using fluid and gravity allow detection of significant lesions of the stomach and intestines sonographically. Real-time imaging provides the ability to assess the presence or absence of peristalsis. Ultrasound can be used as a first diagnostic measure in cases of palpable abdominal masses if involvement of the GI tract is suspected.[9] In many instances, ultrasound should not replace contrast studies and endoscopy.[50] Ultrasound of the upper GI tract is extremely operator dependent, and it takes time and experience to become adept at making a proper diagnosis.[26]

REFERENCES

1. Dubbins PA. Gastrointestinal tract and peritoneum. In: Goldberg BB, ed. Textbook of abdominal ultrasound. Baltimore: Williams & Wilkins, 1993:221.
2. Holm HH. Ultrasonic scanning in the diagnosis of space-occupying lesions of the upper abdomen. Br J Radiol 1971;44:24.
3. Dubbins PA. The gastrointestinal tract. In: Kurtz AJ, ed. Clinics in diagnostic ultrasound: gastrointestinal ultrasonography. New York: Churchill Livingstone, 1988:195.
4. Evans HE, Christensen GC. The digestive apparatus and abdomen. In: Evans HE, Christensen GC, eds. Miller's anatomy of the dog. 2nd ed. Philadelphia: WB Saunders, 1979:411.
5. Rosenzweig LJ. The Organization of the coelom and the digestive and respiratory systems. In: Rosenzweig LJ, ed. Anatomy of the cat: text and dissection guide. Dubuque: William C Brown, 1990:140.

6. Ellenport CR. Carnivore digestive system. In: Getty R, ed. Sisson and Grossman's the anatomy of the domestic animals. 5th ed. Philadelphia: WB Saunders, 1975:1538.
7. Biller DS, Partington BP, Miyabayashi T, Leveille R. Ultrasonographic appearance of chronic hypertrophic pyloric gastropathy in the dog. Vet Radiol Ultrasound 1994;35:30.
8. Dimling GM. Right lower quadrant pain. In: Sanders RC, ed. Clinical sonography: a practical guide. 2nd ed. Boston: Little, Brown and Co, 1991:201.
9. Mittlestaedt CA. Gastrointestinal tract. In: Mittlestaedt CA, ed. General ultrasound. New York: Churchill Livingstone, 1992:449.
10. Worlicek H, Dunz D, Engelhard K. Ultrasonic examination of the wall of the fluid-filled stomach. J Clin Ultrasound 1989; 17:15.
11. Penninck DG, Nyland TG, Fisher PE, Kerr LY. Ultrasonography of the normal canine gastrointestinal tract. Vet Radiol 1989;30:272.
12. Botet JF, Lightdale C. Endoscopic ultrasonography of the upper gastrointestinal tract. In: Silver B, ed. The radiologic clinics of North America: ultrasonography of small parts. Philadelphia: WB Saunders, 1992;30:1067.
13. Leopold GR, Asher WM. Deleterious effects of gastrointestinal contrast material on abdominal echography. Radiology 1971;98:637.
14. Sarti DA, Lazere A. Reexamination of the deleterious effects of gastrointestinal contrast material on abdominal echography. Radiology 1978;126:231.
15. Bolondi L, Casanova P, Santi V, et al. The sonographic appearance of the normal gastric wall: an in vivo study. Ultrasound Med Biol 1986;12:991.
16. Penninck DG, Nyland TG, Kerr LY, Fisher PE. Ultrasonographic evaluation of gastrointestinal diseases in small animals. Vet Radiol 1990;31:134.
17. Kimmey MB, Martin RW, Haggitt RC, et al. Histologic correlates of gastrointestinal ultrasound images. Gastroenterology 1989;96:433.
18. Fleischer AC, Muhletaler CA, James AE. Sonographic patterns arising from normal and abnormal bowel. In: James AE, ed. Radiologic clinics of North America: symposium on advances in ultrasonography, vol 18. Philadelphia: WB Saunders, 1980:145.
19. Tidwell AS, Penninck DG. Ultrasonography of gastrointestinal foreign bodies. Vet Radiol Ultrasound 1992;33:160.
20. Goldberg BB, Liu JB, Merton DA, Kurtz AB. Endoluminal US: experiments with nonvascular uses in animals. Radiology 1990;175:39.
21. Fleischer AC, Muhletaler CA, James AE. Sonographic assessment of the bowel wall. Am J Roentgenol 1981;136:887.
22. Fakhry JR, Berk RN. The "target" pattern: characteristic sonographic feature of stomach and bowel abnormalities. Am J Roentgenol 1981;137:969.
23. Bluth EI, Merritt CRB, Sullivan MA. Ultrasonic evaluation of the stomach, small bowel, and colon. Radiology 1979;133: 677.
24. Bozkurt T, Richter F, Lux G. Ultrasonography as a primary diagnostic tool in patients with inflammatory disease and tumors of the small intestine and large bowel. J Clin Ultrasound 1994;22:85.
25. Twedt DC, Magne ML. Diseases of the stomach. In: Ettinger SJ, ed. Textbook of veterinary internal medicine: diseases of the dog and cat. 3rd ed. Philadelphia: WB Saunders, 1983:1289.
26. Haller JO, Cohen HL. Hypertrophic pyloric stenosis: diagnosis using US. Radiology 1986;161:335.
27. Spevak MR, Ahmadjian JM, Kleinman PK, et al. Sonography of hypertrophic pyloric stenosis: frequency and cause of nonuniform echogenicity of the thickened pyloric muscle. Am J Roentgenol 1992;158:129.
28. Goff WB, Kilcheski TS. A gastric bezoar causing a target lesion as revealed by ultrasound. J Ultrasound Med 1984;3: 275.

29. Hayden CK, Swischuk LE, Rytting JE. Gastric ulcer disease in infants: US findings. Radiology 1987;164:131.
30. Grooters AM, Miyabayashi T, Biller DS, Merryman J. Sonographic appearance of uremic gastropathy in four dogs. Vet Radiol Ultrasound 1994;35:35.
31. Chew DJ, DiBartola SP. Diagnosis and pathophysiology of renal disease. In: Ettinger SJ, ed. Textbook of veterinary internal medicine: diseases of the dog and cat. 3rd ed. Philadelphia: WB Saunders, 1989:1893.
32. Johnson BA. A proposed new sonographic sign to aid in further differentiation of gastric neoplasms. J Diagn Med Sonogr 1987;3:21.
33. Bolondi L, Casanova P, Caletti GC, et al. Primary gastric lymphoma versus gastric carcinoma: endoscopic US evaluation. Radiology 1987;165:821.
34. Saunders HM, Pugh CR, Rhodes WH. Expanding application of abdominal sonography. J Am Anim Hosp Assoc 1992;28:369.
35. Morgan CL, Trought WS, Oddson TA, et al. Ultrasound patterns of disorders affecting the gastrointestinal tract. Radiology 1980;135:129.
36. Tennenhouse JE, Wilson SR. Sonographic detection of a small-bowel bezoar. J Ultrasound Med 1990;9:603.
37. Spaulding KA, Bunch SE, Hardie EM, Flynn MF. Veterinary case of the day. J Ultrasound Med 1990;9:S103.
38. Bowerman RA, Silver TM, Jaffe MH. Real-time ultrasound diagnosis of intussusception in children. Radiology 1982;143:527.
39. Verbanck JJ, Rutgeerts LJ, Douterlungne PH, et al. Sonographic and pathologic correlations in intussusception of the bowel. J Clin Ultrasound 1986;14:393.
40. Holt S, Samuel E. Multiple concentric ring sign in the ultrasonographic diagnosis of intussusception. Gastrointest Radiol 1978;3:307.
41. Montali G, Croce F, De Pra L, Solbiati L. Intussusception of the bowel: a new sonographic pattern. Br J Radiol 1983;56:621.
42. Miller JH, Kemberling CR. Ultrasonic scanning of the gastrointestinal tract in children: subject review. Radiology 1984;152:671.
43. Sherding RG. Diseases of the small bowel. In: Ettinger SJ, ed. Textbook of veterinary internal medicine: diseases of the dog and cat. 3rd ed. Philadelphia: WB Saunders, 1989:1323.
44. Dubbins PA. Ultrasound demonstration of bowel wall thickness in inflammatory bowel disease. Clin Radiol 1984;35:227.
45. Richter KP. Diseases of the large bowel. In: Ettinger SJ, ed. Textbook of veterinary internal medicine: diseases of the dog and cat. 3rd ed. Philadelphia: WB Saunders, 1989:1397.
46. Wang KY, Kimmey MB, Nyberg DA, et al. Colorectal neoplasms: accuracy of US in determining the depth of invasion. Radiology 1987;165:827.
47. St Ville EW, Jafri SZH, Madrazo BL, et al. Endorectal sonography in the evaluation of rectal and perirectal diseases. Am J Roentgenol 1991;157:503.
48. Penninck DG, Crystal MA, Matz ME, Pearson SH. The technique of percutaneous ultrasound guided fine-needle aspiration biopsy and automated microcore biopsy in small animal gastrointestinal diseases. Vet Radiol Ultrasound 1993;34:433.
49. Crystal MA, Penninck DG, Matz ME, et al. Use of Ultrasound-guided fine-needle aspiration biopsy and automated core biopsy for the diagnosis of gastrointestinal diseases in small animals. Vet Radiol Ultrasound 1993;34:438.
50. Bartolozzi C, Menchi I, Pozzo CD, et al. Radiologic exploration of the upper gastrointestinal tract: the usefulness of ultrasonography and computed tomography. J Belge Radiol 1984;67:377.

Small Animal Ultrasound, edited by Ronald W. Green.
Lippincott-Raven Publishers, Philadelphia © 1996.

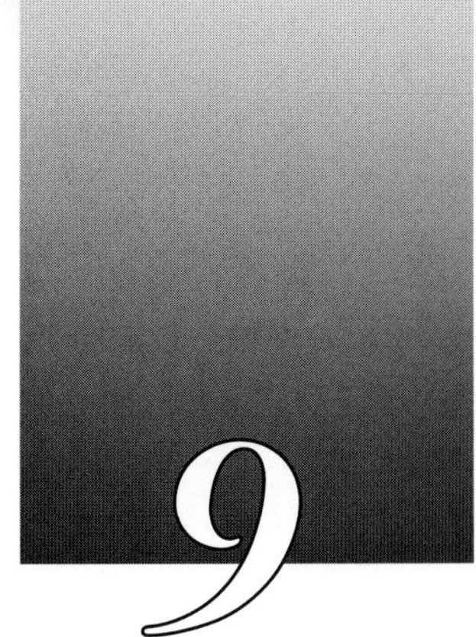

PANCREAS

Linda D. Homco

The pancreas has only recently become a part of most routine abdominal sonographic examinations. Advances in ultrasound imaging systems, which provide improved resolution and gray scale, allow us to image even the normal pancreas in dogs and cats. The pancreas, because of its similar echogenicity with surrounding tissues and the interference of gas from nearby gastrointestinal viscera, was once thought to be unidentifiable ultrasonographically unless it was diseased. Knowledge of the anatomy of the pancreas and surrounding organs in the dog and cat is essential for sonographic identification of the normal and the abnormal pancreas.

NORMAL ANATOMY AND LOCATION

The pancreas is a V-shaped organ consisting of two long lobes or limbs that meet at an acute angle caudal to the pylorus (Fig. 9-1).[1] The right lobe is medial and slightly dorsal to the descending duodenum, extends caudally in this plane, and usually terminates at the duodenal loop just beyond the caudal pole of the right kidney. This limb is ventral to the right kidney and dorsal to the ileum and cecum. Loops of jejunum and the ascending colon may lie ventral to this limb and often interfere with imaging.[2] The left lobe lies in the greater omentum and passes from the right to left cranial abdomen along the greater curvature of the stomach. It is bounded dorsally by the liver and splenic vein, cranioventrally by the stomach, and caudoventrally by the transverse colon. This limb terminates near the hilus of the spleen at or near the cranial pole of the left kidney.

The body of the pancreas, also referred to as the pancreatic angle, joins the two limbs and lies within the gastroduodenal angle ventral to the portal vein and caudomedial to the pylorus.[2] The body of the pancreas is located in the right cranial quadrant in the dog, and in the cat, it is located nearer midline because of the position of the pyloric portion of the cat's stomach. The anatomic relation of the pancreas with cranial abdominal viscera is otherwise similar in the cat (Fig. 9-2).[3,4]

The right limb is typically long, thin, and somewhat slender compared with the left limb, which is thicker and only two thirds as long.[2] There are usually two pancreatic ducts in the dog, the larger of which opens into the duodenum with or within proximity to the bile duct.[1,2] The cat typically has only one pancreatic duct, although an accessory duct has been described in 20% of cats.[5] The main pancreatic duct runs centrally throughout the length of each limb.[2]

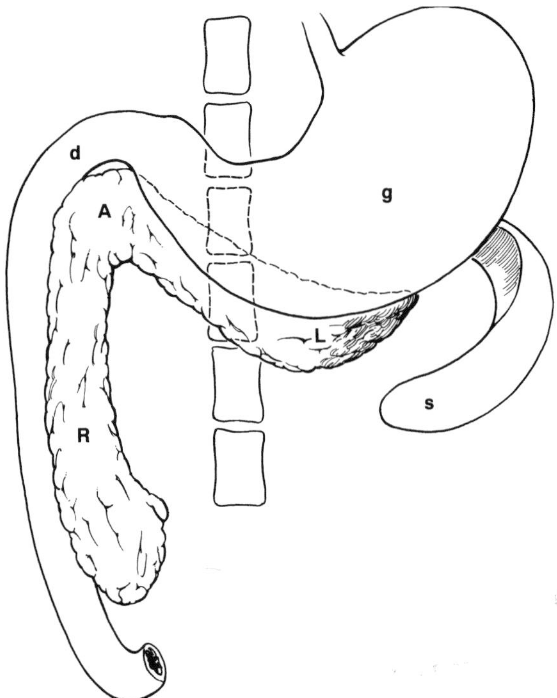

Figure 9-1. Line drawing illustrating the normal location and shape of the pancreas in the dog. *R*, right limb; *A*, angle (body); *L*, left limb; *d*, duodenum; *g*, stomach; *s*, spleen.

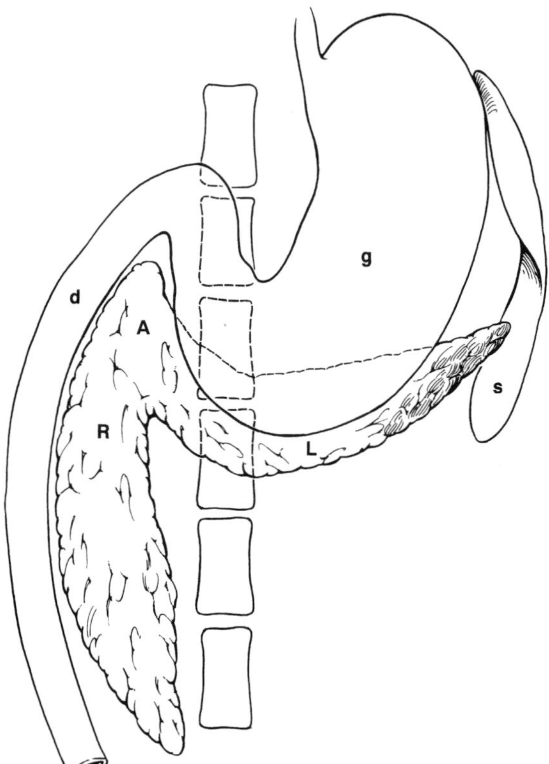

Figure 9-2. Line drawing illustrating the normal location and shape of the pancreas in the cat. *R*, right limb; *A*, angle (body); *L*, left limb; *d*, duodenum; *g*, stomach; *s*, spleen.

SCANNING TECHNIQUES

It is best to perform an ultrasound examination of the pancreas in a fasted animal, because an empty stomach is less likely to interfere with imaging of the body and left limb and because fasting reduces the overall amount of bowel gas. A cleansing enema is helpful in removing material from the transverse colon, but it should not be done within 2 hours of scanning because it introduces gas into the gastrointestinal tract.

An ultrasound examination of the pancreas can be done with the patient in almost any position. It is important to consider the organization of gastrointestinal structures in relation to the pancreas and consider the abdominal discomfort of animals with pancreatic disease. Bowel and bowel gas can be displaced from the near field by using a small-footprint transducer and by applying slight abdominal compression with the scanhead.

As with most examinations that are performed with the patient in dorsal recumbency, the location of various anatomic structures and landmarks are predictable. Right lateral recumbency places fluid within the pyloric antrum and duodenum, but the gastric fundus and body may distend with gas, which may limit the visibility of the left limb. Left lateral recumbency fills the descending duodenum with gas and "carries" it closer to the right lateral body wall, allowing imaging of the pancreas from a ventral midline approach. If sufficient free peritoneal fluid is present in the abdomen, the patient should be positioned so the pancreatic area is dependent and surrounded by the fluid. A technique for pancreatic imaging by introduction of fluid into the peritoneal space has been described but is not recommended on a routine basis.[6] Additional detailed descriptions of scanning techniques for the pancreas have been published.[7,8]

As with any ultrasound examination, the highest-frequency transducer possible should be used, and the focal zone of the transducer chosen should be matched to the depth of the pancreas. In large dogs, a 5.0-MHz medium- to short-focal-length transducer can be used, and a 7.5-MHz transducer is optimal for small dogs and cats.

After the pancreas has been identified, scanning should be performed along the short and long axis of the gland. A complete examination of the pancreas must include the body and both limbs. This examination is often technically difficult when evaluating a normal pancreas because of the lack of an acoustic window caused by bowel gas artifact. The descending duodenum is a reliable landmark for following the right limb. By keeping a transverse image of the duodenum in the field of view at all times, the right limb usually can be scanned from the body to the tail. The organ landmarks for the left limb are less predictable, but systematic scanning of the area immediately caudal to the greater curvature of the stomach often is rewarding. If disease of the pancreas has been identified, the adjacent small bowel and the gallbladder should also be evaluated for abnormalities that may be the result or the cause of pancreatic disease.

NORMAL SONOGRAPHIC APPEARANCE

The normal pancreas is isoechoic with the surrounding mesenteric tissues, isoechoic or slightly hyperechoic to adjacent liver lobes, and less echogenic than the spleen.[9] In humans, the degree of echogenicity is determined by the amount of fat between lobules and the amount of interlobular fibrous tissue.[10] The pancreas is homogeneous in echotexture, and even with higher-frequency transducers, it is not well delineated from the surrounding tissues (Figs. 9-3 and 9-4). A tubular, anechoic structure can often be seen in the middle of the parenchyma of the right limb, which has been reported by one researcher to correspond to the pancreaticoduodenal vein (Fig. 9-5).[7] A similar structure seen in the pancreas in humans represents the main pancreatic duct.[10,11] If spectral Doppler is available, a venous waveform can be detected in the pancreaticoduodenal vein but not in the pancreatic duct.

In the dog, the right lobe is approximately 1 cm thick and varies in length and width according to the size of the dog (Fig. 9-6).[2] The left lobe is similar in thickness, but it is typically wider and shorter than the right limb. The

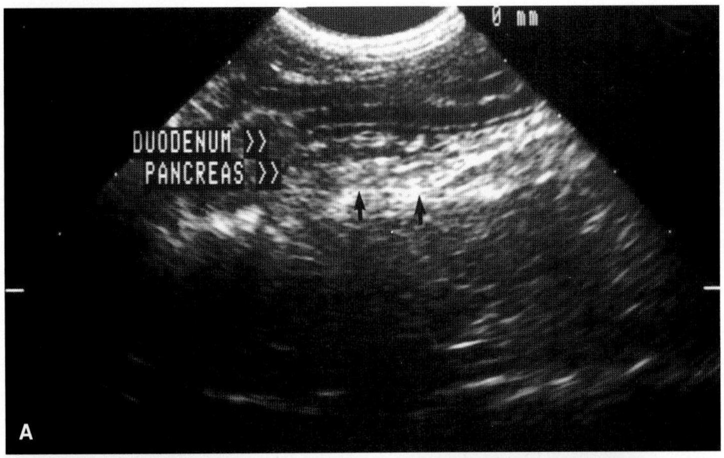

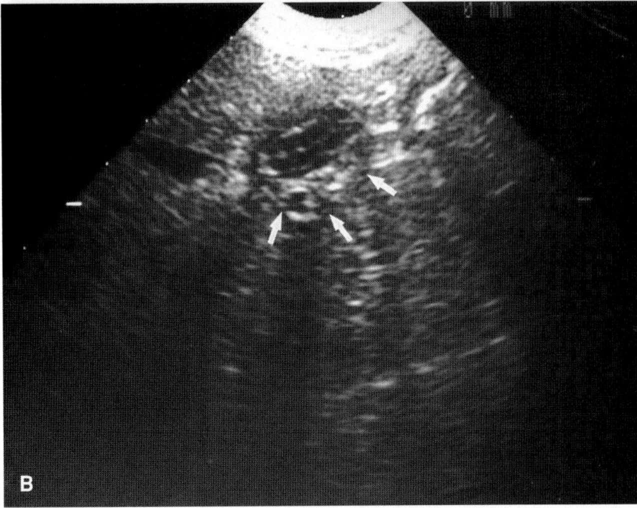

Figure 9-3. (**A**) Sagittal and (**B**) transverse sonograms of the normal right limb of the pancreas (*arrows*) in a dog demonstrate the isoechoic appearance and show the surrounding mesentery and the proximity of the right limb to the duodenum.

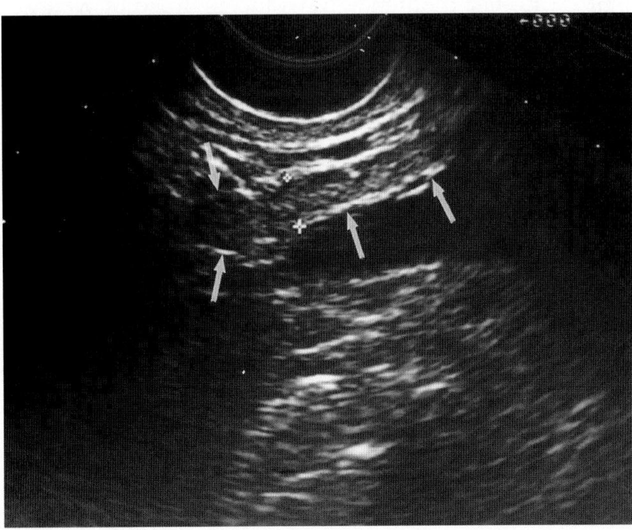

Figure 9-4. Endoscopic ultrasound image of the left limb of the normal canine pancreas (*arrows*) as viewed through the stomach wall.

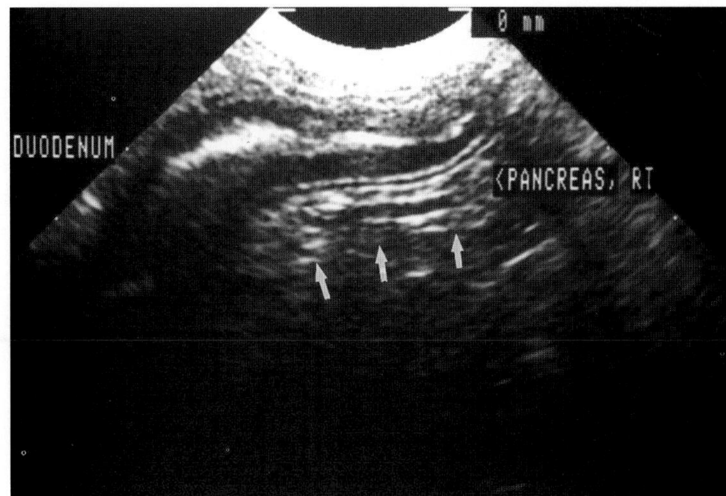

Figure 9-5. The sagittal sonogram of the right limb of the normal canine pancreas (*arrows*) shows a tubular, anechoic structure within the middle of the parenchyma that represents the main pancreatic duct or the pancreaticuduodenal vein. (Doppler was not available.)

body or angle of the pancreas is approximately 1 × 3 cm, depending on the size of the animal. Dimensions for the normal pancreas of the cat have not been reported (Fig. 9-7).

DISEASES OF THE PANCREAS

Most diseases of the pancreas can be categorized as inflammatory or neoplastic. There are many subclassifications of the inflammatory diseases, and the inflammatory changes may result in a variety of complications or sequelae. The various forms of pancreatitis are discussed separately, although some overlap of the sonographic appearance can occur.

Pancreatitis

Acute Edematous Pancreatitis

The sonographic appearance of experimentally induced canine pancreatitis has been described.[8,12–14] The sonographic appearance of acute pancreatitis varies with the severity of the

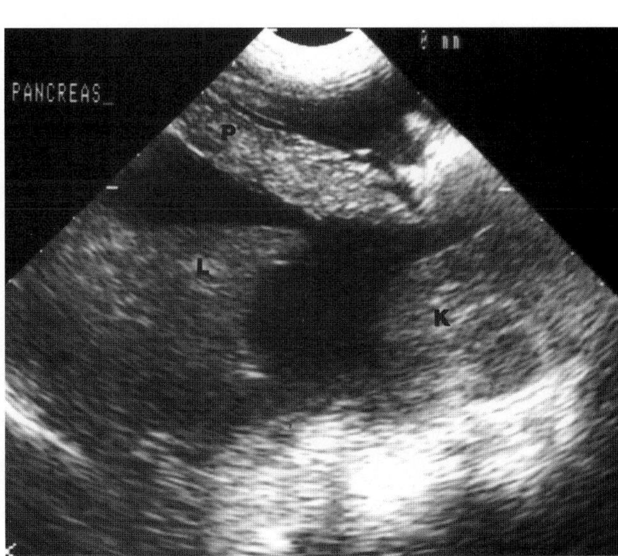

Figure 9-6. Sagittal sonogram of the normal right limb of the pancreas (*P*) in a dog with ascites. Notice that the echogenicity of the pancreas is slightly hyperechoic to the liver lobe (*L*) and the right kidney (*K*).

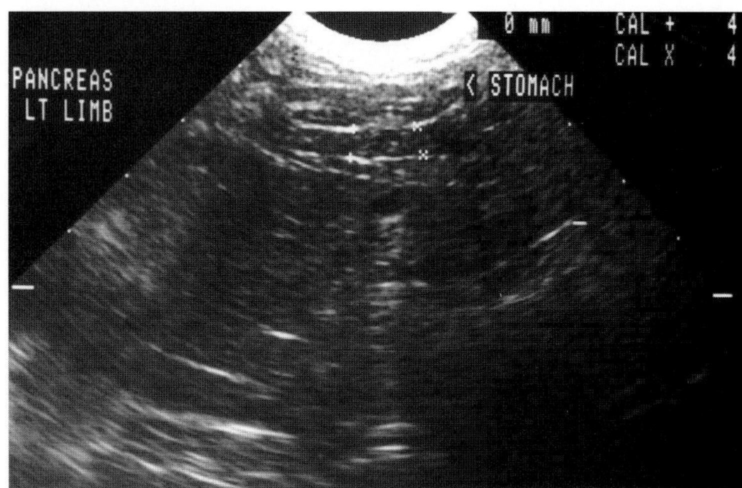

Figure 9-7. Sagittal sonogram of the normal left limb of the pancreas in a cat, identified with caliper marks (+). This limb was 4 mm thick.

inflammatory response and the time of onset of disease relative to the ultrasound examination. With mild or low-grade inflammation, the pancreas may appear as a distinct, well-defined hypoechoic tissue surrounded by normal to slightly hyperechoic mesentery (Figs. 9-8 through 9-10).[14] In more severe cases, the pancreatic parenchyma remains hypoechoic, but the margins are less distinct (Figs. 9-11 through 9-13). Because of the edema that occurs in inflamed tissue, distant enhancement causes the mesentery in the far field to appear brighter than that in the near field (Figs. 9-14 and 9-15).[14] As the disease progresses over the next few days, the mesentery in the near field may increase in echogenicity because of saponification of the fat.[12]

The literature contains few reports about the ultrasonographic appearance of acute feline pancreatitis (Fig. 9-16).[15–17] Because of nonspecific clinical signs and the subclinical nature of

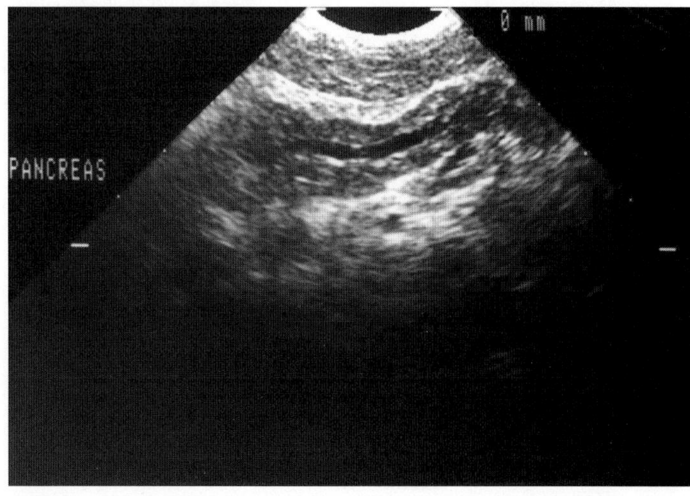

Figure 9-8. Sagittal sonogram of the right limb of the pancreas in a dog with mild or low-grade acute pancreatitis. The margins of the pancreas are well defined, and the parenchyma is hypoechoic relative to the surrounding mesentery. The central anechoic, tubular structure may be the pancreaticoduodenal vein or the main pancreatic duct.

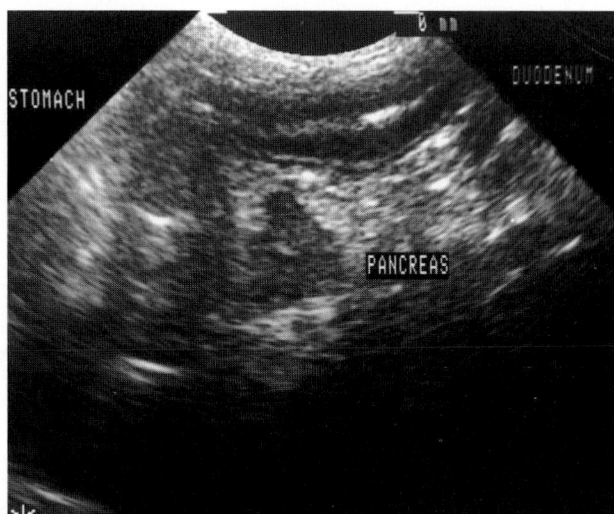

Figure 9-9. Transverse sonogram of the body (angle) of the pancreas in a dog with mild, acute pancreatitis. The margins are well defined, and the parenchyma is less echogenic than the surrounding mesentery.

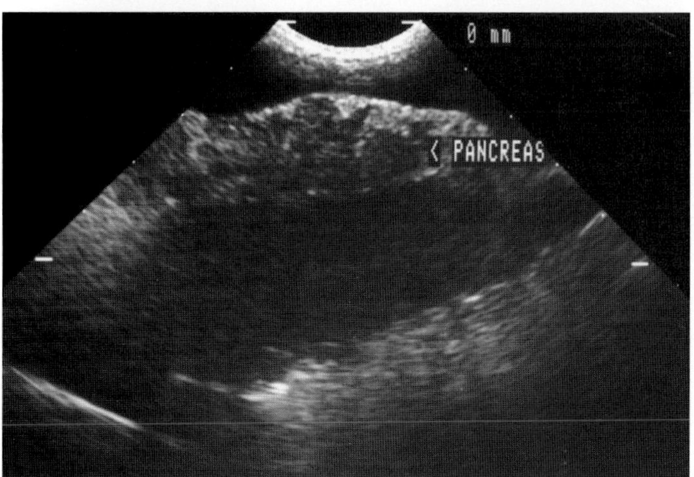

Figure 9-10. Sagittal sonogram of the right limb of the pancreas in a dog with ascites and mild acute pancreatitis. The margins of the pancreas are distinct within the hyperechoic mesentery, which is surrounded by anechoic fluid.

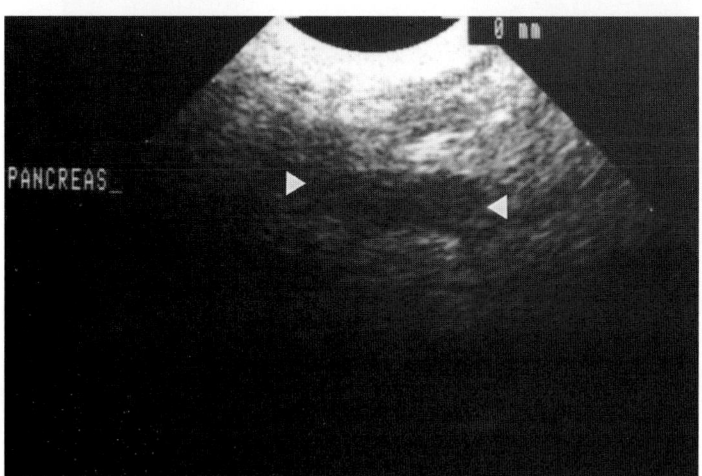

Figure 9-11. The sonogram of the pancreas in a dog with acute pancreatitis demonstrates hypoechoic parenchyma with ill-defined margins (*arrowheads*).

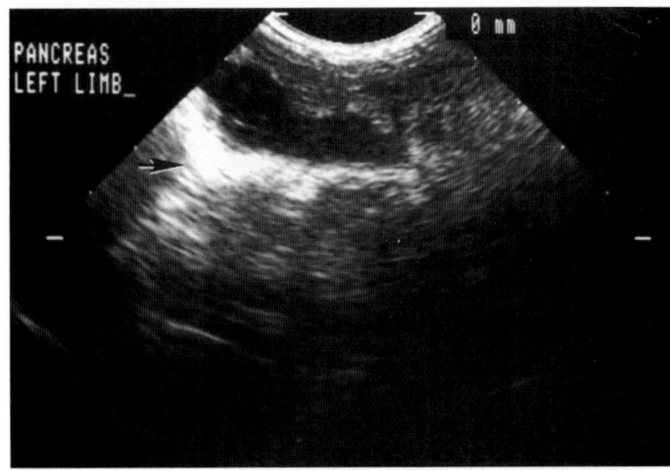

Figure 9-12. The sonogram of the left limb of the pancreas in a dog with acute edematous pancreatitis shows hypoechoic parenchyma and enhancement in the far field (*arrow*) caused by parenchymal edema.

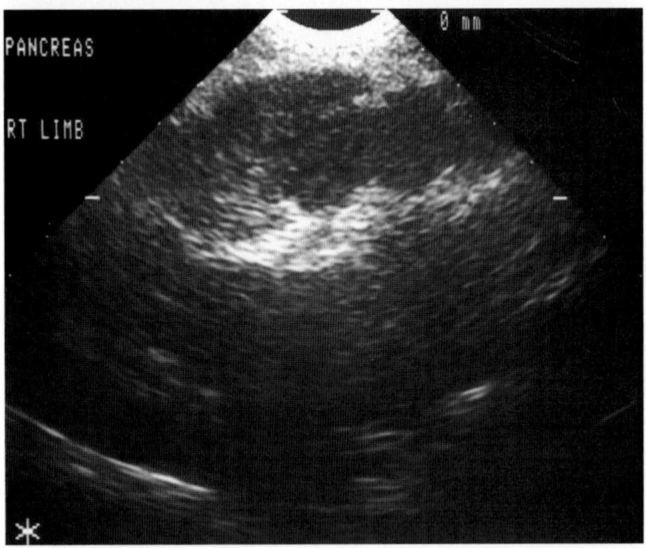

Figure 9-13. Sagittal sonogram of the right limb of the pancreas in a dog with acute edematous pancreatitis. Notice the hypoechoic parenchyma with indistinct margins and the distant enhancement caused by edema.

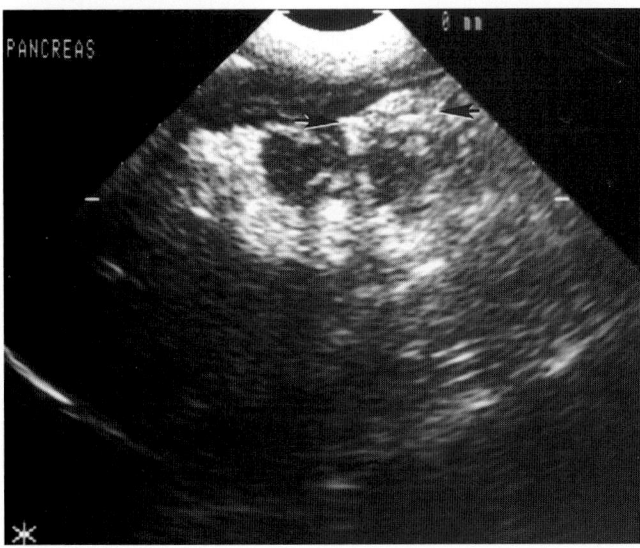

Figure 9-14. Sagittal sonogram of the right limb of the pancreas of the dog shown in Figure 9-13 3 days later. The mesentery in the near field (*arrows*) has increased in echogenicity because of saponification of the fat.

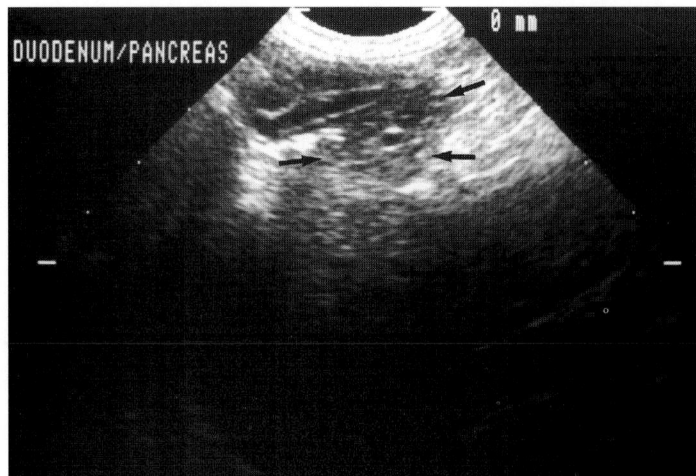

Figure 9-15. Transverse sonogram of the right limb of the pancreas in a dog with resolving, mild, acute edematous pancreatitis. The parenchyma (*arrows*) is hypoechoic without distant enhancement, and the mesentery adjacent to the pancreas is hyperechoic.

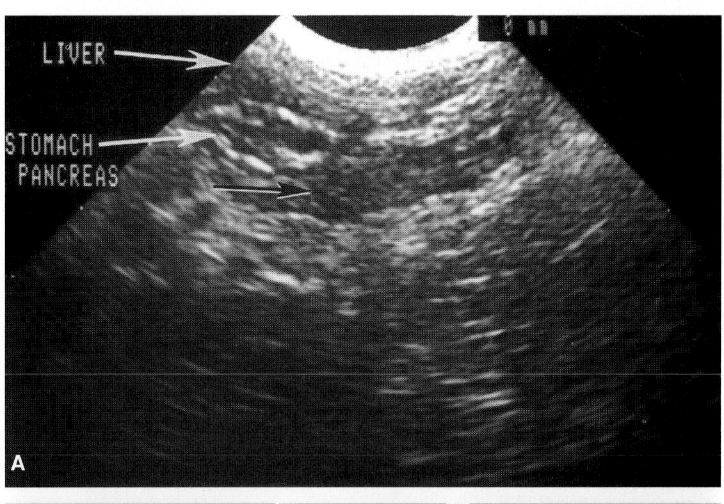

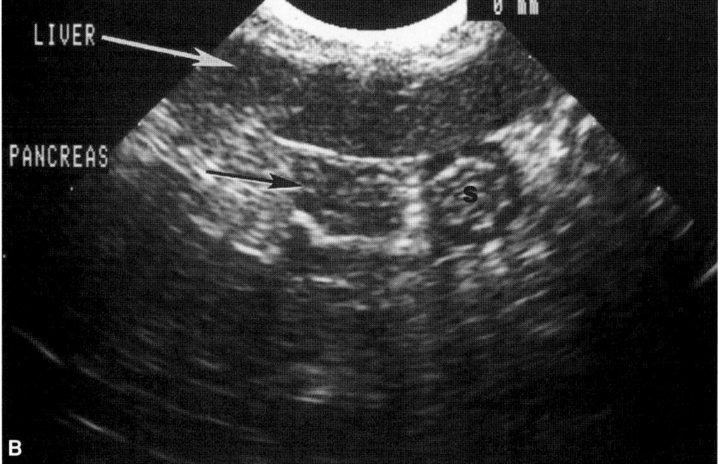

Figure 9-16. (**A**) Sagittal and (**B**) transverse sonograms of the pancreas (*black arrows*) in a cat with acute pancreatitis, which was surgically confirmed. The parenchyma is hypoechoic relative to the surrounding mesentery. *S*, stomach.

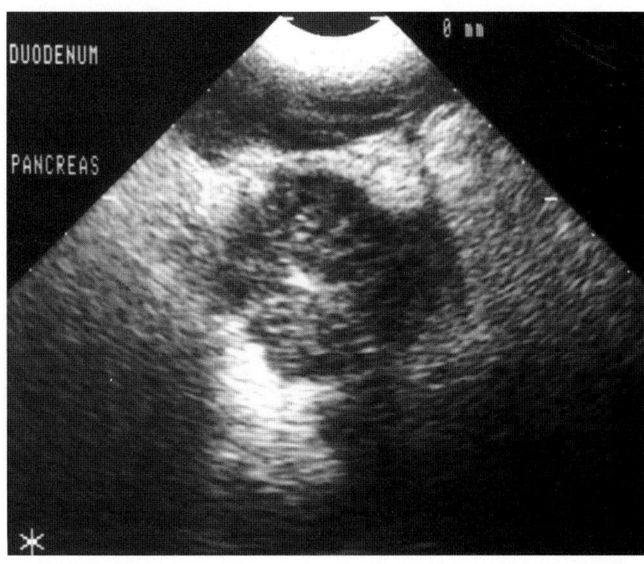

Figure 9-17. The sonogram of the pancreas in a dog with acute hemorrhagic pancreatitis shows a decrease in parenchymal echogenicity, loss of normal texture, distant enhancement, and an increase in size.

this disease in many cats, chronic pancreatitis is more commonly diagnosed with ultrasound than the acute forms of the disease.[5,18]

Acute Hemorrhagic Pancreatitis

This severe form of acute pancreatitis is caused by intracellular activation of pancreatic enzymes, resulting in hemorrhage and diffuse parenchymal destruction. The pancreas becomes hypoechoic to anechoic, loses its normal texture and margination, and increases in size because of swelling (Figs. 9-17 and 9-18). The pancreas may appear as an inhomogeneous mass that may displace the duodenum (Figs. 9-19 and 9-20).[8,13] The peripancreatic changes seen with this form of pancreatitis are minimal focal to extensive regional peritoneal effusion with duodenal wall thickening and ileus (Figs. 9-21 and 9-22).[8] The fluid that surrounds the pancreas in this disorder is the result of hemorrhage and liquefaction necrosis rather than edema as seen in milder forms of acute pancreatitis.[19]

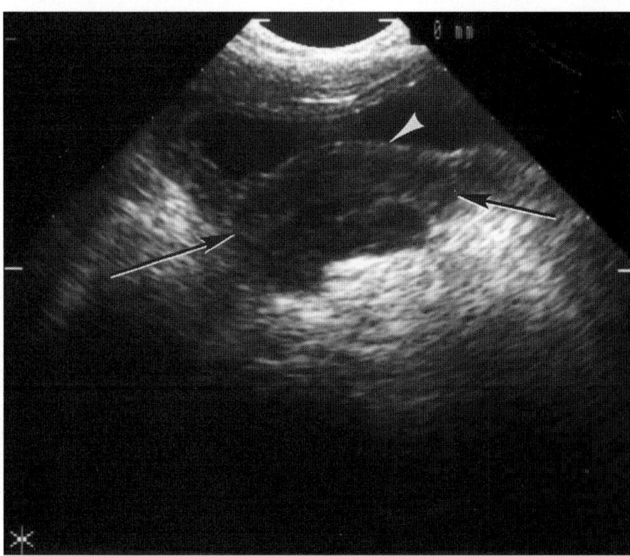

Figure 9-18. Sagittal sonogram of the left limb of the pancreas in a dog with acute hemorrhagic pancreatitis. Notice the hypoechoic to near-anechoic parenchyma (*black arrows*) and the ill-defined margins, distant enhancement, and thickening with displacement of the stomach wall (*white arrowhead*).

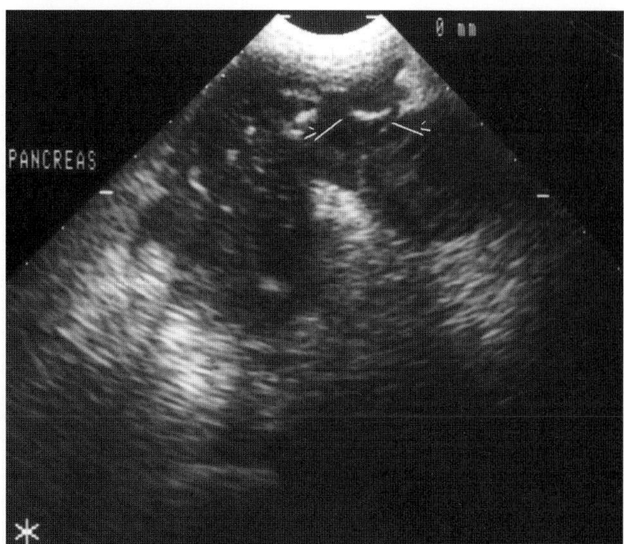

Figure 9-19. Sonogram of the pancreas in a dog with acute hemorrhagic pancreatitis. The pancreas appears as an inhomogeneous mass that displaces the duodenum (*arrows*).

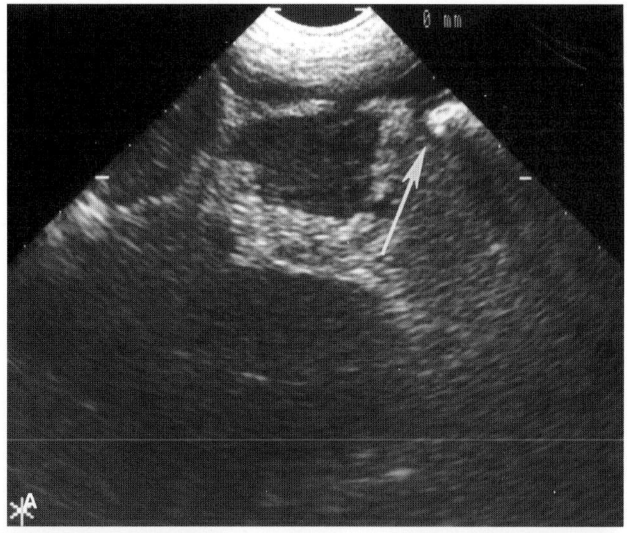

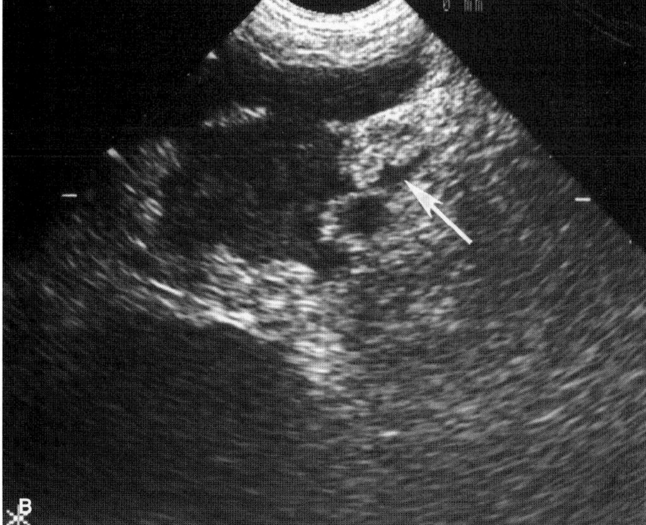

Figure 9-20. Sonograms of the right limb of the pancreas in a dog with acute hemorrhagic pancreatitis. (**A**) The transverse sonogram of the angle demonstrates an overall increase in size and displacement of the duodenum (*arrow*). (**B**) The sagittal sonogram of the right limb shows a loss of margination and peripancreatic fluid (*arrow*).

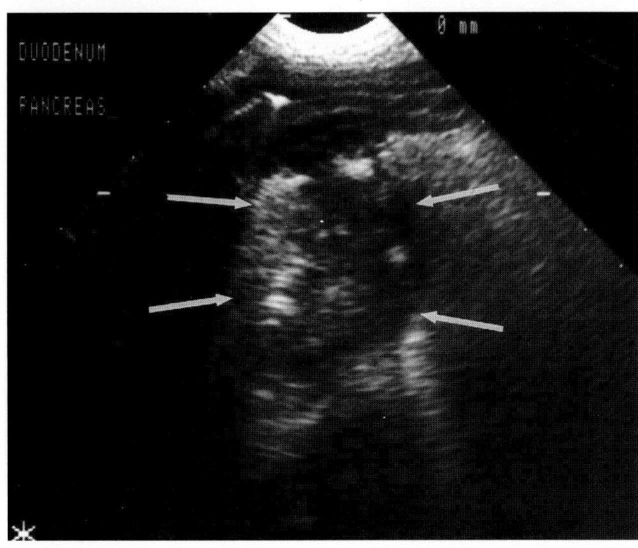

Figure 9-21. Sagittal sonogram of the right limb of the pancreas in a dog with acute hemorrhagic pancreatitis. The pancreas appears as an inhomogeneous mass (*arrows*). The duodenal wall is thickened, and ileus was apparent on real-time imaging.

Chronic Pancreatitis

This form of pancreatitis represents a chronic recurrent disease process that is the result of repeated insults or progressive subclinical acute pancreatitis.[10] With chronic inflammatory disease, little to no edema is present, and the pancreas develops an increased amount of fibrous stroma. The tissue may vary from a mixed to a uniform echo pattern (Fig. 9-23). Typically, there is an overall increase in the parenchymal echogenicity because of fibrotic or fatty changes or both. The echotexture loses its smooth appearance, and the limbs may appear thickened (Figs. 9-24 and 9-25). At times, it may even be difficult to identify the pancreas because of the similarity in echogenicity with surrounding fat (Fig. 9-26). Calcification, which gives a stippled appearance with tiny foci of acoustic shadowing, has been described in the pancreas and surrounding peripancreatic tissue (Figs. 9-27 and 9-28).[10,11]

Complications of Pancreatitis

Several other sonographic changes can be seen as a result of severe acute or chronic recurrent pancreatitis. *(text continues on p. 191)*

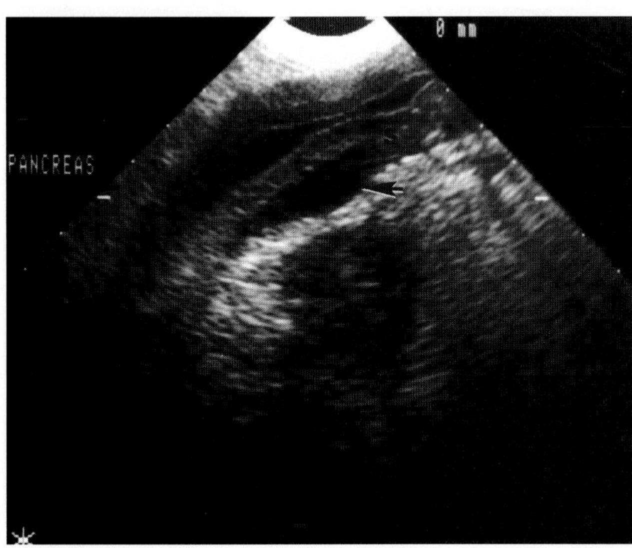

Figure 9-22. The sagittal sonogram of the left limb of the pancreas in a dog with acute hemorrhagic pancreatitis demonstrates peripancreatic fluid (*arrow*) and thickening of the stomach wall (*s*).

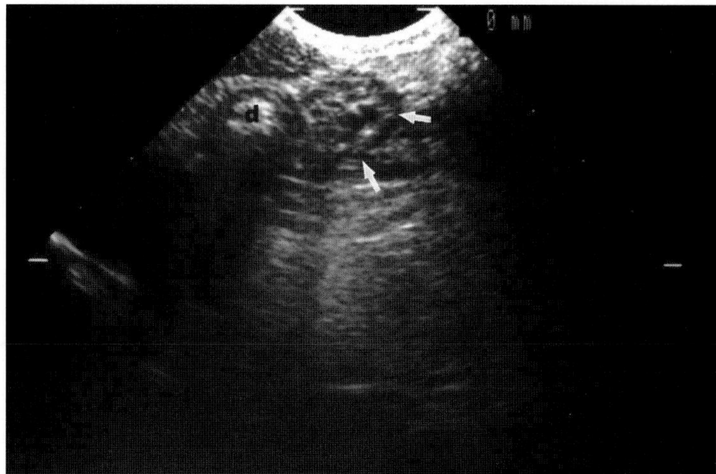

Figure 9-23. The transverse sonogram of the right limb of the pancreas (*arrows*) in a cat with chronic pancreatitis shows a mixed echo pattern. *d*, duodenum.

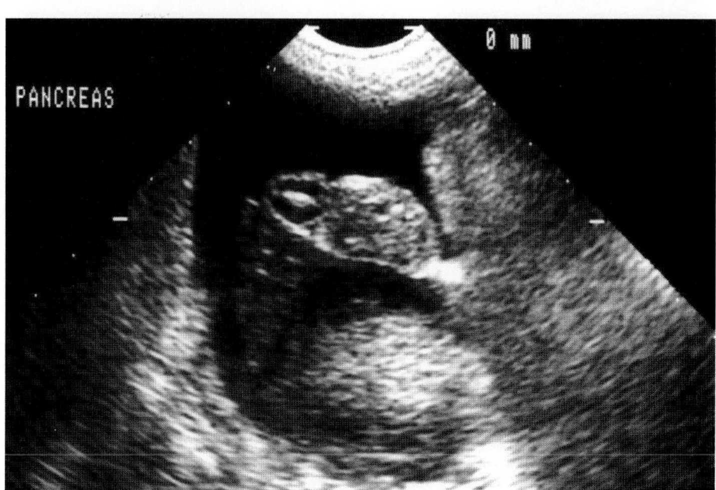

Figure 9-24. Transverse sonogram of the right limb of the pancreas in a dog with ascites and chronic pancreatitis. The limb is thickened, and the echotexture is no longer smooth.

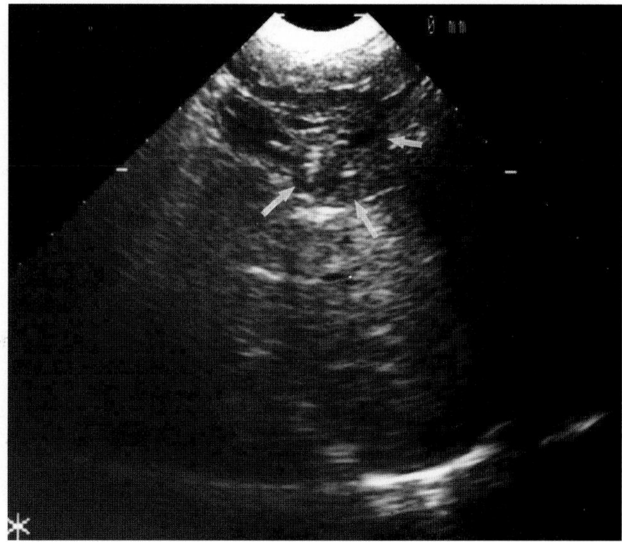

Figure 9-25. Transverse sonogram of the right limb of the pancreas (*arrows*) in a dog with chronic pancreatitis. The limb is thickened, and the parenchyma has a mixed echo pattern with echodense foci, suggesting parenchymal fibrosis.

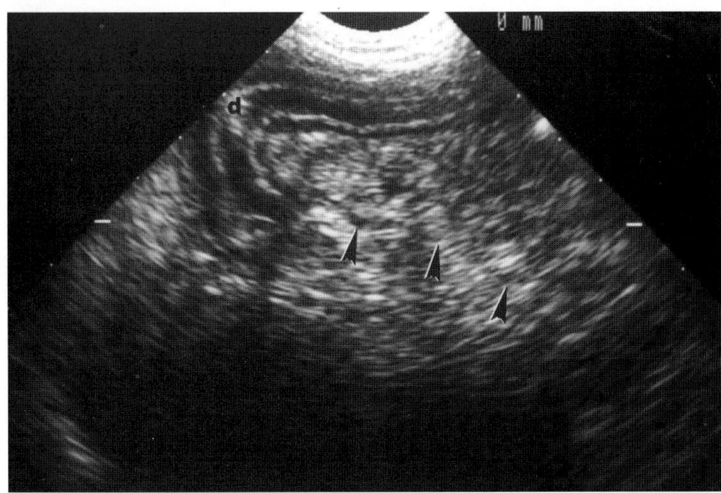

Figure 9-26. Sagittal sonogram of the right limb of the pancreas in a dog with chronic pancreatitis. The limb is thickened, and it is difficult to delineate the margins (*arrows*) from the surrounding mesentery. *d*, duodenum.

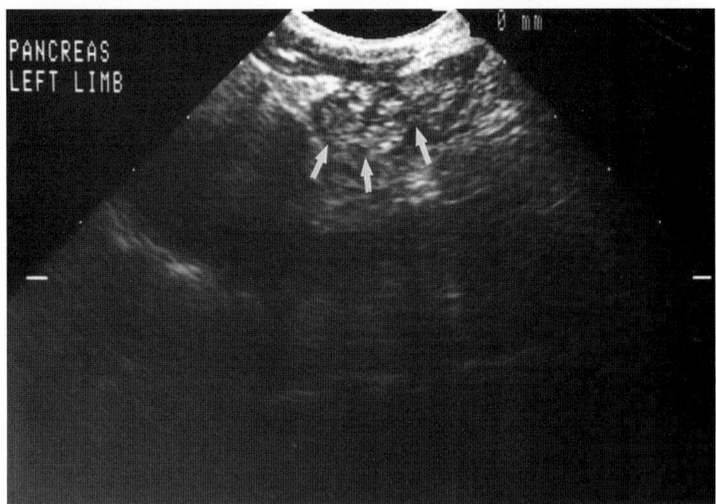

Figure 9-27. The sagittal sonogram of the left limb of the pancreas (*arrows*) in a dog with chronic pancreatitis shows tiny echodense foci of mineralization within the parenchyma.

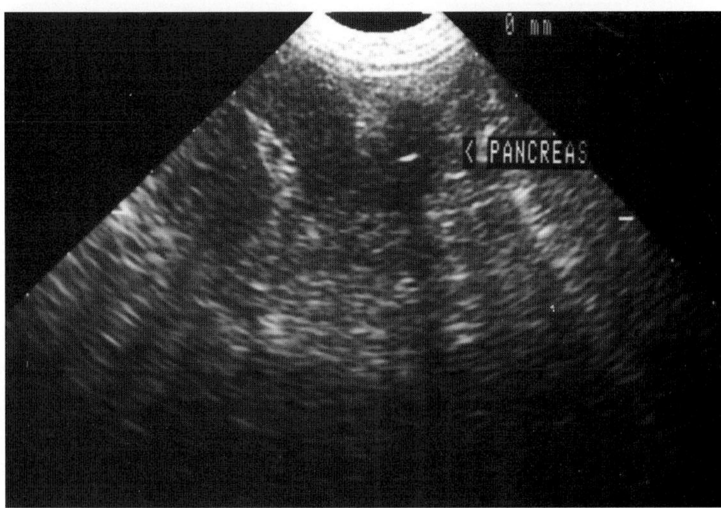

Figure 9-28. The sonogram shows a thickened hypoechoic pancreas in a dog with chronic pancreatitis. The echodense area with acoustic shadowing is the result of parenchymal mineralization.

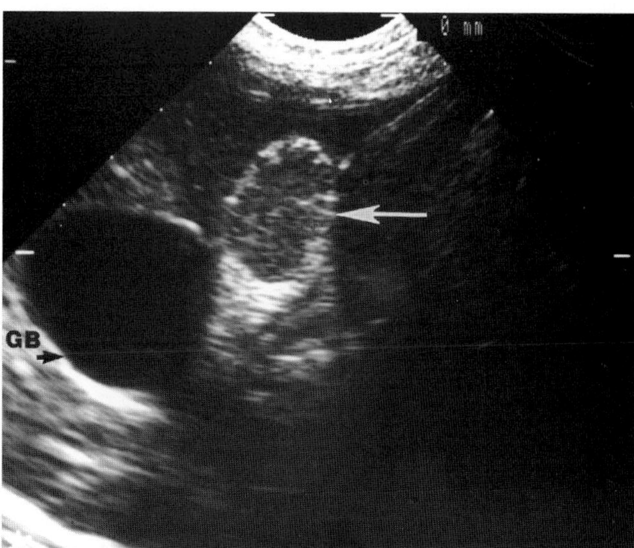

Figure 9-29. Sonogram of a unilocular pancreatic abscess (*arrow*) within the pancreatic body near the gallbladder (*GB*) in a dog. The abscess is smoothly marginated and shows distant enhancement.

Abscess. Pancreatic abscess is an uncommon sequela of acute pancreatitis.[20] It should be considered in any case of unresolving acute pancreatitis. Abscesses develop as a result of superinfection of necrotic pancreatic or peripancreatic tissues.[10,21] The abscess may be unilocular (Fig. 9-29) or multilocular (Fig. 9-30). The mass is often hypoechoic with a smooth to irregular shape and few or no internal echoes (Fig. 9-31). Distant or far-field enhancement aids in the identification of fluid within the mass. Gas is rarely seen, possibly because of interference with or difficulty in differentiating it from bowel gas.

Phlegmon. Pancreatic phlegmons are solid masses that develop within days of an episode of severe pancreatitis and are the result of edema, inflammation, and necrosis.[19] They consist of indurated pancreatic and other adjacent tissues. The sonographic appearance of a phlegmon is that of a hyperechoic to mixed echogenicity mass that does not contain fluid (Fig.

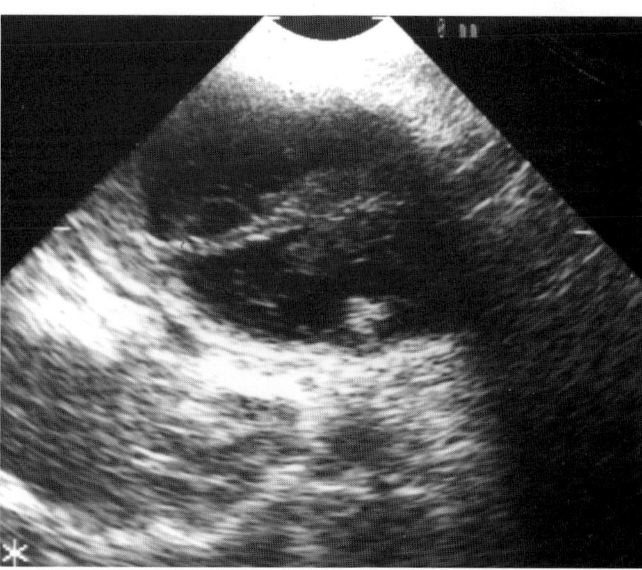

Figure 9-30. Sonogram of a multiloculated pancreatic abscess in a dog. The shape of the abscess is very irregular, and mixed internal echoes and far-field (distant) enhancement are evident.

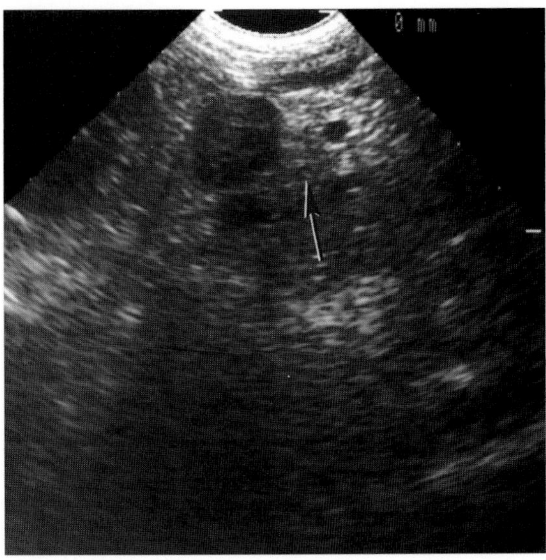

Figure 9-31. Sonogram of a pancreatic abscess in a dog. This abscess has smooth margins and moderate internal echoes, and it is similar in size to the thickness of the adjacent normal pancreas (*arrow*).

9-32). Most phlegmons resolve spontaneously.[19] One potential complication of phlegmons is bile duct obstruction, which may require surgery.

Pseudocyst. Pseudocysts represent collections of fluid that arise from localized inflammation, hemorrhage, or necrosis. They are almost always associated with or are the result of pancreatitis.[21] Pseudocysts are usually solitary, oval to round, and vary in size (Fig. 9-33). The walls are discrete and well-defined, and acoustic enhancement is nearly always demonstrated. Although percutaneous drainage or surgery is often recommended in people because of the high incidence of rupture into the peritoneal cavity,[22] spontaneous regression of pseudocysts does occur and has been reported in animals.[13,21]

Extrahepatic Biliary Obstruction. The complication of extrahepatic biliary obstruction, also called obstructive pancreatitis, is the result of stricture or stenosis of the bile duct with subsequent dilatation as a sequela to chronic or recurrent pancreatitis or a mass near the bile duct (Fig. 9-34). If severe or chronic pancreatic disease is recognized during ultrasonography, scanning of the gallbladder and the bile duct should be done. If the patient has been anorexic or intentionally fasted for the sonographic study, the gallbladder often is distended. The bile duct must be evaluated for dilatation, and serial sonograms may be necessary over a few days to evaluate increasing size of the gallbladder and distention and tortuosity of the bile duct.[7]

Pancreatic Neoplasia

Two types of primary pancreatic neoplasia have been described in companion animals: carcinoma, which involves the exocrine portion of the gland, and islet cell tumors, the most com-

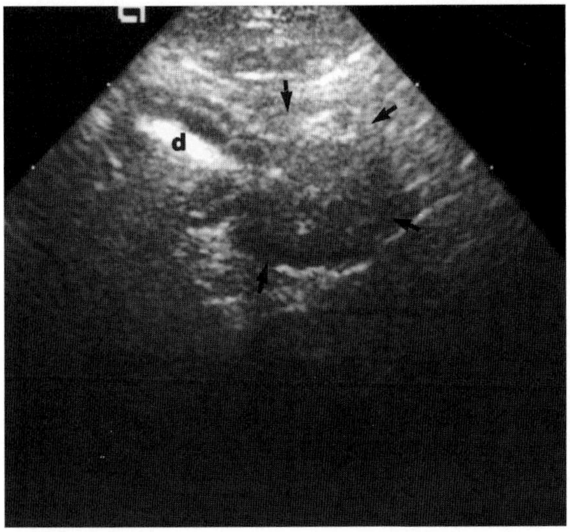

Figure 9-32. The transverse sonogram of the right limb of the pancreas in a dog recovering from severe pancreatitis shows a mixed-echogenicity mass (*arrows*). This mass developed within the angle near the bile duct, causing extrahepatic biliary obstruction. *d*, duodenum.

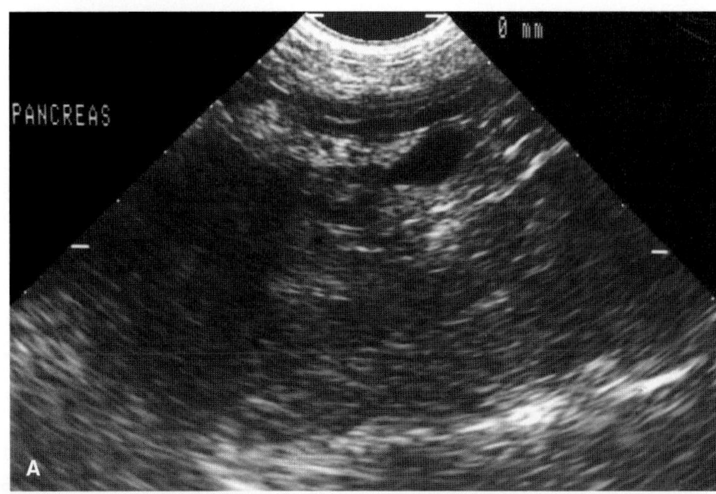

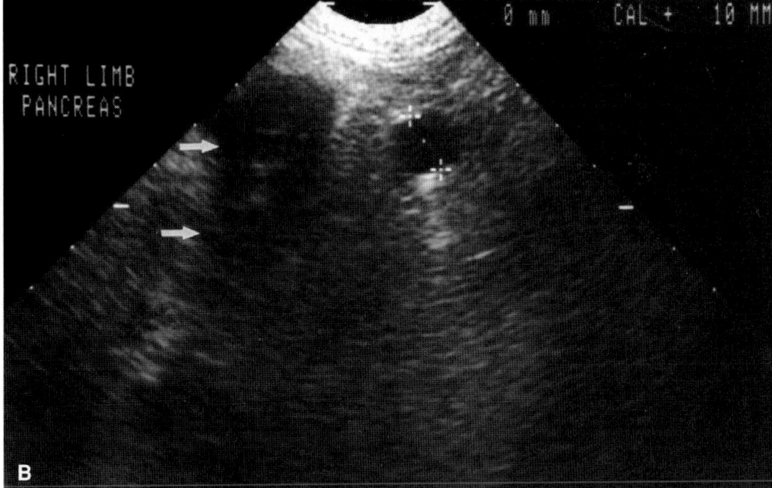

Figure 9-33. Sonograms of pancreatic pseudocysts that developed after episodes of severe pancreatitis in two dogs. (**A**) The pancreatic pseudocyst is oval and has discrete well-defined walls. The duodenum is seen in the near field. (**B**) The pancreatic pseudocyst shows some distant enhancement. Abnormal pancreatic parenchyma is still evident (*arrows*) in this recovering dog.

mon one being the insulinoma. Metastasis of intraabdominal lymphomas and extramedullary gastrointestinal plasmacytomas to the pancreas have been reported in people, but metastases are rare. Secondary involvement of the pancreas is usually a result of direct extension from gastric, colonic, duodenal, or biliary tumors.[10]

Sonography for pancreatic neoplasia is difficult, because some tumor nodules are solitary and small, with no preferred site within the organ.[23] If a complete examination of the entire pancreas has not been performed, a malignancy may go undetected. Pancreatic insulinomas have been described as discrete spherical or lobulated hypoechoic nodules that are typically small (Fig. 9-35).[7,24,25] Pancreatic carcinomas vary in echogenicity, size, and location (Fig. 9-36).[10] Carcinomas and insulinomas can metastasize within the abdomen to regional lymph nodes and the liver.[7] If a tumor is suspected, these organs should be evaluated for metastatic disease.

BIOPSY TECHNIQUES

Pancreatic biopsy is typically a procedure performed during exploratory laparotomy, because the pancreas in companion animals is a very narrow structure and ultrasound target. I have performed ultrasound-guided fine-needle aspiration in at least three cases of mixed-echogenicity masses at least 1.5 cm in diameter and confirmed pancreatic adenocarcinoma in all three. Ultrasound-guided pancreatic biopsy and

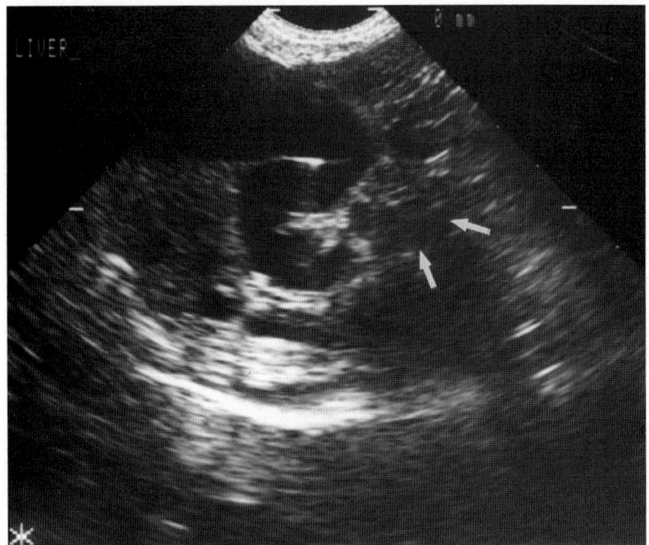

Figure 9-34. Sonogram of the gallbladder and bile duct in a dog with extrahepatic biliary obstruction as a result of a pancreatic mass (ie, phlegmon) that formed near the bile duct (see Fig. 9-32). The gallbladder and bile duct are distended, and the bile duct is tortuous. A portion of this mass is also evident (*arrows*).

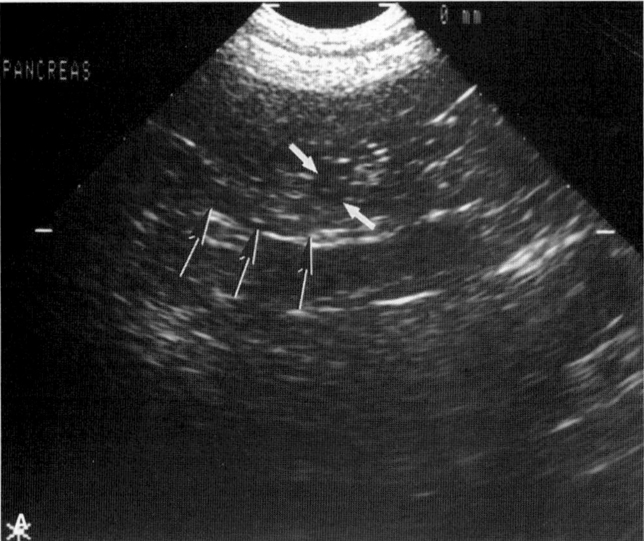

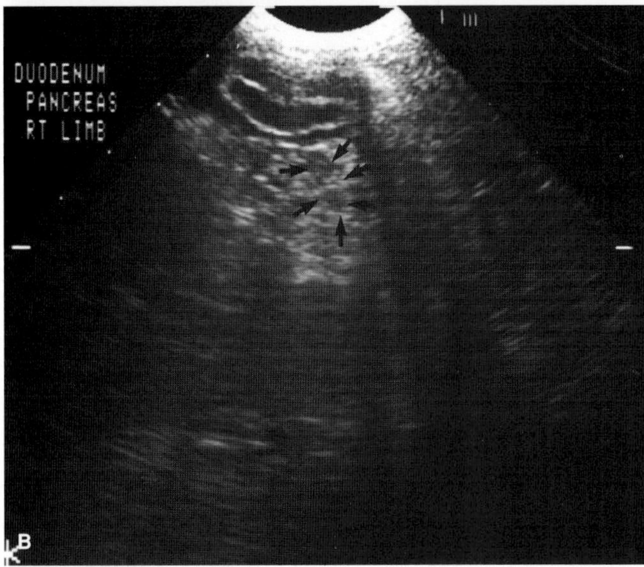

Figure 9-35. Sonograms of surgically confirmed pancreatic insulinomas in two dogs. (**A**) A 4-mm ill-defined hypoechoic nodule (*white arrows*) within the distal aspect of the right limb (*black arrows*). (**B**) A lobulated, mixed-echogenicity mass was 3 × 7 mm and contained two discrete hypoechoic nodules within the right limb.

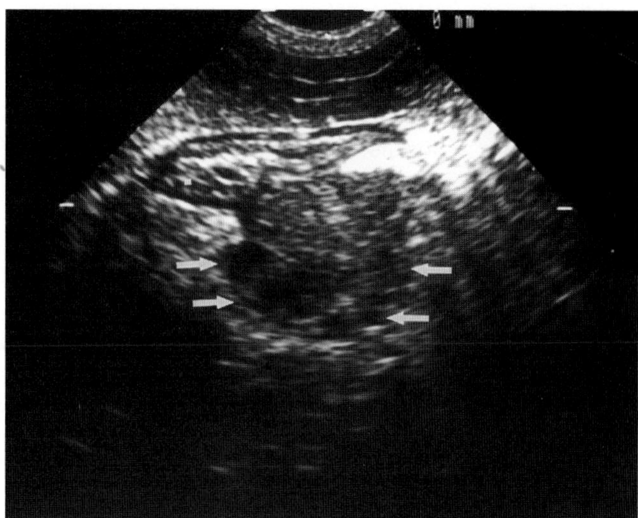

Figure 9-36. Sonogram of the pancreas of a dog with pancreatic carcinoma confirmed with ultrasound-guided fine-needle aspiration. The mass has mixed echogenicity and margins that are indistinct from the normal parenchyma. Notice the lack of enhancement deep to the hypoechoic areas of this tumor (*arrows*), suggesting cellular infiltrates rather than fluid.

percutaneous drainage of pancreatic pseudocysts or abscesses are fairly common but high-risk procedures in human medicine.[22,26] Laparotomy is preferred over ultrasound-guided drainage of pancreatic abscesses in animals, especially because imaging of the entire gland is often not possible.

CONCLUSION

The pancreas of small animals can be imaged and evaluated by ultrasound. Ultrasound also provides a way to obtain biopsies from an enlarged pancreas. Biopsy and imaging of the pancreas is not easy, but with patience, anatomic knowledge, good scanning technique, and good ultrasound equipment, the sonographic examination of the pancreas can become a regular sonographic procedure.

REFERENCES

1. Ellenport CR. Carnivore digestive system. In: Getty R, ed. Sisson and Grossman's the anatomy of the domestic animals. 5th ed. Philadelphia: WB Saunders, 1975:1538.
2. Evans HE, Christensen GC. The digestive apparatus and abdomen. In: Evans HE, Christensen GC, eds. Miller's anatomy of the dog. 2nd ed. Philadelphia: WB Saunders, 1979:411.
3. Rosenzweig LJ. The organization of the coelom and the digestive and respiratory systems. In: Rosenzweig LJ, ed. Anatomy of the cat: text and dissection guide. Dubuque: William C Brown, 1990:140.
4. Waters DJ. Endocrine system. In: Hudson LC, Hamilton WP, eds. Atlas of feline anatomy for veterinarians. Philadelphia: WB Saunders, 1993:127.
5. Smith FW. Feline pancreatitis: a review. Comp Anim Pract 1987;9:4.
6. Miles KG, Lattimer JC, Krause GF, et al. The use of intraperitoneal fluid as a simple technique for enhancing sonographic visualization of the canine pancreas. Vet Radiol 1988;29:258.
7. Saunders HM. Ultrasonography of the pancreas. In: Kaplan PM, ed. Problems in veterinary medicine: ultrasound. Philadelphia: JB Lippincott, 1991:583.
8. Nyland TG, Mulvany MH, Strombeck DR. Ultrasonic features of experimentally induced, acute pancreatitis in the dog. Vet Radiol 1983;24:260.
9. Saunders HM, Pugh CR, Rhodes WH. Expanding applications of abdominal ultrasonography. J Am Anim Hosp Assoc 1992;28:369.

10. Mittlestaedt CA. Pancreas. In: Mittlestaedt CA, ed. General ultrasound. New York: Churchill Livingstone, 1992: 371.
11. Sanders RC, Ling MM. Epigastric pain (upper abdominal pain). In: Sanders RC, ed. Clinical sonography: a practical guide. 2nd ed. Boston: Little, Brown and Co, 1991:201.
12. Murtaugh RJ, Herring DS, Jacobs RM, DeHoff WD. Pancreatic ultrasonography in dogs with experimentally induced acute pancreatitis. Vet Radiol 1985; 26:271.
13. Maier W. Echographic patterns of just evolving acute pancreatitis: an experimental study. Eur J Radiol 1990;11:145.
14. Schelling CG. Abdominal imaging: gastrointestinal, pancreas and adrenal. In: Syllabus of the second annual American Institute of Ultrasound in Medicine animal ultrasound seminar and wet-lab. Bethesda: American Institute of Ultrasound in Medicine, 1990:59.
15. Kitchell BE, Strombeck DR, Cullen J, et al. Clinical and pathological changes in experimentally induced acute pancreatitis in cats. Am J Vet Res 1986;47:1170.
16. Akol KG, Washabau RJ, Saunders HM, Hendrick MJ. Acute pancreatitis in cats with hepatic lipidosis. J Vet Intern Med 1993;7:205.
17. Hill RC, Van Winkle TJ. Acute necrotizing pancreatitis and acute suppurative pancreatitis in the cat: a retrospective study of 40 cases (1976–1989). J Vet Intern Med 1993;7:25.
18. Simpson KW. Current concepts of the pathogenesis and pathophysiology of acute pancreatitis in the dog and cat. Compend Contin Ed 1993;15:247.
19. Edwards DF, Bauer MS, Walker MA, et al. Pancreatic masses in seven dogs following acute pancreatitis. J Am Anim Hosp Assoc 1990;26:189.
20. Salisbury SK, Lantz GC, Nelson RW, Kazacos EA. Pancreatic abscess in dogs: six cases (1978–1986). J Am Vet Med Assoc 1988;193:1104.
21. Rutgers C, Herring DS, Orton EC. Pancreatic pseudocyst associated with acute pancreatitis in a dog: ultrasonographic diagnosis. J Am Anim Hosp Assoc 1985;21:411.
22. D'Agostino HB, vanSonnenberg E, Sanchez RB, et al. Treatment of pancreatic pseudocysts with percutaneous drainage and octreotide: work in progress. Radiology 1993;187:685.
23. Howard TJ, Stabile BE, Zinner MJ, et al. Anatomic distribution of pancreatic endocrine tumors. Am J Surg 1990;159:258.
24. Gorman B, Charboneau JW, James EM, et al. Benign pancreatic insulinoma: preoperative and intraoperative sonographic localization. Am J Roentgenol 1986; 147:929.
25. Gunther RW. Ultrasound and CT in the assessment of suspected islet cell tumors of the pancreas. Semin Ultrasound CT MR 1985;6:261.
26. Brandt KR. Charboneau JW, Stephens DH, et al. CT- and US-guided biopsy of the pancreas. Radiology 1993;187:99.

Small Animal Ultrasound, edited by Ronald W. Green.
Lippincott-Raven Publishers, Philadelphia © 1996.

KIDNEYS

Ronald W. Green

The kidneys are relatively easy to image with ultrasound. Other than clipping the hair, no special patient preparation is required, and most dogs and cats can be scanned without the use of tranquilizers. With knowledge of renal anatomy, good scanning techniques, and modern ultrasound equipment, the practitioner can use ultrasound to obtain useful clinical information concerning the kidneys.

RENAL ANATOMY

The kidneys are bean-shaped retroperitoneal organs surrounded by fat. They are located between the last thoracic and third lumbar vertebrae. The right kidney lies in the renal fossa of the caudate liver lobe and is cranial to the left kidney. The kidneys are loosely attached to the body wall, which allows them to move with respiration; to be displaced by enlargement of the stomach, liver, or spleen; and to move in accordance with changes in abdominal recumbency (ie, dorsal, ventral, and lateral recumbencies).[1] Feline kidneys are more loosely attached to the body wall than those of dogs and are located caudal to the last ribs.[2]

The right kidney is lateral to the vena cava and dorsal to the duodenum and right limb of the pancreas. The right adrenal gland is medial to the right kidney. The left kidney lies medial to the spleen and caudal to the greater curvature of the stomach. The left adrenal gland and pancreas are just cranial to the left kidney.

The kidney is composed of the renal capsule, renal cortex, renal medulla, diverticula, branches of the renal arteries and veins, renal pelvis, and renal sinus. The renal capsule is a fibrous membrane that covers the kidney. With the exception of a few ectopic glomeruli, all glomeruli are located within the renal cortex. The cortex and medulla contain renal tubules, vessels, and connective tissue. Most tubules of the collecting system are in the renal medulla. The renal diverticula are made of fibrous connective tissue that divide the medulla into segments. The interlobular vessels lie within the diverticula. The renal arteries enter and the renal vein and ureter exit the kidney at the renal sinus. The renal sinus also contains fat. Urine collects in the renal pelvis then enters the ureter.

The size of the normal canine kidney varies with the size of the dog. A normal canine kidney can be 6 to 9 cm long, 4 to 5 cm high, and 3 to 4 cm wide.[1] Feline kidneys are more uniform in size and are 3.8 to 4.4 cm long, 2.7 to 3.1 cm high, and 2.0 to 2.5 cm wide.[3] The cortex is 2 to 5 mm thick in the cat and 3 to 8 mm thick in the dog.[3,4]

SONOGRAPHIC ANATOMY

The renal capsule produces a thin bright specular echo.[5] The cortex is hyperechoic to the medulla because it is more cellular and the medulla contains more fluid (Fig. 10-1). The normal canine and feline kidney should have a distinct demarcation between the cortex and medulla. The lack of echoes in the medulla may be mistakenly diagnosed as hydronephrosis, dilation of the renal pelvis, or a polycystic kidney. A patient receiving intravenous fluids before sonography should have a prominent, well-demarcated, nearly anechoic medulla.[3,5,6] The diverticula are hyperechoic to the medulla and divide the medulla into segments. The renal sinus contains fat, which produces very bright echoes and acoustic shadowing.[6] These echoes may be mistaken for calculi in the renal pelvis. The renal pelvis is not normally visualized with ultrasound.[3,7] The echotexture of the renal cortex is hyperechoic to the renal medulla but hypoechoic to the liver and spleen.[5] Efforts should be made to compare the echogenicity of the right kidney with the liver and the echogenicity of the left kidney with the spleen. Some normal cats deposit fat in the cortices of their kidneys. This deposition of fat causes the cortex to produce bright echoes, which make the cortices of these animals isoechoic or hyperechoic to the liver and spleen.[8]

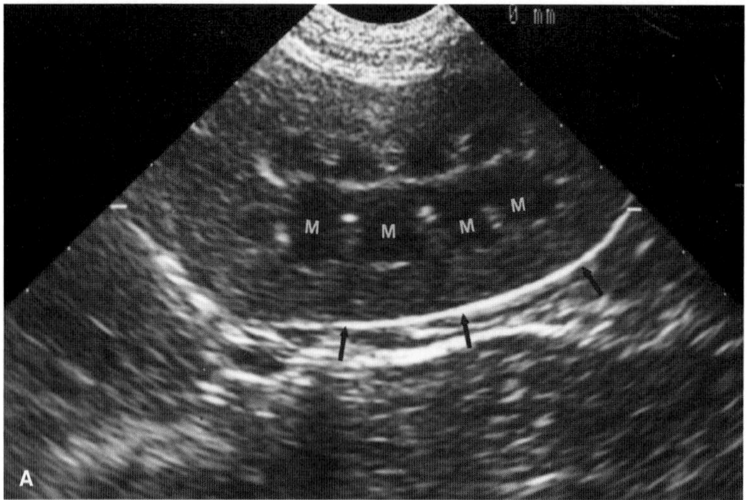

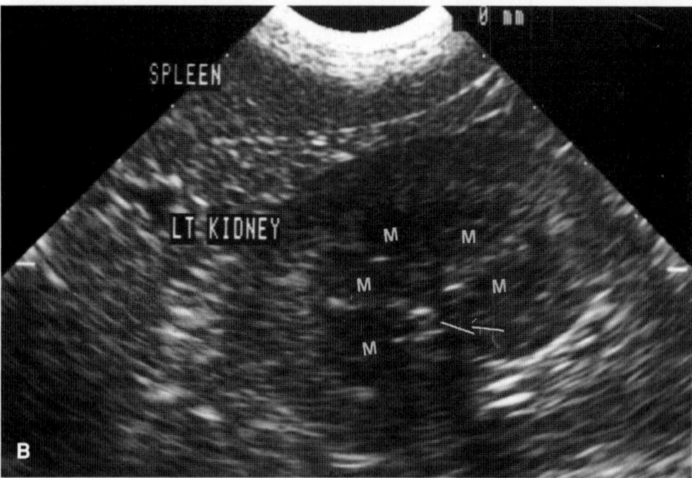

Figure 10-1. (**A**) The sagittal view of the normal kidney shows the medulla (*M*) to be hypoechoic to the cortex. The renal capsule produces a bright specular echo (*arrows*). (**B**) A frontal view of the normal left kidney shows the medulla (*M*) to be hypoechoic to the cortex. The cortex is hypoechoic to the spleen. Fat in the renal sinus produces a bright echo (*arrow*).

SCANNING TECHNIQUES

Techniques for scanning the kidneys are described in Chapter 3. High-quality images are needed for an accurate diagnosis. The quality of the sonogram may be altered by fluid or gas in the abdomen. Problems encountered by gas-filled loops of bowel are often overcome by changing the patient's position or changing the scanning plane. Ascites is a good acoustic window for imaging the kidneys; however, ascites may cause displacement of the kidneys and make the kidneys appear hyperechoic due to distant enhancement (ie, through transmission artifact).

RENAL DISEASES

Acute Renal Failure

Acute renal failure (ARF) is a syndrome characterized by azotemia attributable to renal disease that has occurred within the last 2 weeks. Acute tubular necrosis, cortical necrosis, acute interstitial nephritis, and diseases of the glomeruli are common causes of ARF.[9]

The sonographic findings of ARF are usually unremarkable. The kidneys may become slightly enlarged. The echogenicity of kidneys in acute renal failure may range from hypoechogenic to hyperechogenic. The main role of ultrasound in acute renal failure is to exclude hydronephrosis.[9]

Chronic Renal Failure

Chronic renal failure (CRF) is a result of progressive loss of nephrons that occur over a few months to several years. CRF is recognized clinically when uremia develops. Many diseases such as glomerulonephritis, chronic pyelonephritis, diabetes mellitus, polycystic renal disease, autoimmune diseases, and diseases caused by exposure to nephrotoxins can cause CRF.

The sonographic findings of CRF are nonspecific. The findings may range from normal kidneys to small, hyperechoic, irregularly shaped kidneys (Figs. 10-2 through 10-5). Renal function cannot be directly correlated with kidney size or with echogenicity.[9]

Ethylene Glycol Toxicity

Ethylene glycol, a component of antifreeze, is nephrotoxic. Ingestion of ethylene glycol results in microscopic oxalate crystal deposition in various organs, including the brain, liver, and kidneys. Crystals in the kidneys are deposited in the cortex and medulla. In the medulla, the

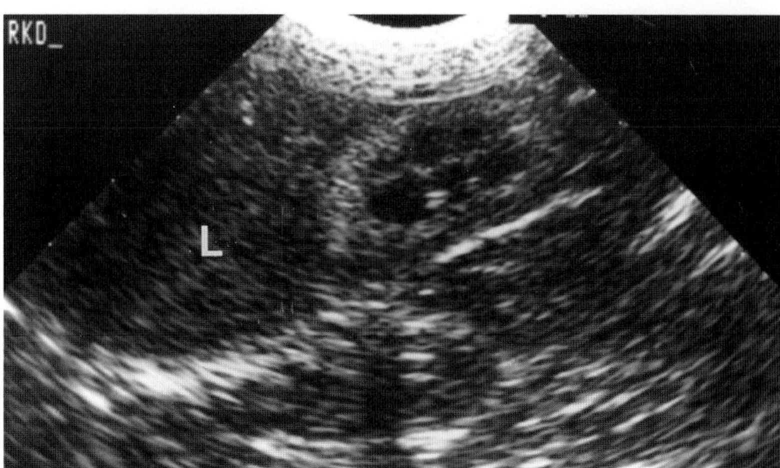

Figure 10-2. Sagittal view of a kidney in chronic renal failure due to nephrotoxin. The renal cortex is hyperechoic to the liver (*L*).

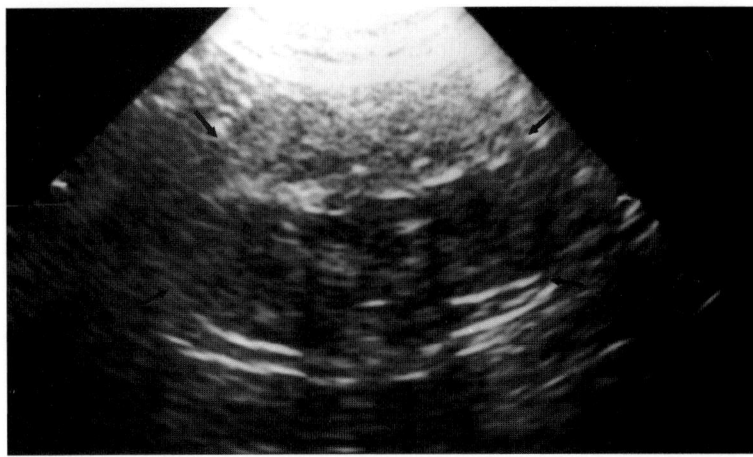

Figure 10-3. Sagittal view of a kidney in chronic renal failure caused by systemic lupus erythematosus. The margins of the kidney are marked by arrows. Notice the patchy hyperechoic cortex and poor demarcation between the cortex and medulla.

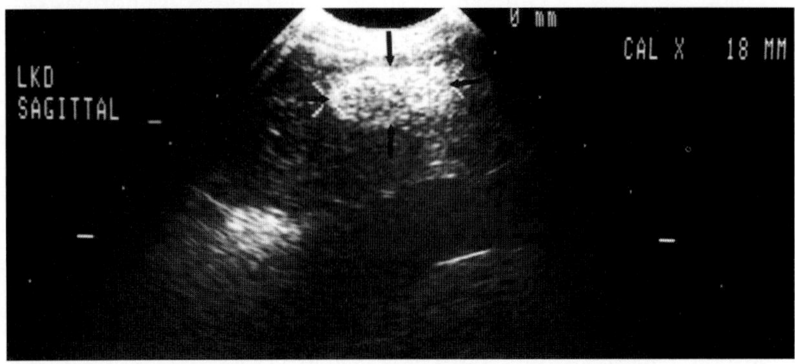

Figure 10-4. Sagittal view of a kidney in chronic renal failure due to an unknown cause. The margins of the hyperechoic kidney are marked by arrows. The kidney is only 18 mm long, and there is no demarcation between the cortex and medulla.

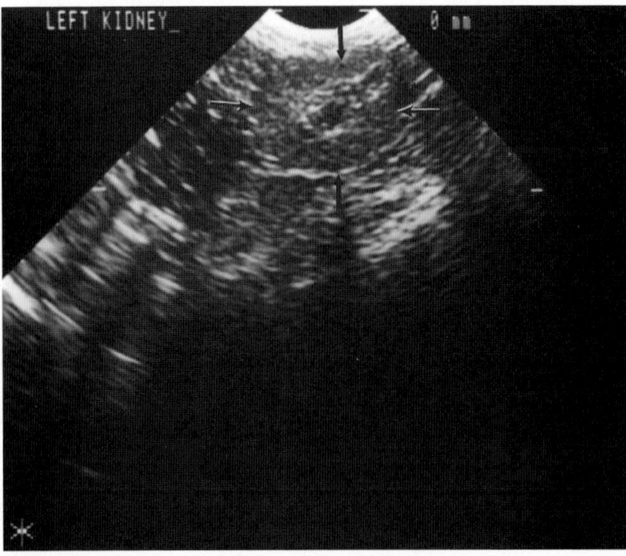

Figure 10-5. Sagittal view of a kidney of a 4-year-old shih tzu in chronic renal failure due to familial nephropathy. The margins of the kidney are marked by arrows. The kidney is small and hyperechoic.

calcium oxalate salts are deposited within the tubules and their epithelial lining.[10] In acute ethylene glycol toxicity, the renal cortex becomes hyperechoic to the liver and isoechoic to the spleen. This finding may be seen within 4 hours of ingestion of antifreeze.[11] The medulla becomes hyperechoic after the cortical changes occur.

The *medullary rim sign* and the *halo sign* are seen within the medulla. The medullary rim sign is an echogenic line in the outer zone of the renal medulla that parallels the corticomedullary junction. The halo sign is a thin hypoechoic zone at the corticomedullary junction. Both of these sonographic signs have been seen in patients with ethylene glycol toxicity. These sonographic signs are nonspecific and are seen with other renal diseases (Fig. 10-6).[12]

Pyelonephritis

Pyelonephritis is inflammation of the renal pelvis and renal parenchyma. Ascending infec-

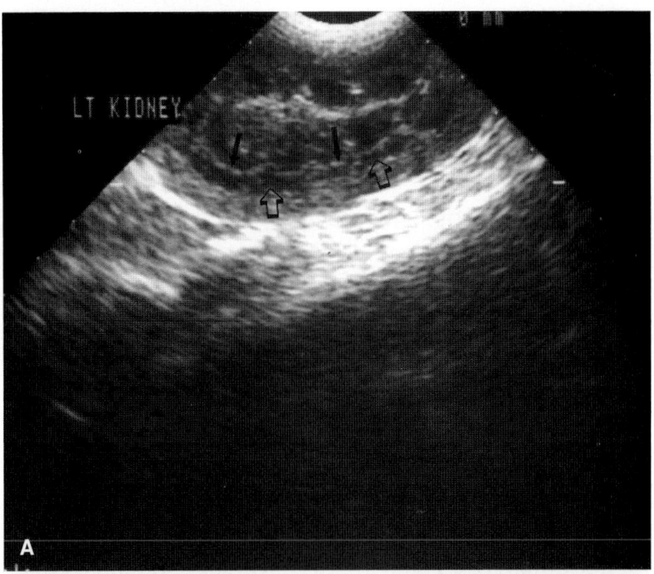

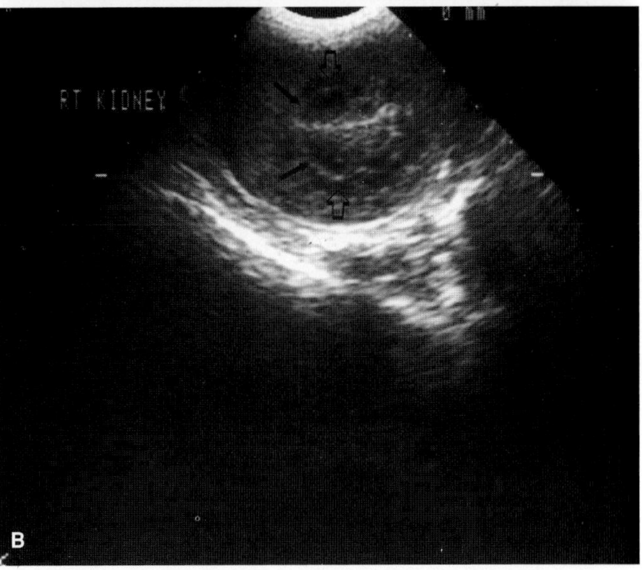

Figure 10-6. (**A**) Sagittal view of a left kidney affected by ethylene glycol toxicity. Notice the medullary rim sign (*solid arrows*) and halo sign (*open arrows*). (**B**) Transverse view of the right kidney. Notice the medullary rim sign (*solid arrows*) and halo sign (*open arrows*).

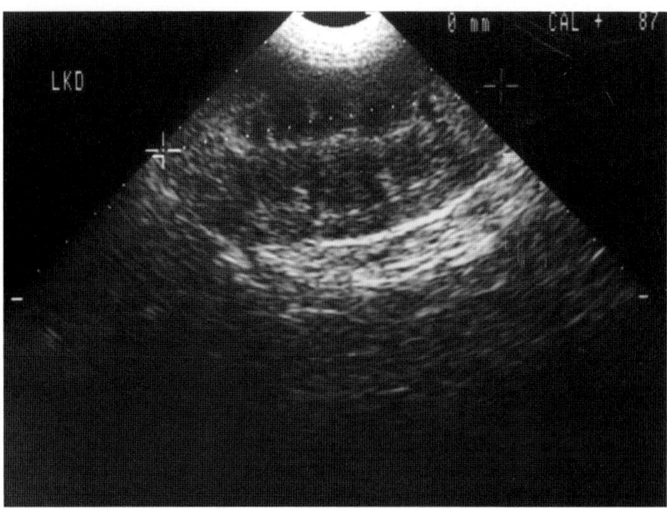

Figure 10-7. Sagittal view of a kidney with acute pyelonephritis. Notice patchy hyperechoic cortex.

tion from the lower urinary tract is the most common cause of pyelonephritis.

Sonographic findings of acute pyelonephritis may include renomegaly, increased echogenicity of the renal cortex and medulla, patchy, ill-defined areas of hyperechogenicity in the cortex, and lack of visualization of the corticomedullary junction (Figs. 10-7 and 10-8).[13] The renal pelvis may be dilated and hyperechoic debris may be present (Fig. 10-9). In mild cases, there are no visible sonographic abnormalities.[14]

Chronic pyelonephritis results in fibrosis of the kidney. Sonographic findings of chronic pyelonephritis include increased echogenicity of the renal cortex and medulla, dilated renal pelvis, and small, irregularly shaped kidneys (Fig. 10-10).

Renal Abscess

Renal abscesses are not common in dogs or cats. Sonographically, abscesses appear as well-marginated, round to oval anechoic masses with irregular walls. Distant enhancement is a characteristic feature of abscesses. Debris within an abscess may produce specular echoes.[3] If an abscess contains a large amount of inspissated material, it can be echogenic and not demonstrate distant enhancement.[9]

Polycystic Kidneys

Polycystic kidneys contain multiple, fluid-filled cavities derived from renal tubules. This condi-

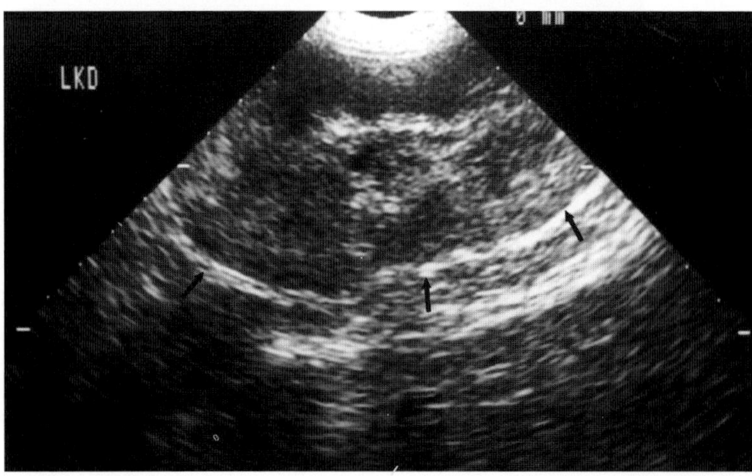

Figure 10-8. Sagittal view of a kidney with acute pyelonephritis. Notice the patchy hyperechoic cortex and poor demarcation between the cortex and medulla. Arrows mark the irregular margin of the renal capsule.

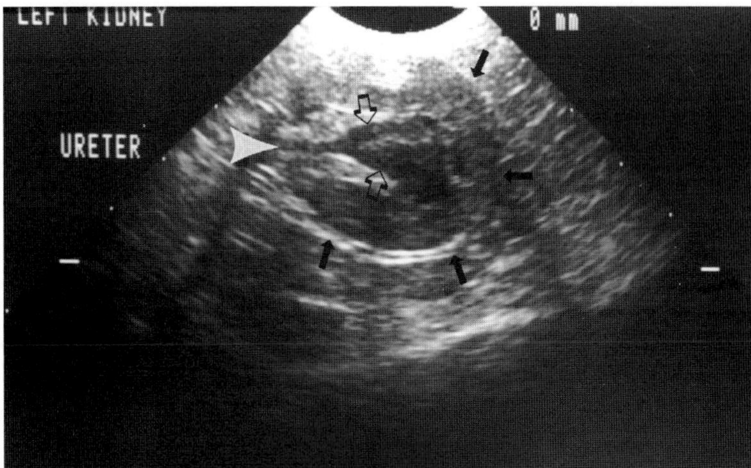

Figure 10-9. Transverse view of a kidney with acute pyelonephritis. Notice the dilated hypoechoic ureter (*white arrowhead*) and dilated pelvis (*open arrows*). The margins of the kidney are marked by black arrows.

tion can be inherited (eg, cairn terriers, longhaired cats) or can be acquired secondary to inflammation or obstruction of the renal tubules.[15] Obstruction of the renal tubules may result in urine-filled cysts.[9] Clinical signs are the result of chronic renal failure. Polycystic renal disease is more common in cats than in dogs. In dogs, solitary cysts may be incidental findings.[16] Shih tzu and Lhasa apso dogs with familial nephropathy may have focal areas of numerous cortical cysts. People with polycystic kidney disease often have polycystic liver disease. Polycystic kidney disease with concurrent hepatic cysts has been reported in cats.[17]

Sonographically, cysts are anechoic masses of variable size that have distant enhancement (Fig. 10-11). Most cysts occur in the medulla. Cysts can become secondarily infected and may show small internal echoes due to cellular debris. In severe cases, the renal architecture may be disrupted, but the echogenic fat in the renal sinus should still be present. Renomegaly is a common finding.

Hydronephrosis

Hydronephrosis is the result of complete or partial obstruction of urine flow from the affected kidney. Obstruction of urine outflow causes dilation of the renal pelvis and diverticula. As the condition progresses, the parenchyma of the kidney atrophies. The extent of the pelvic dilation and the parenchymal atrophy depends on

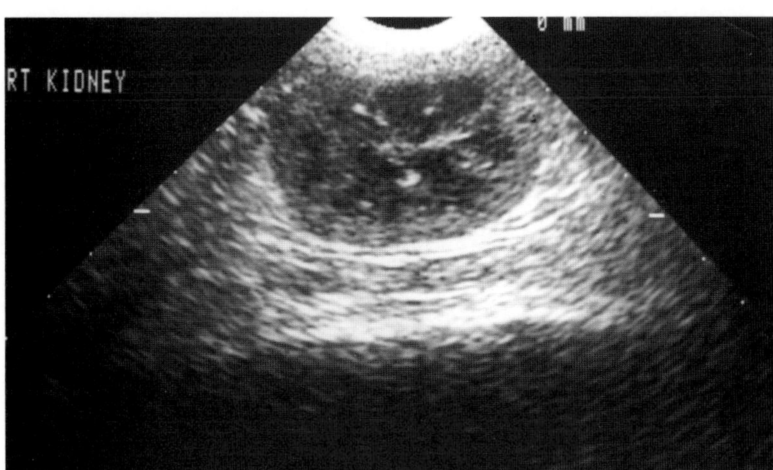

Figure 10-10. Feline kidney with chronic pyelonephritis. The kidney is small, with a patchy, hyperechoic cortex and medulla.

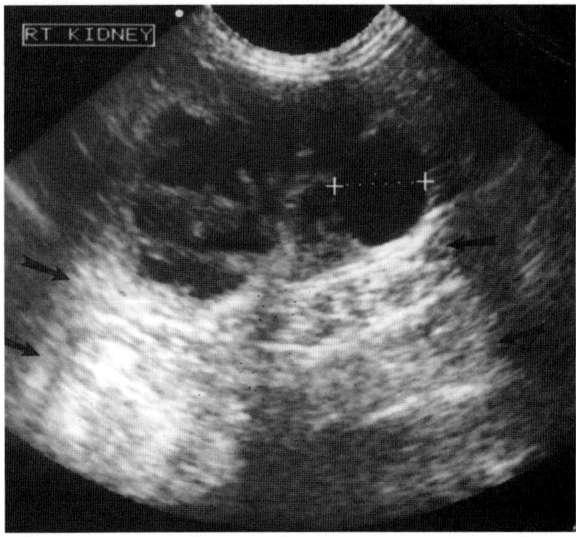

Figure 10-11. Kidney with polycystic disease. Notice the large, anechoic cyst marked by calipers and distant enhancement produced by the polycystic kidney (*arrows*).

the stage of the disease. Hydronephrosis may be unilateral or bilateral, depending on the cause and extent of the obstruction. Moderate to severe hydronephrosis is easily diagnosed with ultrasound.[18] The sonographic features of hydronephrosis include a dilated anechoic pelvis with distant enhancement, an alteration of the medullary and cortical architecture, and an enlarged anechoic ureter (Fig. 10-12). The renal vein may appear similar to a dilated ureter, but it can be differentiated from the ureter by following it to the vena cava. Mild hydronephrosis is best seen on the transverse view of the renal pelvis.

Perirenal Pseudocyst

A perirenal pseudocyst is an encapsulated accumulation of fluid surrounding the cortex of the kidney. Perirenal pseudocysts can be caused by trauma, neoplasia, ureteral obstruction, and infections. Sonographically, they often appear as elliptical anechoic or hypoechoic structures with distant enhancement (Fig. 10-13).[9]

Urinoma

Urine that leaks outside of the kidney and becomes encapsulated in the retroperitoneal space is called a urinoma. Parauteral pseudocyst, uriniferous perirenal pseudocyst, and paraureteral pseudocyst are synonyms for this condition. This condition can be caused by ureteral obstruction, tumor, renal injury, a complication of surgery, or spontaneous occurrence.

Sonographically, urinomas appear to be an anechoic or hypoechoic mass. They are usually elliptical, but may be indented by adjacent organs. They tend to have sharp margins and may contain thin septa.[19]

Renal Calculi

Both contrast radiography (ie, excretory urogram) and ultrasonography are useful for detecting renal calculi. Sonography can be the better choice because it is noninvasive, usually does not require tranquilization, does not depend on kidney function, does not produce emesis, and does not have the potential to produce an anaphylactic reaction.

Sonographically, radiopaque and radiolucent calculi are hyperechoic with acoustic shadowing (Fig. 10-14).[20] Careful control of the machine's overall gain setting is needed to optimize the detection of acoustic shadowing. Usually, lowering the overall gain increases the detection of shadowing. The intensity of the echo does not depend on the size or the compo-

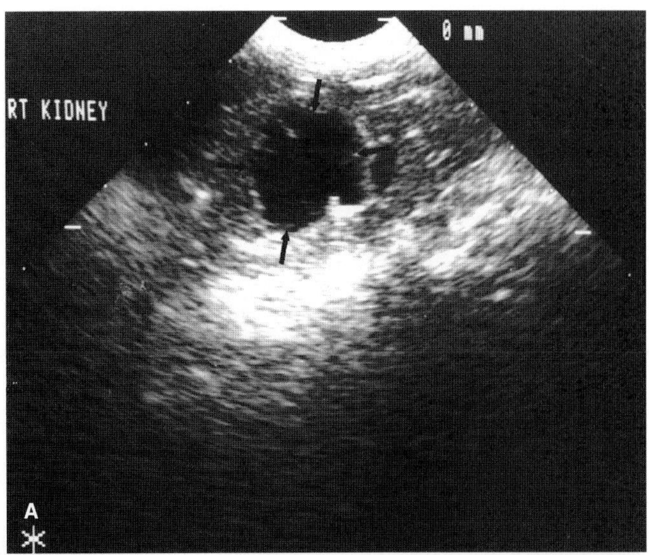

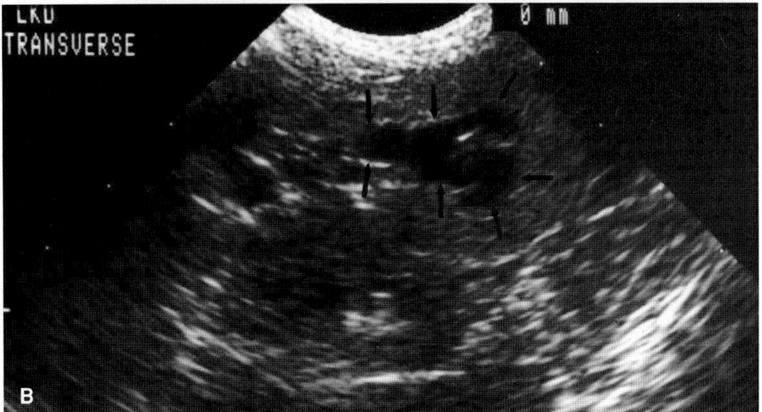

Figure 10-12. (**A**) Sagittal view of a hydronephrotic kidney. Notice the dilated, anechoic pelvis (*arrows*). (**B**) Transverse view of a hdronephrotic kidney. The dilated, anechoic pelvis and medulla are marked by arrows.

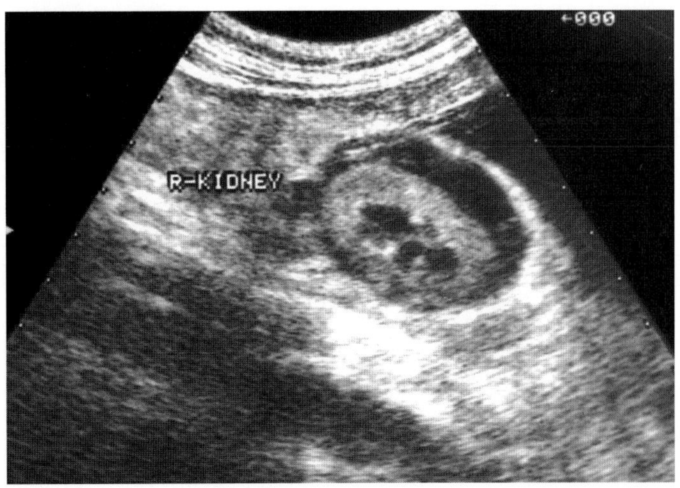

Figure 10-13. Sagittal view of a kidney with a perirenal pseudocyst. The hypoechoic cyst surrounds the hyperechoic cortex.

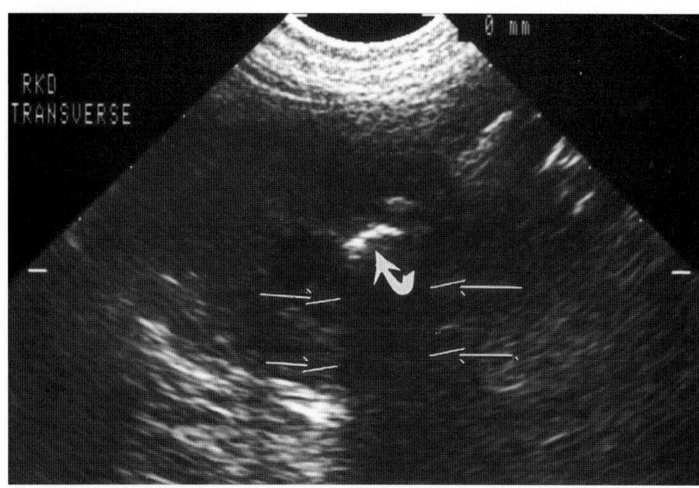

Figure 10-14. Transverse view of a kidney with a calculus (*white arrow*) in the renal pelvis. Notice the acoustic shadow (*black arrows*).

sition of the calculus. At times, the echoes produced by a calculus in the collecting system may be difficult to differentiate from the echoes created by fat in the renal sinus. Dilation of the renal pelvis is a common finding associated with renal calculi.

Nephrocalcinosis

Nephrocalcinosis is a pathologic condition characterized by deposition of calcium salts in the renal parenchyma and is usually secondary to hypercalcemia.[21] Hypercalcemia may be caused by neoplasia, bone disease, renal disease, and endocrine disease. Sonographically, a thin hyperechoic band in the outer zone of the renal medulla that runs parallel to the corticomedullary junction can be seen in patients with nephrocalcinosis (Fig. 10-15). This sonographic finding is referred to as the medullary rim sign, which is a nonspecific finding seen in nephrocalcinosis, ethylene glycol toxicity, chronic interstitial nephritis, feline infectious peritonitis, and some normal cats. The medullary rim sign in nephrocalcinosis is thought to be caused by deposition of calcium salts in the tubules. Acoustic shadowing does not occur with the medullary rim sign.[12]

Renal Infarct

An infarct is an area of coagulation necrosis due to local ischemia resulting from obstruction of circulation to the area. Renal infarcts are most often caused by emboli such as those produced by bacterial endocarditis. An infarct produces a characteristic wedge-shaped or triangular lesion. The base of the lesion is located at the capsular surface, and the apex of the lesion points toward the medulla (Fig. 10-16).[22] Experimentally, a renal infarct in a dog produced a hypoechoic lesion 24 hours after arterial occlusion, and the lesion remained hypoechoic for 5 to 7 days. After 7 days, internal echoes were seen, and the infarct gradually became a hyperechoic lesion by day 17.[23] Because renal tumors and infarcts produce focal hyperechoic lesions, fine-needle aspirates or biopsies are often required to differentiate them.

Feline Infectious Peritonitis

The coronavirus that causes feline infectious peritonitis (FIP) infects many organs including the kidneys. The infection results in pyogranulomatous vasculitis. Sonographic findings include focal hyperechogenicity of the renal cortex and medulla (Fig. 10-17) and possibly the halo and medullary rim signs.[24]

Renal Neoplasia

Renal neoplasms in dogs and cats are uncommon. Adenocarcinoma is the most common primary kidney tumor of the dog. This tumor usually begins in one pole of the kidney and

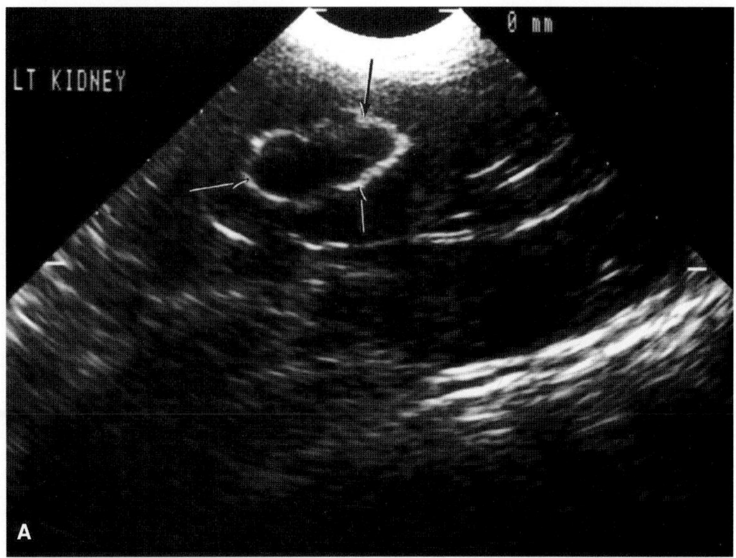

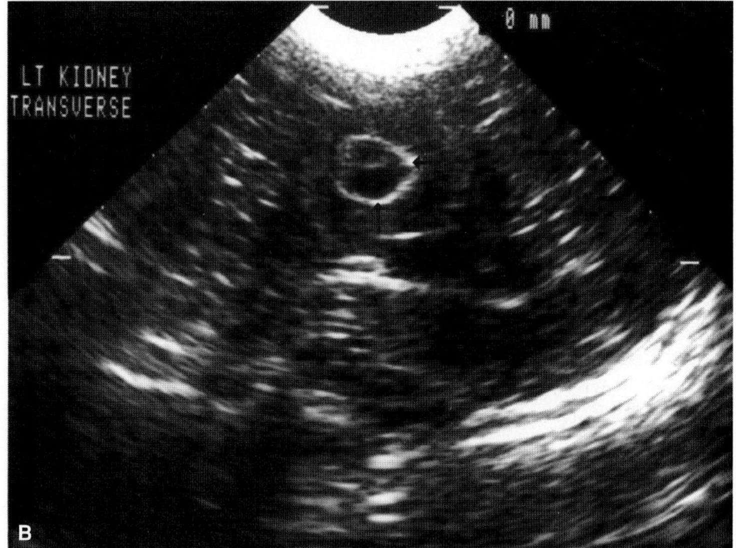

Figure 10-15. (**A**) Sagittal view of a kidney with the medullary rim sign (*arrows*) caused by hypercalcemia. (**B**) Transverse view of the kidney shows a hyperechoic medullary rim sign (*arrows*). There is no acoustic shadowing.

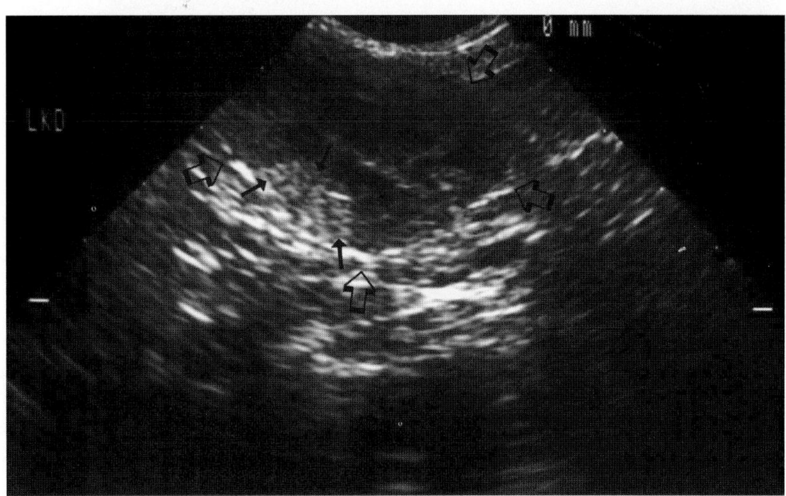

Figure 10-16. Sagittal view of a kidney with a hyperechoic infarct in the cortex (*solid arrows*). The margins of the kidney are marked with open arrows.

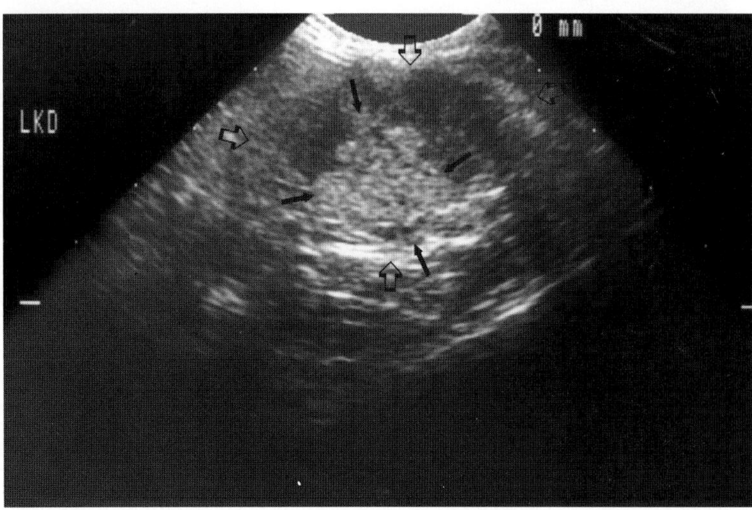

Figure 10-17. Transverse view of a feline kidney with hyperechoic lesions (*solid arrows*) caused by feline infectious peritonitis. The margins of the kidney are marked with open arrows.

sonographically produces focal hyperechoic lesions. Some tumors can be hypoechoic or have a complex echo pattern produced by a mixture of anechoic, hypoechoic, and hyperechoic structures (Fig. 10-18).[16] The echogenicity of neoplasms have been correlated with cell type, the amount of vascularity, the degree of hemorrhage, and the degree of necrosis. Tumors with large amounts of fibrous connective tissue and tumors with mineral deposition are hyperechoic. Poorly vascularized tumors such as lymphosarcoma are hypoechoic. Any renal neoplasm may result in renomegaly. Neoplasms are often expansile and disrupt the architecture of the kidney.[25]

Lymphosarcoma is the most common kidney neoplasm in the cat. Sonographically, lymphosarcoma generally produces hypoechoic to anechoic lesions that do not have distant enhancement. Lymphosarcoma can produce a focal or diffuse lesion and may involve one or both kidneys (Fig. 10-19).[17]

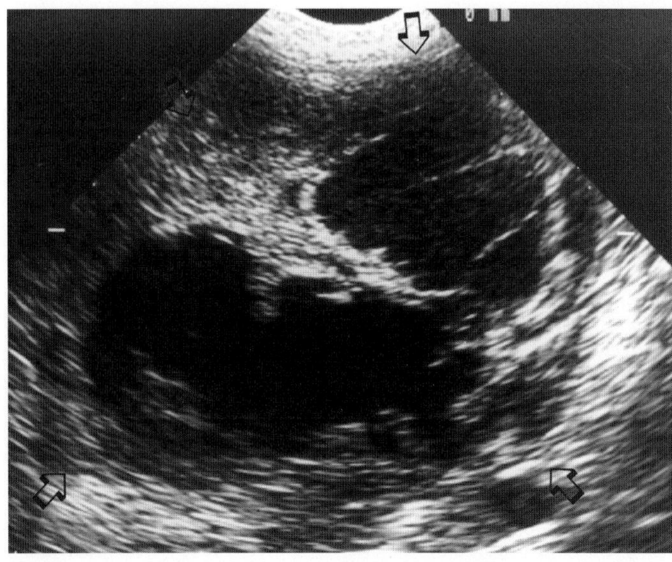

Figure 10-18. Sagittal view of a kidney with disrupted architecture and a mixed echogenic pattern. The margins of the kidneys are marked by open arrows. The diagnosis was fibrosarcoma.

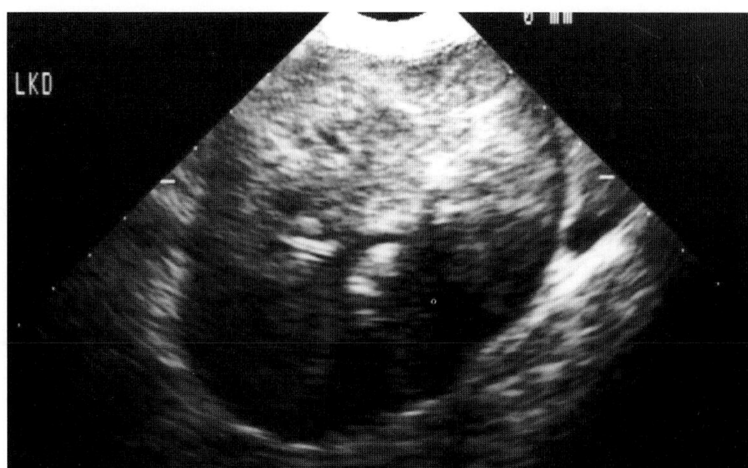

Figure 10-19. Sagittal view of a kidney that has a mixed echogenic pattern and irregular margins. The diagnosis was lymphosarcoma.

RENAL BIOPSIES

A renal biopsy is often required to obtain a definitive diagnosis of kidney disease. Heavy sedation or anesthesia is recommended for renal biopsies. Biopsy techniques are described in Chapter 3. Because kidneys are not in a fixed position, biopsies are best obtained by spring-loaded biopsy instruments. For a sample of the cortex, the caudal pole or lateral cortex of the kidney is recommended. Some sonographers prefer to use a free-hand technique, and others prefer to use a biopsy guide.

CONCLUSION

As a diagnostic tool, ultrasound is often nonspecific. One study showed that 69% of kidneys with nonneoplastic disease were hypoechoic and 31% were normal.[25] Compared with the nonspecificity of survey radiographs and excretory urography, ultrasonography is advantageous in narrowing the spectrum of differential diagnoses.

REFERENCES

1. Christensen G. The urogenital system and mammary glands. In: Miller M, ed. Anatomy of the dog. Philadelphia: WB Saunders, 1964:741.
2. Osborne C, Lowe D, Finco D. Canine and feline urology. Philadelphia: WB Saunders, 1972:3.
3. Walter PA, Johnston GR, Fenny DA, et al. Renal ultrasonography in healthy cats. Am J Vet Res 1987;48:600.
4. Lamb C. A critical review of ultrasonography in small animal renal disease. American Institute of Veterinary Medicine small animal ultrasound seminar, New Orleans, 1990.
5. Konde LJ, Wrigley R, Park R, et al. Ultrasonographic anatomy of the normal canine kidney. Vet Radiol 1984;25:173.
6. Marchal G, Verbeken E, Oyen R, et al. Ultrasound of the normal kidney: a sonographic anatomic and histologic correlation. Ultrasound Med Biol 1986;12:999.
7. Wood, AK, McCarthy PH. Ultrasonographic-anatomic correlation and imaging protocol of the normal canine kidney. Am J Vet Res 1990;51:103.
8. Yeager AE, Anderson WI. Study of association between histologic features and echogenicity of architecturally normal cat kidneys. Am J Vet Res 1989;50:860.
9. Mittlestaedt C. General ultrasound. New York: Churchill Livingstone, 1992:833.
10. Adams WH, Toal RL, Breider MA. Ultrasonographic findings in dogs and cats with oxalate nephrosis attributed to ethylene glycol intoxication: 15 cases (1984–1988). J Am Vet Med Assoc 1991;199:492.

11. Adams WH, Toal RL, Walker MA, et al. Early renal ultrasonographic findings in dogs with experimentally induced ethylene glycol nephrosis. Am J Vet Res 1989;50:1370.
12. Biller DS, Bradley GA, Partington BP. Renal medullary rim sign: ultrasonographic evidence of renal disease. Vet Radiol 1992;33:286.
13. Konde LJ. Renal sonography. Semin Vet Med Surg (Small Anim) 1989;4:32.
14. Neiman HL. Ultrasound of the kidneys. In: Goldberg BB, ed. Textbook of abdominal ultrasound. Baltimore: Williams & Wilkins, 1993:362.
15. Lulich JP, Osborne CA, Walter PA, et al. Feline idiopathic polycystic kidney disease. Compendium on Continuing Education for the Practicing Veterinarian. 1988; 10:1030.
16. Konde LJ. Sonography of the kidney. Vet Clin North Am Small Anim Pract 1985; 15:1149.
17. Walter PA, Johnston GR, Fenny DA, et al. Applications of ultrasonography in the diagnosis of parenchymal kidney disease in cats: 24 cases (1981–1986). J Am Vet Med Assoc 1988;192:92.
18. Cartee RE, Selcer BA, Patton CS. Ultrasonographic diagnosis of renal disease in small animals. J Am Vet Med Assoc 1980;176:426.
19. Tidwell A, Ullman S, Shelling S. Urinoma (para-ureteral pseudocyst) in a dog. Vet Radiol 1990;31:203.
20. Stafford S, Jenkins J, Staab E, et al. Ultrasonic detection of renal calculi: accuracy tested in an in vitro porcine kidney model. J Clin Ultrasound 1981;9: 359.
21. Barr FJ, Patterson MW, Lucke VM, et al. Hypercalcemic nephropathy in three dogs: sonographic appearance. J Vet Radiol 1989;30:169.
22. Biller DS, Schenkman DI, Bortnoski H. Ultrasonographic appearance of renal infarcts in a dog. J Am Anim Hosp Assoc 1991;27:370.
23. Spies JB, Hricak H, Slemmer TM, et al. Sonographic evaluation of experimental acute renal atrial occlusion in dogs. Am J Roentgenol 1984;142:341.
24. Walter PA, Fenny DA, Johnston GR, et al. Feline renal ultrasonography: quantitative analyses of imaged anatomy. Am J Vet Res 1987;48:596.
25. Walter PA, Fenny DA, Johnston GR, et al. Ultrasonographic evaluation of renal diseases in dogs: 32 cases (1981–1986). J Am Vet Med Assoc 1987;191:999.

Small Animal Ultrasound, edited by Ronald W. Green.
Lippincott-Raven Publishers, Philadelphia © 1996.

ADRENAL GLANDS

Linda D. Homco

Sonography of the normal adrenal gland has been generally unsuccessful because of the small size of the normal gland, insufficient knowledge of the anatomy, the limitations of veterinary ultrasound equipment, and the lack of patient compliance. Advances in ultrasound equipment have facilitated imaging of the adrenal glands in companion animals. A sonographer who has good knowledge of abdominal anatomy and good scanning techniques can image the normal and the diseased adrenal gland.

NORMAL ANATOMY AND LOCATION

Canine adrenal glands differ in shape from those of humans.[1] The right canine adrenal gland is triangular, with the apex pointing caudally.[2] Some practitioners refer to the right adrenal gland as having a wedge or harpoon shape, but its true shape is not always appreciated with ultrasound because of an acute angular bend in the cranial part of the gland and its proximity to the right kidney.[3,4] The right adrenal gland is retroperitoneal and dorsolateral to the vena cava, to which it has firm connective tissue attachments.[3] The right adrenal gland is medial to the cranial pole of the right kidney and is near the hilus (ie, pelvis) of this kidney (Fig. 11-1). The cranial two thirds of this adrenal gland is covered by the caudal extension of the right lateral liver lobe. The phrenicoabdominal vein crosses the ventral aspect of the gland.[3]

The left adrenal gland is more caudal than the right (see Fig. 11-1). This gland is craniomedial to the cranial pole of the left kidney and is farther from this renal hilus than the right adrenal gland is from the right renal hilus. The left adrenal gland, which is long and cylindrical, has been described as a figure-eight or dumbbell shape.[2,4] This gland is also retroperitoneal and is loosely bound by connective tissue to the aorta.[3] The left adrenal gland is located lateral to the aorta, between the origins of the cranial mesenteric and the renal arteries. The phrenicoabdominal vein crosses the adrenal gland's ventral surface, creating the central constriction that gives this gland its characteristic shape. The left adrenal gland is dorsal to the left limb of the pancreas.

Both adrenal glands in the cat have a flattened oval or elliptical shape.[5] The right adrenal gland is close to the vena cava and is not in contact with the right kidney, as may occur in the dog (Fig. 11-2). The feline adrenal glands may be surrounded by various degrees of retroperitoneal fat.

Each gland is composed of an outer cortex and an inner medulla. The glands were reported to be 2 to 3 cm long, 1 cm wide, and 0.5 cm thick

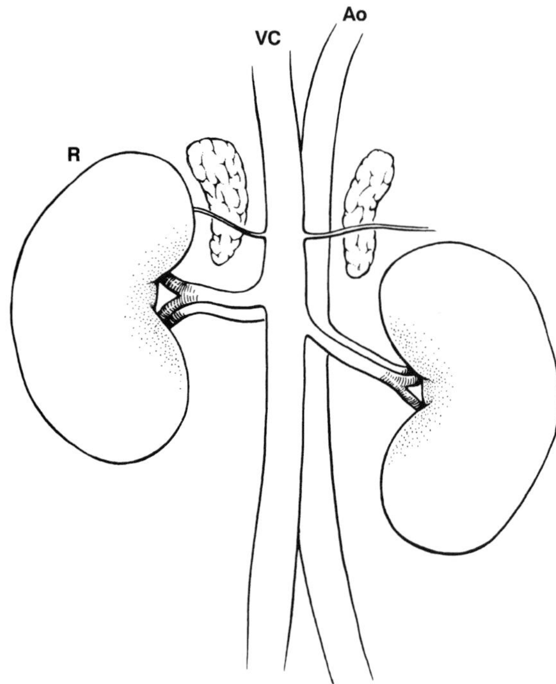

Figure 11-1. Line drawing of the normal locations and shapes of the adrenal glands in the dog. *R*, right kidney; *VC*, vena cava; *Ao*, aorta.

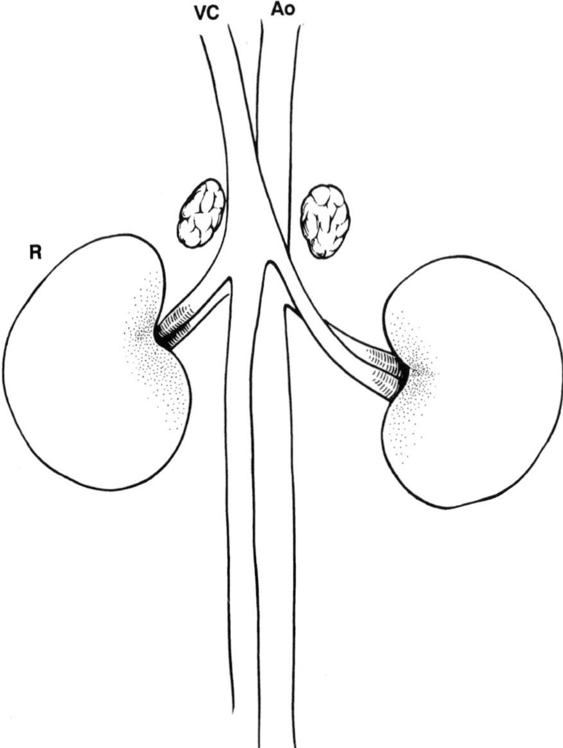

Figure 11-2. Line drawing of the normal locations and shapes of the adrenal glands in the cat. *R*, right kidney; *VC*, vena cava; *Ao*, aorta.

in mature dogs, although neither the breed nor the weight of the dogs were reported in this study.[2] The exact size of normal adrenal glands in various breeds of dogs and cats has yet to be reported.

SCANNING TECHNIQUES

Imaging of the normal adrenal glands is extremely difficult and time consuming. The success rate of imaging the normal adrenal gland depends on the quality of the gray-scale image, the resolution of the transducer, the size and cooperation of the patient, and the skill and effort of the sonographer.

The adrenal gland can be visualized in many planes and from many approaches. In general, the best approach to the adrenal gland is to have the patient in dorsal recumbency while scanning longitudinally or sagittally from a ventral paramedian or a lateral oblique approach. Lateral recumbency, which is also used by some, facilitates dorsal intercostal imaging of the right adrenal gland.[6]

A small-footprint transducer (sector) is ideal for compression and intercostal scanning. A 5.0-MHz transducer with good lateral resolution suffices for most medium to large dogs. A 7.5-MHz sector transducer is ideal for small dogs and cats. In very-deep-chested large-breed dogs, a 3.5-MHz transducer may be needed for penetration, but because of poorer resolution of this frequency transducer, the normal adrenal gland may not be identified. In general, obesity, panting, or poor patient cooperation limit the sonographer's ability to identify the adrenal gland. Another limitation to scanning the adrenal glands is the lack of an acoustic window because of interference by bowel gas, a distended stomach, and a full transverse colon.

NORMAL SONOGRAPHIC APPEARANCE

The adrenal gland, because of its small size and the small difference in acoustic impedance between it and the surrounding tissues, may be definable as a distinct structure in only a few individuals. The normal adrenal gland is hypoechoic within the surrounding echogenic retroperitoneal fat and fibrous tissue (Fig. 11-3), although at times, the adrenal glands may appear only

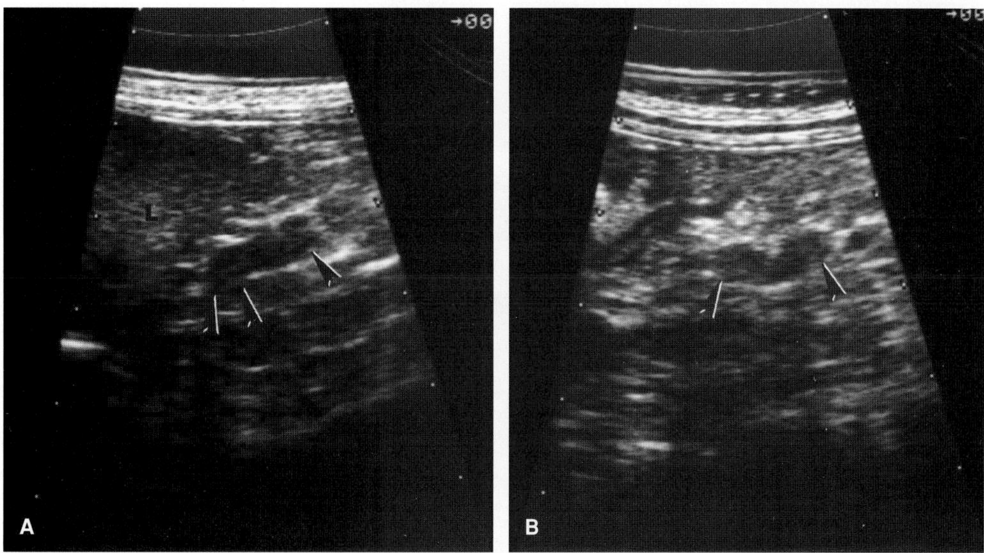

Figure 11-3. Sagittal sonogram of the **(A)** normal right and **(B)** left adrenal glands (*arrows*) in a dog. Both glands are hypoechoic to the surrounding retroperitoneal fat. Notice the difference in shape between the two glands. *L*, liver.

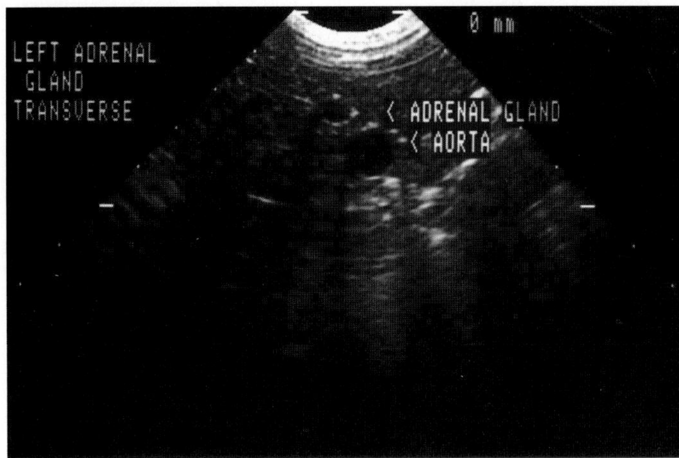

Figure 11-4. Dorsal plane transverse sonogram of the cranial pole of the normal left adrenal gland in a dog. Notice the anechoic appearance of the aorta relative to the adrenal gland parenchyma and the proximity of this adrenal gland to the aorta.

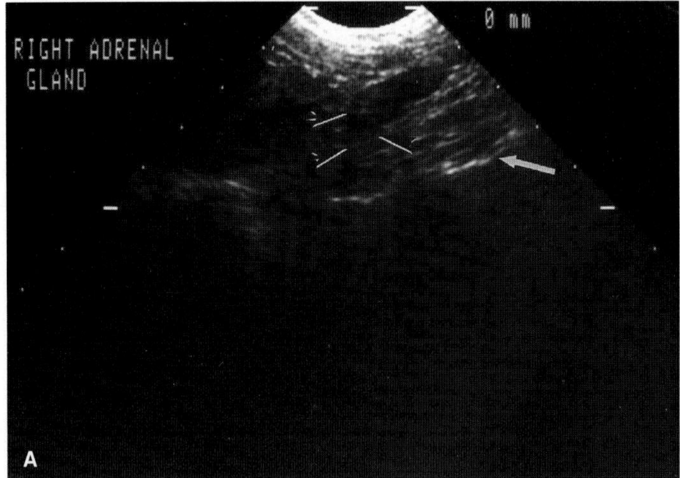

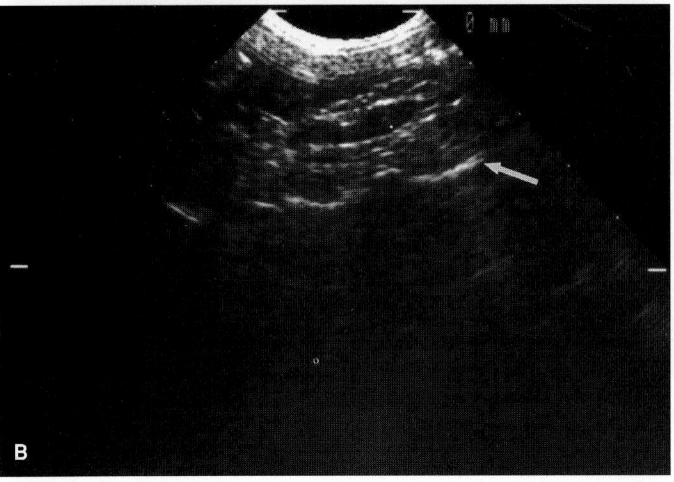

Figure 11-5. (**A**) Sagittal sonogram of a normal right adrenal gland in a dog. The cranial pole (*arrowheads*) is broader than the caudal pole, which gives this adrenal gland a wedge shape. Compare this with the normal left adrenal gland in **B** with its long figure-eight shape. The echodense scalloped lines (*white arrows*) deep to each adrenal gland in **A** and **B** are the ventral aspects of the lumbar vertebral bodies.

slightly less echoic than the surrounding tissue.[7] If the kidney is imaged in the same plane, the adrenal gland typically is slightly more echoic than the renal cortex. Adjacent blood vessels are anechoic by comparison (Fig. 11-4).

Normal canine and feline adrenal glands should appear relatively thin, with no distortion of their characteristic shape (Figs. 11-5 and 11-6). When imaging in a longitudinal plane, the left canine adrenal gland is shaped like a dumbbell or a peanut in a shell, with prominent symmetric cranial and caudal poles and a constriction in the center (Fig. 11-7). The right adrenal gland is triangular or shaped like an arrowhead, with the cranial third appearing wider when imaged from a frontal long-axis or dorsal plane (Fig. 11-8).[8] When viewed in a longitudinal plane from the ventral aspect, the right adrenal gland may appear comma shaped or somewhat like a bent arrow (Fig. 11-9).[7,9]

DISEASES OF THE ADRENAL GLANDS

Most of the diseases of the adrenal glands that can be evaluated with ultrasound fall into two categories: pituitary- or adrenal-dependent hyperadrenocorticism and neoplasia. Other causes of adrenal gland enlargement in humans have been reported.[10]

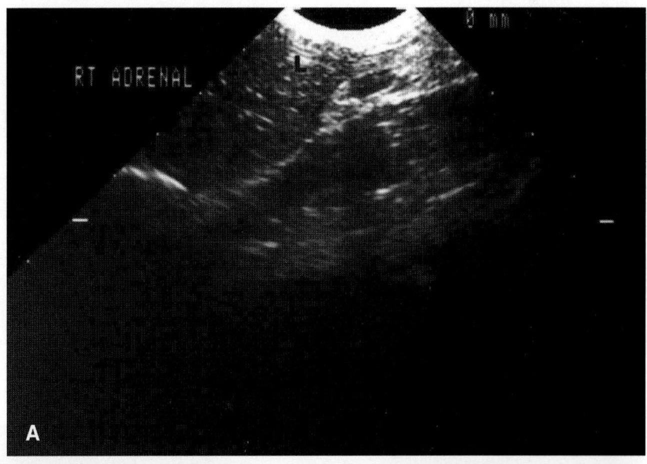

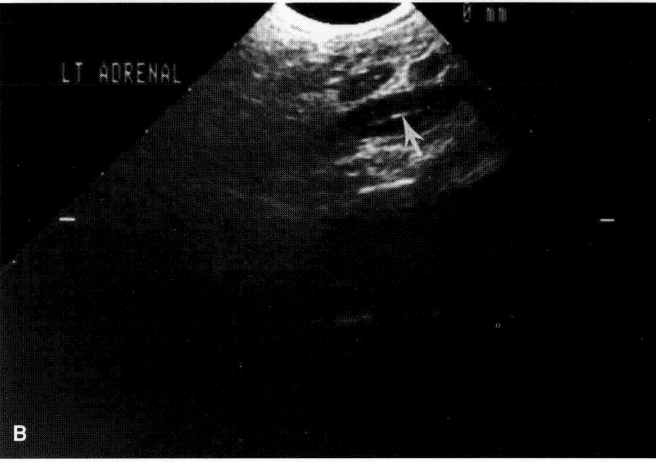

Figure 11-6. Sagittal sonogram of the normal adrenal glands in a cat. Notice that both are thin and ovoid. **(A)** The right adrenal gland is surrounded by echogenic retroperitoneal fat. *L*, liver. **(B)** The left adrenal gland is also surrounded by echodense retroperitoneal fat and is close to the aorta (*arrow*).

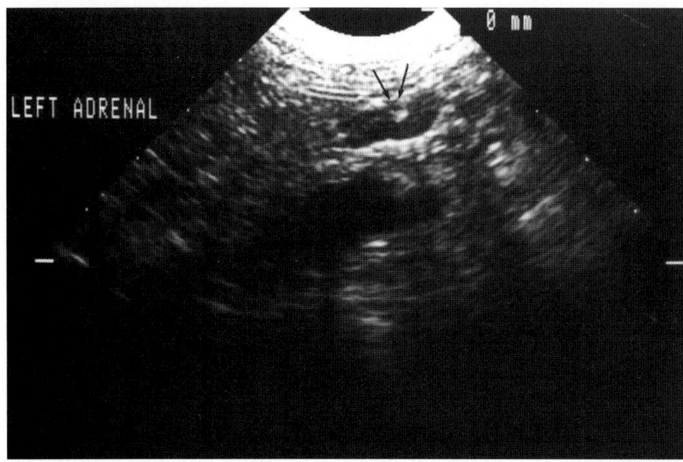

Figure 11-7. Sagittal sonogram of a normal canine left adrenal gland shows the characteristic peanut-in-a-shell shape. The central constriction is created by the phrenicoabdominal vein, which can be seen crossing the ventral surface of this gland (*arrows*).

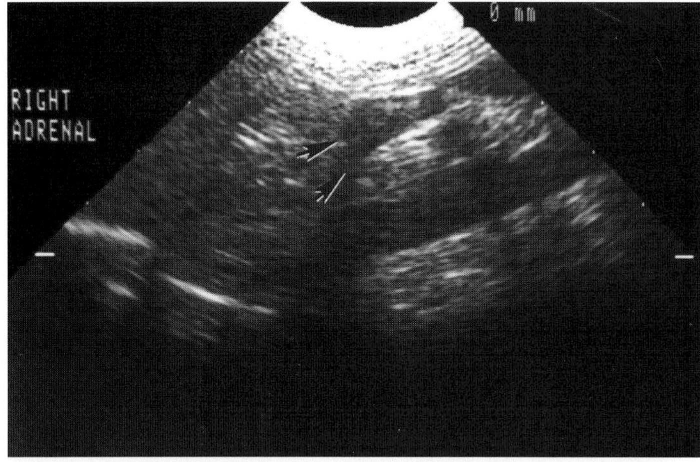

Figure 11-8. Dorsal plane long-axis sonogram of a normal canine right adrenal gland. This adrenal gland demonstrates the characteristic arrowhead shape, with the cranial pole (*arrows*) wider than the caudal pole in this image plane.

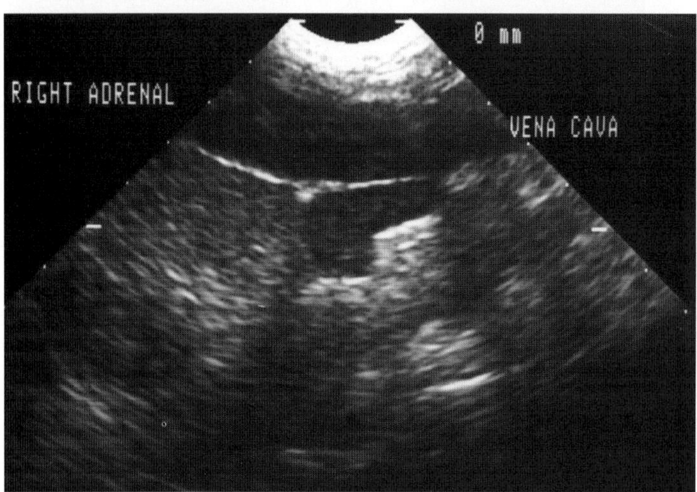

Figure 11-9. A comma-shaped appearance of the right adrenal gland was best demonstrated in this dog in a dorsal long-axis plane imaged from the left side. This is the reason the vena cava is seen in the near field. (If the right kidney were included in this scan plane, it would be displayed deep to the adrenal gland in the far field.)

Pituitary-Dependent Hyperadrenocorticism

In pituitary-dependent hyperadrenocorticism (PDH), both adrenal glands hypertrophy as a result of overstimulation from the pituitary gland. Both adrenal glands enlarge symmetrically (Fig. 11-10). Because both adrenal glands are normally thin structures, an increase in thickness or a plump appearance is characteristic of adrenal gland hypertrophy (Fig. 11-11). This assessment is more reliable than measuring the length of the gland, because the normal length of adrenal glands in various breeds and sizes of dogs has yet to be reported. The adrenal gland cross-sectional area has been compared with the cross-sectional area of the aorta, but this measurement overlaps that of dogs with normal and neoplastic glands (Fig. 11-12*C, D*).[11] Because of their increase in size, both adrenal glands are easier to identify and often appear isoechoic or hypoechoic to the renal cortex. Occasionally, distinct layers of alternate echogenicity are seen in some PDH glands (see Fig. 11-12). The reason for this is unknown, although I think the change may be caused by hypertrophy of the adrenal cortex. As a result of this change, a thick outer hypoechoic zone contrasts with the echogenic medulla, an appearance similar to that described for the normal neonatal adrenal gland in which the cortex is normally 13 times the size of the adult adrenal cortex.[12]

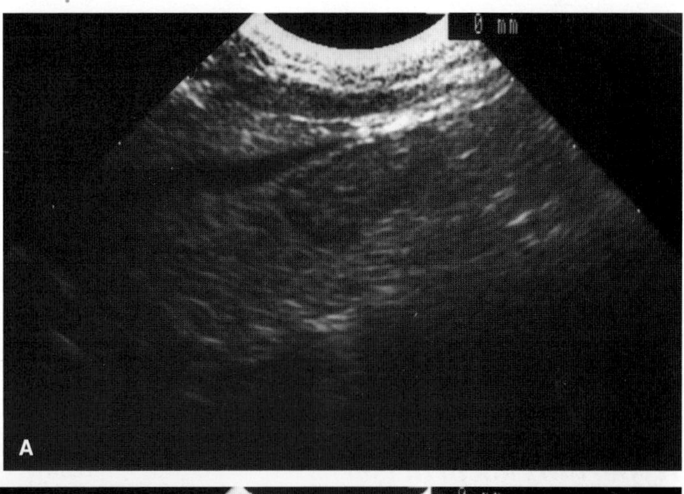

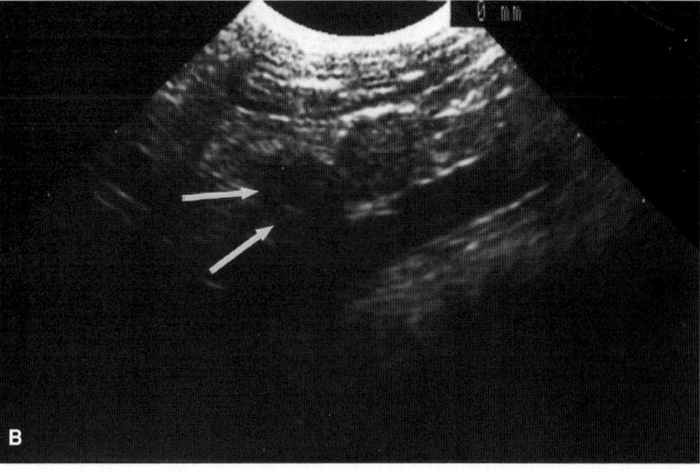

Figure 11-10. Sagittal sonograms of the (**A**) right and (**B**) left adrenal glands from a dog with pituitary-dependent hyperadrenocorticism. Both adrenal glands are enlarged and appear somewhat plump but have maintained their respective shape. The borders of the cranial aspect of the left adrenal gland in **B** are defined with arrows.

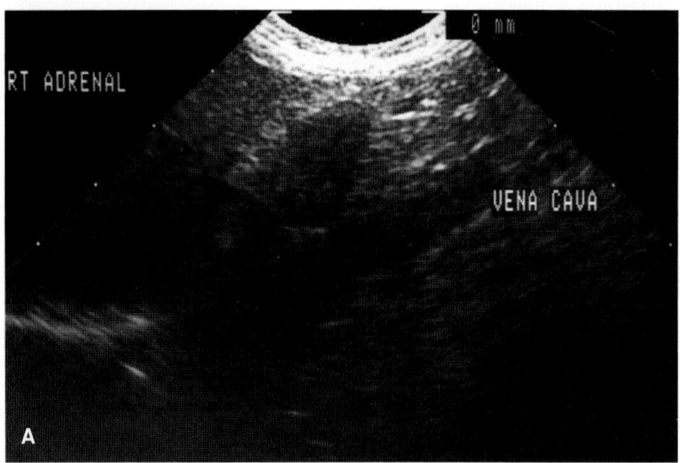

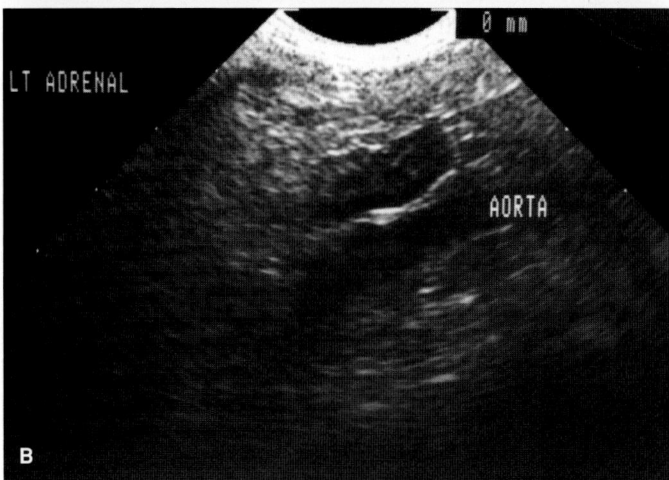

Figure 11-11. Sagittal sonograms of the (**A**) right and (**B**) left adrenal glands from a dog with pituitary-dependent hyperadrenocorticism. Notice the increased thickness of each gland compared with the size of the abdominal vessels.

Adrenal-Dependent Hyperadrenocorticism

In adrenal-dependent hyperadrenocorticism (ADH), a functional unilateral mass is present. The lesion can vary in size and location within either gland, and the mass may appear hyperechoic or hypoechoic relative to the remaining normal parenchyma (Figs. 11-13 and 11-14).[7,9,13,14] The contralateral gland typically atrophies and appears reduced in size or may not be imaged at all (Fig. 11-15).[7,15]

Adrenal Masses or Neoplasia

Adrenal masses may be unilateral or bilateral, functional or nonfunctional, benign or malignant, and primary or metastatic.

Primary adrenocortical neoplasia can be the result of an adenoma or a carcinoma (Fig. 11-16).[14,16] The comparative ultrasonographic characteristics of benign and malignant neoplasms have not been described for the dog or cat. Adrenal tumors may be hypoechoic or hyperechoic, and because of a uniform cellular structure, their texture theoretically should be homogeneous.[17] However, as tumors enlarge, focal necrosis causing hyperechoic foci, cystic cavitations, and eventually mixed or complex echo patterns may occur.[17,18] Mineralization in the canine adrenal gland has been reported in cases of adrenal carcinoma and adenoma, and mineralization in the feline adrenal gland is normal in up to 30% of the population.[11,19] Tumors may occur anywhere in the adrenal gland and are often recognized because of the distorted

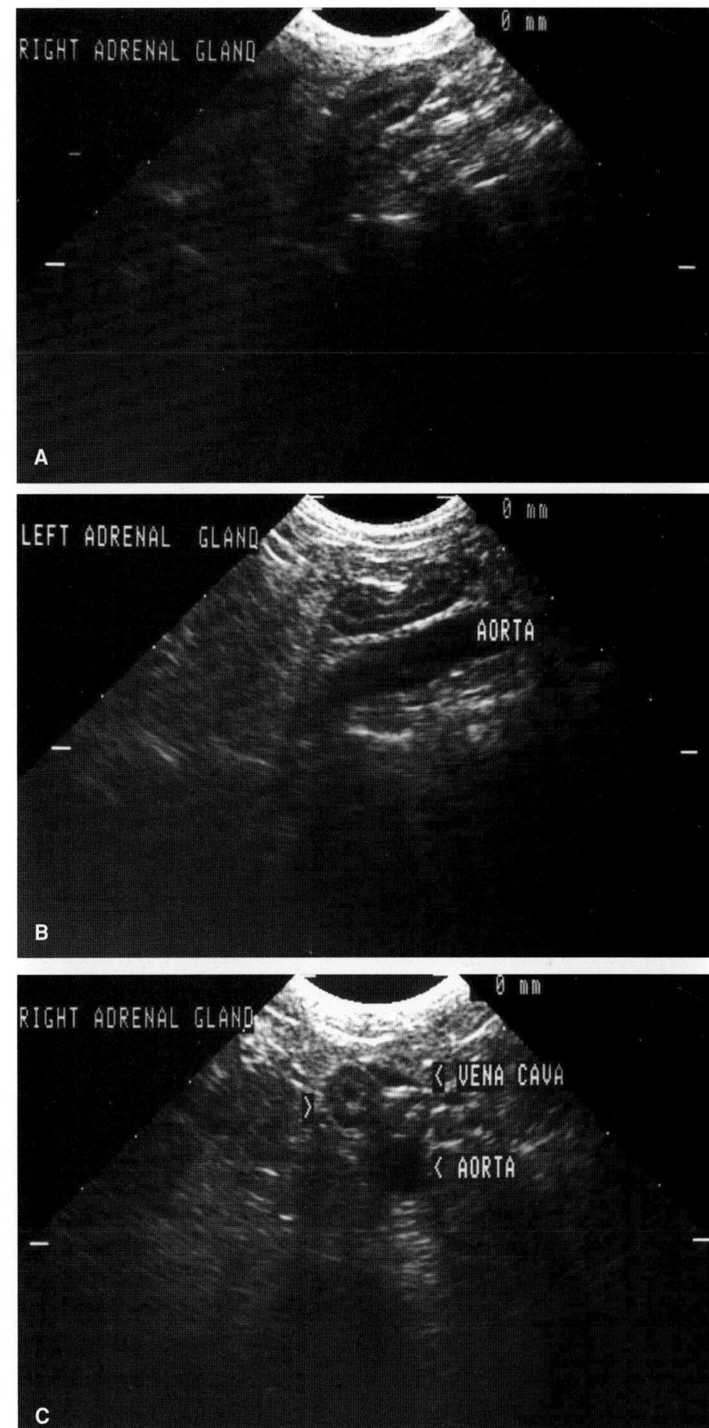

Figure 11-12. (**A and B**) Sagittal and (**C and D**) transverse sonograms show distinctly different echogenic layers of the adrenal glands from a dog with pituitary-dependent hyperadrenocorticism. *(continued)*

shape of the individual gland. Large adrenal masses may displace or deform adjacent organs or vessels. The smallest human adrenal tumors reported have been 0.8 cm in diameter.[20] Microadenomas may not be seen.

Unilateral functional adrenal tumors suppress the contralateral gland, causing atrophy that is apparent during routine sonographic examination. Other adrenal neoplasms that are

(text continues on p. 223)

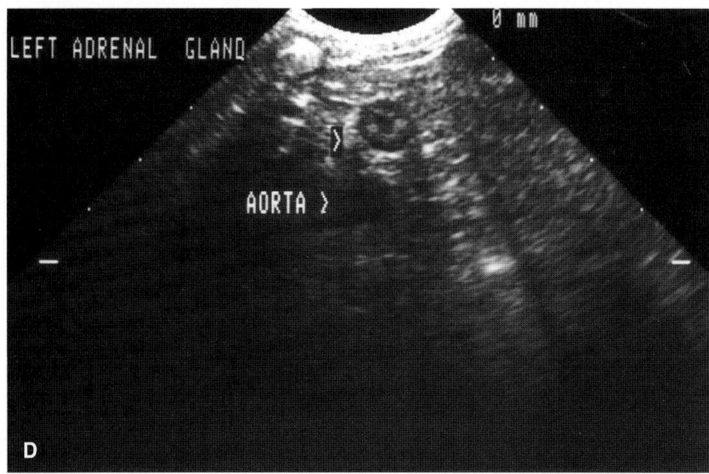

Figure 11-12. *(Continued)* Compare the cross-sectional area of each adrenal gland with the aorta in **C** and **D** and to the normal adrenal gland shown in Figure 11-4. The vena cava appears flat in **C** because of the graded compression used to displace the small intestine from the imaging plane.

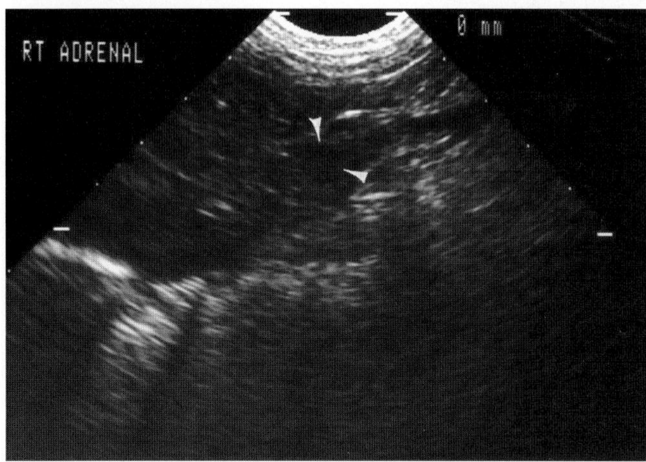

Figure 11-13. Sagittal sonogram of the right adrenal gland in a dog with adrenal-dependent hyperadrenocorticism. The mass in the cranial pole (*arrowheads*) is hypoechoic relative to the adrenal parenchyma and does not distort the normal arrowhead-shape of this gland. The left adrenal gland in this dog was atrophied.

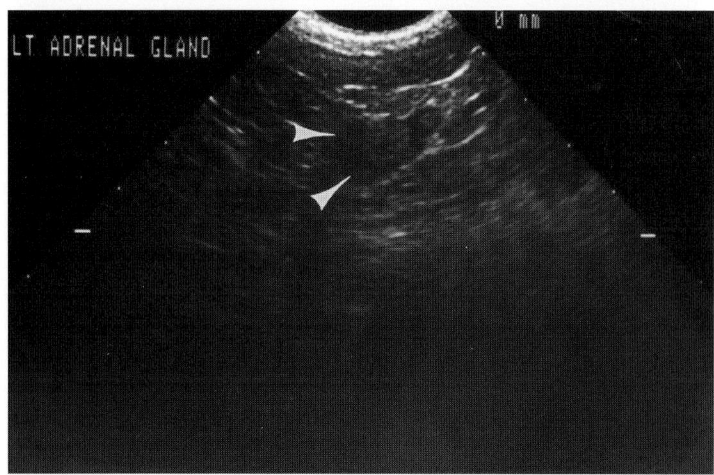

Figure 11-14. Sagittal sonogram of the left adrenal gland in a dog with adrenal-dependent hyperadrenocorticism. The mass is hyperechoic and distorts the entire cranial aspect (*arrows*) of this adrenal gland. The right adrenal gland in this dog was not located sonographically.

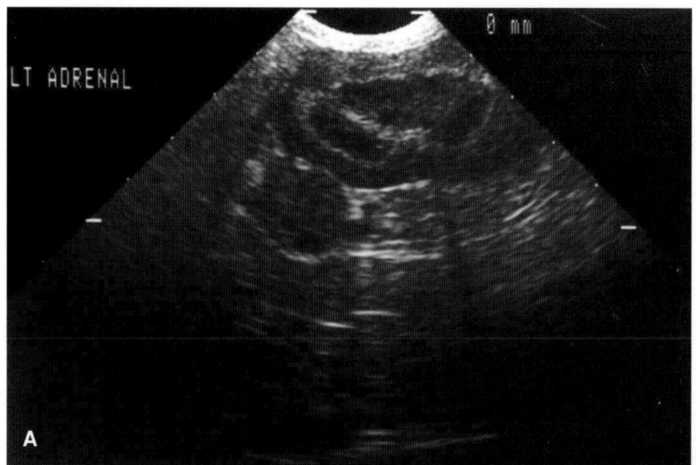

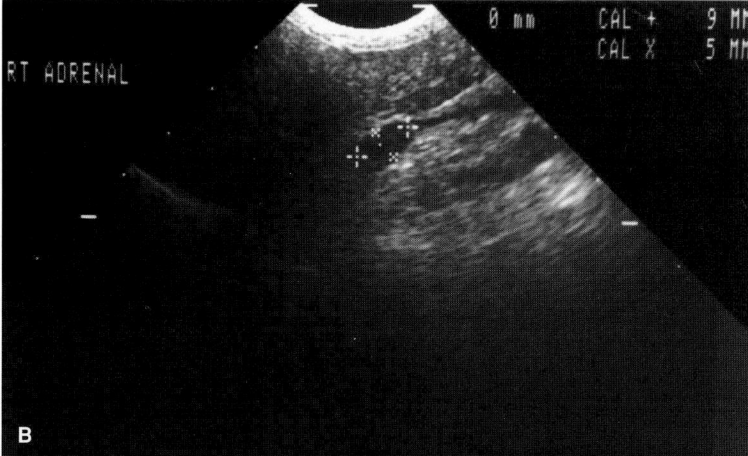

Figure 11-15. (**A**) Dorsal plane long-axis sonogram of the left adrenal gland and kidney in a dog with adrenal-dependent hyperadrenocorticism. The mass, which is nearly isoechoic to the renal cortex, distorts all but the caudal pole of this adrenal gland. (**B**) Sagittal sonogram of the atrophied right adrenal gland in the dog.

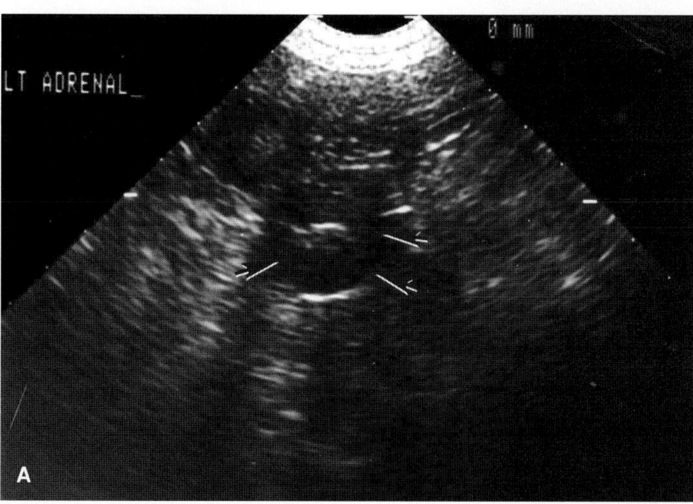

Figure 11-16. (**A**) Sagittal and (**B**) dorsal long-axis sonograms of a primary adrenocortical carcinoma in a dog. This mass (*arrows*) is hypoechoic, with a central echogenic zone resulting from parenchymal mineralization, which was also evident on abdominal radiographs. A portion of the left kidney (*LKD*) is seen in **B**.

(continued)

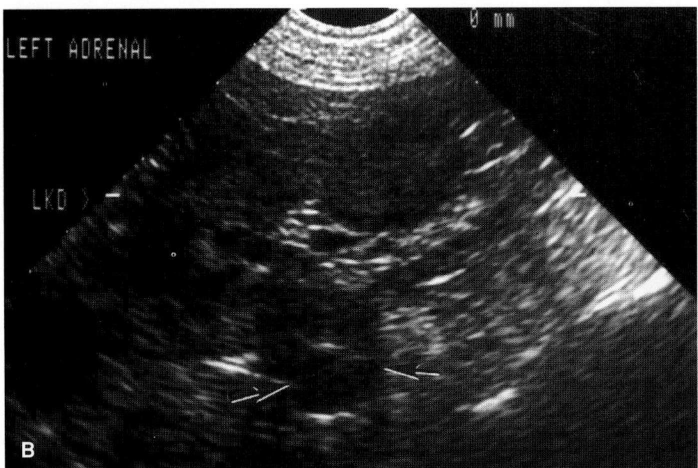

Figure 11-16. *(Continued)*

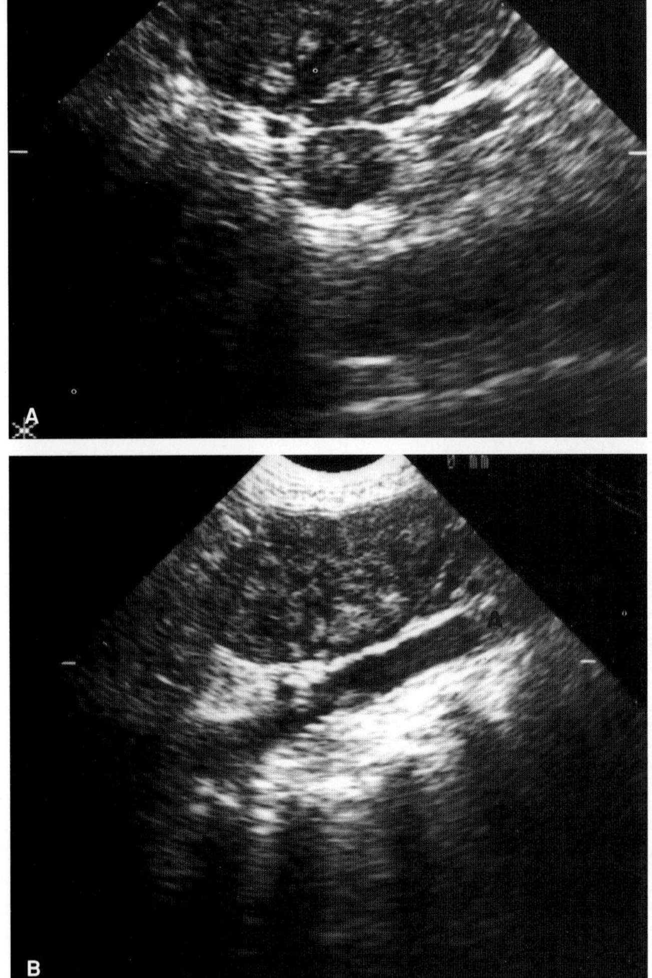

Figure 11-17. Sagittal sonograms of a pheochromocytoma of the left adrenal gland in a dog. (**A**) This tumor displays a mixed-echo pattern and an irregular shape. (**B**) It is close to the aorta *A*, with no local vascular invasion evident.

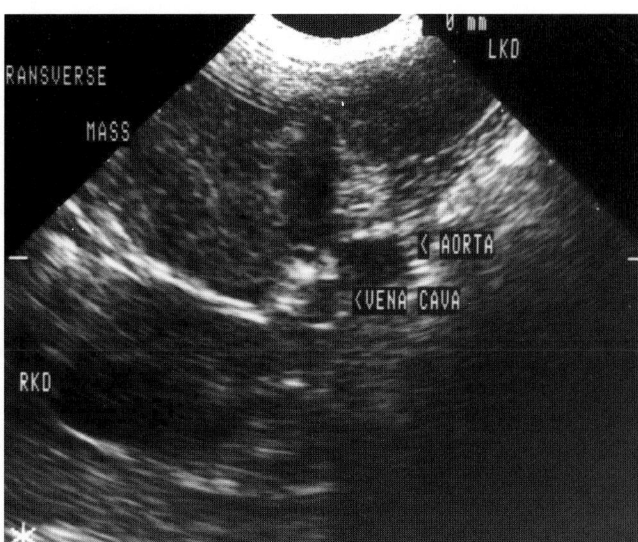

Figure 11-18. Transverse sonogram of a pheochromocytoma of the right adrenal gland in a dog. Local tumor invasion of the vena cava is apparent. Notice the increased echogenicity in the lumen of the vena cava compared with the aorta. Portions of the right (*RKD*) and left (*LKD*) kidneys are also included in this image.

often unilateral are nonfunctional adrenocortical tumors, adrenal medullary tumors (eg, pheochromocytoma, neuroblastoma, ganglioneuromas), and metastatic tumors. Pheochromocytomas are characterized by a mixed-echo pattern, large size, irregular shape, and invasiveness (Fig. 11-17).[17,21] They often surround and invade vascular structures in the area, particularly of the vena cava (Fig. 11-18).[22]

Bilateral primary adrenal tumors have been reported (Fig. 11-19).[16] Metastases to both adrenal glands can occur simultaneously.[18,23] After an adrenal mass has been identified, a thorough ultrasound examination of the liver for metastatic disease is highly recommended.

Other Causes of Adrenal Gland Enlargement

The human literature reports that diffuse enlargement of both adrenal glands can occur with systemic fungal diseases such as histoplasmosis.[10] The glands often enlarge symmetrically and may be increased in echogenicity (Fig. 11-20).

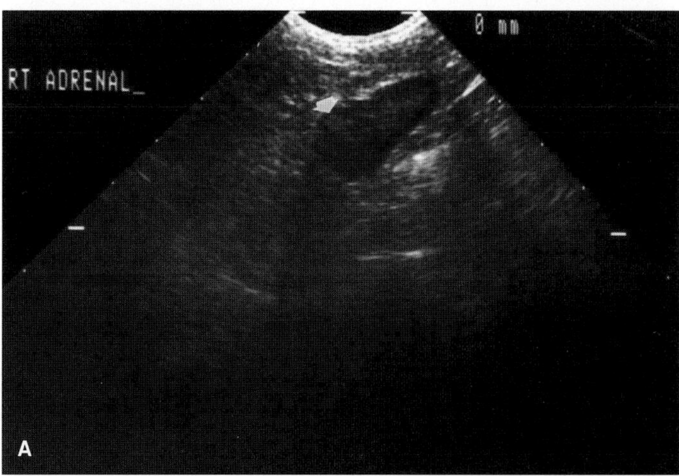

Figure 11-19. Sagittal sonograms of the (**A**) right and (**B**) left adrenal glands in a dog with bilateral primary adrenal adenomas. Small, hyperechoic nodules (*arrows*) are seen within the ventral aspect of the cranial pole of the right adrenal gland and the mid-ventral aspect of the left adrenal gland. *(continued)*

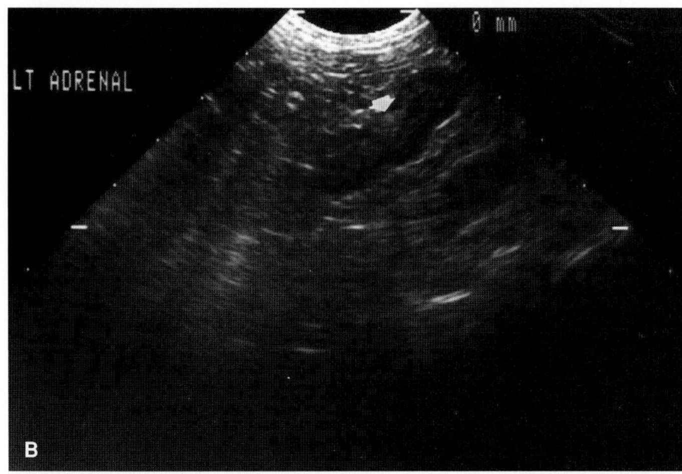

Figure 11-19. *(Continued)*

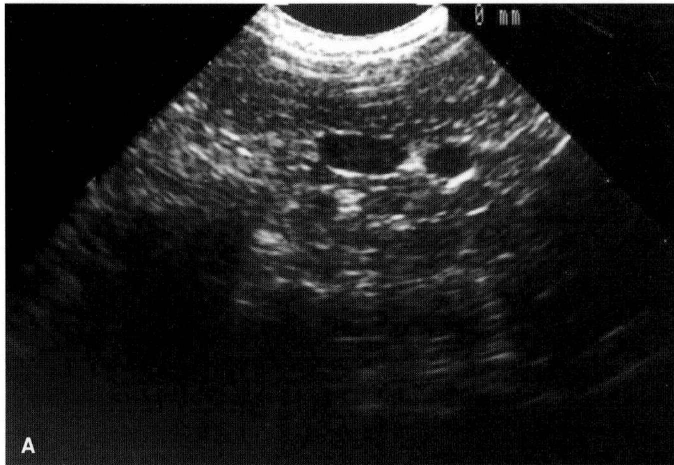

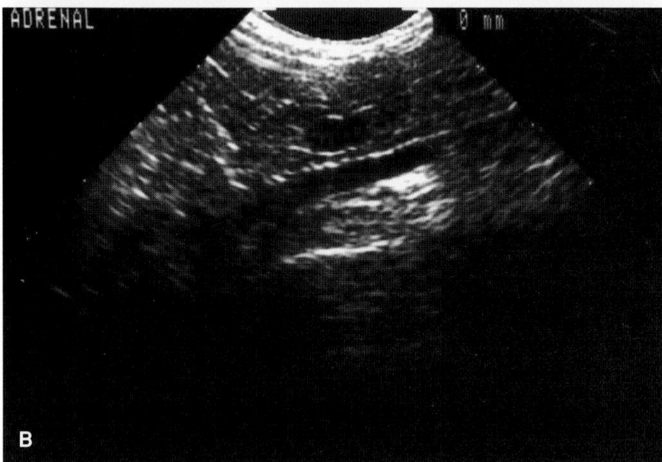

Figure 11-20. Sagittal sonograms of the (**A**) right and (**B**) left adrenal glands in a cat with feline infectious peritonitis. Both adrenal glands are thickened. In a transverse scan plane (not shown), the cross-sectional area of the left adrenal gland was larger than the aorta, as is apparent in **B**.

BIOPSY TECHNIQUES

Biopsy of enlarged adrenal glands or masses is not routinely done in veterinary medicine, primarily because of the relatively small size of the organ and the proximity to major abdominal vessels. Manipulation of a pheochromocytoma carries the additional risk of blood pressure alterations during guided biopsy.[22]

CONCLUSION

Routine sonography of the adrenal glands has become possible because of improvements in technology and operator skills. The differentiation of PDH and ADH can be aided by sonography. Ultrasound can also be helpful in the detection of tumors of the adrenal glands.

REFERENCES

1. Yeh HC. Sonography of the adrenal glands: normal glands and small masses. Am J Roentgenol 1980;135:1167.
2. Venzke WG. Carnivore endocrinology. In: Getty R, ed. Sisson and Grossman's the anatomy of the domestic animals. 5th ed. Philadelphia: WB Saunders, 1975: 1590.
3. Hullinger RL. The endocrine system. In: Evans HE, Christensen GC, eds. Miller's anatomy of the dog. 2nd ed. Philadelphia: WB Saunders, 1979:602.
4. Baker DD. Studies of the suprarenal glands of dogs. Am J Anat 1936;60:231.
5. Waters DJ. Endocrine system. In: Hudson LC, Hamilton WP, eds. Atlas of feline anatomy for veterinarians. Philadelphia: WB Saunders, 1993:127.
6. Voorhout G. X-ray computed tomography, nephrotomography, and ultrasonography of the adrenal glands of healthy dogs. Am J Vet Res 1990;51:625.
7. Saunders HM, Pugh CR, Rhodes WH. Expanding applications of abdominal ultrasonography. J Am Anim Hosp Assoc 1992;28:369.
8. Schelling CG. Abdominal imaging: gastrointestinal, pancreas and adrenal. In: Syllabus of the second annual American Institute of Ultrasound in Medicine animal ultrasound seminar and wet-lab. Bethesda: American Institute of Ultrasound in Medicine, 1990:59.
9. Schelling CG. Ultrasonography of the adrenal gland. In: Kaplan PM, ed. Problems in veterinary medicine: ultrasound. Philadelphia: JB Lippincott, 1991:604.
10. Dubbins PA. Retroperitoneum. In: Goldberg BB, ed. Textbook of abdominal ultrasound. Baltimore: Williams & Wilkins, 1993:261.
11. Emms SG, Wortman JA, Johnston DE, Goldschmidt MH. Evaluation of canine hyperadrenocorticism using computed tomography. J Am Vet Med Assoc 1986; 189:432.
12. Oppenheimer DA, Carroll BA, Yousem S. Sonography of the normal neonatal adrenal gland. Radiology 1983;146:157.
13. Kantrowitz BM, Nyland TG, Feldman EC. Adrenal ultrasonography in the dog: detection of tumors and hyperplasia in hyperadrenocorticism. Vet Radiol 1986; 27:91.
14. Reusch CE, Feldman EC. Canine hyperadrenocorticism due to adrenocortical neoplasia: pretreatment evaluation of 41 dogs. J Vet Intern Med 1991;5:3.
15. Nelson RW, Feldman EC, Smith MC. Hyperadrenocorticism in cats: seven cases (1978–1987). J Am Vet Med Assoc 1988; 193:245.
16. Ford SL, Feldman EC, Nelson RW. Hyperadrenocorticism caused by bilateral adrenocortical neoplasia in dogs: four cases (1983–1988). J Am Vet Med Assoc 1993;202:789.
17. Poffenbarger EM, Feeney DA, Hayden DW. Gray-scale ultrasonography in the diagnosis of adrenal neoplasia in dogs: six cases (1981–1986). J Am Vet Med Assoc 1988;192:228.
18. Mittelstaedt CA. Retroperitoneum. In: Mittelstaedt CA, ed. General ultrasound. New York: Churchill Livingstone, 1992: 749.

19. Mahaffey MB, Barber DL. The adrenal glands. In: Thrall DE, ed. Textbook of veterinary diagnostic radiology. Philadelphia: WB Saunders, 1986:405.
20. Gunther RW, Kelbel C, Lenner V. Real-time ultrasound of normal adrenal glands and small tumors. J Clin Ultrasound 1984;12:211.
21. Bowerman RA, Silver TM, Jaffe MH, et al. Sonography of adrenal pheochromocytomas. Am J Roentgenol 1981;137:1227.
22. Bouayad H, Feeney DA, Caywood DD, Hayden DW. Pheochromocytoma in dogs: 13 cases (1980–1985). J Am Vet Med Assoc 1987;191:1610.
23. Silverman SG, Mueller PR, Pinkney LP, et al. Predictive value of image-guided adrenal biopsy: analysis of results of 101 biopsies. Radiology 1993;187:715.

Small Animal Ultrasound, edited by Ronald W. Green.
J. B. Lippincott Company, Philadelphia © 1996.

URINARY BLADDER

Ronald W. Green

Ultrasound (ie, cystosonography) is a simple noninvasive means of evaluating the urinary bladder. The urinary bladder is the easiest of the abdominal organs to examine with ultrasound because of its superficial location and ideal acoustic properties. The urinary bladder is a good acoustic window for adjacent organs such as the uterus, caudal vena cava, aorta, and iliac lymph nodes.

Indications for ultrasound examination of the urinary bladder include lower urinary tract disease such as strangury, pollakiuria, and dysuria; clinical laboratory results indicating hematuria, crystalluria, and pyuria; localization of nonpalpable bladders; hydronephrosis or hydroureter; and as part of a complete abdominal ultrasound examination.[1]

ANATOMY

The urinary bladder is a hollow musculomembranous organ that varies in size, shape, and position, depending on the urine volume. The normal canine bladder is oval and lies in the caudal abdomen just cranial to the pubis and may be partially within the pelvic canal. The normal feline bladder is ellipsoid, has a longer neck than the canine bladder, and lies 2 to 3 cm cranial to the pubis. The bladder wall consists of the mucosa, submucosa, three muscle layers, and serosa. The bladder wall is 2.0 to 5.0 mm thick, depending on its degree of distention.[2] The urinary bladder of a 25-pound dog has the capacity to hold approximately 125 mL of urine without being overly distended. The distended bladder is approximately 17.5 cm in diameter and 18.0 cm long, but when empty, it is approximately 2.0×3.2 cm.[3]

Other structures near the bladder include the ureters, urethra, aorta, vena cava, medial iliac lymph nodes, colon, the prostate in male dogs, and the uterus in intact females. The ureters empty into the urinary bladder at the trigone, and the urethra originates at the neck of the bladder. The caudal abdominal aorta and vena cava are dorsal to the urinary bladder. The medial iliac lymph nodes are located on either side of the aorta between the branches of the deep circumflex iliac and external iliac arteries. The colon is dorsal to the urinary bladder. In the male dog, the prostate surrounds the proximal urethra, and in the intact female dog and cat, the uterus is dorsal to the urinary bladder and ventral to the colon.

SONOGRAPHIC ANATOMY

The sonographic appearance of the normal bladder is an oval or ellipsoid, anechoic structure with thin, hyperechoic walls. With high-frequency transducers (7.5 MHz or higher), the bladder wall may have three distinct layers: hyperechoic serosa, hypoechoic muscle layer, and hyperechoic mucosa (Fig. 12-1).[4] The thickness of the urinary bladder wall is 2 to 5 mm, depending on the urine volume.[2] As the bladder is distended, the layers become ill defined. The ureters enter the bladder at the trigone, but unless they are dilated, they are not seen with ultrasound.[5] The caudal urinary bladder tapers into the tubular urethra, which has an anechoic lumen. In male dogs, the urethra can be seen as it passes through the prostate.

SCANNING TECHNIQUE

Scanning should begin with the patient in dorsal recumbency. The hair on the ventrocaudal abdomen should be clipped or shaved. Copious amounts of coupling gel should be placed on both the skin and transducer to eliminate any air between them. Depending on the size of the patient, a 5.0-MHz or 7.5-MHz transducer should be used. The urinary bladder is normally found on the midline, cranial to the pubis. An empty urinary bladder may require catheterization and filling with sterile saline to locate ultrasonographically. After the bladder is located, the entire bladder should be examined in sagittal and transverse planes. The colon is dorsal to the urinary bladder and may displace or distort the urinary bladder. If the colon is distended with gas, reverberation artifacts can create an illusion of a cystic calculus (Fig. 12-2 and see Fig. 8-14). By rotating the transducer 90°, thoroughly scanning the entire bladder, and possibly changing the patient's position, hyperechoic structures can be identified as being in the urinary bladder or colon (see Chap. 3).

BLADDER DISEASES AND ABNORMALITIES

Strangury, pollakiuria, dysuria, hematuria, pyuria, and crystalluria may be signs of bladder disease. Most cystosonograms are performed on patients with one or more of these signs.

Cystitis

Bacterial cystitis is a common disease of dogs but is less common in cats. Ascending microbial migration from the lower urinary and genital tract is the most common route of infection.[6] Acute cystitis may not produce any noticeable sonographic change in the bladder wall. However, if free blood, pus, or cellular debris are present in the urine, multiple small echoes may be seen in the normally anechoic urine (Fig. 12-3). In severe or chronic cases of cystitis, the bladder wall becomes hyperechoic, thick, and irregular (Fig. 12-4).

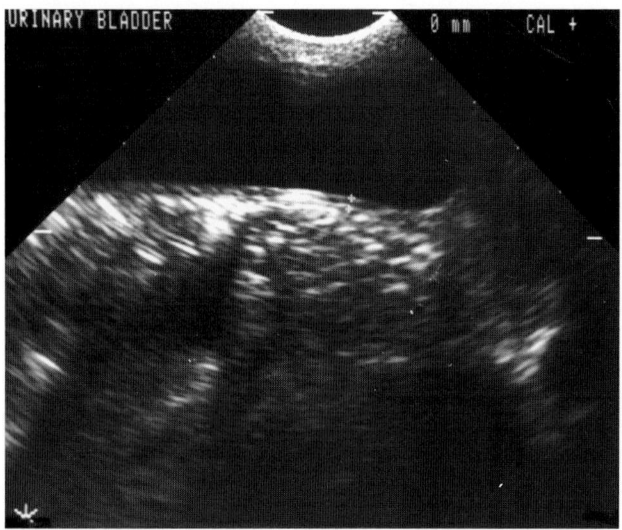

Figure 12-1. Sagittal view of a normal bladder. Notice the anechoic urine, three layers of the bladder wall (*between calipers*), and the 2-mm thickness of the bladder wall (*between calipers*).

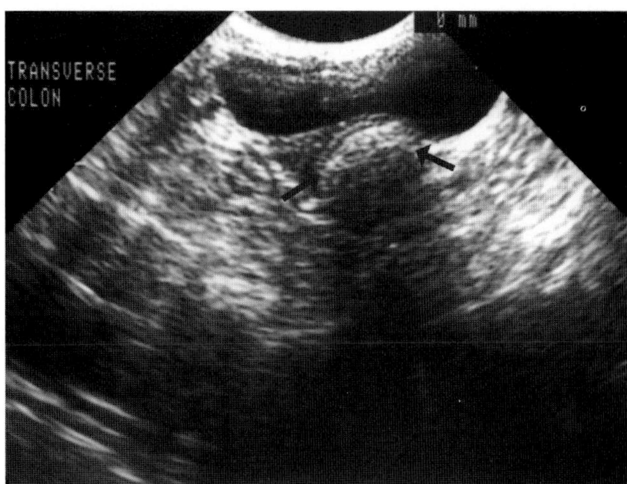

Figure 12-2. Transverse view of a normal bladder. The colon is producing a bright echo with acoustic shadowing (*arrows*) at the middorsal aspect of the urinary bladder.

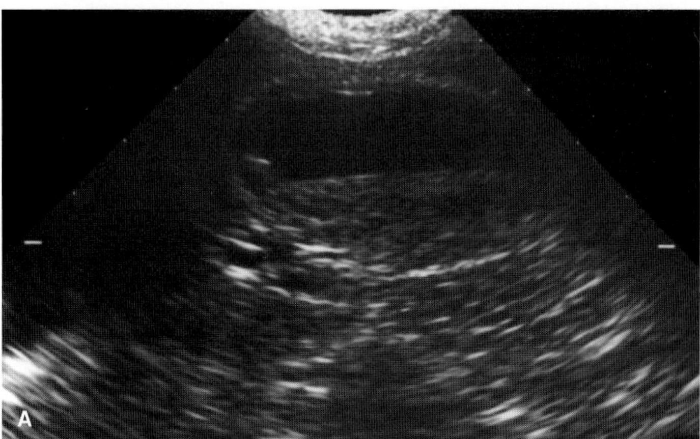

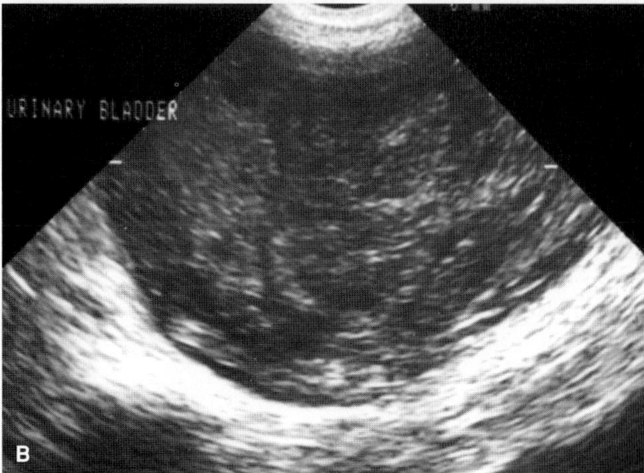

Figure 12-3. (**A**) Sagittal view of a bladder half filled with blood and cellular debris. Notice the sediment is isoechoic, and the bladder wall is thickened. The diagnosis was cystitis with hematuria. (**B**) Sagittal view of the apex of a bladder with multiple bright echoes uniformly suspended in urine. The diagnosis was hemorrhagic cystitis.

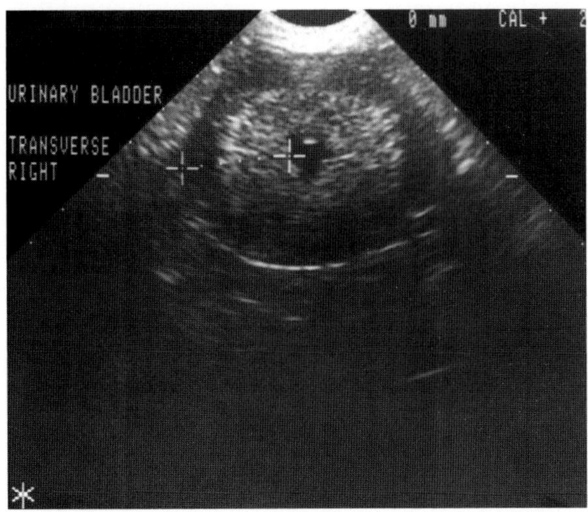

Figure 12-4. Transverse view of a bladder with chronic cystitis. The bladder wall thickness is 23 mm, and the mucosa is hyperechoic. The diagnosis was chronic cystitis.

Urolithiasis

Urolithiasis (ie, urocystolithiasis) is a common urinary tract disorder in dogs and cats.[7] The cause of urolithiasis varies with the urolith (eg, struvite, urate, oxalate, cystine). Cystosonography is sensitive in detecting calculi. Some examiners report 100% accuracy in detecting the presence of calculi in the urinary bladder with ultrasound.[1] An acoustic shadow is created distal to the interface of the sound beam with a calculus (Fig. 12-5). Radiolucent calculi (eg, urate, cystine, xanthine) create acoustic shadows and are more easily detected with sonography than with noncontrast radiography. Calculi may range in size from a few millimeters to several centimeters. They are usually mobile and change position as the position of the bladder changes (Fig. 12-6). Ballotting the bladder and scanning with the patient in various positions (eg, dorsal recumbency, lateral recumbency, standing) aids the detection of cystic calculi.

Cellular Debris and Crystalline Matrix

Small calculi, crystalline particles (ie, sand), and cellular debris will settle in the dependent portion of the bladder and create an acoustic inter-

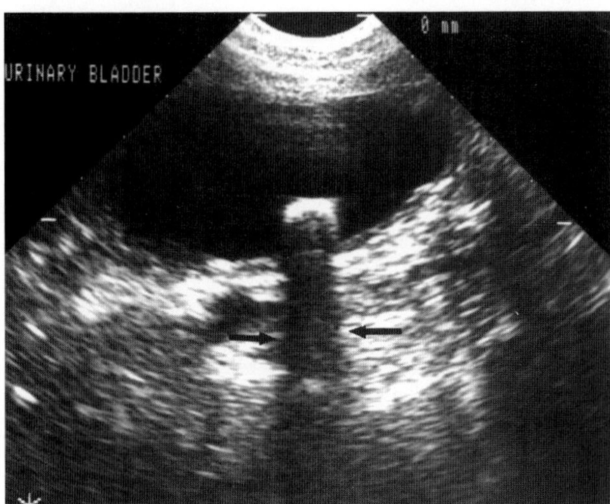

Figure 12-5. Sagittal view of a bladder with a calculus. The acoustic shadow (*arrows*) was caused by the echogenic calculus.

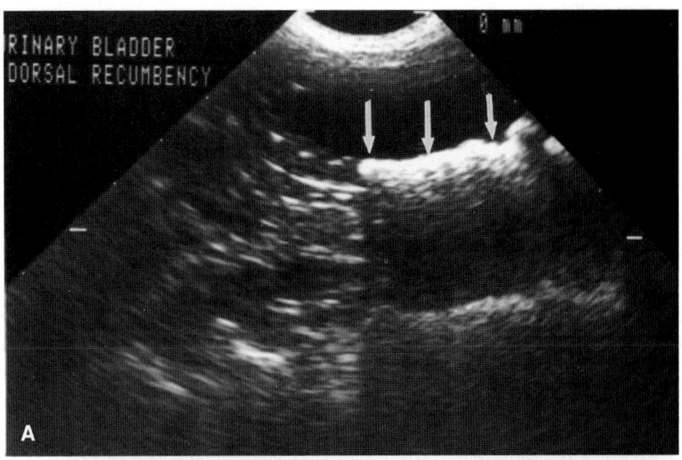

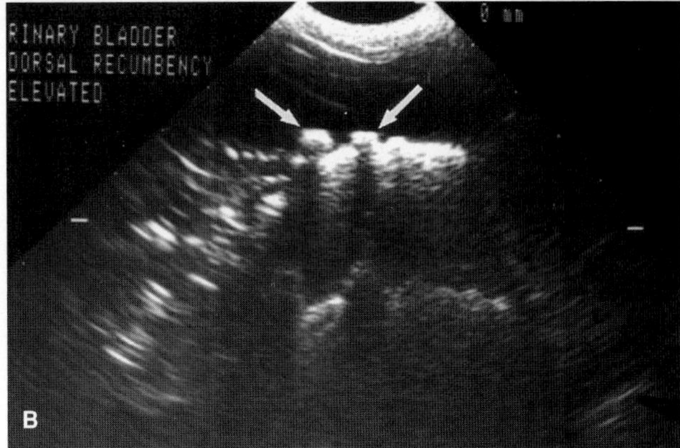

Figure 12-6. (**A**) Sagittal view of a urinary bladder with multiple calculi (*arrows*). By changing the position of the patient, (**B**) the calculi also change position (*arrows*).

face that resembles a calculus (Fig. 12-7*A*). If the urinary bladder is ballotted or agitated, the small hyperechoic densities become suspended in the anechoic urine and then slowly settle to the dependent portion of the bladder again. This appearance is similar to a liquid-filled toy or paperweight that, when turned upside down, creates a "snow scene" (Fig. 12-7*B*).

Neoplasia

Transitional cell carcinoma is the most common bladder tumor in dogs and cats.[8,9] Other epithelial tumors, such as squamous cell carcinoma, are frequently encountered.[10] Adenocarcinoma, undifferentiated carcinoma and botryoid rhabdomyosarcoma also have been reported in the urinary bladder.[8]

Three sonographic patterns of bladder tumors have been described: echogenic or complex focal filling defects arising from the mucosal surface of the urinary bladder (Fig. 12-8); massive tumor obliterating the bladder lumen (Fig. 12-9); and infiltrative tumor in the bladder wall producing thickening of the wall with little loss of intraluminal space (Fig. 12-10).[11] The transition between the tumor and normal mucosa is usually abrupt.[8] Ninety-five percent of tumors larger than 2 cm are readily detected by ultrasound, but tumors smaller than 5 mm and those in the neck of the bladder are difficult to find.[12,13] Neoplasia involving the caudal urinary bladder and trigone occur more commonly than tumors involving the cranial half of the bladder. Bladder tumors, urinary polyps, blood clots, hemorrhagic cystitis, and granulomatous cystitis have similar sonographic patterns. Fine-needle aspirates and ul-

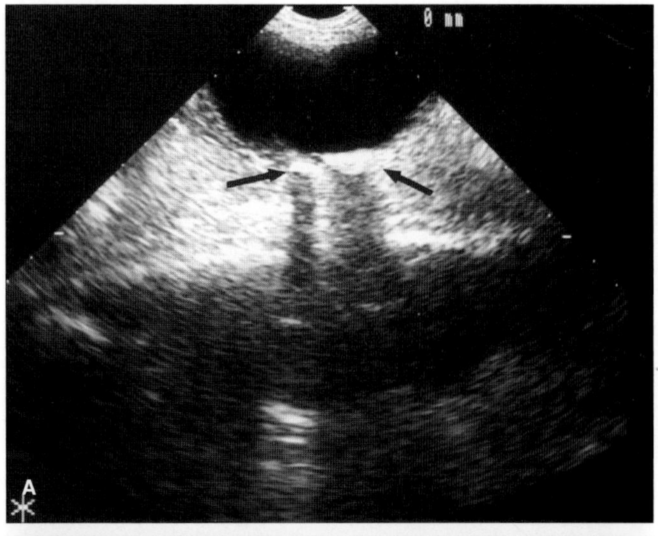

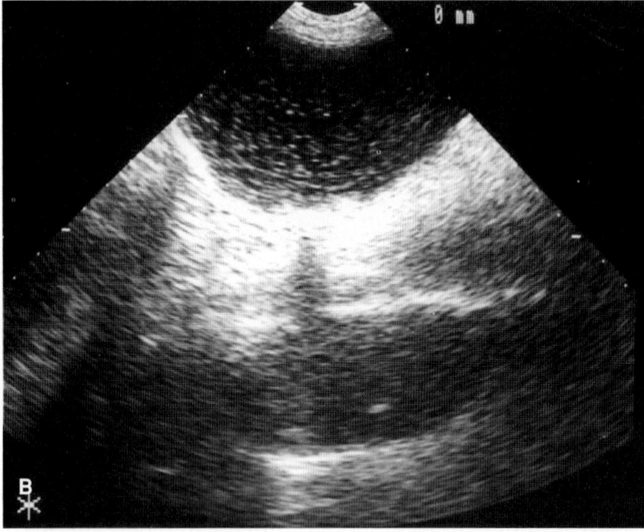

Figure 12-7. (**A**) Sagittal view of a bladder with anechoic urine and hyperechoic sediment (*arrows*), which is creating acoustic shadows. (**B**) Sagittal view of the bladder in **A** after ballottement. Notice the hyperechoic particles are now suspended in the urine.

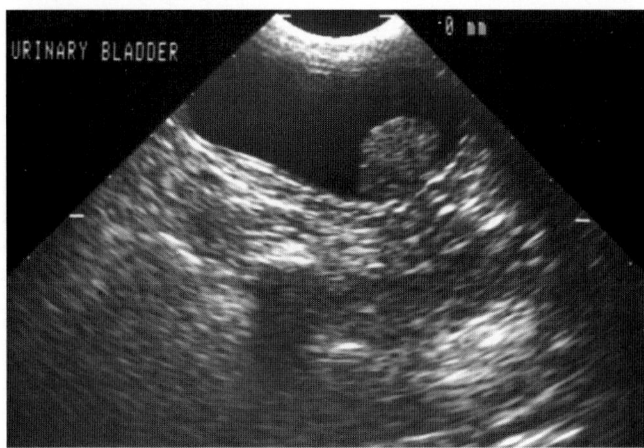

Figure 12-8. Sagittal view of a urinary bladder. Notice the hyerechoic mass arising from the dorsal bladder wall. The diagnosis was transitional cell carcinoma.

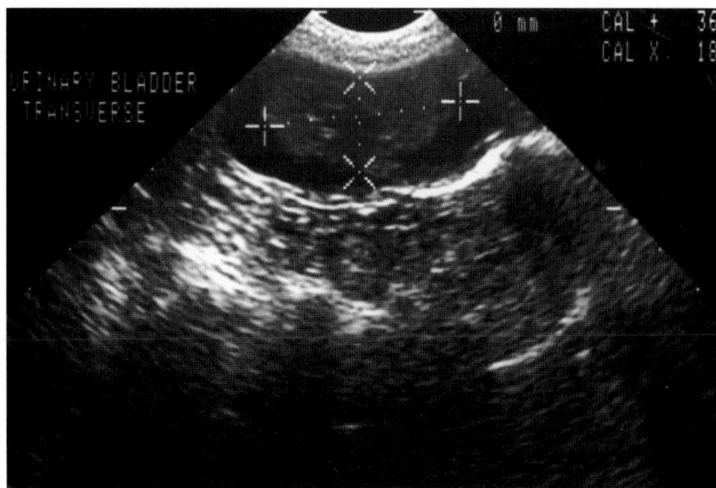

Figure 12-9. Transverse view of a urinary bladder with a massive tumor (18 × 36 mm) obliterating most of the lumen of the bladder. The diagnosis was transitional cell carcinoma.

trasound-guided biopsies of the bladder wall should be used to confirm the diagnosis.

Hemorrhage and Blood Clots

Trauma, infection, inflammation, and toxins can cause hemorrhage and blood clots in the urinary bladder. Blood clots are usually mobile and settle to the dependent portion of the urinary bladder. Scanning with the patient in various positions can differentiate blood clots from bladder neoplasia or polyps. Blood clots are hyperechoic to the urine but usually do not create an acoustic shadow (Fig. 12-11).

Ectopic Ureters

Excretory urography is superior to sonography in detecting ectopic ureters because ectopic ureters must be dilated before they can be identified by ultrasound.[2]

Ruptured Urinary Bladder

Positive contrast cystography is superior to sonography in diagnosing a ruptured urinary bladder. Free fluid in the abdomen may be the only abnormal sonographic finding.

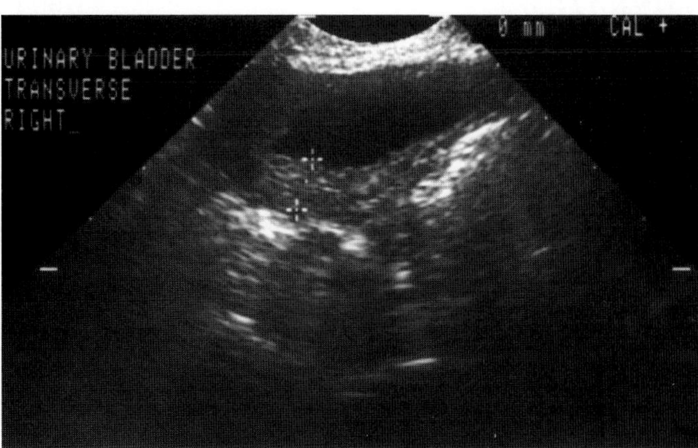

Figure 12-10. Transverse view of a urinary bladder with a diffusely thickened and irregular bladder wall. The diagnosis was transitional cell carcinoma.

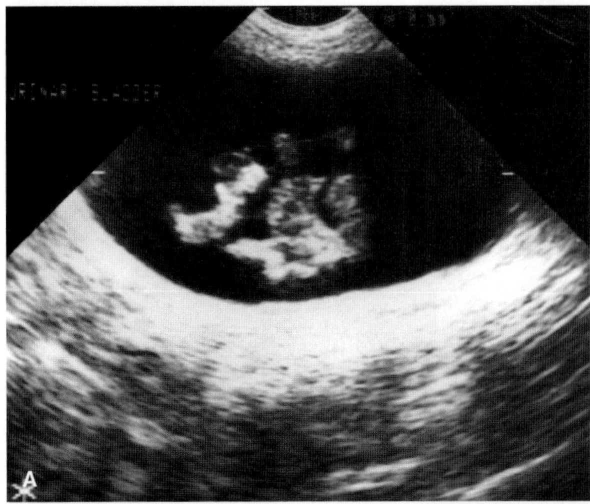

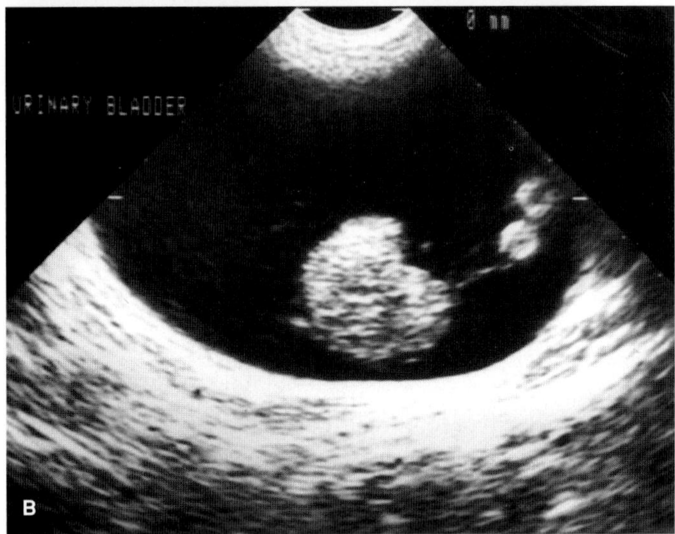

Figure 12-11. (**A**) Sagittal view of a bladder shows a mixed echogenic, irregular mass in the lumen. There is no acoustic shadow. (**B**) Sagittal view of the bladder shows a hyperechoic mass in the lumen with no acoustic shadow. The diagnosis was blood clots.

BIOPSY AND FINE-NEEDLE ASPIRATES

Ultrasound-guided biopsies and fine-needle aspirates of the urinary bladder are relatively easy to obtain because of the superficial location of the bladder (see Chap. 3). Ultrasound-guided cystocentesis can be performed in most animals without the use of chemical restraint.

CONCLUSION

A distended urinary bladder is easy to examine with ultrasound. Changes in the bladder wall and urine due to disease can be readily detected. Aspirates of the urine or biopsies of the bladder wall may be required to obtain a definitive diagnosis. The distended urinary bladder is also a good acoustic window that can be used to sonographically view other structures in the caudal abdomen (see Chaps. 3, 15, and 17).

REFERENCES

1. Biller D, Kantrowitz B, Partington B, Miyabayashi T. Diagnostic ultrasound of the urinary bladder. J Am Anim Hosp Assoc 1990;26:397.
2. Finn-Bodner S. Nephrosonography and cystosonography in veterinary medicine.

In: Diagnostic Ultrasound Seminar. American College of Veterinary Radiology, Orlando, August 1992.

3. Christensen G. The urogenital apparatus. In: Christensen G, Evans H, eds. Miller's anatomy of the dog. Philadelphia: WB Saunders, 1979:552.
4. Finn-Bodner S, Cartee R, Gray B, Williams J. Sonographic architecture and morphometric evaluation of the normal feline urinary bladder wall. American College of Veterinary Radiology annual meeting proceedings. Orlando, August 1992.
5. Mittlestaedt C. General ultrasonography. New York: Churchill Livingstone, 1992: 1043.
6. Osborne C, Low D, Finco D. Canine and feline urology. Philadelphia: WB Saunders, 1972:355.
7. Lees G. Diagnosis and treatment of canine urolithiasis. In: Lees G, ed. Diseases of the urinary system. College Station, TX: Texas A&M Press, 1992: 148.
8. Léveillé R, Biller D, Partington B, Miyabayashi T. Sonographic investigation of transitional carcinoma of the urinary bladder in small animals. Vet Radiol 1992;33:103.
9. Susaneck S. Neoplastic diseases In: Norsworthy G, ed. Feline practice. Philadelphia: JB Lippincott, 1993:435.
10. O'Brien T. Radiology of the urinary bladder and urethra. In: O'Brien T, ed. Radiographic diagnosis of abdominal disorders of the dog and cat. Philadelphia: WB Saunders, 1978:543.
11. Cronan J, Simeone J, Pfister R, et al. Cystosonography in the detection of bladder tumors. J Ultrasound Med 1982;1:237.
12. Itzchak Y, Singer D, Fishelovitch Y. Ultrasonographic assessment of bladder tumors. I. Tumor detection. J Urol 1981; 126:31.
13. Abu-Yousef M, Narayana A, Franken E, Brown R. Urinary bladder tumors studied by cystosonography. Radiology 1984; 153:223.

Small Animal Ultrasound, edited by Ronald W. Green.
Lippincott-Raven Publishers, Philadelphia © 1996.

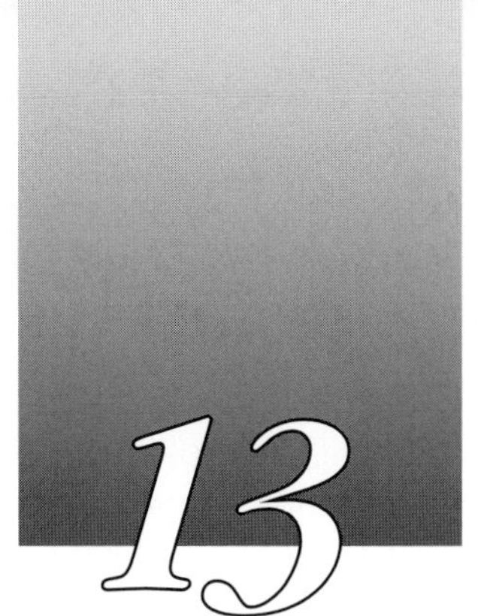

PROSTATE GLAND

Ronald W. Green and Linda D. Homco

Prostatic enlargement is common in dogs older than 5 years of age. Benign hyperplasia, prostatitis, abscesses, cysts, and neoplasia all cause prostatomegaly. Before the development of ultrasound, the prostate gland was evaluated primarily by digital palpation or radiography. Both of these methods can be used to detect prostatomegaly, but ultrasound can detect organ enlargement and changes in the internal architecture of the organ. Although changes in the internal architecture are easily detected, a fine-needle aspirate or biopsy may be required for a definitive diagnosis.

NORMAL ANATOMY AND LOCATION

The canine prostate gland is a bilobed musculoglandular organ that surrounds the proximal urethra between the membranous portion of the urethra and the neck of the urinary bladder.[1,2] The prostate gland is located in the retroperitoneal space caudal to the urinary bladder, ventral to the rectum, dorsal to the pubic symphysis, and ventral abdominal wall.[2] A prominent median septum divides the gland into two ovoid lobes that are dorsally flattened.[2] The prostatic portion of the urethra passes through the middle to middorsal portion of the gland. The entire gland is surrounded by a thick capsule, and a layer of fat usually covers its ventral surface.[2]

The location of the prostate gland is affected by the degree of distention of the urinary bladder.[3] When the bladder is empty, the prostate gland may be entirely within the pelvic canal, but urinary bladder distention results in an intraabdominal location.[4] Age, breed, sexual maturity, and disease may also influence the location of the prostate gland.[1,2] Progressive enlargement of the prostate gland occurs with aging.[1,2] Shrinkage of the prostate gland occurs after castration.

The feline prostate gland is very similar in location to that of the dog, although the size of the gland is much smaller.[5]

SCANNING TECHNIQUES

Sonographic imaging of the prostate gland can be accomplished by a transabdominal approach through a prepubic or suprapubic window, a transperineal approach, an endorectal or transrectal approach, or an endourethral or transurethral approach.[6–8]

The transabdominal approach is the one most often used in small animal ultrasonography. Other than clipping hair from the caudoventral abdomen, no special preparation of the patient is necessary, although some examiners recommend cleansing enemas.[3] A full urinary bladder is beneficial, because it "pulls" the prostate gland forward to the cranial edge of the pelvic canal and facilitates scanning. A full bladder also displaces gas-filled viscera from the pubic area.[3,9]

The animal can be imaged in dorsal, dorsal oblique, or lateral recumbency. Sector or convex-phased–array transducers with smaller footprints are more desirable than linear-array transducers, because a smaller transducer provides easier access to a prostate gland that may be partially or completely within the pelvic inlet. Scanning of most prostate glands can be accomplished with 5.0- or 7.5-MHz transducers, although 3.5-MHz transducers may be required for very large dogs. The transducer is placed on either side of the prepuce, just cranial to the pubis. Fanning of the transducer allows visualization of both lobes of the prostate gland from one transducer site. The prostate gland should be scanned in sagittal (ie, longitudinal) and transverse imaging planes. If the prostate gland remains within the pelvic canal, a finger can be inserted into the rectum to displace the prostate gland cranially.[10,11]

The techniques for transrectal ultrasonography of the prostate gland in the dog have been reported.[9,12] The most practical transducers available for canine transrectal scanning are smaller versions of the linear-array transducers designed for equine endorectal pregnancy diagnosis (see Fig. 3-14).[9] The 7.5- and 5.0-MHz linear-array transducers provide the best image resolution.[3] Specially designed endocavity transducers with single and biplane capabilities can be used.[6] The oblique and end-fire probes designed for endovaginal and endorectal use in humans are relatively expensive probes and have had limited use in veterinary medicine.

Patients can be positioned for scanning in lateral or sternal recumbency or standing. A full urinary bladder is not necessary for transrectal scanning. To ensure good transducer contact with the rectal wall, a cleansing enema is recommended 1 to 2 hours before the ultrasound examination. The transducer should be protected with an ultrasound probe cover or a condom. The probe cover or condom should be filled with warm water or ultrasound gel, and tape or an elastic band should be used to secure the end of the cover to the probe.[6–8] Ultrasound gel is placed on the outside for lubrication and coupling, and the transducer is inserted slowly into the rectum to the level of the neck of the urinary bladder. The transducer is then withdrawn, enabling imaging of the entire length of the prostate gland. With the linear-array single-plane transducers typically used in veterinary medicine, sagittal views of each lobe of the prostate gland can be obtained by slowly rotating the transducer from side to side.

Transperineal imaging of the prostate gland uses the same transducers as those used for transabdominal ultrasound.[6] Hair may need to be clipped from the perineum. The transducer is placed on the perineum ventral to the anus and angled cranially.

Transducers used for endourethral or transurethral imaging are very expensive and are not commonly used in veterinary medicine.

NORMAL SONOGRAPHIC APPEARANCE

The sonographic appearance of the normal prostate gland has been described as uniformly coarse and moderately echoic, with an echogenicity similar to that of the spleen (Fig. 13-1*A*).[9,13,14] The gland is bilobed and spherical to ovoid with smooth margins (Fig. 13-1*B*).[10,14] The capsule is echoic but difficult to detect with transabdominal imaging because it is a specular reflector.[9,15,16] The prostatic urethra is not seen sonographically unless the bladder is distended or the patient sedated. The cranial portion of the prostatic urethra is distensible and may appear wider than the caudal portion (Fig. 13-2).[11] With transverse imaging, a hyperechoic central area is seen. This area, called the hilar echo, represents the prostatic urethra and the periurethral ducts (see Fig. 13-1*B*).[13,15] The hilar echo is often surrounded by a hypoechoic zone, which may be caused by the smooth muscle.[11] To help identify the urethra during scanning, a fluid or air-filled catheter can be placed in the urethra.[10]

The size of the normal prostate gland varies with age, breed, body weight, sexual maturity, and hormonal influences.[10,15] One study reported the cranial-to-caudal and dorsal-to-ventral ultrasonographic measurements of the

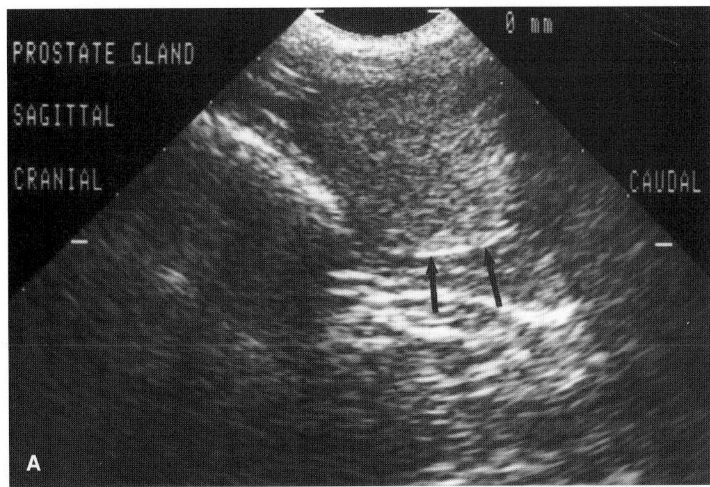

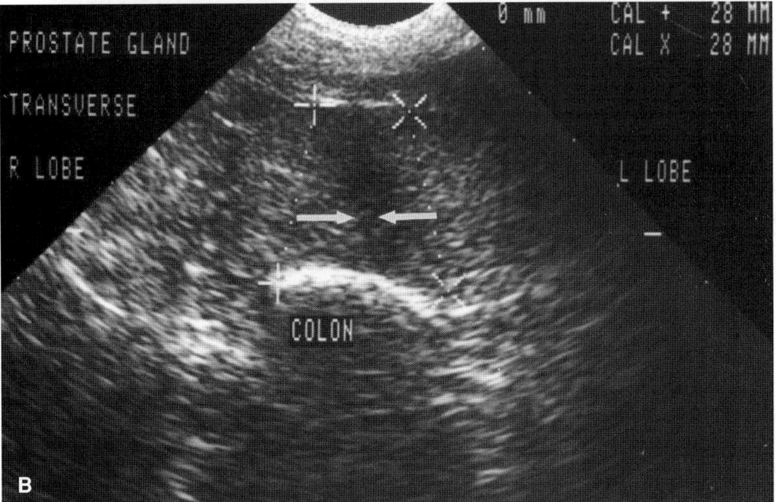

Figure 13-1. (**A**) The sagittal sonogram of the prostate gland in a sexually mature mixed-breed dog. The parenchyma is coarse and moderately echoic. Notice that only the portion of the capsule (*arrows*) that is perpendicular to the ultrasound beam is detected. (**B**) Transverse sonogram of both lobes of the prostate gland. The hilar echo (*arrows*) is seen within the middorsal aspect of the gland.

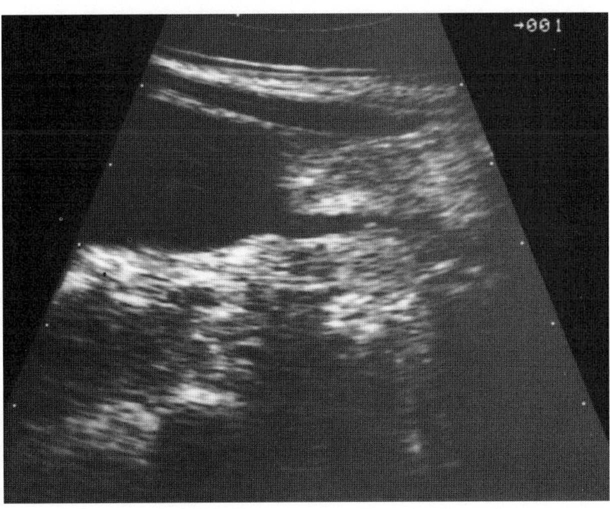

Figure 13-2. Sagittal sonogram of the prostate gland in a male poodle. The distended cranial portion of the prostatic urethra is apparent.

prostate gland in sexually mature 7- to 30-kg dogs to be 22 and 22 mm, with a range of 13 to 30 mm in both planes.[14] Because the capsule of the prostate gland is a specular reflector and the adjacent tissues are often isoechoic, measurement of the prostate gland by the transabdominal method is difficult.[14,17] Size assessment of the prostate gland is more objective using abdominal radiography, because the entire gland is usually visualized.[9,15,17,18]

The castrated dog should have a small prostate gland with no distinct lobes (Fig. 13-3). The echogenicity should be slightly hypoechoic to surrounding fat and adjacent tissues.[11] The prostate gland in the cat is of little clinical significance, and the sonographic appearance of the normal feline prostate gland has not been reported.

DISEASES OF THE PROSTATE GLAND

Diseases of the prostate gland are common in older male dogs and are the result of aging changes, inflammation, and neoplasia.[1] Prostatic disease is rare in the cat, and the only literature reports are those of neoplasia.[19,20]

Reports indicate trends in the response of the prostate gland to pathologic conditions.[13,14,21,22] An increase in echogenicity of the gland occurs with hyperplasia, chronic inflammation, fibrosis, and neoplasia, and a decrease in echogenicity often occurs with acute inflammation, parenchymal edema, abscesses, and retention cysts.

Benign Prostatic Hyperplasia

Benign prostatic hyperplasia (BPH) is an aging change that is reported only for dogs and humans.[1] The prostate gland in the intact male dog undergoes a benign hyperplastic process that begins uniformly within the epithelial portion of the gland as early as 2.5 years of age.[1]

With benign hyperplasia, the prostate gland may be mildly or moderately enlarged and remains symmetric with smooth margins.[15] The parenchymal echogenicity is normal to slightly increased (Fig. 13-4). The central hilar echo may not be detected, probably because of the surrounding increase in echogenicity. Small, anechoic cavitations of variable size with smooth internal margins and distant enhancement may be seen within the parenchyma (Figs. 13-5 and 13-6).[3] These result from the retention of prostatic secretions and are called retention cysts. Cystic hyperplasia frequently accompanies BPH.[11] BPH begins in the younger animal as glandular hyperplasia, which tends to become cystic with age.[1] If large cysts occur in the periphery, the shape of the prostate gland may be altered (Fig. 13-7). If the cysts exceed 1.5 cm in diameter, cystic hyperplasia, hematocysts, and prostatic hematomas are considerations.[3] The differential diagnoses for BPH and cystic hyperplasia include bacterial prostatitis and bacterial prostatitis with abscesses.[3]

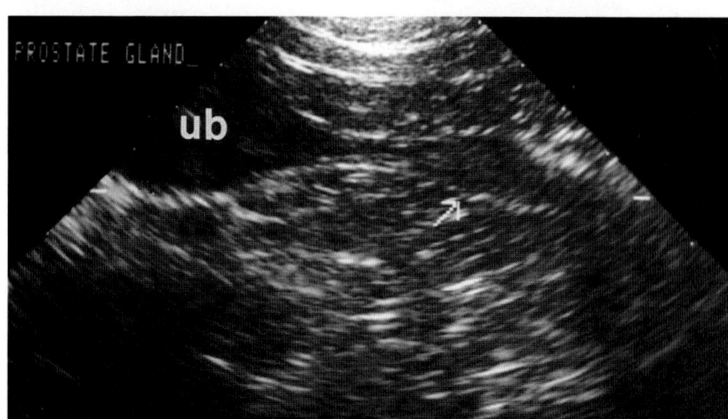

Figure 13-3. Sagittal sonogram of the prostate gland (*white arrow*) in a castrated male Labrador retriever. Notice that the parenchyma is slightly less echoic than the surrounding fat. *ub*, urinary bladder.

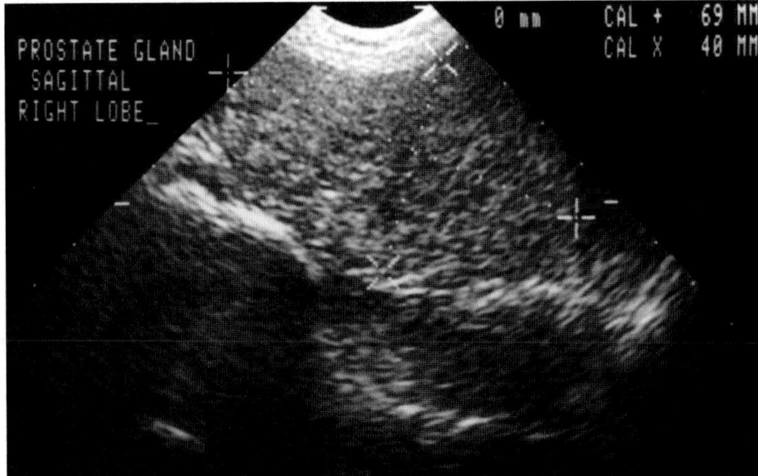

Figure 13-4. Sagittal sonogram of the left lobe of the prostate gland in a male Labrador retriever with benign prostatic hyperplasia. The gland is moderately enlarged, and the parenchyma is hyperechoic.

Prostatitis

Acute Bacterial Prostatitis

The classic appearance of the prostate gland with acute bacterial prostatitis is an overall hypoechoic parenchyma (Fig. 13-8).[6,9] However, the parenchyma may appear coarsely hyperechoic, with small cavitations representing focal edema.[3] A mottled texture, presumably caused by areas of hemorrhage or necrosis, may be seen.[10] The gland is usually enlarged and symmetric during early or acute inflammation.[10,15]

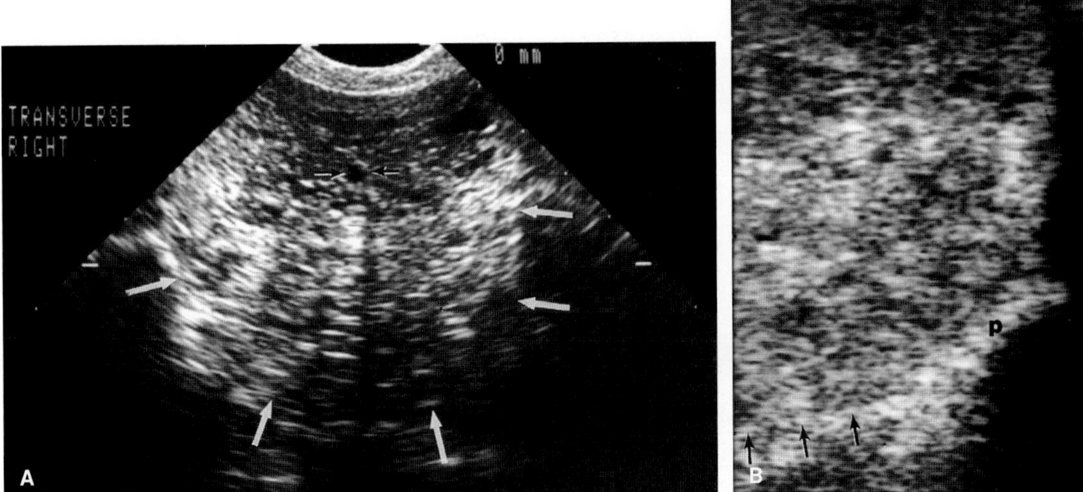

Figure 13-5. (**A**) Transabdominal transverse sonogram of the prostate gland in a male Labrador retriever with benign prostatic hyperplasia. The central hilar echo is not seen, and refraction artifacts originate from the urethra (*small arrows*). Tiny cavitations are seen within the parenchyma. Large arrows delineate the margins of each lobe because the capsule is not detected. (**B**) Transrectal sagittal sonogram of the same prostate gland shows multiple cavitations throughout the dorsal aspect in the near field. Notice the capsule (*arrows*), which is not seen with transabdominal imaging. *p*, pubis.

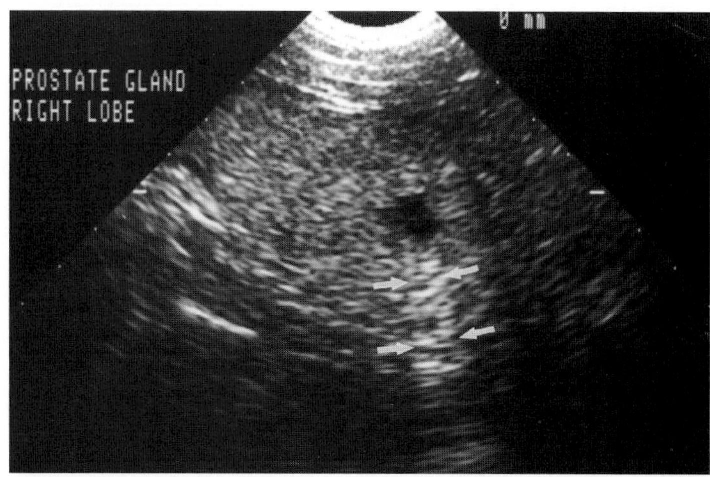

Figure 13-6. Sagittal sonogram of the right lobe of the prostate gland in a male giant schnauzer with benign prostatic hyperplasia. A retention cyst shows distant enhancement (*arrows*).

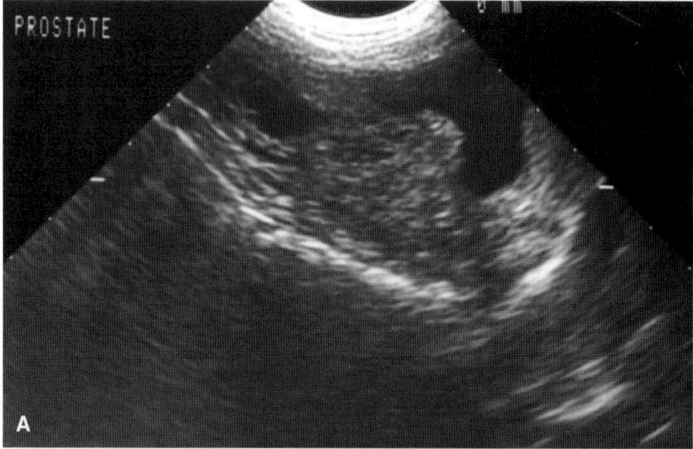

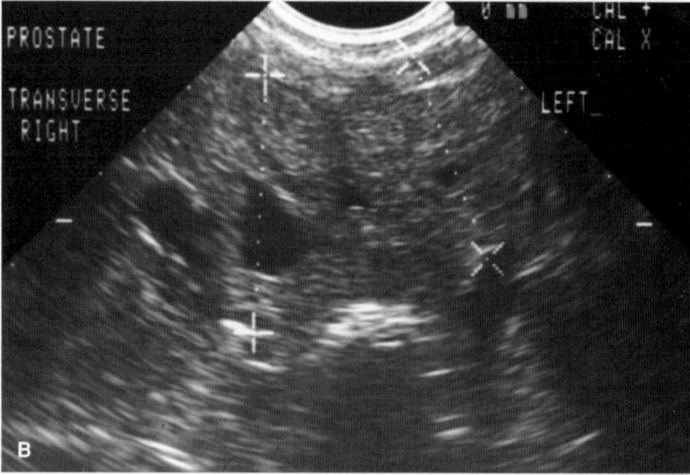

Figure 13-7. (**A**) Sagittal and (**B**) transverse sonograms of the prostate gland in a male Rhodesian ridgeback with cystic hyperplasia. Notice the smooth margins of the anechoic cavitations and the asymmetric shape of the gland.

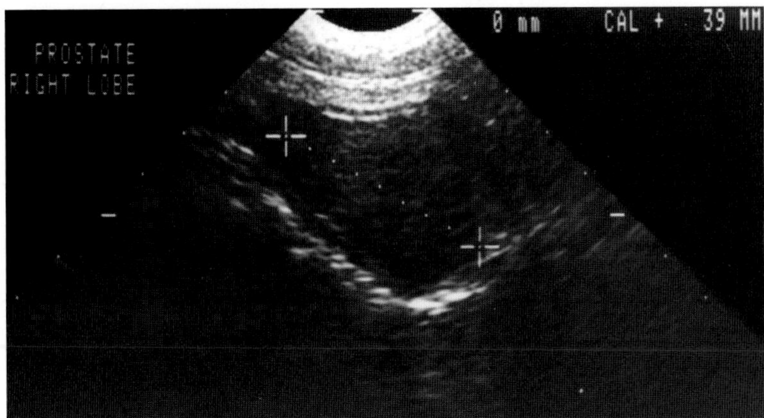

Figure 13-8. Sagittal sonogram of the prostate gland in a male Labrador retriever with acute bacterial prostatitis. The parenchyma is hypoechoic and slightly mottled, and the gland is enlarged. The hyperechoic capsule is easily seen because of the decrease in parenchymal echogenicity.

The differential diagnoses include BPH and prostatic neoplasia.

Chronic Bacterial Prostatitis

The sonographic appearance of chronic bacterial prostatitis is that of a coarsely hyperechoic parenchyma with a heterogenous echotexture due to irregular hyperechoic foci throughout the parenchyma (Figs. 13-9 and 13-10).[11,15] The increased echogenicity is thought to be caused by the fibrosis resulting from chronic inflammation.[3] Mineralization may also be seen, but this is uncommon with inflammation and is much more characteristic of carcinoma (Fig. 13-11).[3,15] Small hypoechoic to anechoic intraparenchymal cavitations, probably representing areas of abscessation, may be seen.[11,15] The internal margins of the cavitations may be irregular, and these areas exhibit distant enhancement. The prostate gland is often small in a patient with chronic inflammation because of fibrosis and contraction.[15] The shape may be symmetric or irregular. The differential diagnoses are cystic hyperplasia and prostatic neoplasia.

Granulomatous Prostatitis

Chronic granulomatous prostatitis is uncommon, but it has been associated with blastomy-

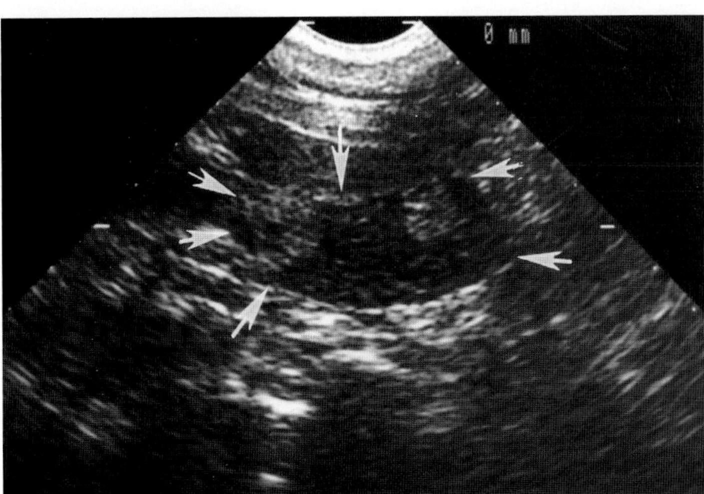

Figure 13-9. Sagittal sonogram of the prostate gland in a male Doberman pinscher with chronic bacterial prostatitis. Irregular hyperechoic foci are seen within the parenchyma, and the gland's shape is irregular (*arrows*).

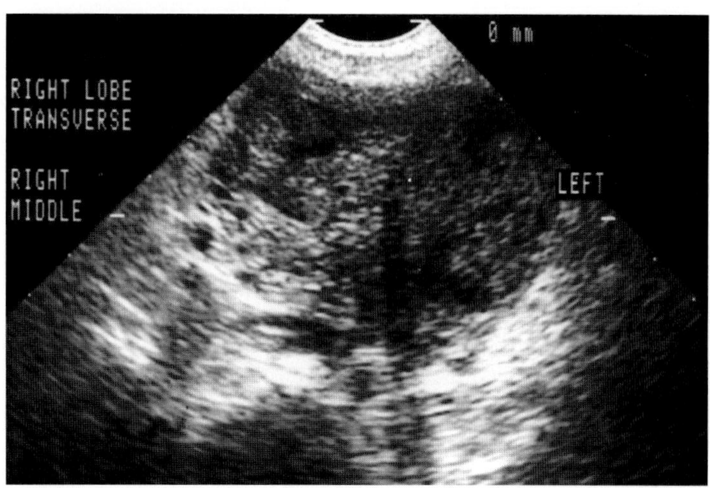

Figure 13-10. Transverse sonogram of the prostate gland in a male Staffordshire terrier with chronic bacterial prostatitis. Irregular hyperechoic foci are seen within the right lobe, and small, irregularly shaped hypoechoic intraparenchymal cavitations exist within both lobes.

cosis and cryptococcosis.[1] Granulomatous prostatitis, such as that seen in blastomycosis, may result in a prostate gland with an irregular, hyperechoic parenchyma.

Prostatic Abscess

Abscessation in the prostate gland is a result of severe chronic bacterial prostatitis in which pockets of exudate develop within the parenchyma.[1] The echogenicity of the prostate gland is usually increased because of chronic inflammation.[15] Abscesses appear as hypoechoic or anechoic cavitations that exhibit distant enhancement (Fig. 13-12). Prostatic abscesses are often lobulated with irregular and occasionally septated internal margins. Most clinically significant prostatic abscesses are larger than

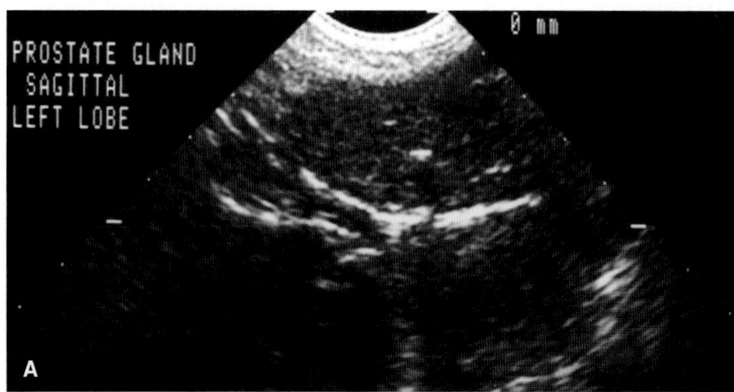

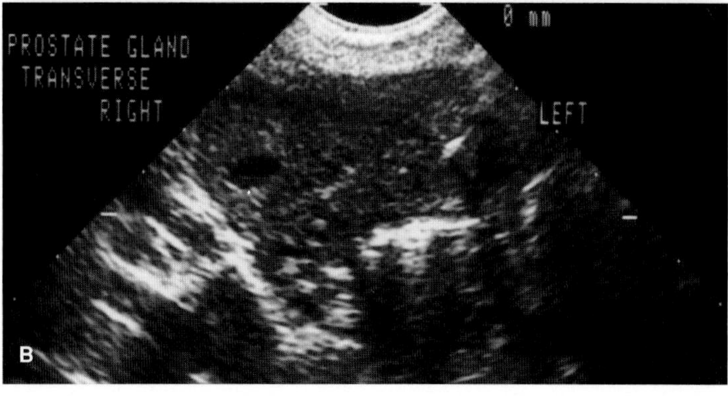

Figure 13-11. (**A**) Sagittal and (**B**) transverse sonograms of the prostate gland in the same dog as in Figure 13-10 after 2 months of antibiotic therapy. The prostate gland is smaller and asymmetric. Mineralization and at least one cavitation are seen within the mixed-echogenicity parenchyma.

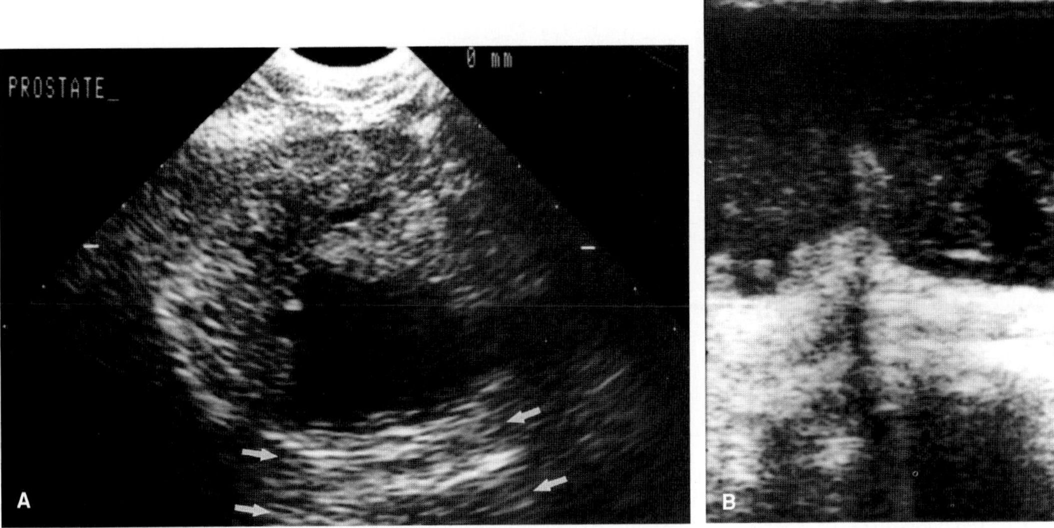

Figure 13-12. (**A**) Transabdominal and (**B**) transrectal sagittal sonograms of the prostate gland in a male rottweiler with a prostatic abscess. Notice the irregular internal margins and the distant enhancement (*arrows*) of the dorsally located abscess in **A** and the irregular wall and echogenic material within the abscess in **B**.

1.5 cm.[15] The prostate gland usually is enlarged and has an irregular asymmetric shape (Figs. 13-13 and 13-14).[1,15] The differential diagnoses include prostatic hematomas, hematocysts, and cystic prostatic neoplasia.[10,15]

Prostatic Neoplasia

Adenocarcinoma is the most common primary prostatic neoplasm in dogs.[1] Transitional cell carcinoma, primary and metastatic squamous cell carcinoma, and leiomyosarcoma have also been reported.[1] Benign neoplasms of the prostate gland have not been reported. A few cases of prostatic adenocarcinoma have been reported in the cat.[19]

An irregularly shaped prostate with multifocal, poorly defined, and coalescing hyperechoic foci is the common sonographic finding of prostatic neoplasia in the dog (Fig. 13-15).[11,15] Irregularly distributed foci of mineralization

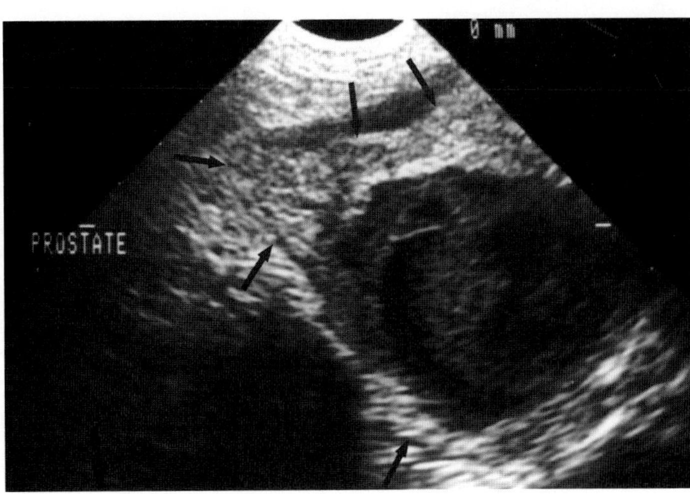

Figure 13-13. Sagittal sonogram of the prostate gland in a male German shepherd with a prostatic abscess. Notice the large and irregular shape of the gland and the hyperechoic parenchyma (*arrows*) surrounding the hypoechoic, septated abscess.

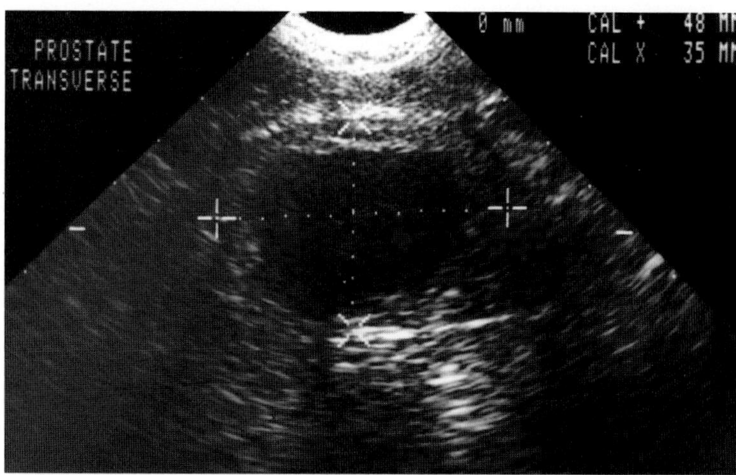

Figure 13-14. Transverse sonogram of the prostate gland in a male mixed-breed dog with a prostatic abscess. There is loss of distinct lobation, and the internal margin of the cavity is irregular.

with acoustic shadowing are also typical of prostatic neoplasia (Fig. 13-16).[3,11,15] Very early prostatic tumors may be hypoechoic.[11,15] Parenchymal cavitations are uncommon in prostatic neoplasia.[15,23] Capsular disruption has been reported as an indicator of prostatic neoplasia (Fig. 13-17).[15] However, this may be difficult to detect with transabdominal imaging, and

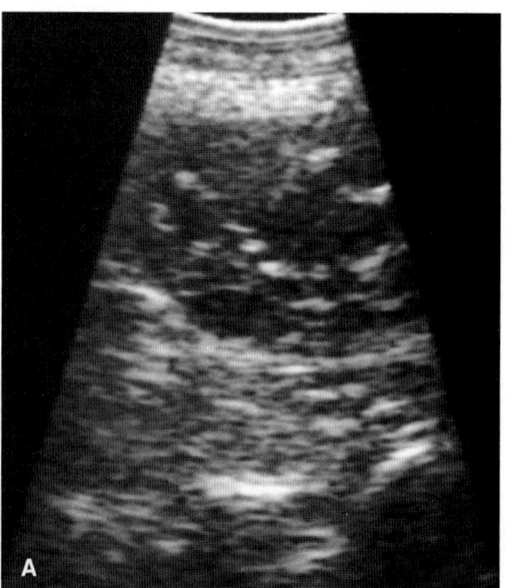

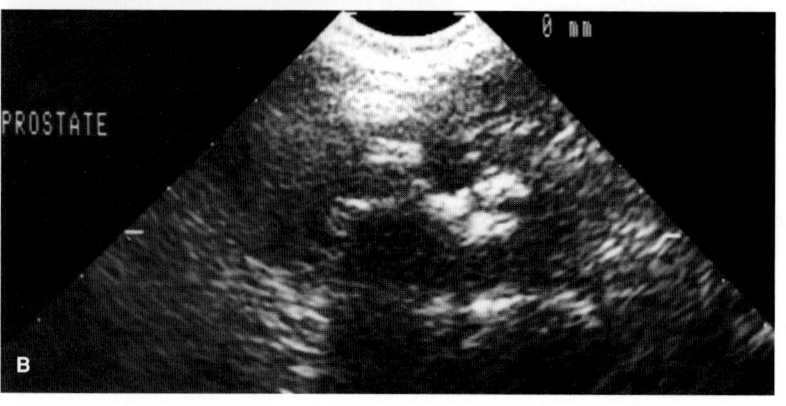

Figure 13-15. (**A**) Sagittal sonogram of the prostate gland in a castrated male Lhasa apso with prostatic adenocarcinoma. Multiple tiny hyperechoic foci are apparent. (**B**) Sagittal sonogram of the prostate gland in a castrated male mixed-breed dog with prostatic adenocarcinoma. Poorly defined coalescing hyperechoic foci and acoustic shadowing are seen.

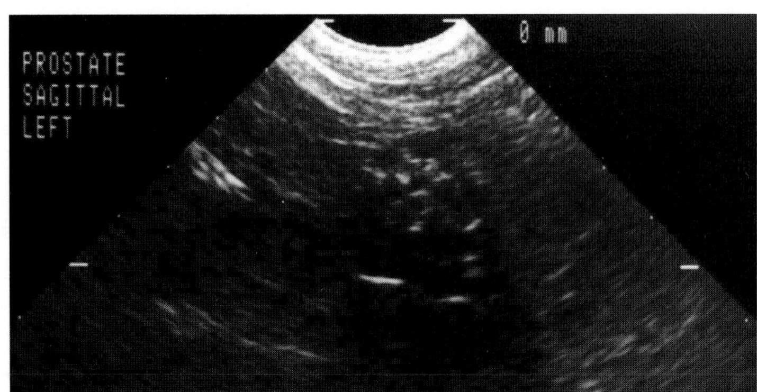

Figure 13-16. Sagittal sonogram of the prostate gland in a castrated male mixed-breed dog with prostatic adenocarcinoma. Tiny foci of parenchymal mineralization are visible.

transrectal ultrasonography should be used to confirm this finding. Chronic bacterial prostatitis is almost impossible to differentiate from prostatic neoplasia without a biopsy.[13]

Paraprostatic Cysts

Canine paraprostatic cysts are uncommon.[24] Paraprostatic cysts may result from a remnant of the müllerian duct, a prostatic retention cyst extending beyond the margins of the prostate gland, or a prostatic hematoma.[13,24]

Paraprostatic cysts vary in size, shape, and location.[10] Most cysts are located cranial or dorsal to the prostate gland or the trigone of the urinary bladder (Fig. 13-18).[24] They may extend cranially, displacing the bladder, or caudally into the pelvic canal (Fig. 13-19).[24] Paraprostatic cysts are usually large, well-circumscribed, ovoid structures with anechoic or hypoechoic fluid content (see Fig. 13-18). Various amounts of solid tissue may be present, and the cyst may contain single to multiple, thin, hyperechoic septa (see Fig. 13-19).[24] The prostate gland is usually identified as a separate structure, and it may be sonographically difficult to identify the stalk-like connection between the cyst and the prostate gland.[10,24] It is not possible to differentiate infected from noninfected cysts with ultrasound. The mixed-echo patterns in some paraprostatic cysts may represent infection, hematoma, or neoplasia.[10,24]

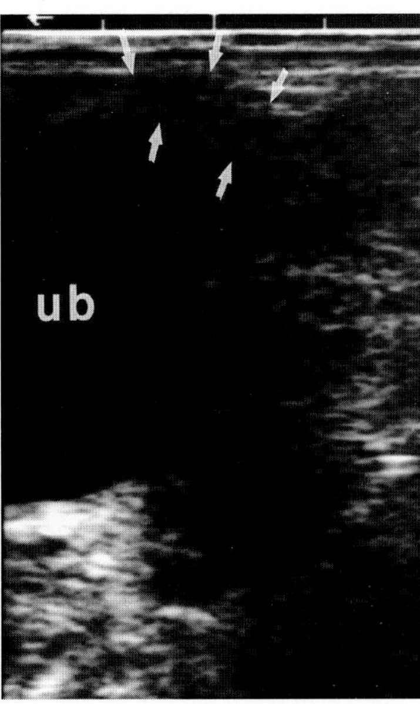

Figure 13-17. Transrectal sagittal sonogram of the prostate gland and caudal urinary bladder in a male mixed-breed dog with prostatic neoplasia. There is capsular disruption (*arrows*) and extension of the tumor dorsal to the trigone of the urinary bladder (*ub*).

Prostatic Calculi

Prostatic calculi are much less common in dogs than humans.[13] Prostatic calculi form along the urethra or in periurethral areas secondary to chronic inflammation.[6,20] They are generally composed of calcium phosphate or calcium carbonate and are usually located in cyst-like cavitations associated with inflammation (Fig. 13-20).[20] Sonographically, prostatic calculi of various sizes create acoustic shadows.

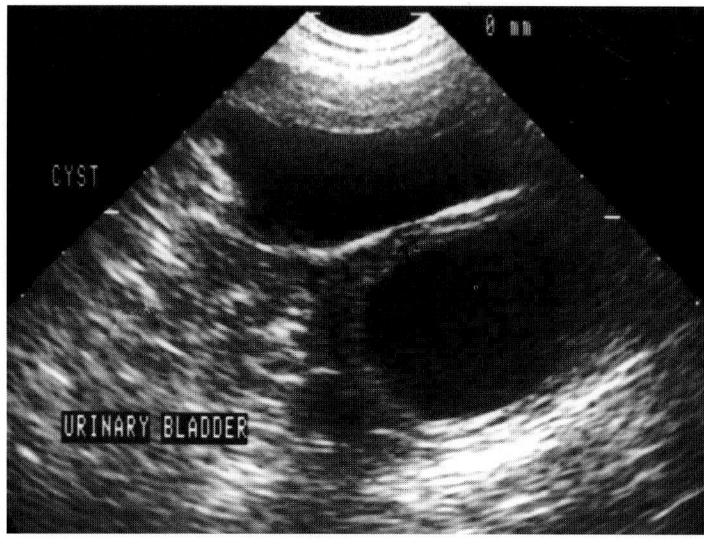

Figure 13-18. Sagittal sonogram of the caudal abdomen in a male golden retriever with a paraprostatic cyst. Notice that this cyst is ventral to the urinary bladder, displacing it dorsally. The large, well-circumscribed cyst is filled with anechoic fluid.

BIOPSY TECHNIQUES

Ultrasound-guided fine-needle aspiration or biopsy is a safe procedure for obtaining a cytologic sample from the prostate gland. Although general anesthesia is usually unnecessary, sedation is recommended to improve the sampling accuracy of smaller prostate glands or intraparenchymal lesions. After preparation of the skin surface, the transducer is placed to the right or left of the prepuce and aimed caudally.[25] A fluid- or air-filled catheter can be preplaced within the urethra before core biopsy sampling to mark the exact location of and avoid damage to the prostatic urethra (Fig. 13-21).[26] Transient hematuria may occur after prostatic biopsy.[26]

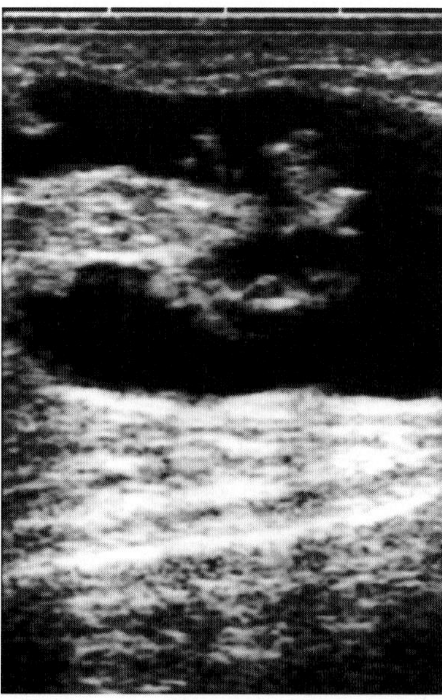

Figure 13-19. Transrectal sagittal sonogram at the level of the pelvic inlet in a male Labrador retriever with a paraprostatic cyst that extends caudally into the pelvic canal. Notice the hyperechoic septa and the solid tissue.

In addition to transabdominal ultrasound-guided prostatic aspirates and biopsies, ultrasound-guided urethral catheter aspirates can be performed.[9] The animal is catheterized, and the opening of the urethral catheter is sonographically guided to the region of interest before external suction is applied.

CONCLUSION

Prostatic ultrasound in indicated for prostatomegaly, glandular asymmetry, a caudal abdominal mass, or nonspecific lower urinary tract signs in the male dog. Unlike radiography, ultrasound is helpful in defining the internal architecture of the prostate gland and in differentiating cavitary from noncavitary prostatic diseases. Although ultrasound may be able to identify abnormal areas of echogenicity within the prostate gland, these findings are not

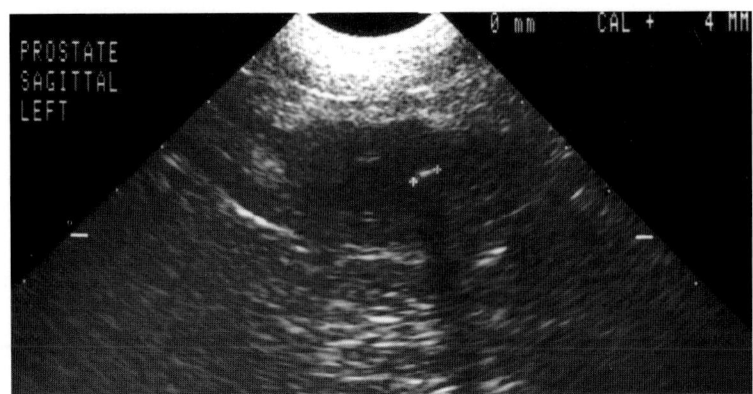

Figure 13-20.

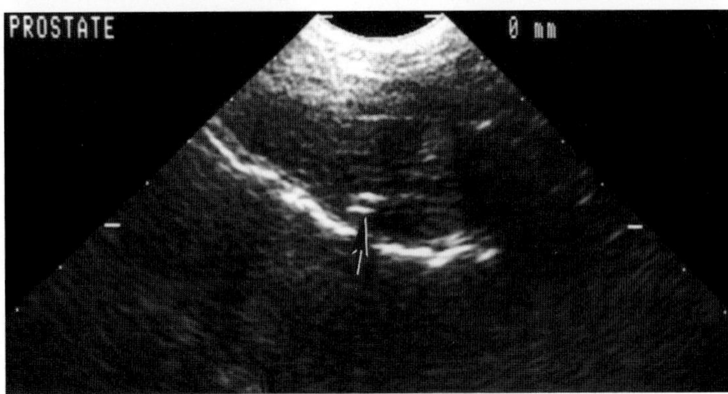

Figure 13-21.

Figure 13-20. Sagittal sonogram of the prostate gland in a castrated male mixed-breed dog with a prostatic calculus, indicated by the calipers (+), within a cyst-like cavitation in the parenchyma.

Figure 13-21. Sagittal sonogram of the prostate gland shows the tip of a fluid-filled urinary catheter (*arrow*) placed to identify the eccentric prostatic urethra before ultrasound-guided biopsy.

pathognomonic for a specific disease, and ultrasound-guided biopsies should be performed.

REFERENCES

1. Barsanti JA, Finco DR. Canine prostatic diseases. In: Ettinger SJ, ed. Textbook of veterinary internal medicine: diseases of the dog and cat. 3rd ed. Philadelphia: WB Saunders, 1989:1859.
2. Christensen GC. The urogenital apparatus. In: Evans HE, Christensen GC, eds. Miller's anatomy of the dog. 2nd ed. Philadelphia: WB Saunders, 1979:544.
3. Johnston GR, Feeney DA, Rivers B, Walter PA. Diagnostic imaging of the male canine reproductive organs. The veterinary clinics of North America: small animal practice. Philadelphia: WB Saunders, 1991;21:553.
4. Ellenport CR. Carnivore urogenital apparatus. In: Getty R, ed. Sisson and Grossman's the anatomy of the domestic animals. 5th ed. Philadelphia: WB Saunders, 1975:1576.
5. Lattimer JC. The prostate gland. In: Thrall DE, ed. Textbook of veterinary diagnostic radiology. 2nd ed. Philadelphia: WB Saunders, 1994:479.
6. Rifkin MD. Prostate. In: Goldberg BB, ed. Textbook of abdominal ultrasound. Baltimore: Williams & Wilkins, 1993:418.
7. Thickman D, Parker SH. Prostate. In: Mittlestaedt CA, ed. General ultrasound.

New York: Churchill Livingstone, 1992: 1147.

8. Sanders RC, Casey J. Prostate. In: Sanders RC, ed. Clinical sonography: a practical guide. 2nd ed. Boston: Little, Brown and Co, 1991:333.
9. Feeney DA, Badertscher RR, Klausner JS, Bell FW. Imaging of the canine prostate gland. Proceedings of the American Institute of Ultrasound in Medicine advanced small animal imaging seminar. New Orleans, LA, 1990.
10. Barr F. Imaging of the urinary tract. In: Barr F. Diagnostic ultrasound in the dog and cat. Oxford: Blackwell Scientific Publications, 1990:46.
11. Spaulding K. Ultrasound of the reproductive tract in the dog and cat. Proceedings of the American Institute of Ultrasound in Medicine animal ultrasound seminar and wet-lab. Raleigh, NC, 1989.
12. Miyashita H, Watanabe H, Ohe H, et al. Transrectal ultrasonotomography of the canine prostate. Prostate 1984;5:453.
13. Feeney DA, Johnston GR, Klausner JS. Two-dimensional, gray-scale ultrasonography: applications in canine prostatic disease. The veterinary clinics of North America: small animal practice. Philadelphia: WB Saunders, 1985:1159.
14. Cartee RE, Rowles T. Transabdominal sonographic evaluation of the canine prostate. Vet Radiol Ultrasound 1983; 24:156.
15. Feeney DA, Johnston GR, Klausner JS, Bell FW. Canine prostatic ultrasonography—1989. Semin Vet Med Surg (Small Anim) 1989;4:44.
16. Cartee RE, Rumph PF, Kenter DC, et al. Evaluation of drug-induced prostatic involution in dogs by transabdominal B-mode ultrasonography. Am J Vet Res 1990;51:1773.
17. Feeney DA, Johnston GR, Walter PA. Ultrasonography of the kidney and prostate gland. In: Kaplan PM, ed. Problems in veterinary medicine: ultrasound. Philadelphia: JB Lippincott, 1991:619.
18. Feeney DA, Johnston GR. Urogenital imaging: a practical update. Semin Vet Med Surg (Small Anim) 1986;1:144.
19. Carpenter JL, Andrews LK, Holzworth J. Tumors and tumor-like lesions. In: Holzworth J, ed. Diseases of the cat. Philadelphia: WB Saunders, 1987:406.
20. Bartels JE. Radiology of the genital tract. In: O'Brien TR, ed. Radiographic diagnosis of abdominal disorders in the dog and cat. Philadelphia: WB Saunders, 1978: 615.
21. Feeney DA, Johnston GR, Klausner JS, et al. Canine prostatic disease—comparison of ultrasonographic appearance with morphologic and microbiologic findings: 30 cases (1981–1985). J Am Vet Med Assoc 1987;190:1027.
22. Foss RR, Wrigley RH, Park RD, et al. A new frontier—veterinary ultrasound: the prostate, part II. Med Ultrasound 1984; 8:15.
23. Llewellyn CH, Holthaus LH. Cystic carcinoma of the prostate: findings on transrectal sonography. Am J Roentgenol 1991;157:785.
24. Stowater JL, Lamb CR. Ultrasonographic features of paraprostatic cysts in nine dogs. Vet Radiol Ultrasound 1989;30 :232.
25. Hager DA, Nyland TG, Fisher P. Ultrasound-guided biopsy of the canine liver, kidney, and prostate. Vet Radiol Ultrasound 1985;26:82.
26. Barr F. Ultrasound-guided biopsy techniques. In: Barr F, ed. Diagnostic ultrasound in the dog and cat. Oxford: Blackwell Scientific Publications, 1990:178.

Small Animal Ultrasound, edited by Ronald W. Green.
Lippincott-Raven Publishers, Philadelphia © 1996.

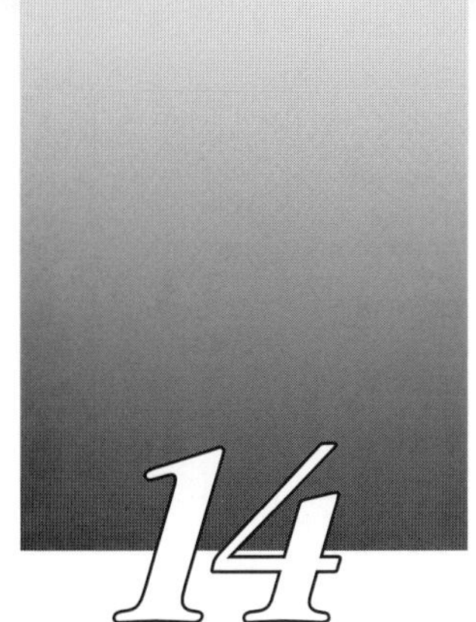

TESTES

Charles R. Pugh

Ultrasonography is an accurate and easy method for investigation of scrotal abnormalities.[1,2] The external location of the testes within the scrotum render them accessible to palpation; however, palpation alone is frequently unsatisfactory for the successful detection of abnormalities. By physical examination alone, it is frequently difficult to determine if a palpable abnormality is of testicular or extratesticular origin, and the diagnostic palpation of the scrotal content may be hindered by pain or swelling. Testicular tumors that are completely nondetectable by palpation have been located with diagnostic ultrasound.

SCANNING TECHNIQUE

Sonographic scrotal evaluation usually is performed as a part of the routine abdominal ultrasound examination.[1] The dogs are usually positioned and restrained in dorsal or lateral recumbency; however, the scrotal examination can be performed with the patient standing. Chemical restraint is rarely required. The scrotal hair is clipped only when necessary. Because of the usual glabrous nature of the scrotal skin, acoustic coupling gel can often be applied directly to the scrotum without any prior preparation.

Intrascrotal structures are superficial and relatively small, and highly detailed images can be obtained using higher-frequency transducers. Although transducers of 7.5 MHz or greater are recommended for scrotal ultrasonography, satisfactory images can be obtained with 5.0-MHz transducers. Scanning can be performed with direct coupling of the transducer to the scrotal skin or with an interfacing ultrasound standoff pad. The standoff pad improves imaging of the skin and the more superficial structures.

The most frequently used scan planes for testicular imaging are the sagittal and the transverse (Fig. 14-1).[1] Transverse imaging allows direct comparison of one testicle with the other on the same image. Slightly oblique dorsal plane imaging with the transducer oriented in a craniocaudal or caudocranial direction can be used as needed for supplementary imaging of the epididymal tail or head. A lateromedial dorsal imaging plane can be used to obtain true dorsal planar image of the testicle. This imaging plane can also be employed when using lower-frequency transducers because the near-field testicle serves as an anatomic standoff device for the distal testicle. This technique is sometimes useful for imaging small testes.

NORMAL SONOGRAPHIC ANATOMY

Normal testicular parenchyma has a medium-coarse, homogeneous sonographic texture with a thin, hyperechoic surrounding capsule (Fig. 14-2). The parenchymal pattern tends to appear

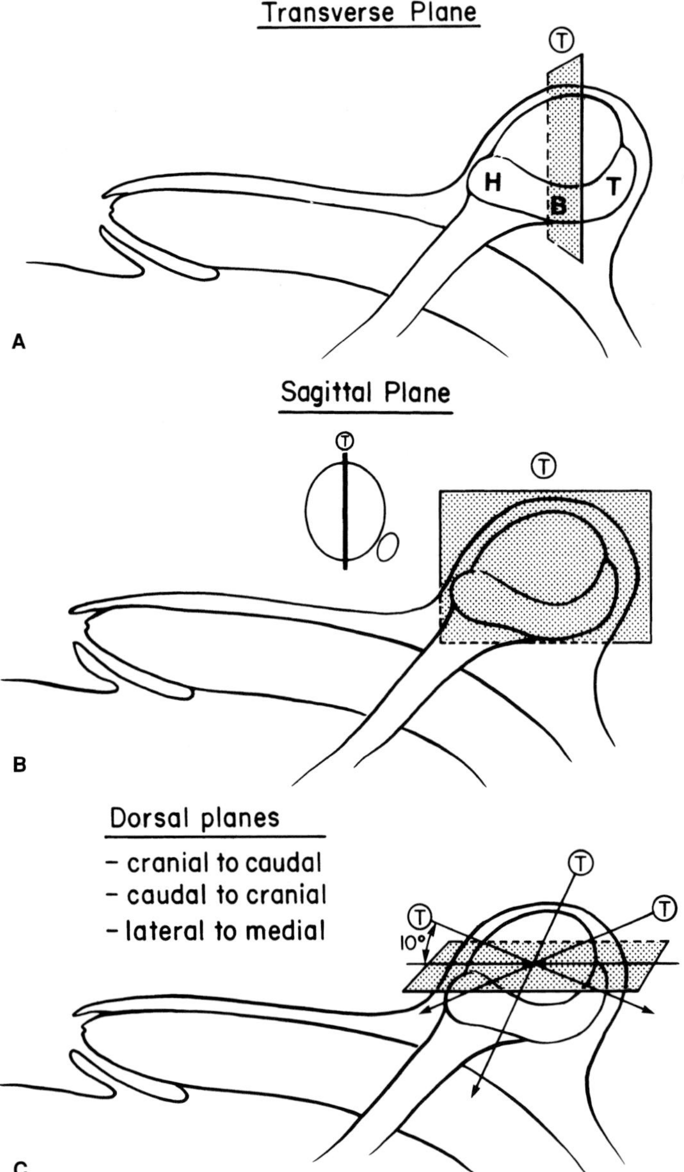

Figure 14-1. The male canine reproductive anatomy illustrated with the dog in dorsal recumbency. The circled T shows the transducer position. The stippled rectangles represent scan planes. (**A**) Transverse plane through the midtesticle (at maximum width) and epididymis. The head (*H*), body (*B*), and tail (*T*) of the epididymis are labeled. (**B**) Sagittal plane through the testicle, with the epididymis located medially. (**C**) Dorsal plane through the testicle is the stippled field, but this was angled 10° dorsocranially or dorsocaudally to facilitate imaging of the head or the tail of the epididymis. The lateral-to-medial scan is in the true dorsal plane. (From Pugh CA, Konde LJ, Park RD. Testicular ultrasound in the normal dog. Vet Radiol 1990;31:195.)

more coarse when using lower-frequency transducers because of decreased axial resolution. The evenly homogeneous, echotexture of the testicular parenchyma serves as an excellent background for the detection of abnormalities.[1]

A thin, central, linear hyperechogenicity is consistently seen within the testicle oriented longitudinally in a cranial to caudal direction (see Fig. 14-2). This hyperechoic structure is the mediastinum testis and has a diameter of about 2 mm on longitudinal and transverse sonograms. The mediastinum testis is a fibrous extension of the tunica albuginea that extends along the long axis of the testis and gives off radiating sheets of connective tissue between testicular parenchymal segments.[3,4] Small, linear, hyperechoic flecks representing portions of this radiating connective tissue occasionally are detected within the testicular parenchyma.

The canine epididymis is closely attached to the testis and anatomically described as lying along the dorsolateral surface of the testicle.[3]

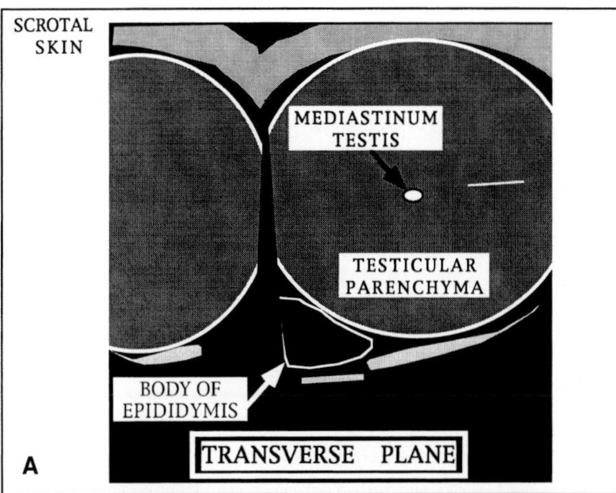

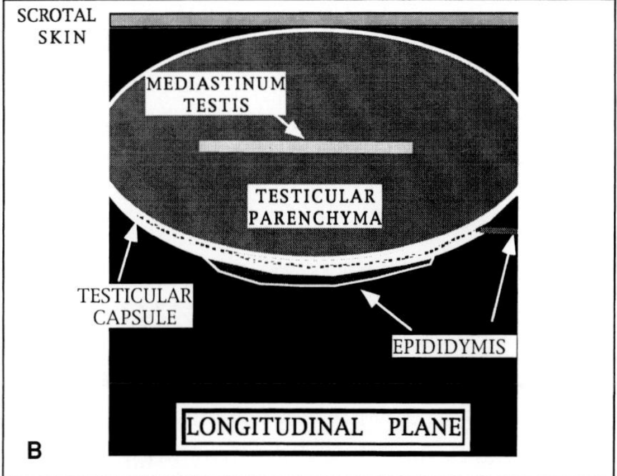

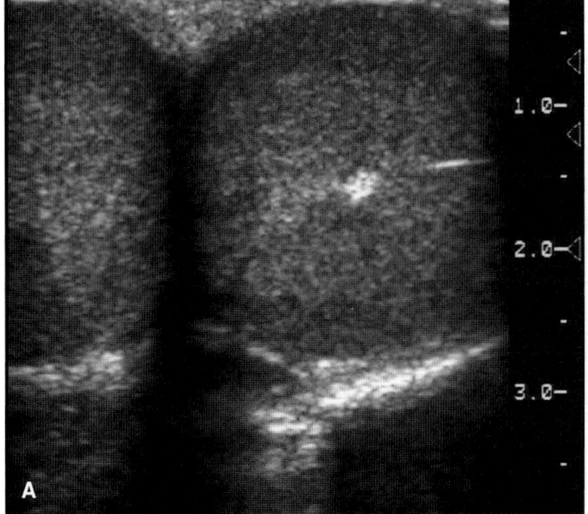

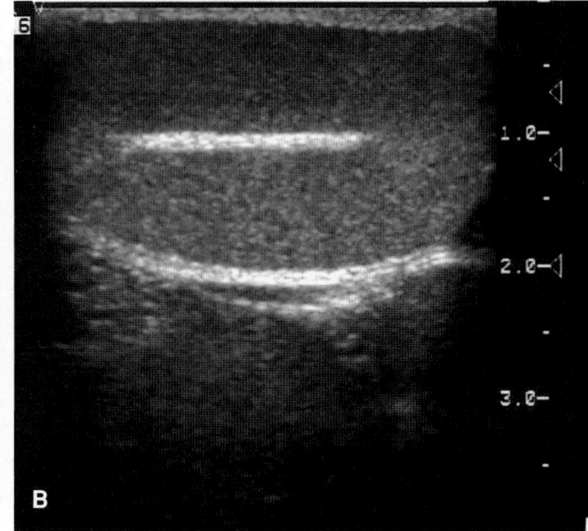

Figure 14-2. Normal testicular 7.5-MHz sonograms and accompanying graphics. (**A**) Transverse plane. (**B**) Longitudinal plane.

The epididymis is divided into a head, tail, and body segment (see Fig. 14-1). The epididymal structures appear hypoechoic to anechoic.[1]

The tail is the largest and most consistently imaged part of the canine epididymis. The epididymal tail is firmly attached to the caudal testicular pole by the proper ligament of the testis.[1,3,4] The head of the epididymis is smaller than the tail and located adjacent to the cranial testicular pole.

The body is the smallest part of the epididymis. Because the testes are mobile within the scrotum, the relative position of the epididymal body may vary as the scrotum is manipulated during examination. During routine sonographic scanning, the epididymal body is most frequently encountered in a dorsomedial location relative to its testicle.

A small amount (0–1 mm) of peritesticular fluid has been described as a normal finding in men.[5,6] This does not appear to be a feature common to canine testicular ultrasonography.[1]

The scrotal wall is thin and normally appears hyperechoic relative to testicular echogenicity. Scrotal wall detail is frequently lost in the near field when scanning with transducers directly coupled to the scrotal skin surface. Scrotal wall sonographic investigation can be enhanced by using an ultrasound standoff device.

Testicular size has been correlated with body size, and the utility of ultrasound as a tool for assessment of testicular size has also been described.[7] A possible correlation between size and fertility has been investigated using ultrasound measurements.[8]

ULTRASONOGRAPHY OF TESTICULAR ABNORMALITIES

Ultrasonography has proven to be a highly reliable and widely accepted diagnostic tool in human medicine.[5,9,10] Although external location renders scrotal structures readily accessible to palpation, palpation alone has proven to be grossly inaccurate in assessing human scrotums, particularly in differentiating testicular from extratesticular abnormalities.[11,12] The physical examination of abnormal scrotums is frequently hindered by pain or swelling. Scrotal ultrasonography approaches 100% accuracy in differentiating testicular from extratesticular structures.[10,13] Ultrasound has proved useful for detection of nonpalpable tumors and abnormalities.[11] Sonography is a sensitive method for the detection of testicular abnormalities, with a conspicuous absence of false-negative findings reported for human patients.[12]

For the purpose of discussion, the testicular and scrotal abnormalities are sorted into neoplastic disorders, infectious disorders, and nonneoplastic, noninfectious disorders.

NEOPLASTIC DISORDERS

Testicular neoplasia is the second most common neoplasm of male dogs, accounting for 5% to 15% of all tumors.[14,15] Testicular neoplasia is more common in the dog than in any other species, including humans. Although testicular tumors in men are often malignant, they are usually benign in animals.[16,17] Testicular neoplasia is extremely rare in the cat.[18]

One review reports no breed predilection for testicular neoplasia.[14,17] One study places the Shetland sheepdog, German shepherd, Siberian husky, boxer, weimaraner, Chihuahua, Pomeranian, Yorkshire terrier, poodle, and miniature schnauzer breeds at excessive risk and Labrador retrievers, beagles and mixed-breed dogs at low risk.[16,19]

Testicular tumors occur bilaterally in as many as 50% of affected dogs, although the tumor in the opposite testicle is clinically detectable in only 12% of the dogs.[20] More than one histologic tumor type may occur in a single or pair of testicles.[21,22] The right testicle is reported to be affected 80% more frequently than the left, which is the same proportion of occurrence as for right and left cryptorchidism.[15]

Most testicular tumors are Sertoli cell tumors, seminomas, or interstitial (Leydig) cell tumors. Each of these histologic tumor types occurs with approximately equal overall frequency.[14,21] Testicular neoplasia tends to affect older dogs, and the reported average ages for Sertoli cell, seminoma, and interstitial cell tumors are 9, 10, and 11.5 years, respectively.[14,17]

Other histologic tumor types affecting the testes are rare. These include granulosa cell tumor, hemangioma, embryonal carcinoma, and sarcoma.[15,19]

The frequency of testicular tumors in descended testicles is approximately 40% interstitial cell tumors, 40% seminomas, and 20% Sertoli cell tumors.[15] Because interstitial cell tumors do not usually cause testicular or scrotal enlargement, a scrotal testicular tumor that is detected on physical observation is twice as likely to be a seminoma as a Sertoli cell tumor.[15]

Approximately 60% of the tumors of undescended testes are Sertoli cell tumors and approximately 40% are seminomas.[15] Cryptorchid males are reported to be at 13.6 times the risk for developing neoplasia than males with descended testes.[14,19] Teratoma and dermoid cysts have also been reported in undescended testicles. Tumors in undescended testicles tend to occur at a younger age than occurrence in normal dogs.[20] It has also been reported that tumor incidence is twice as high in inguinal undescended testicles as in abdominal nondescended testicles.[20]

Sertoli Cell Tumor

Sertoli cell tumor tends to be the most clinically significant tumor type in dogs. Approximately

25% to 60% of dogs with Sertoli cell tumor show some clinical signs, and clinical abnormalities are more likely manifested when the tumor involves an abdominal or inguinally located testicle.[21,23,24] Dogs with Sertoli cell tumors may show a variety of clinical signs, which are apparently related to elevated levels of estrogen. The amount of estrogen production appears to be proportional to the tumor size.[24] The most common presenting sign is scrotal or inguinal enlargement, but some dogs present with abdominal distention, signs of feminization, or hematologic disorders. A bilaterally symmetric alopecia with hyperpigmentation may occur. Signs of feminization may occur with gynecomastia, pendulous prepuce, and penile and contralateral testicular atrophy.[21,23,24] Prostatic enlargement may occur as a result of squamous metaplasia secondary to hyperestrogenism.[23] Approximately 25% of male dogs with feminization may attract other male dogs, similar to a bitch in estrus.[24]

Estrogen-induced myelotoxicity is occasionally reported in dogs with Sertoli cell tumor. The hematologic response may include a nonregenerative anemia, granulocytopenia, and thrombocytopenia. Orchiectomy is beneficial for some dogs, but death from hematopoietic failure can occur, especially if the diagnosis is delayed.[25,26]

Sertoli cell tumors have the highest metastatic rate of all testicular tumors. The estimated metastatic rate for canine Sertoli cell tumors ranges from 2% to 20%.[22,24] Lymphatic spread to regional lymph nodes is the most common course of metastasis. Further dissemination to more distal lymph nodes, liver, lung, spleen, pancreas, and kidney rarely occurs.[22,24]

Testicular removal is the usual treatment of choice. In the absence of metastasis or myelotoxicity, the prognosis for Sertoli cell tumor is excellent. Improvement of hematologic parameters usually occurs in 2 to 3 weeks.[17,25]

Seminoma

Seminomas are not usually associated with secondary clinical signs. Seminomas occasionally have been associated with increased estrogen levels, but associated abnormal clinical signs are unusual. In one study, an array of concurrent clinical signs associated with seminoma included prostatic disease, alopecia, perineal hernia, perianal gland adenoma, and perianal gland adenocarcinoma.[23,27] These signs were thought to be hormonally mediated. The seminoma metastatic rate is low, with an estimated incidence of 5% to 10%.[16,28] Metastasis may occur to the spermatic cord, regional lymph nodes, lungs, and other visceral sites. The prognosis for seminoma is generally good.[17]

Interstitial Cell Tumor

There are usually no clinical signs associated with interstitial cell tumors. They most frequently do not even cause detectable scrotal enlargement. One study reported associated clinical signs that included perineal hernias, perianal tumors, prostatic disease, and alopecia.[23] An association of these clinical signs with elevated testosterone levels was suggested. Nodular hyperplasia of Leydig cells is a frequent finding in older dogs. The differentiation of hyperplasia and benign tumor is arbitrarily based on an ability to grossly visualize the nodule.[15] Metastasis does not occur, and the prognosis is uniformly excellent.[23]

Sonography of Testicular Tumors

Although some typical sonographic patterns have been reported for testicular tumors in men, there does not appear to be a consistent predictable pattern of sonographic change to characterize different tumor types in dogs (Figs. 14-3 and 14-4).[2,5,6] Testicular tumors vary from anechoic or hypoechoic solitary nodules to complex mixed-echogenic patterns.

A small or early tumor may appear as a small nodule within an otherwise normal-appearing testicular parenchymal background, discovered incidentally during routine ultrasound examination (see Fig. 14-3). These nodules usually have a decreased echogenicity relative to the adjacent normal parenchyma. The sonographic appearance of these neoplastic nodules may be similar, regardless of histopathologic tumor type (see Fig. 14-3).

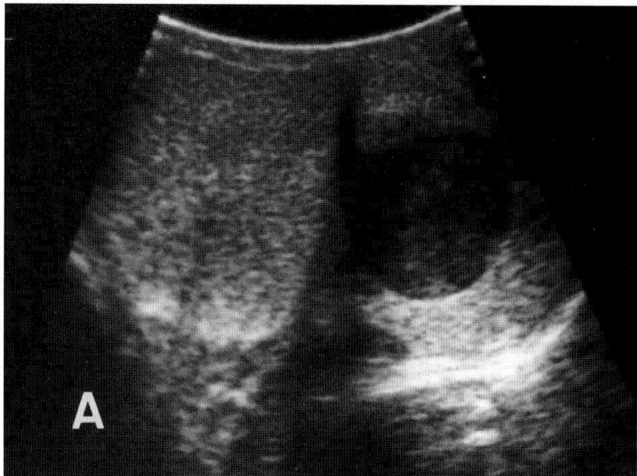

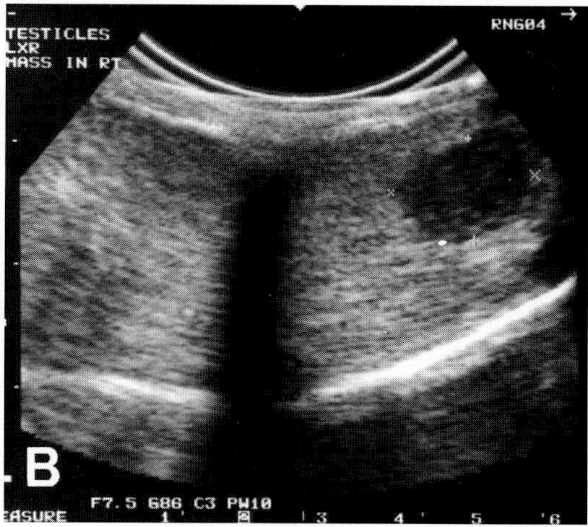

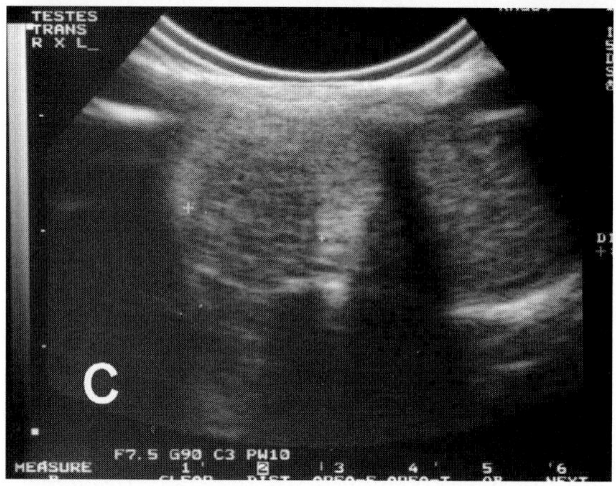

Figure 14-3. Transverse sonograms of three different dogs with focal, unilateral testicular tumors that were not detected on physical examination. (**A**) Seminoma in an 8-year-old mixed-breed dog. (From Pugh CR, Konde LJ. Sonographic evaluation of canine testicular and scrotal abnormalities: a review of 26 case histories. Vet Radiol 1991;32:243.) (**B**) Interstitial cell tumor in a 7-year-old Afghan hound. (**C**) Sertoli cell tumor in an 11-year-old Scottish terrier. The sonographic pattern of each tumor is remarkably similar and hypoechoic relative to the adjacent normal testicular parenchyma. Each dog presented for ultrasound examination with palpable prostatomegaly.

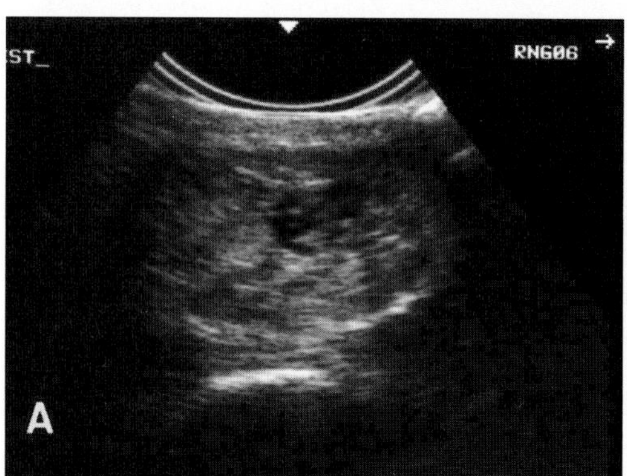

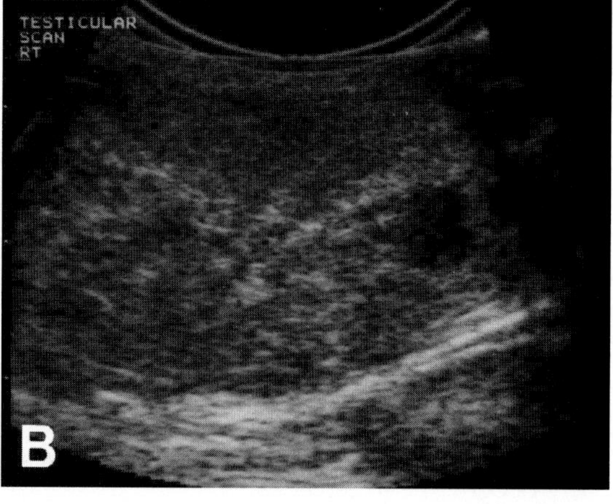

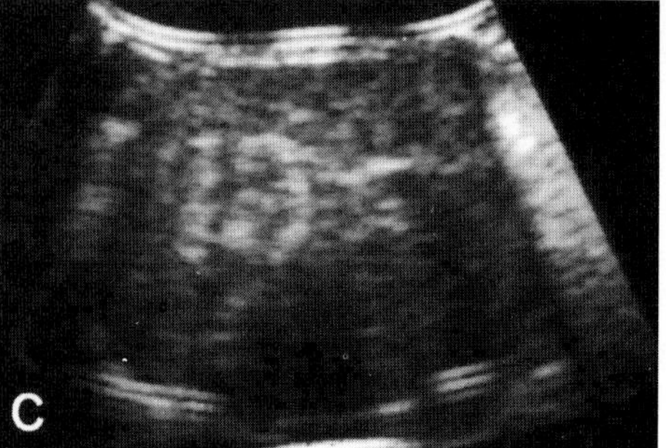

Figure 14-4. Sagittal sonograms of diffusely infiltrative neoplasms causing marked disruption of the normal testicular sonographic architecture in three different dogs with three different histopathologic tumor types. (**A**) Seminoma in an 8-year-old Labrador retriever. (**B**) Interstitial cell tumor in a 15-year-old mixed-breed dog. (**C**) Sertoli cell tumor in an 16-year-old collie. (From Pugh CR, Konde LJ. Sonographic evaluation of canine testicular and scrotal abnormalities: a review of 26 case histories. Vet Radiol 1991;32:243.)

In canine patients presenting with clinically detectable scrotal enlargement, testicular involvement can be extensive and advanced. The sonographic pattern is usually a mixed echoic pattern with considerable disruption of the normal testicular architecture, frequently including partial or complete destruction of the mediastinum testis (see Fig. 14-4). Concurrent extratesticular fluid has been reported, but it appears to be an infrequent finding.[2] Bilateral testicular involvement is not uncommon, and two or more histopathologic tumor types may occur in the same dog or same testis (Fig. 14-5). Histologically different testicular neoplasms may produce similar sonographic findings (see Fig. 14-4).

Nondescended (retained) testes can frequently be located with ultrasound. These testicles may appear normal, atrophic, or grossly altered (Fig. 14-6). Atrophic testicles are typically small and normal to hypoechoic, with retention of internal architectural features (see Fig. 14-6*A*). Abdominal retained testicles that have undergone neoplastic transformation frequently manifest as large, complex abdominal masses (see Fig. 14-6*B*). Small nodular neoplasms within retained testes are an uncommon finding (see Fig. 14-6*C*).

It has been reported that testicular lesions that are uniformly hyperechoic are usually benign.[29] This also appears to be a trend in dogs with small, hyperechoic foci in otherwise normal-appearing testicular parenchyma.

Ultrasound is a very sensitive diagnostic tool for detection of testicular parenchymal neoplasms. However, as is shown by the case examples shared in this chapter, the sonographic appearance of a testicular neoplasm does not specifically correlate to the histopathologic tumor type. If a cause of neoplasia is suspected, the ultrasonographic appearance coupled with the aforementioned epidemiologic characteristics may be used to attempt to predict the tumor type. The final diagnosis is ultimately determined by histopathologic analysis.

INFECTIOUS DISORDERS

The sonographic appearance of five cases of active orchitis and epididymitis have been previously described.[2] In each of five dogs, the affected testicle was characterized with a diffuse, patchy, hypoechoic pattern. The testicle was enlarged in four dogs, and the epididymis was enlarged in all five. One dog had bilateral involve-

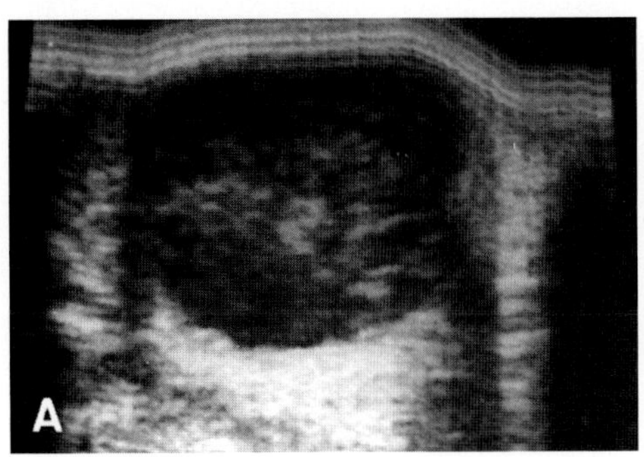

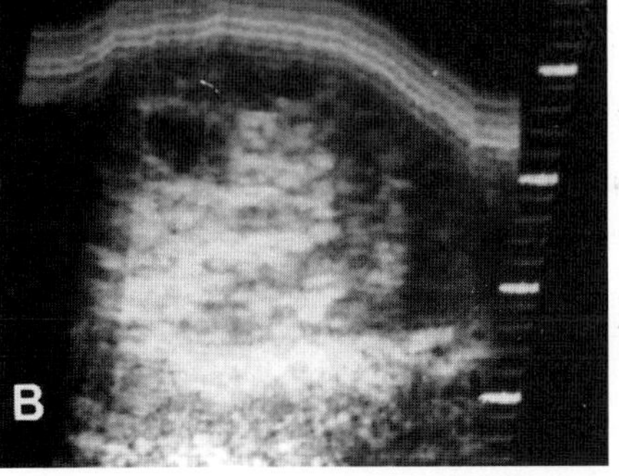

Figure 14-5. Sagittal testicular static B-scans of an 11-year-old golden retriever that presented for routine dentistry. Hard, enlarged testes were detected on physical examination. (**A**) The left testicle shows an overall decreased echogenicity with multiple hypoechoic to anechoic foci of various sizes and shapes. A well-defined central hyperechoic focus with a hypoechoic rim is identified. (**B**) The right testicle shows an overall increased echogenicity with total disruption of the normal architecture. A well-defined anechoic focus with a hyperechoic rim is also seen. Seminoma of the left testicle and Sertoli cell tumor and interstitial cell tumor of the right were diagnosed by histopathologic analysis. (From Pugh CR, Konde LJ. Sonographic evaluation of canine testicular and scrotal abnormalities: a review of 26 case histories. Vet Radiol 1991;32:243.)

ment. Extratesticular fluid was detected in three of the five. One dog had scrotal thickening. Disruption of the internal testicular parenchyma with partial or complete loss of the mediastinum testes was observed in dogs with advanced stages of infection. Additional cases reviewed for this chapter reflected changes similar to those previously reported (Figs. 14-7 and 14-8).

Any time orchitis or epididymitis is the suspected diagnosis, *Brucella canis* should be considered as the possible etiologic agent. Possible zoonotic implications should be considered and appropriate serologic and cultural testing should be performed.

NONNEOPLASTIC, NONINFECTIOUS DISORDERS

Patients may present with scrotal enlargement from causes other than neoplasia or infection. The cause of the enlargement may be testicular or extratesticular. Ultrasound is a particularly helpful diagnostic tool in these cases.

Scrotal enlargement may occur from enlargement of the scrotal wall itself. Intrascrotal fluid accumulation or an inguinal-scrotal hernia may also cause extratesticular scrotal enlargement.[2] Scrotal wall enlargement may be caused by edema, inflammation, or infiltration (Fig. 14-9). Scrotal wall thickening can be accompanied by accumulation or extratesticular fluid. Ultrasound permits direct visualization of the wall and extratesticular space and enables a differential evaluation of the testes and epididymis, which are frequently rendered nonpalpable by the scrotal abnormality.

Extratesticular fluid accumulation may result from serous fluid (ie, hydrocele), blood (ie, hematocele), pus (ie, pyocele), or possibly urine.[2] Hydrocele is the most common cause of extratesticular fluid accumulation in men and is usually painless. Hydrocele appears to be less common in dogs.[2] Human hydrocele may result from trauma, neoplasia, infarction, torsion, infection, inguinal hernia, or be secondary to ascites; it is often idiopathic.[30,31] Hematoceles in humans are the result of trauma, neoplasia, or

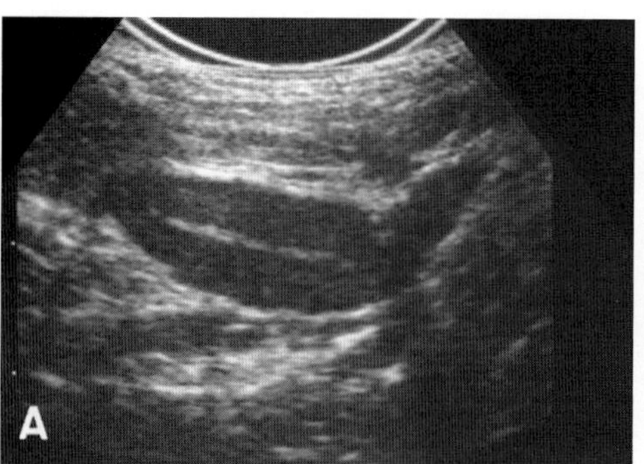

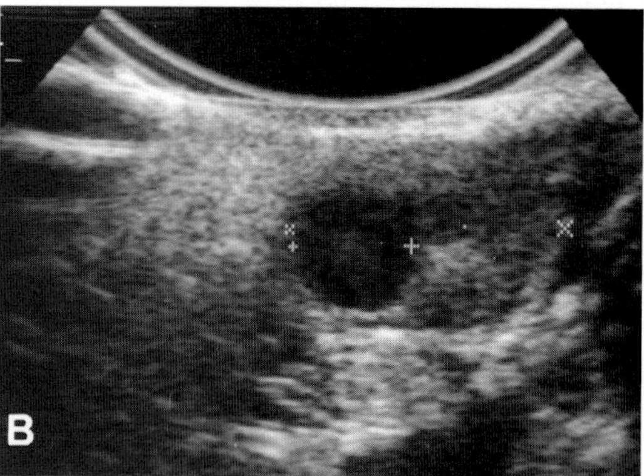

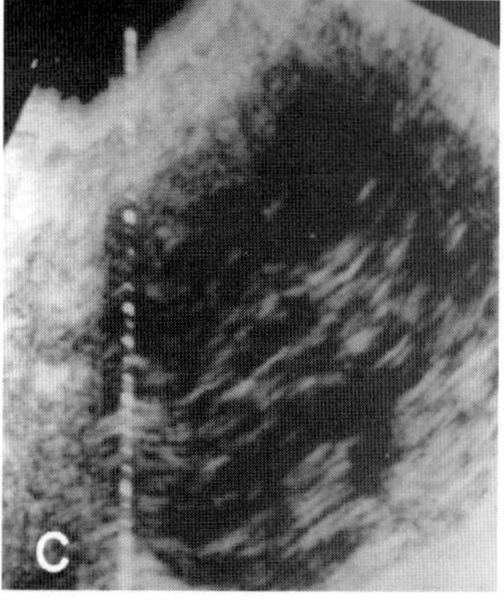

Figure 14-6. Sagittal sonograms of three different dogs with retained testicles. (**A**) Small atrophic testicle in an 1-year-old Shetland sheepdog. (**B**) Small retained testicle with a 0.7-cm hypoechoic, well-defined nodule in a 14-year-old mixed-breed dog. The histopathologic diagnosis was interstitial cell tumor. (**C**) Static B-scan of a large, abdominal Sertoli cell tumor in a dog of unknown age. (**A** and **C** from Pugh CR, Konde LJ. Sonographic evaluation of canine testicular and scrotal abnormalities: a review of 26 case histories. Vet Radiol 1991;32:243.)

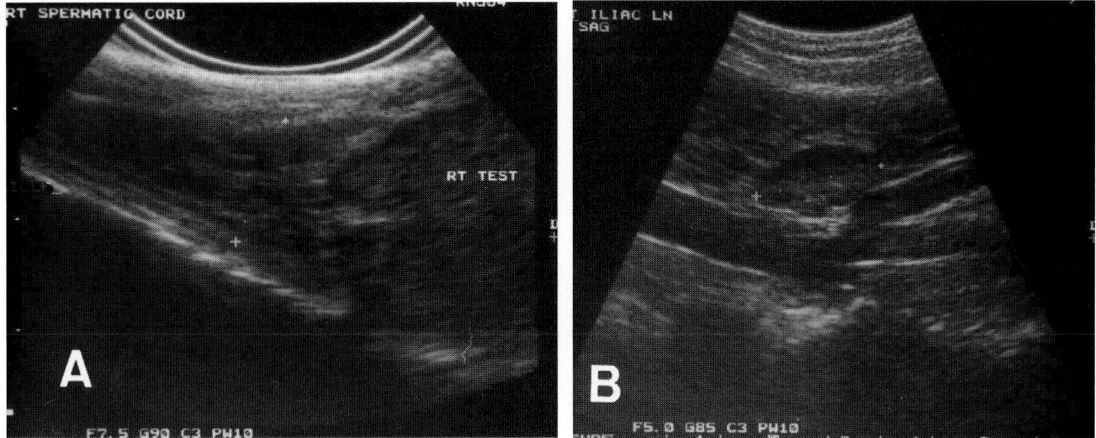

Figure 14-7. (**A**) Right sagittal sonogram of a spermatic cord and cranial half of the testicle of a 7-year-old Labrador retriever with bacterial orchitis and epididymitis (between + cursor marks). (**B**) The right medial iliac lymph node (between + cursor marks) is enlarged, irregular, and hypoechoic to mixed echoic (ie, secondary lymphatic reaction). The dog has a 6-week history of nonpainful scrotal swelling and leukocytosis. The condition was bilateral, with more severe sonographic changes in the right testis and epididymis.

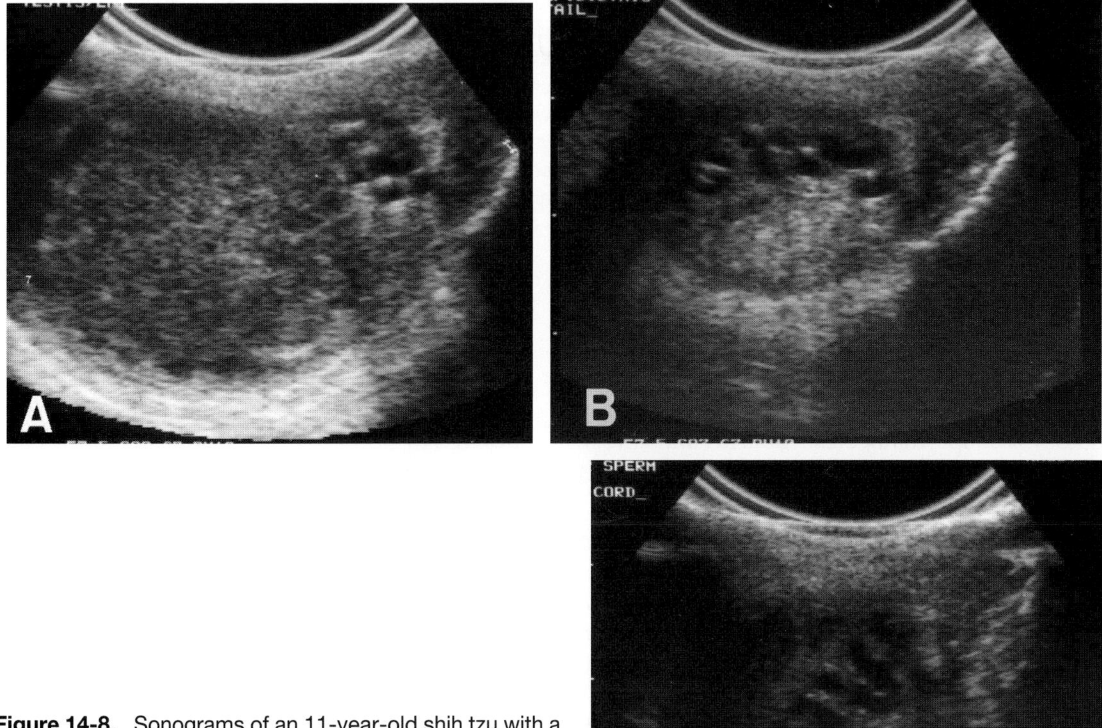

Figure 14-8. Sonograms of an 11-year-old shih tzu with a 4-day history of firm, nonpainful scrotal swelling. (**A**) The sagittal testicular sonogram shows mixed-echoic testicular enlargement with complete disruption of the parenchymal architecture. The epididymis (**B** and **C**) is enlarged, with multiple serpentine, anechoic, tubular structures. The histopathologic diagnosis was testicular abscessation.

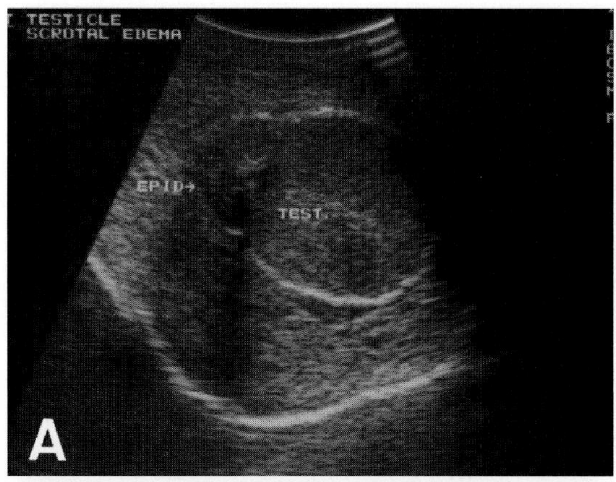

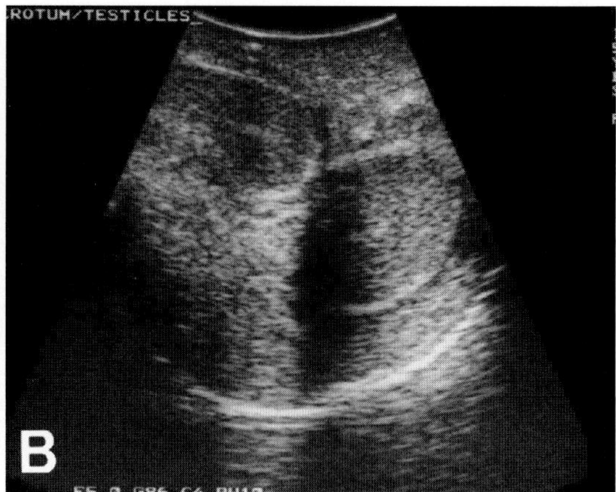

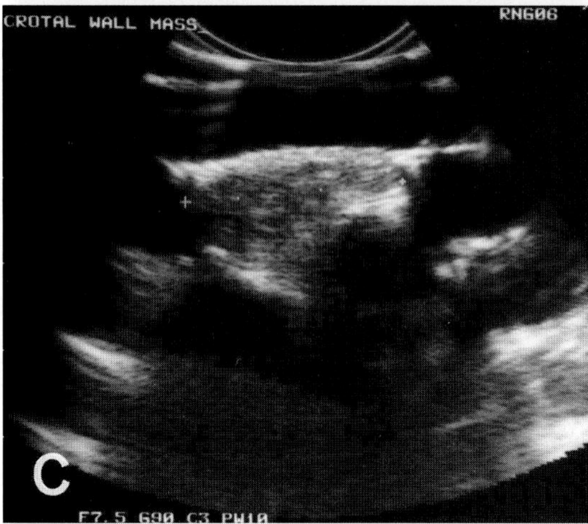

Figure 14-9. Sonograms of extratesticular scrotal enlargement due to scrotal wall abnormalities. (**A**) The grossly thickened scrotal wall with even, coarse echogenicity was caused by edema in a 5-year-old Scottish deerhound that presented with fever and hindlimb edema. The testes were normal. (**B**) Asymmetrically thickened scrotum in a 5-year-old bull mastiff that presented with a scrotal mass. Sonographic characteristics are remarkably similar to **A**. The testes were normal. The histopathologic diagnosis was a varicose tumor of the scrotum. (**C**) Mixed-echoic, focal scrotal mass in an 11-year-old Siberian husky. The histopathologic diagnosis was a mast cell tumor.

diabetes mellitus. Pyoceles result from abscess rupture, often into a preexisting hydrocele.[30]

Testicular epididymal lesions of the nonneoplastic, noninfectious category include spermatocysts, spermatoceles, epididymal cysts, varicoceles, torsion, infarct, sterile necrosis, and hematoma.

The sonographic appearance of two dogs with vascular compromise (ie, torsion and infarction) of the testes has been reported.[2] In both cases, an accumulation of fluid was detected surrounding a hypoechoic testicular parenchyma that was characterized by an irregular peripheral border (Fig. 14-10*A*). In both cases, the mediastinum testis was still intact, which would not be expected with a similarly destructive disorder that resulted from neoplasia or advanced infection. The sonographic appearance in a case of testicular infarction first reported in this chapter differed from the previous description (Fig. 14-10*B*). There was neither peritesticular fluid nor an irregular peripheral testicular border, and the mediastinum testis was interrupted. All of these dogs with testicular infarction had nonpainful, swollen scrotums at the time of presentation. One was documented to have been painful two days prior to presentation. In one case involving a potentially valuable breeding dog, ultrasound allowed for a rapid and accurate assessment and prognosis of both testes. One testicle was considered to be normal, while the other was considered essentially destroyed relative to function. Unilateral castration was elected.

Ultrasound is a useful tool for detection of nondescended, nonneoplastic testicles. Often the testes are atrophic and characterized by small size and are slightly hypoechoic or nor-

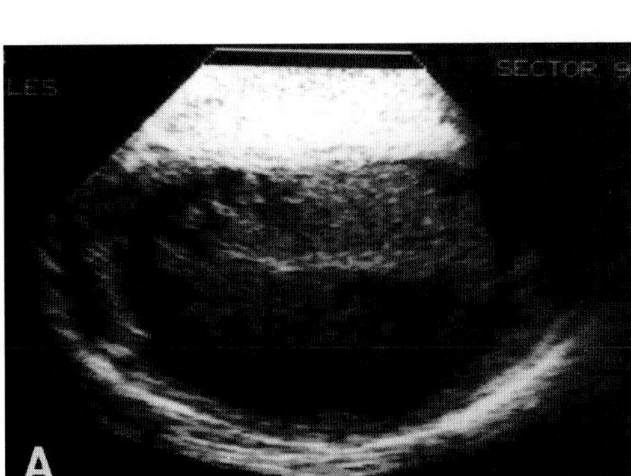

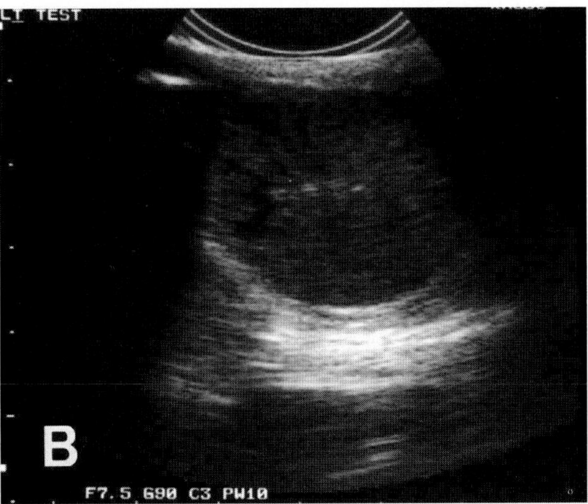

Figure 14-10. (**A**) Sagittal sonogram of an 11-month-old Labrador retriever with a nonpainful asymmetric scrotal swelling of 2 weeks' duration. At the onset of swelling, the testicle had been painful. Ultrasound revealed a grossly swollen left testicle with a disrupted, irregular peripheral contour surrounded by anechoic fluid. The testicular capsule or scrotal wall appeared thickened, with an irregular inner margin adjacent to the fluid. The overall parenchymal echogenicity was decreased. The mediastinum testis was seen. The right testicle was normal. The histopathologic diagnosis was acute necrotizing orchitis, suggesting testicular infarction. The epididymis was unremarkable. No evidence of torsion was shown, and there was no growth from the culture of testicular fluid. (From Pugh CR, Konde LJ. Sonographc evaluation of canine testicular and scrotal abnormalities: a review of 26 case histories. Vet Radiol 1991;32:243.) (**B**) Sagittal sonogram of a 9-year-old boxer with a 2-month history of lameness and a large retroperitoneal mass (hemangiosarcoma). The left testicle is enlarged, with patchy hypoechoic areas appearing to radiate linearly from an interrupted mediastinum. Histopathologic analysis showed the testicular parenchyma was necrotic secondary to obliteration of the vascular supply. The adjacent epididymis and capsule were normal. The final pathologic diagnosis was left testicular infarction.

moechoic (see Fig. 14-6*A*). Atrophic cryptorchid testes are frequently inguinally located, but could be found anywhere along the normal pathway of descent.

BIOPSY TECHNIQUES

Diagnosis of testicular disorders by interventional methods such as aspiration or biopsy are inherently risky. The immunologic consequences from breaching the testes-blood barrier can lead to transient infertility, granuloma formation, or permanent infertility. Sonography can be used to screen patients selectively for whom interventional methods are being considered. Because of its high specificity and accuracy, with a near absence of false-negative results, testicular sonography allows for clear differentiation of unilateral disease disorders. If interventional techniques are selected, ultrasound can be used to direct a needle precisely into the diseased portion of the testicle or epididymis.

CONCLUSION

Ultrasound is a very sensitive diagnostic tool for detection of testicular parenchymal abnormalities. As case experience has been gained, the value of its application has become increasingly apparent. However, it also has become apparent that attempts to predict the underlying histologic cause of a sonographically detected lesion should be made with great caution. The case examples shared in this chapter illustrate that the sonographic appearance of a testicular neoplasm does not correlate with the histopathologic tumor type. If a cause of neoplasia is suspected, the ultrasonographic appearance, coupled with the aforementioned epidemiologic characteristics, may be used to attempt to predict the tumor type. The final diagnosis is ultimately determined by histopathologic examination.

It appears that mixed or hypoechoic disruption of the testicular parenchyma, accompanied by loss of mediastinum testis integrity, is characteristic of aggressive testicular disease. This pattern is usually caused by neoplasia or advanced infection, although one case of testicular infarction demonstrated similar sonographic features.

Ultrasound is becoming an accepted, requested, and valuable tool in diagnostic veterinary medicine. Ultrasonography is a sensitive, rapid, and accurate method for assessing scrotal contents and for detecting lesions of the testes. Scrotal ultrasonography should be included as a routine part of the abdominal ultrasound examination of every intact male dog.

REFERENCES

1. Pugh CR, Konde LJ, Park RD. Testicular ultrasound in the normal dog. Vet Radiol 1990;31:195.
2. Pugh CR, Konde LJ. Sonographic evaluation of canine testicular and scrotal abnormalities: a review of 26 case histories. Vet Radiol 1991;32:243.
3. Sisson S. Urogenital system: male genitalia. In: Getty R, ed. Sisson and Grossman's the anatomy of the domestic animals. Philadelphia: WB Saunders, 1975: 939.
4. Christensen GC. The reproductive organs: the male genital organs. In: Evans HE, Christensen GC, eds. Miller's anatomy of the dog. Philadelphia: WB Saunders, 1979:554.
5. Arger PH, Mulhern CB, Coleman BG, et al. Prospective analysis of the value of scrotal ultrasound. Radiology 1981;141: 763.
6. Leopold GR, Woo VL, Scheible FW, et al. High-resolution ultrasonography of scrotal pathology. Radiology 1979;131:719.
7. Pugh CR. Canine testicular ultrasound. Proceedings of the 34th annual convention of the American Institute of Ultrasound in Medicine. New Orleans, 1990.
8. England GCW. Relationship between ultrasonographic appearance, testicular size, spermatozoal output and testicular lesions in the dog. J Small Anim Pract 1991;32:306.
9. Sample WF, Gottesman JE, Skinner DG, Ehrich RM. Gray scale ultrasound of the scrotum. Radiology 1978;127:225.
10. Willscher MH, Conway JF, Daly KJ, et al. Scrotal ultrasonography. J Urol 1983; 130:931.
11. Peterson LJ, Catalona WJ, Koehler RE. Ultrasonic localization of non-palpable testis tumor. J Urol 1979;122:843.
12. Nachtsheim DA, Scheible FW, Gosink BB. Ultrasonography of testis tumors. J Urol 1983;129:978.
13. Rifkin MD, Kurtz AB, Goldberg BB. Epididymis examined by ultrasound. Radiology 1984;151:187.
14. Hayes HM, Pendergrass TW. Canine testicular tumors: epidemiologic features of 410 dogs. Int J Cancer 1976;18:482.
15. Loan AS. Tumors of the genital system and mammary glands. In: Ettinger SJ, ed. Textbook of veterinary internal medicine. Philadelphia: WB Saunders, 1989: 1814.
16. Madewell BR, Theilen GH. Tumors of the genital system. In: Theilen GH, Madewell BR, eds. Veterinary cancer medicine. 2nd ed. Philadelphia: Lea & Febiger, 1987:583.
17. Postorino NC. Tumors of the male reproductive tract. In: Withros SJ, MacEwen EG, eds. Clinical veterinary oncology. Philadelphia: JB Lippincott, 1989;305.
18. Carpenter JL, Andrews LK, Holzworth J. Tumors and tumor-like lesions. In: Holzworth, J, ed: Diseases of the cat. Philadelphia: WB Saunders, 1987:517.

19. Pendergrass TW, Hayes HM. Cryptorchidism and related defects in dogs: epidemiologic comparisons with man. Teratology 1975;12:51.
20. Reif JS, Maguire TG, et al. A cohort study of canine testicular neoplasia. J Am Vet Med Assoc 1979;175:719.
21. Cotchin E. Testicular neoplasms in the dog. J Comp Pathol 1960;70:232.
22. Brodey RS, Matin JE. Sertoli cell neoplasms in the dog—the clinicopathological and edocrinological findings in thirty-seven dogs. J Am Vet Assoc 1958;133:249.
23. Lipowitz AJ, Schwartz A, et al. Testicular neoplasms and concomitant clinical changes in the dog. J Am Vet Med Assoc 1973;163:1364.
24. Pulley LT. Sertoli cell tumor. Vet Clin North Am 1979;9:145.
25. Morgan RV. Blood dyscrasias associated with testicular tumors in the dog. J Am Anim Hosp Assoc 1982;18:971.
26. Sherding RG, Wilson GP, et al. Bone marrow hypoplasia in eight dogs with Sertoli cell tumor. J Am Vet Med Assoc 1982; 178:497.
27. Comhaire F, Mattheuws D, Vermeulen A. Testosterone and oestradiol in dogs with testicular tumors. Acta Endocrinol 1974;77:408.
28. Weller RE, Palmer B. Metastatic seminoma in a dog. Mod Vet Pract 1983; 64:275.
29. Vick CW, Bird KI, Viscomi GN, Taylor KJW. Scrotal masses with uniformly hyperechoic pattern. Radiology 1983;148: 209.
30. Krone KD, Carroll BA. Scrotal ultrasound. Radiol Clin North Am 1985; 23: 121.
31. Johnston GR, Feeney DA, Rivers B, Walter PA. Diagnostic imaging of the male reproductive organs. Vet Clin North Am 1991;21:553.

Small Animal Ultrasound, edited by Ronald W. Green.
Lippincott-Raven Publishers, Philadelphia © 1996.

UTERUS

Amy E. Yeager and Patrick W. Concannon

SCANNING TECHNIQUE FOR THE UTERUS

The uterus of small animals can be difficult to detect, because the middle portions of the uterine horns are freely movable within the caudal abdomen; they are normally small in size; and they can easily be obscured by intestinal gas. Uterine horn diameter is typically less than 1 cm, except in cases of pyometra, mass lesions, and the second and third trimesters of pregnancy. The scanning technique must be excellent (see Chap. 3). It is desirable that animals are fasted for 12 hours before an ultrasonographic examination of the uterus, lie cooperatively in recumbency, and breathe without panting.

Positioning the animal in recumbency minimizes animal motion, which improves the ability of the sonographer to detect and follow the small, curving shape of the uterine horns. Positioning the animal in recumbency also enables the sonographer to apply various degrees of abdominal compression with the transducer. This is done to displace intestine out of the scan plane and place segments of the uterus in more superficial locations against the body wall, where the uterus is more likely to be detected. The decision to put the animal in dorsal, oblique dorsal, or lateral recumbency is made according to the preference of the sonographer. However, it may be easier to detect the cranial portion of the right uterine horn when the right side of the animal is positioned upward. Similarly, the left horn may be easier to detect when the left side of the animal is positioned upward. Fasting the animal decreases intestinal gas that may otherwise obscure portions of the uterus beneath acoustical shadows and reverberation artifacts.

A variety of transducer configurations and frequencies are appropriate for scanning the small animal uterus. The choice of sector, linear, or curvilinear transducers is made according to the preference of the sonographer. If a variety of dogs, cats, and other small animal species are scanned, it is advisable to have the use of 5.0- and 7.5-MHz transducers. If scanning is limited to animals that weigh less than 10 to 15 kg, the 5.0-MHz transducer may be unnecessary. Instead, a 10.0-MHz transducer may be of benefit, especially if a substantial number of the animals that are scanned weigh less than 4 kg.

Sonographic evaluation of the uterus includes scanning of the cervix, uterine body, and both uterine horns. The cervix, uterine body, and a variable amount of the uterine horns are located dorsal and to the left or right of the urinary bladder (Fig. 15-1). Although unnecessary, it is advantageous to scan for these structures when the bladder is full, using the bladder as a reference and an acoustic window through which the uterus can be visualized (Fig. 15-2). The bladder cannot be used as a window to

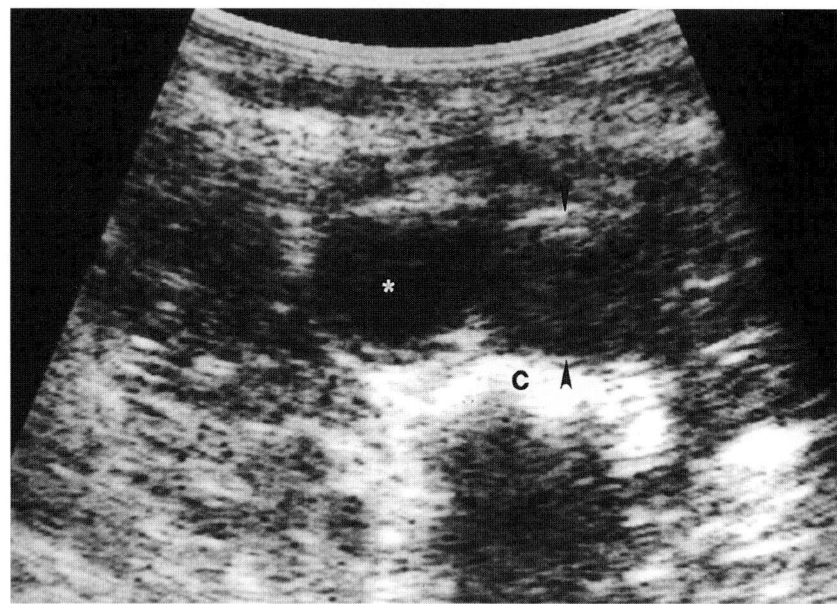

Figure 15-1. Transverse sonogram of the cervix (*arrowheads*), urinary bladder (*), and colon (*c*) of a proestrus beagle. Notice the spatial relations between these structures. In this case, the cervix is located to the right side of the urinary bladder and colon. The cervix has multiple layers, which appear as concentric rings of variable echogenicity.

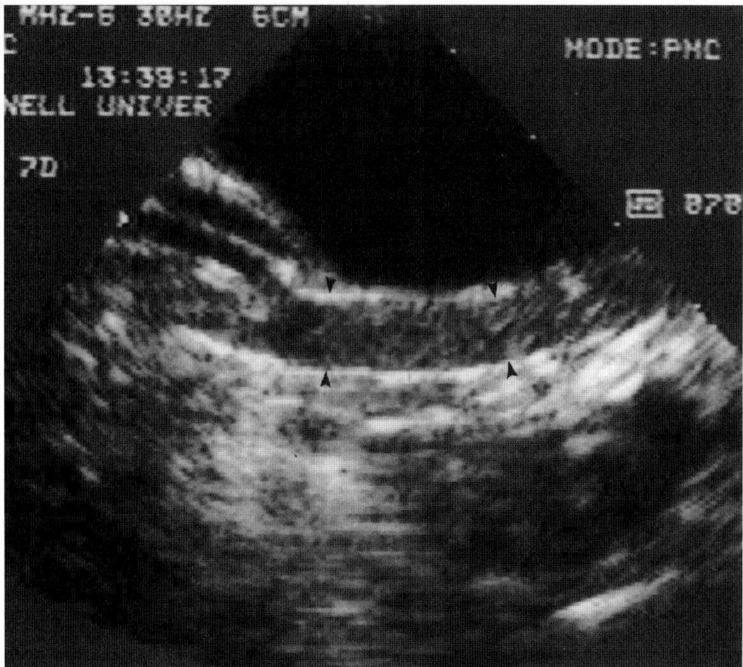

Figure 15-2. Sagittal sonogram of the urinary bladder and uterine horn (*arrowheads*) of a proestrus beagle. In this case, the uterus is dorsal to the bladder, and the bladder is an acoustic window through which a lengthy segment of uterine horn is visible.

visualize the entire uterus, because a substantial portion of each uterine horn is located cranial to the bladder.

When the uterus is not enlarged, the horns are usually located laterally on the left and right sides of the abdomen, caudal to the kidneys and the ovaries. The kidneys provide a second reference point for locating the uterus. When the animal is positioned in dorsal or oblique dorsal recumbency, the cranial end of each uterine horn may be visualized with another technique. The examiner locates the ipsilateral kidney in the sagittal scan plane, places the caudal pole of that kidney on the cranial edge of the image, and searches for the uterus by pointing or sliding the transducer medial and lateral to the kidney. The practitioner searches dorsal and ventral to the kidney if the animal is positioned in lateral recumbency.

A third reference point that may be useful for detection of uterus is the descending colon. The uterine body or a segment of uterine horn must cross ventral to the colon (Fig. 15-3).

When the uterus is not enlarged, it may not be possible to visualize the full extent of both horns, especially during anestrus.[1] It may only be possible to view focal segments of one or both horns, and differentiation from small intestine may be a problem. Typically, when the uterus is pathologically enlarged or enlarged during the

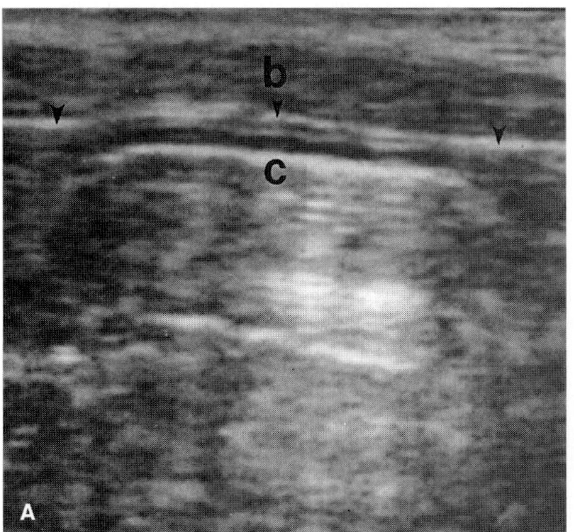

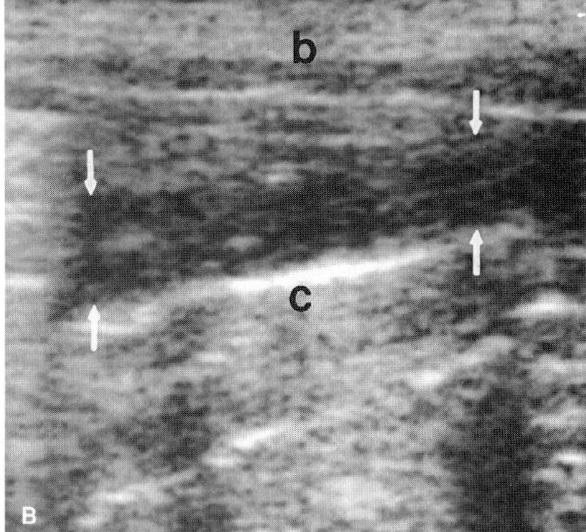

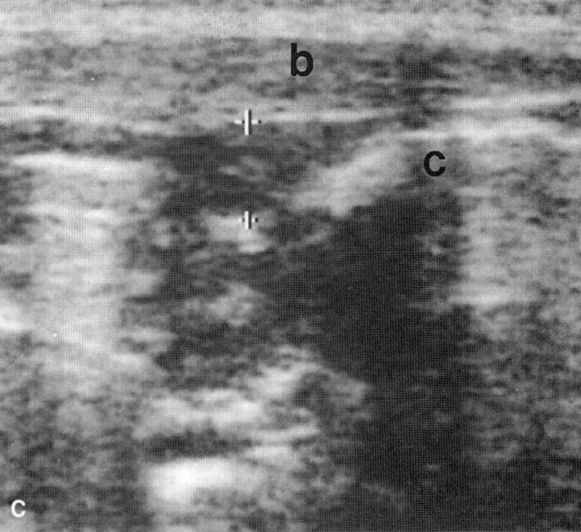

Figure 15-3. Sonograms of a proestrus German shepherd bitch. When the full extent of the descending colon is scanned, a segment of uterine horn is detected crossing ventral to the colon. (**A**) Notice the typical appearance of the gas-filled colon (*c*) in the transverse scan plane. It is located adjacent to the ventral surface of the peritoneal cavity (*arrowheads*) and the body wall (*b*). It has a thin (1.5 mm) wall composed of three layers of distinct echogenicity, and the gas in its lumen creates a hyperechoic interface with reverberation. (**B**) A sagittal segment of uterine horn (*white arrows*) crosses ventral to the colon. In the sagittal plane, the uterus has a tubular shape. (**C**) A transverse segment of uterine horn (*cursors*) is adjacent to the colon. In the transverse plane, the uterus has an oval or circular shape.

latter part of pregnancy, the horns are easily detected. In some cases, the enlarged uterus displaces most of the small intestine out of the caudal abdomen.

SONOGRAPHIC ANATOMY OF THE UTERUS

Nongravid Uterus

The uterus of dogs, cats, and many of the other small mammals typically seen in small animal practice is predominantly composed of two long horns that are oval to circular in the transverse plane and have a curving tubular shape in the sagittal plane (see Figs. 15-2 and 15-3). Primates are an exception. They have a relatively large, pear-shaped uterine body and small uterine horns. The size and echogenicity of the nongravid canine uterus depends on the stage of the estrous cycle. Detection is more difficult during the latter part of diestrus and throughout anestrus, when the horns are flaccid, uniformly hypoechoic compared with adjacent fat, and are 3 to 8 mm in diameter, depending on dog breed (Fig. 15-4). During anestrus, the cervix is difficult to differentiate from the vagina or the uterine body.

Beginning in proestrus and continuing through estrus and early diestrus, the uterus is less difficult to detect, because it is turgid and the uterine horn diameter increases by 1 to 3 mm. The horns may develop a central echo and hypoechoic middle layers (Fig. 15-5). The cervix is easily identified, because it is focally thicker than the vagina or the uterine body and it is composed of multiple layers that appear as a bull's-eye pattern in the transverse plane (see Fig. 15-1). During diestrus, the layered echogenicity of the uterine horns and the prominent cervix regress. The echogenicity of the horns may be decreased compared with anestrus and proestrus, and they temporarily may develop a tortuous contour if viewed in the sagittal plane (Fig. 15-6).

The uterus and small intestine are similar in size and shape, which may result in misidentification of their sonographic images. This is more likely to occur if the sonographic image is "noisy" because of inherent physical characteristic of the animal (eg, obesity, thick skin), poor acoustic contact with the skin (eg, animal's hair coat not clipped, dirty or scabby skin, too little acoustic coupling agent applied to the skin), panting motion, or use of a transducer that has insufficient resolution in the near field of the image. The small intestine is differentiated from the uterus because it contains ingesta or gas in its lumen (see Fig. 15-3), it has peristaltic motion in real-time images, and its wall is composed of muscular (thin and hypoechoic), submucosal

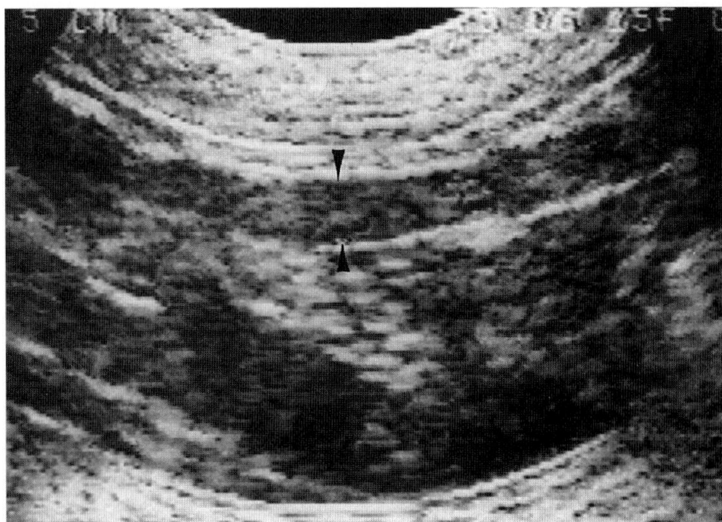

Figure 15-4. Sagittal sonogram of the uterine horn (*arrowheads*) of an anestrus beagle. The uterus has a small diameter (0.5 cm), and it is uniformly hypoechoic compared with the adjacent abdominal fat.

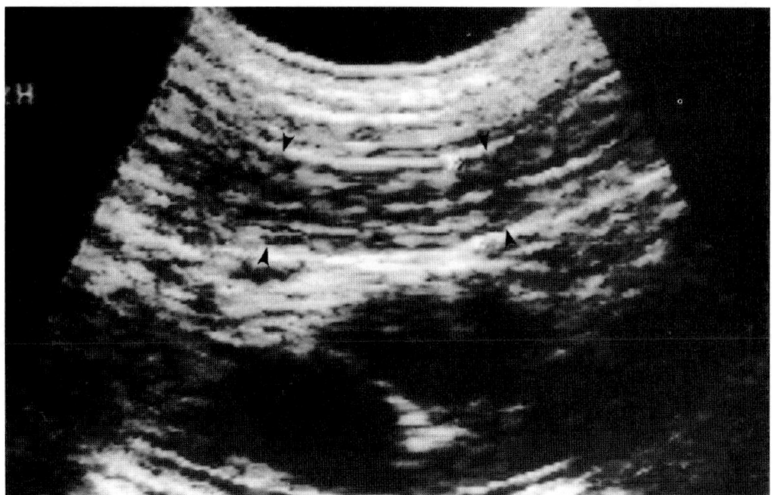

Figure 15-5. Sagittal sonogram of the uterine horn (*arrowheads*) of a proestrus beagle. The uterus is 6 mm in diameter, and it has a central linear echo and thin, hypoechoic middle layers.

(thin and hyperechoic), mucosal (thick and very hypoechoic), and luminal (thin and hyperechoic) layers when it is empty (Fig. 15-7; see Chap. 8). Layers of variable echogenicity are apparent in the uterine wall during proestrus, estrus, and postpartum, but the layer pattern is different from that of the empty small intestine.

Gravid Uterus and Fetus

In the dog and the cat, one of the most common indications for scanning the uterus is for pregnancy detection. Sonography is a highly accurate test for pregnancy in the dog. One study reports that the positive predictive value for pregnancy detection at about 30 days of gestation is 98%, and the negative predictive value is 96%.[2] The gravid and nongravid uterus are indistinguishable before the detection of the gestational sac (ie, chorionic cavity; Fig. 15-8*A*).[1,3] In the dog, these sacs can be detected as early as 17 days after the luteinizing hormone peak (LHP).[4] It is recommended that scanning for accurate diagnosis of pregnancy be performed no earlier than 27 days after the LHP or 25 days after the last breeding, at which time the gestational sac of a viable pregnancy is likely to be 1 cm in

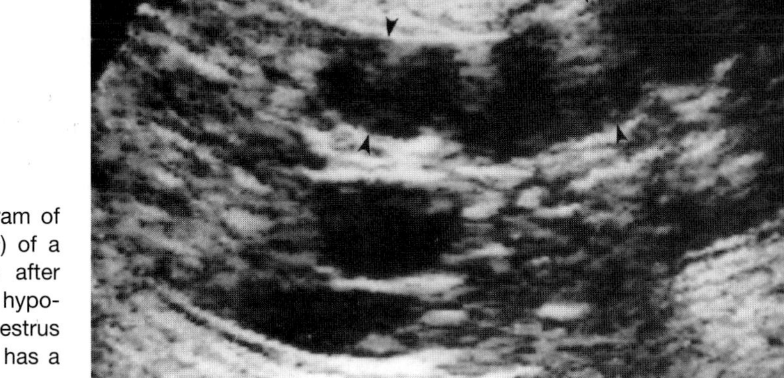

Figure 15-6. Sagittal sonogram of the uterine horn (*arrowheads*) of a diestrus beagle at 22 days after luteinizing hormone peak. It is hypoechoic compared with the anestrus uterus (see Fig. 15-4), and it has a tortuous contour.

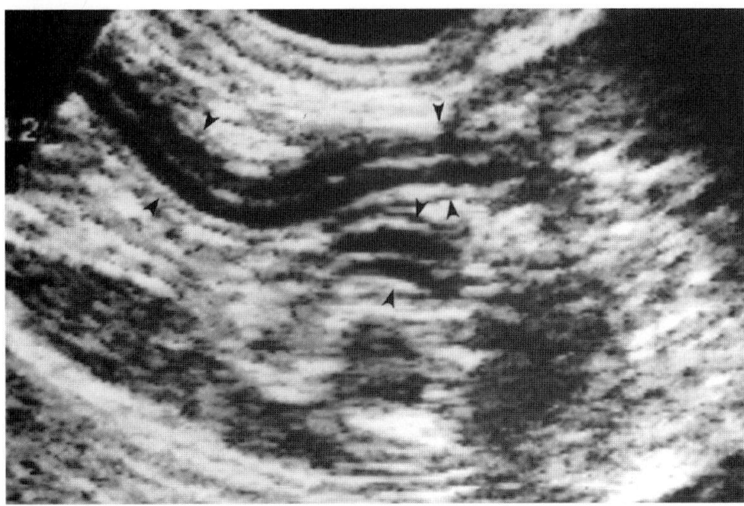

Figure 15-7. Sagittal sonogram of two segments of empty small intestine (*arrowheads*), demonstrating multiple layers within the wall of the intestine. Typically, the most prominent layer is the thick, hypoechoic mucosa.

diameter, and it is likely to contain an embryo with a detectable heartbeat.[5] In the cat, the gestational sac can be detected as early as 11 to 14 days after coitus (Fig. 15-8*B*), and scanning for accurate pregnancy diagnosis is recommended at 16 to 20 days (Fig. 15-8*C*) or later.[6]

Scanning may be used to estimate gestation length based on the size of the pregnancy or its anatomic appearance. These data are available for beagles (Fig. 15-9), retrievers (Table 15-1), and domestic cats (Fig. 15-10)[7]. Figures 15-11 to 15-13 contain sonograms that exemplify the appearance of beagle fetal anatomy at known times after the LHP. The sonographic appearance of the feline fetus is quite similar to the dog. The estimation of the length of gestation is probably more accurate during the second trimester, because at this stage, the breed of dog and the number of fetuses in the litter have less influence on pregnancy size than in the third trimester. The second trimester is also the time when the most obvious changes in fetal anatomy occur. Estimation based on pregnancy size is probably less accurate for toy and giant breeds of dogs and for litters containing only one or two fetuses. The estimation of length of gestation based on anatomic appearance may be influenced by the experience of the sonographer and technical factors (eg, transducer frequency) that affect the resolution of the image.[7]

Scanning may also be used to estimate fetal number. This estimation is more accurate between 27 and 37 days after the LHP (Fig. 15-14).[7] Before this time, litter size may be underestimated because the gestational sacs are small, and a few may go undetected. After this time, counting fetuses is less accurate because as the pregnancy progresses to term the fetuses become confluent; they are surrounded by relatively less fetal fluid; and the fetal length usually becomes greater than the width of the sonographic image. It becomes increasingly difficult to distinguish right from left horns because the elongated horns traverse the abdomen, and the same fetus may be counted more than once. Estimation of fetal number is more accurate if litter size is four or fewer. Fetal number is usually underestimated if there is a large litter.[8–10]

Postpartum Uterus

Layers are apparent in the hypertrophied wall of the postpartum uterus (Fig. 15-15). The endometrium is the thickest layer. It is hypoechoic at placental sites and hyperechoic between placental sites. Placental sites are not distinct after 8 to 12 weeks postpartum. Hyperechoic endometrium persists for as long as 14 weeks postpartum. Initially, the myometrium has three layers of distinct echogenicity. The circular and longitudinal muscle layers are hypoechoic, and a hyperechoic fibrovascular layer is interposed between the two muscle layers. Hypertrophied

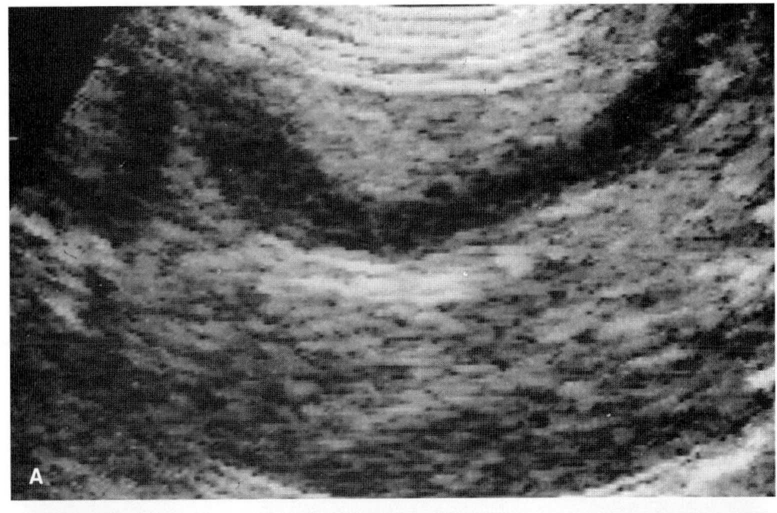

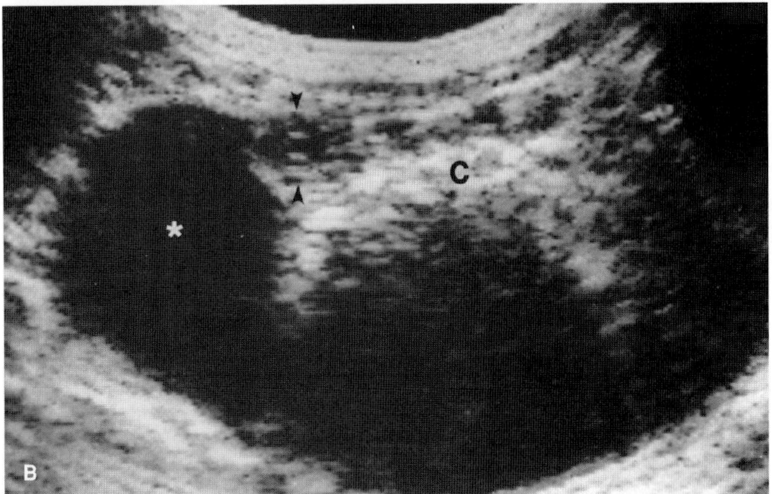

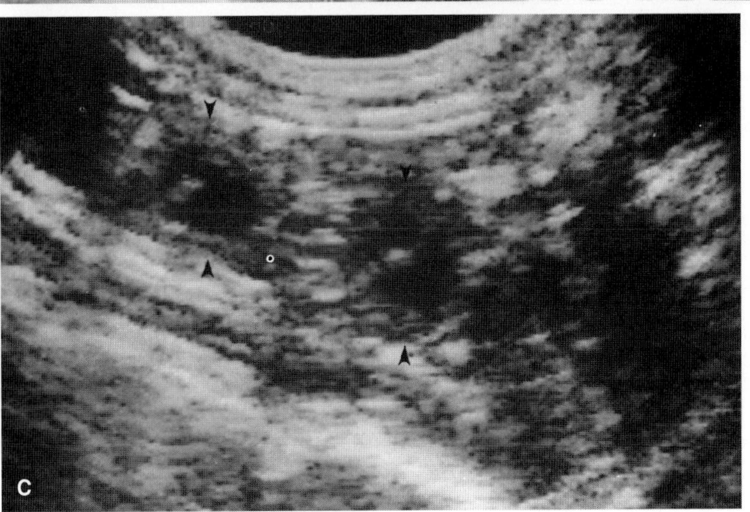

Figure 15-8. Serial sonograms of a pregnant domestic cat. (**A**) This sagittal image of the 0.4-cm-diameter uterine horn obtained at day 10 after coitus is indistinguishable from the nonpregnant day 10 uterus. (**B**) This transverse image of a 1-mm-diameter, anechoic gestational sac (*arrowheads*) was obtained on the earliest day that pregnancy was detected, 11 days after coitus. The gestational sac is adjacent to the urinary bladder (*) and the colon (*c*). (**C**) This transverse image of two 0.6-cm-diameter gestational sacs was obtained at day 16 after coitus. Both gestational sacs contain echogenic embryos attached to the uterine wall. Real-time imaging showed that the embryos had heartbeats.

Estimation of Beagle Gestation Length Based on Sonographic Appearance of Pregnancy

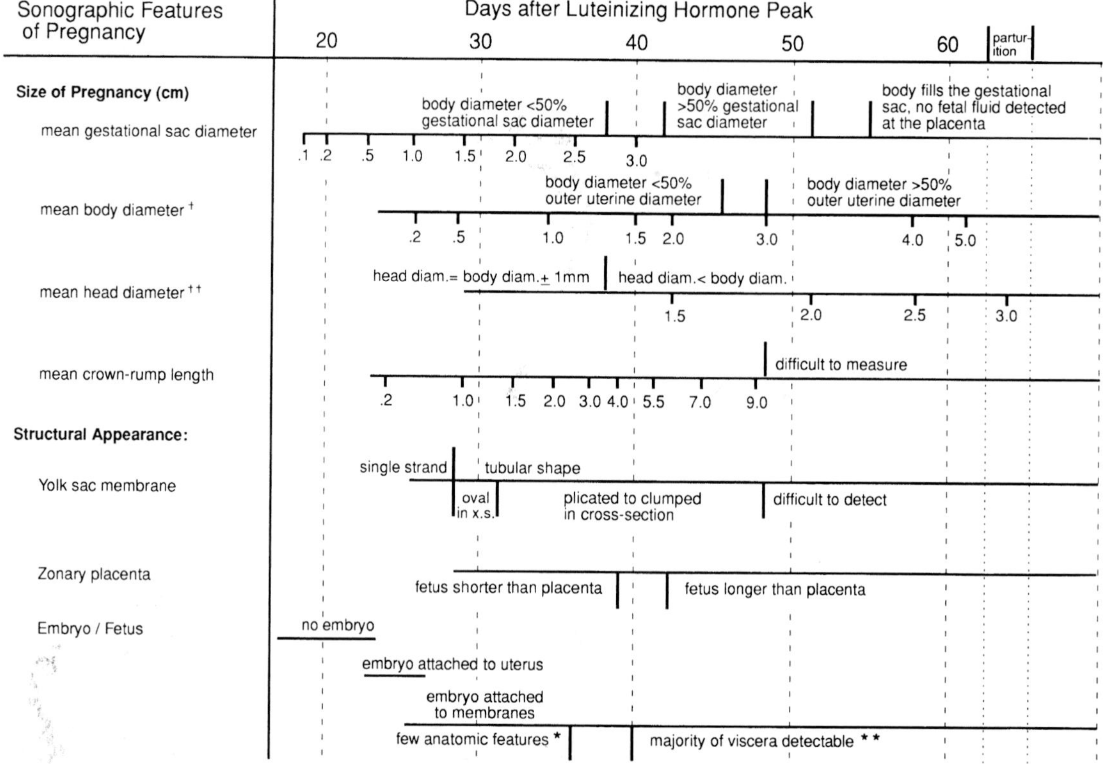

Figure 15-9. Estimation of the length of beagle gestation based on the sonographic appearance of the pregnancy. Body diameter (+) is measured at the level of the liver and stomach. The head diameter (++) is the biparietal diameter. The few anatomic features (*) include the bipolar-shaped embryo, ventricles in the brain, limb buds, fetal motion, face with snout shape, and faintly hyperechoic axial skeleton (mandible and maxilla first). The viscera (**), in order of detection, include the bladder, stomach, lung (hyperechoic compared with the liver), liver (hypoechoic compared with the caudal aspect of the abdomen), hyperechoic appendicular skeleton, kidneys, major blood vessels, skeleton (casts obvious acoustic shadows), intestine, and gallbladder.

blood vessels may be detected in the broad ligament adjacent to the serosal margin of the uterus. Small (<1 cm) focal accumulations of fluid may be present in the uterine lumen for as long as 11 weeks postpartum.[11]

The postpartum uterus rapidly decreases in size in the weeks following parturition. Placental sites, which initially are as large as 4 cm in diameter in beagles, decrease to less than 2 cm in diameter after 3 weeks. Uterine diameter is less than 1 cm after 6 weeks and returns to anestrus diameter by 8 to 12 weeks postpartum.

COMMON DISEASES

Most female pet dogs, cats, and ferrets are neutered, except for those specifically intended for breeding, and many of the common diseases involving the uterus are associated with a problem in reproduction. Commonly, scanning is indicated for diagnosis, prognosis, and therapy planning when there are problems of infertility, vaginal discharge, fetal death, dystocia, or failure to whelp at the expected time.

(text continues on p. 277)

TABLE 15-1
Fetal biparietal head diameter (cm)

Fetal trunk diameter (cm)	1–2	1–3	1–4	1–5	1–6	1–7	1–8	1–9	2–0	2–1	2–2	2–3	2–4	2–5	2–6	2–7	2–8	2–9	3–0	3–1	3–2	3–3
0–6	26	25	24	24	23	23	22	21	21	20	20	19	18	18								
0–8	25	24	24	23	23	22	21	21	20	20	19	18	18	17	17							
1–0	24	24	23	23	22	21	21	20	20	19	19	18	17	17	16	16						
1–2	24	23	23	22	22	21	20	20	19	19	18	17	17	16	16	15	14					
1–4	23	23	22	22	21	20	20	19	19	18	17	17	16	16	15	14	14	13				
1–6	23	22	22	21	20	20	19	19	18	17	17	16	16	15	15	14	13	13	12			
1–8	22	22	21	20	20	19	19	18	17	17	16	16	15	15	14	13	13	12	12	11		
2–0	22	21	20	20	19	19	18	18	17	16	16	15	15	14	13	13	12	12	11	10	10	
2–2	21	21	20	19	19	18	18	17	16	16	15	15	14	13	13	12	12	11	10	10	9	9
2–4	21	20	19	19	18	18	17	16	16	15	15	14	13	13	12	12	11	11	10	9	9	8
2–6	20	19	19	18	18	17	16	16	15	15	14	14	13	12	12	11	11	10	9	9	8	8
2–8	19	19	18	18	17	16	16	15	15	14	14	13	12	12	11	11	10	9	9	8	8	7
3–0	19	18	18	17	17	16	15	15	14	14	13	12	12	11	11	10	9	9	8	8	7	7
3–2	18	18	17	17	16	15	15	14	14	13	12	12	11	11	10	9	9	8	8	7	7	6
3–4	18	17	17	16	15	15	14	14	13	12	12	11	11	10	10	9	8	8	7	7	6	5
3–6	17	17	16	15	15	14	14	13	13	12	11	11	10	10	9	8	8	7	7	6	5	5
3–8	17	16	16	15	14	14	13	13	12	11	11	10	10	9	8	8	7	7	6	5	5	4
4–0	16	16	15	14	14	13	13	12	11	11	10	10	9	8	8	7	7	6	6	5	4	4
4–2	16	15	14	14	13	13	12	11	11	10	10	9	8	8	7	7	6	6	5	4	4	3
4–4	15	14	14	13	13	12	11	11	10	10	9	9	8	7	7	6	6	5	4	4	3	3
4–6	14	14	13	13	12	12	11	10	10	9	9	8	7	7	6	6	5	4	4	3	3	2
4–8	14	13	13	12	12	11	10	10	9	9	8	7	7	6	6	5	4	4	3	3	2	2
5–0		13	12	12	11	10	10	9	9	8	7	7	6	6	5	5	4	3	3	2	2	1
5–2			12	11	10	10	9	9	8	8	7	6	6	5	5	4	3	3	2	2	1	0
5–4				10	10	9	9	8	8	7	6	6	5	5	4	3	3	2	2	1	0	0
5–6					9	9	8	8	7	6	6	5	5	4	3	3	2	2	1	0	0	
5–8						8	8	7	6	6	5	5	4	3	3	2	2	1	1	0		
6–0							7	6	6	5	5	4	4	3	2	2	1	1	0			
6–2								6	5	5	4	4	3	2	2	1	1	0				
6–4									5	4	4	3	2	2	1	1	0					

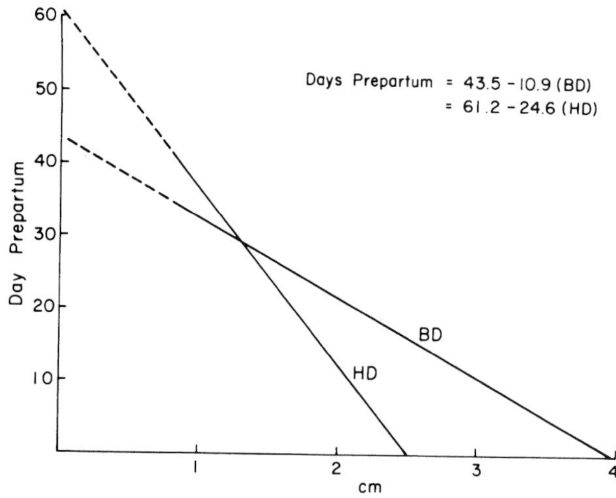

Figure 15-10. Average regression equations and lines for head diameters (*HD*) and body diameters (*BD*) relative to days prepartum. Dashed portions of the lines indicate an inability to differentiate head and body by ultrasound at this early stage of pregnancy.

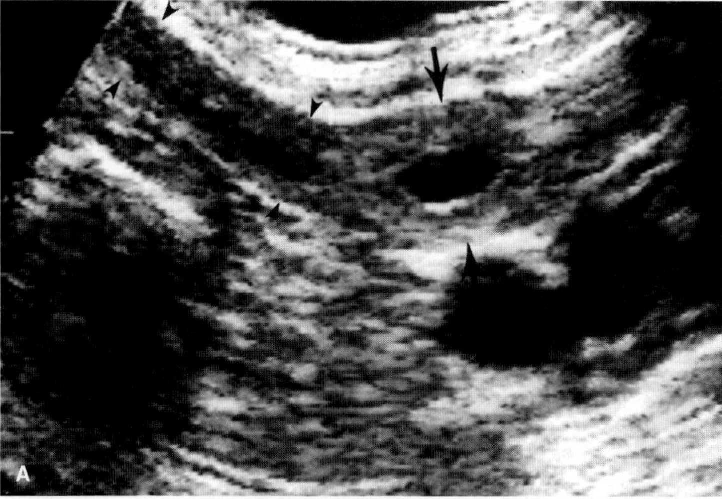

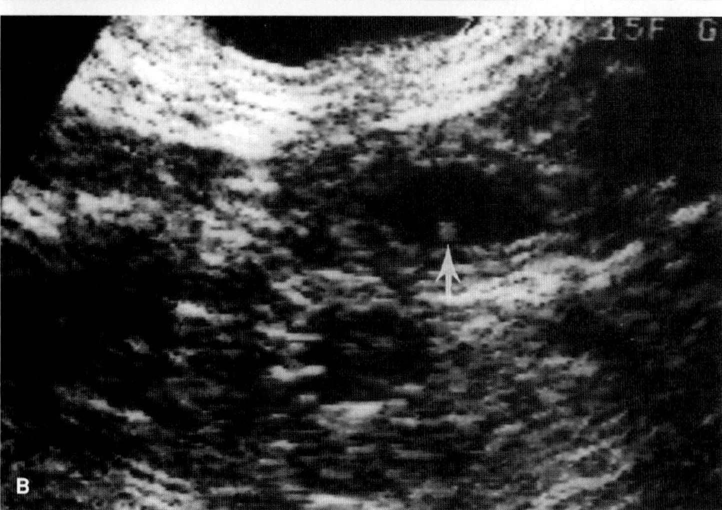

Figure 15-11. Serial sonograms of beagle pregnancy made in the sagittal plane. Day 0 is the day of the luteinizing hormone peak. (**A**) Day 22. A 0.4-cm-diameter gestational sac (*arrows*) without a detectable embryonic mass causes a bulge in the outer contour of the uterine horn (*arrowheads*). (**B**) Day 24. A 0.6-cm-diameter gestational sac contains a 0.2-cm-long embryo that appears to be directly attached to the uterine wall (*arrow*). *(continued)*

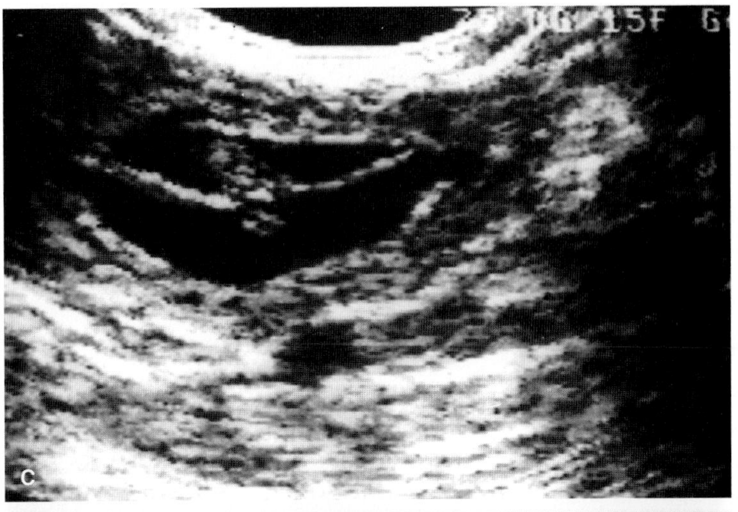

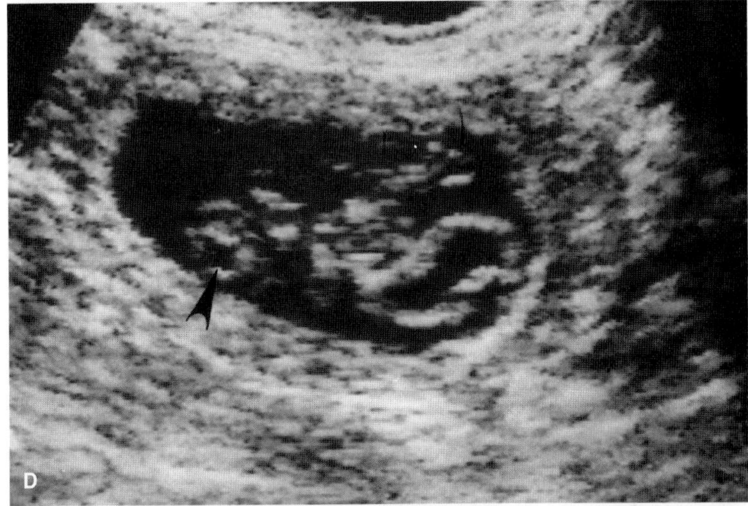

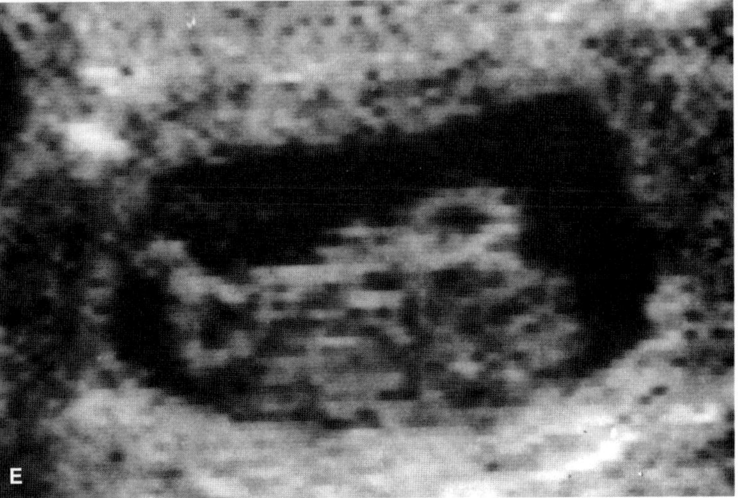

Figure 15-11. *(Continued)* (**C**) Day 28. A 0.8-cm-long embryo is attached to a single-strand yolk sac membrane. (**D**) Day 32. A 1.5-cm-long, bipolar-shaped fetus has few anatomic features. There is a 3-mm anechoic ventricle located in the brain (*arrowhead*). Cranial is to the left in the photograph. Thin allantoic and thick, oval yolk sac membranes are also visible. (**E**) Day 35. A 2.2-cm-long, bipolar-shaped fetus has few anatomic features, and the head and body are approximately the same diameter (the head cannot be distinguished from the body in this image). The echogenic yolk sac membrane has a tubular shape.

(continued)

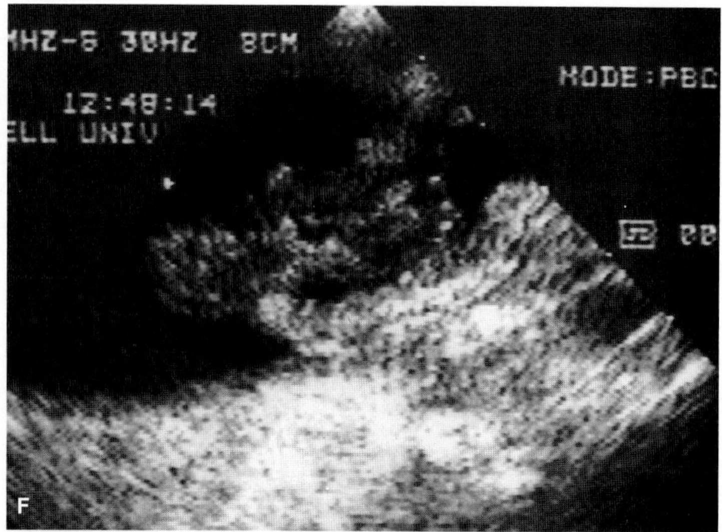

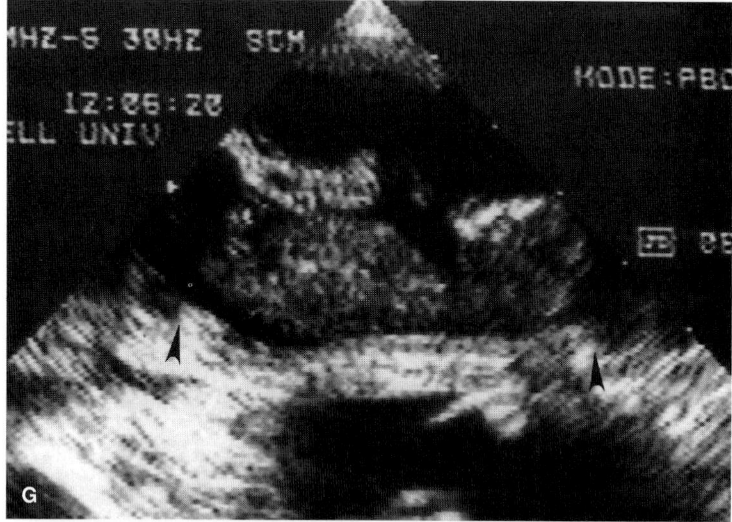

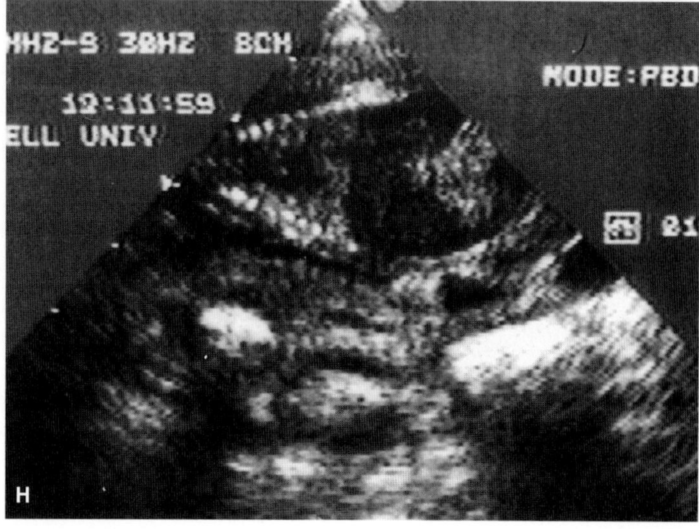

Figure 15-11. *(Continued)* (**F**) Day 39. Viscera are detectable in this 3.5-cm-long fetus. The lung and caudal abdomen are hyperechoic compared with the liver. Anechoic cardiac chambers and urinary bladder are also visualized. The head of the fetus is to the left in the photograph, and the head diameter is less than the body diameter. The fetus is 0.2 cm shorter than the zonary placenta (*arrowheads*). (**G**) Day 39. Hyperechoic foci located in the head of this 4-cm-long fetus cast faint acoustic shadows. These are calcified portions of the mandible, maxilla, and frontal bones. The head of the fetus is to the right in the photograph, and the fetus is several millimeters shorter than the zonary placenta (*arrowheads*). A segment of tubular yolk sac membrane is adjacent to the body of the fetus. (**H**) Day 45. In this image of a fetal body, the viscera are more obvious than in the 39-day fetus (see **G**). Hyperechoic ribs are easily visualized. The length of the fetus exceeds the width of the near field of the 90° sector image. Cranial is to the left in the photograph.

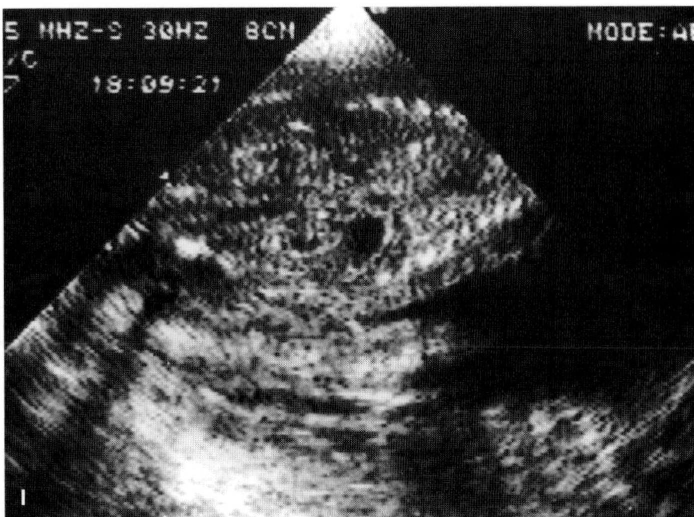

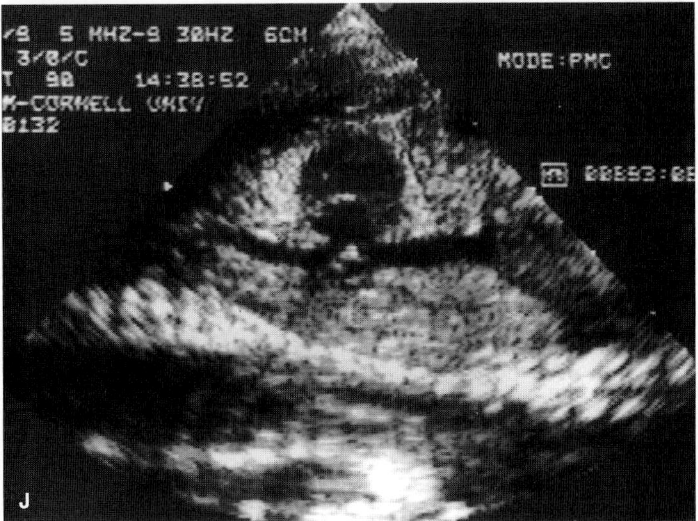

Figure 15-11. *(Continued)* (**I**) Day 47. The image of this fetal body shows some additional anatomy that can be detected at this stage of gestation. Hyperechoic ribs, anechoic stomach, anechoic renal pelves, an anechoic segment of the caudal abdominal aorta, and hyperechoic pelvis casting an acoustic shadow are visible. Cranial is to the right in the photograph. (**J**) Day 59. This image of the fetal thorax and cranial abdomen shows that fetal anatomy is larger and more obvious than it is on day 47 (see **I**). The intensely hyperechoic vertebrae of the thoracic spine, hyperechoic lung, right atrium and ventricle, cranial and caudal vena cava, and hypoechoic liver are visible. Cranial is to the left in the photograph.

Endometritis and Cystic Endometrial Hyperplasia

Endometritis and cystic endometrial hyperplasia are common in older bitches. They often occur concurrently and present as a problem of infertility or vaginal discharge that may progress to pyometra.

Sonography is probably not an accurate test for these diseases, because an affected uterus frequently appears normal and when the uterus appears abnormal, the sonographic findings are nonspecific. Endometrial hyperplasia and metritis may cause mild enlargement of the uterine horns (one to three times the normal diameter). A central hyperechoic layer may be seen (Fig. 15-16), similar to or more extensive than the appearance of the uterus during proestrus and estrus. Alternatively, the uterus may have a blotchy heteroechoic appearance. Occasionally, multiple, small (typically $\leq$3 mm), anechoic cysts are detected within the central hyperechoic layer (Fig. 15-17). Most cysts that develop because of endometrial hyperplasia are microscopic and not detectable by sonography.

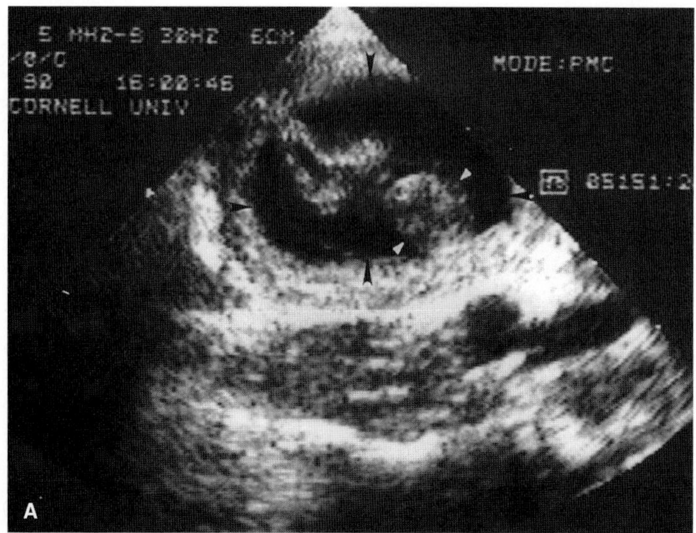

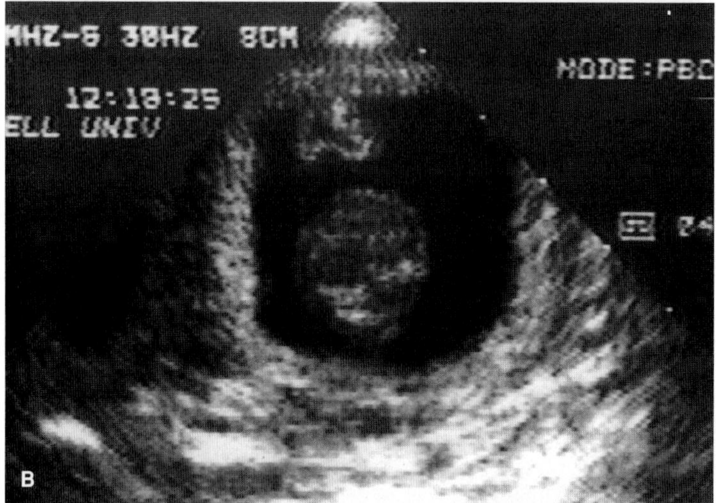

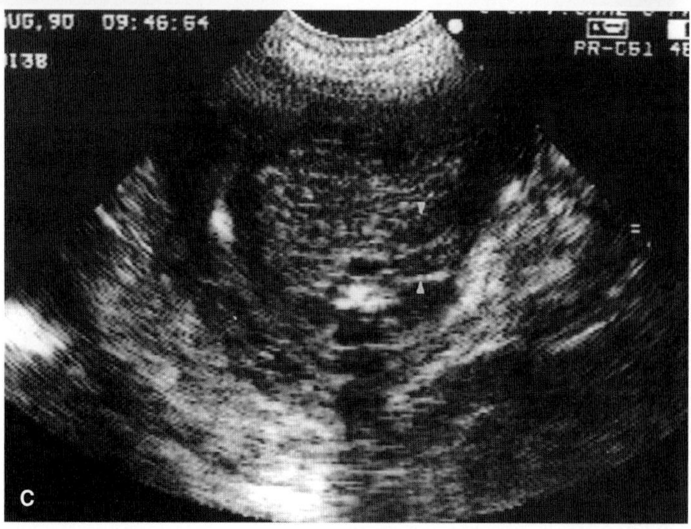

Figure 15-12. Serial sonograms of a beagle pregnancy made in the transverse plane. Day 0 is the day of the luteinizing hormone peak. (**A**) Day 35. In this image, a 1-cm-diameter fetus (*white arrowheads*) and a prominent plicated yolk sac membrane are encircled by a thin allantoic membrane. (**B**) Day 42. The diameter of this fetal body is equal to 50% of the gestational sac diameter. Hypoechoic liver and hyperechoic lung are visible. The plicated yolk sac membrane is located above the fetus in the photograph. (**C**) Day 54. At this stage of gestation, most of the anatomy is detectable. In this particular image of the midabdomen of a fetus, heteroechoic small intestinal segments fill most of the abdomen. Anechoic abdominal aorta, a hypoechoic kidney (*arrowheads*), and an intensely hyperechoic vertebra casting an acoustic shadow are also visible. The dorsum of the fetus is positioned down in the photograph.

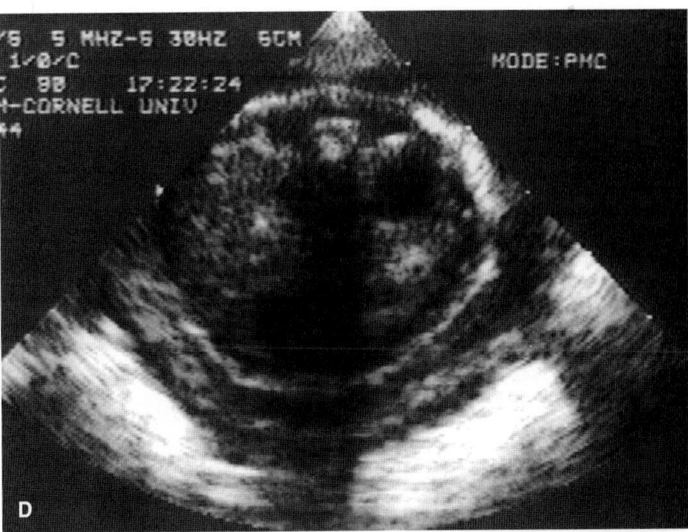

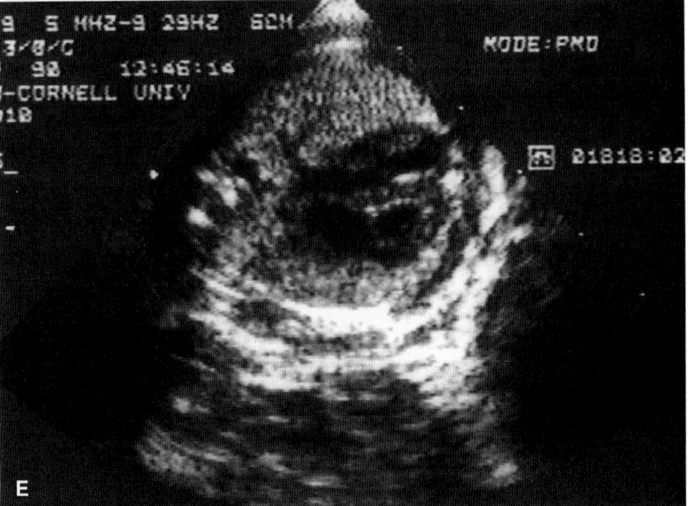

Figure 15-12. *(Continued)* **(D)** Day 57. The 3.8-cm-diameter fetal body fills the lumen of the uterus at the level of the placenta such that no fetal fluid is detectable in this image. The hypoechoic liver, anechoic gastric lumen, and intensely hyperechoic vertebra casting an acoustic shadow are visible. The dorsum of the fetus is positioned up in the photograph. (**E**) Day 61. The fetal thorax shows a hyperechoic lung, right and left atria, right and left ventricles, an anechoic descending thoracic aorta, and an intensely hyperechoic vertebra casting an acoustic shadow. The dorsum of the fetus is positioned to the left in the photograph.

Pyometra

Pyometra is an infection of the uterus that results in the accumulation of pus in the uterine lumen. It most often occurs during late diestrus in bitches with cystic endometrial hyperplasia. Affected bitches typically present with signs of systemic illness such as depression, anorexia, lethargy, fever, vomiting, polydipsia, dehydration, tachycardia, and weight loss. Queens are less likely to show signs of systemic illness. Vaginal discharge may or may not be evident, depending on whether the cervix is open or closed.

Sonography is an accurate diagnostic test for pyometra. The pertinent abnormal finding is obvious anechoic or hypoechoic fluid distention of the uterine horn or horns (Fig. 15-18). Uterine wall thickness and contour depend on the degree of uterine distention. The sonographic appearance of pyometra is not pathognomonic for the disease. Mucometra and hematometra may have the same appearance. The uterine wall should not appear thickened in cases of mucometra (Fig. 15-19). The sonographic appearance of pyometra can always be differentiated from pregnancy.

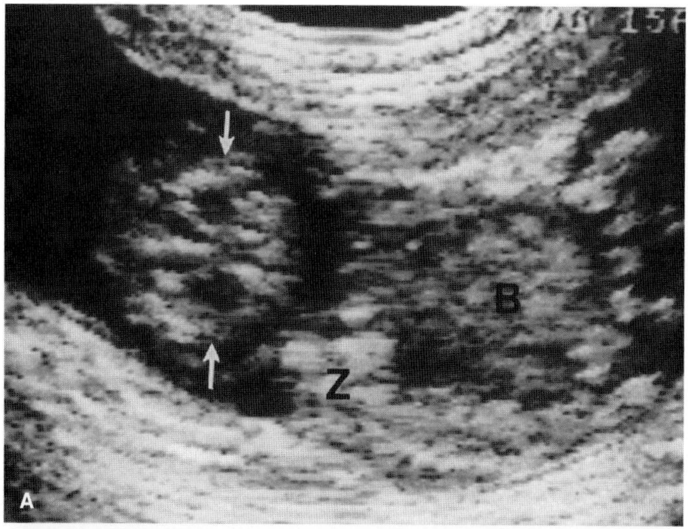

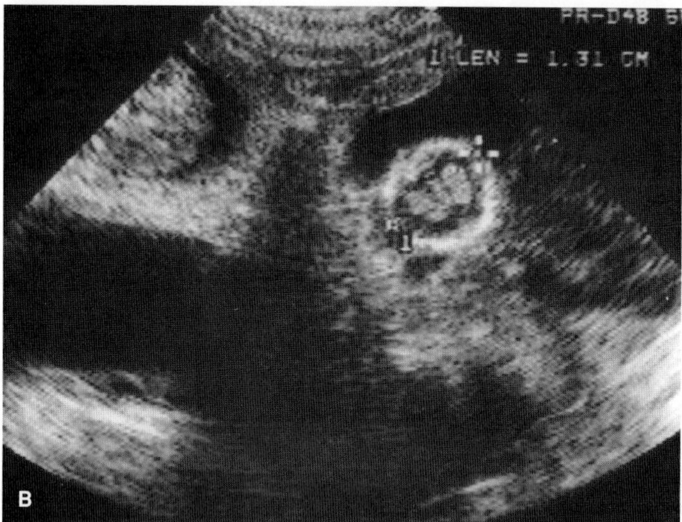

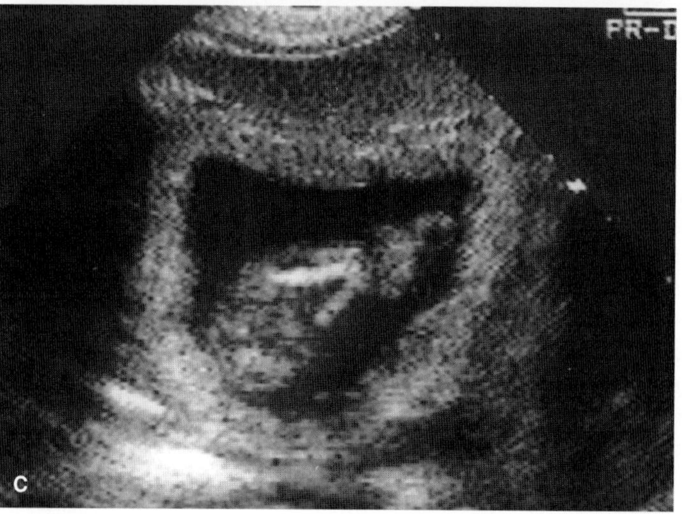

Figure 15-13. Serial sonograms of beagle pregnancy showing the fetal head in coronal and transverse planes. Day 0 is the day of the luteinizing hormone peak. (**A**) Day 37. A 1.2-cm-diameter fetal head (*arrow*) shows anechoic, symmetric lateral ventricles in the brain. The calvarium is not hyperechoic, indicating that it is not yet calcified. The fetal body (*B*) and the edge of the zonary placenta (*Z*) are marked. (**B**) Day 43. Cursors mark the 1.3-cm biparietal diameter of this fetal head. A bilobed, hyperechoic choroid plexus is located in the center of the brain. The calvarium is hyperechoic, indicating that it is calcified. (**C**) Day 43. The V-shaped hyperechoic mandible is visible in the fetal head. A clump-shaped yolk sac membrane is also visible within the 3-cm-diameter gestational sac. It is located to the right of the mandible in the photograph. The maternal spleen is located between the gravid uterus and the ventral body wall of the bitch.

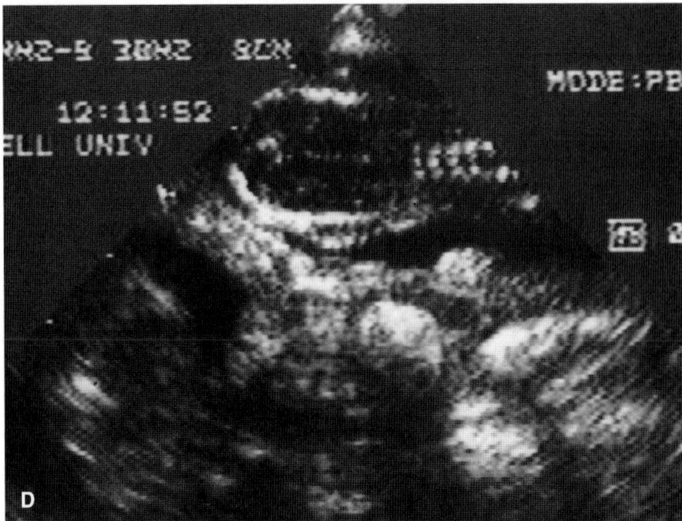

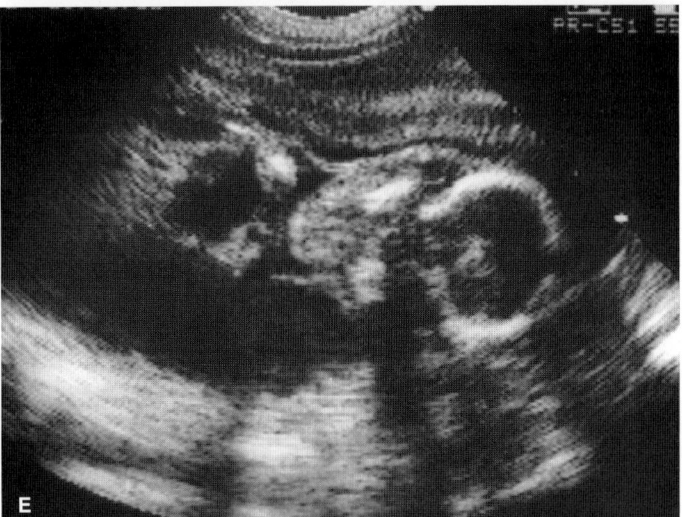

Figure 15-13. *(Continued)* (**D**) Day 45. In this image of a 1.5-cm-diameter fetal head, the intensely hyperechoic calcified calvarium is causing attenuation of the ultrasound beam, which causes the brain to appear hypoechoic and have decreased anatomic definition. The falx cerebri appears as a hyperechoic line visible in the middle of the brain. The hyperechoic cervical vertebrae are located to the right of the fetal head in the photograph. (**E**) Day 51. In this image of a 1.9-cm-diameter fetal head, the nose, anechoic eyes, and intensely hyperechoic maxilla and calvarium, which cast acoustic shadows, are visible. Rostral is to the left in the photograph.

Fetal Death, Distress, and Malformation

Sonographic evaluation for fetal death or distress is indicated if there is infertility, medical complications during pregnancy, dystocia, or other delay in whelping. In cases of infertility, sonography helps to differentiate females that fail to conceive or implant from those that fail to maintain a pregnancy after implantation. Serial sonography ascertains the time of death and the number of fetuses affected. The sonographic findings of fetal death cannot determine the cause. Fetal death is more common during the first half of pregnancy.[12] At this stage, it is not uncommon to observe one or two fetal resorption sites in an otherwise normal dog or cat pregnancy. Sonographic studies suggest that the incidence of spontaneous fetal resorption ranges from 5% to 13% of canine pregnancies before day 40 of gestation.[12,13]

Sonography is accurate for the diagnosis of fetal death after the time in gestation when an embryo with a heartbeat should be detectable (see the previous section on the gravid uterus). Heartbeat and fetal movement are definite evi-

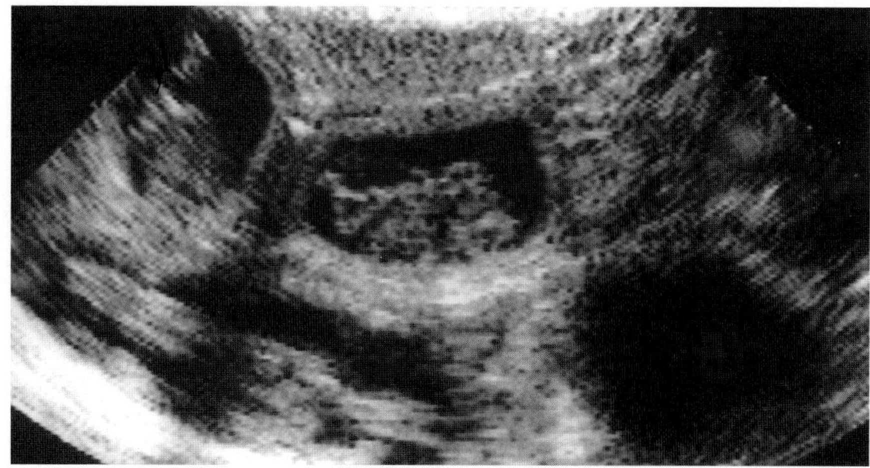

Figure 15-14. Sagittal sonogram of the midabdomen of a pregnant beagle bitch at 35 days after the luteinizing hormone peak. Five gestational sacs are visible. At this stage of gestation, the sacs become confluent, and it becomes more difficult to differentiate individual sacs.

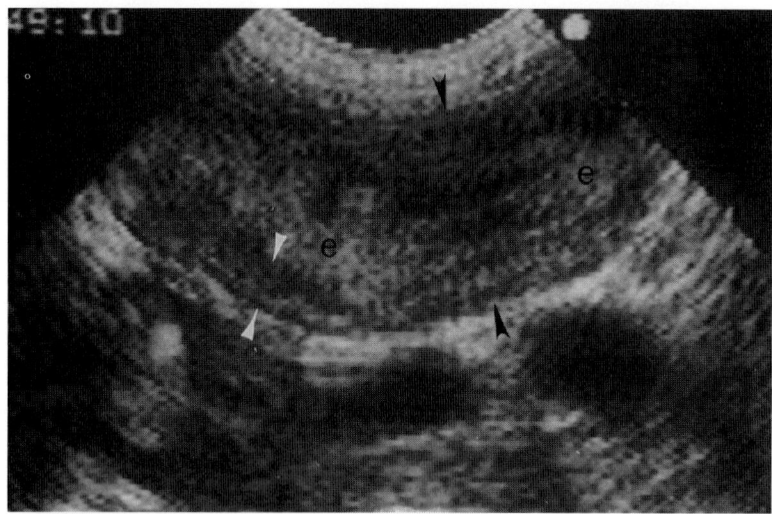

Figure 15-15. Sagittal sonogram of beagle uterine horn at 1 day postpartum. The uterus is enlarged (1.5 cm in diameter). The endometrium (*e*) is hyperechoic except at a hypoechoic placental site (*black arrowheads*). The myometrium is composed of three layers (*white arrowheads*).

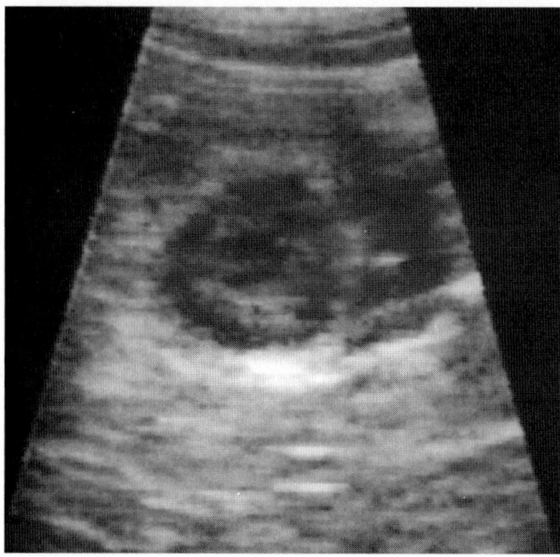

Figure 15-16. Transverse sonogram of the uterine horn of an adult mixed-breed rabbit. The uterus is mildly enlarged (1 cm in diameter), it has hyperechoic endometrium indicative of hyperplasia of inflammation, and there is a 3-mm-diameter accumulation of anechoic fluid in the lumen, which could be mucus, blood, or pus. The histologic diagnosis was severe endometrial hyperplasia and adenomyosis.

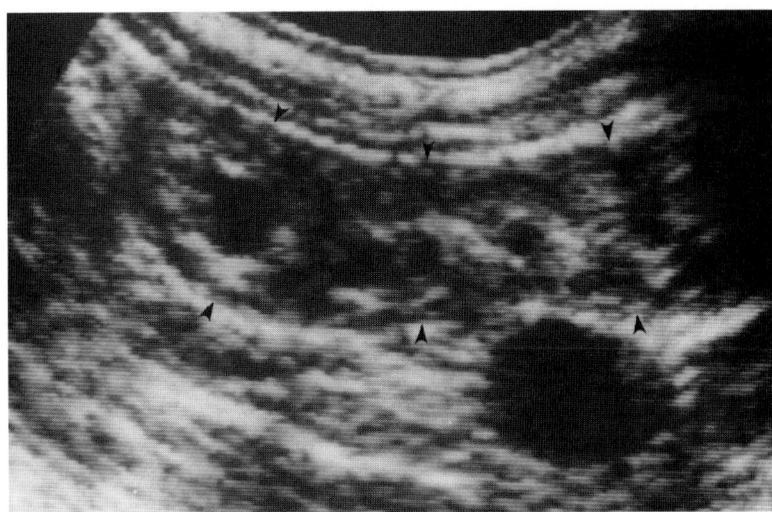

Figure 15-17. Sagittal sonogram of the uterine horn (*arrowheads*) of a 2-year-old border collie with history of depression and a reddish brown vaginal discharge. The uterus is mildly enlarged, ranging up to 1 cm in diameter. The endometrium is hyperechoic, indicating hypertrophy or inflammation. This uterine segment contains five endometrial cysts ranging from 2 to 4 mm in diameter. *Ureaplasma* and *Mycoplasma* were cultured from the vaginal discharge. The bitch had an ovariohysterectomy. The histologic diagnosis was severe cystic endometrial hyperplasia and endometritis.

dence of fetal viability. Lack of heartbeat is highly reliable evidence of fetal death. Technical difficulties could potentially obscure the heartbeat and result in a wrong diagnosis.

When fetal death occurs in bitches before 35 days after the LHP, fetal maceration and resorption are rapid. Within 2 days, the fetus is often not detectable, and the gestational sac is smaller than expected, has an irregular contour, or contains echogenic rather than anechoic fluid (Fig. 15-20). If resorption is complete or if there is abortion, a focal swelling of the uterus is detectable at the implantation site for some length of time. A distinct placental layer may be apparent.

When fetal death and maceration occur in the third trimester, the fetus is usually detectable for at least 1 week or until the pregnancy terminates by whelping or abortion. Maceration causes decrease in the size, echogenicity, and anatomic definition of the fetus (Fig. 15-21). The soft tissues lose definition more rapidly than the skeletal structures. When fetal death occurs during the final trimester, it is more likely to trigger abortion of the entire litter than fetal death and resorption that occur during the first half of pregnancy.

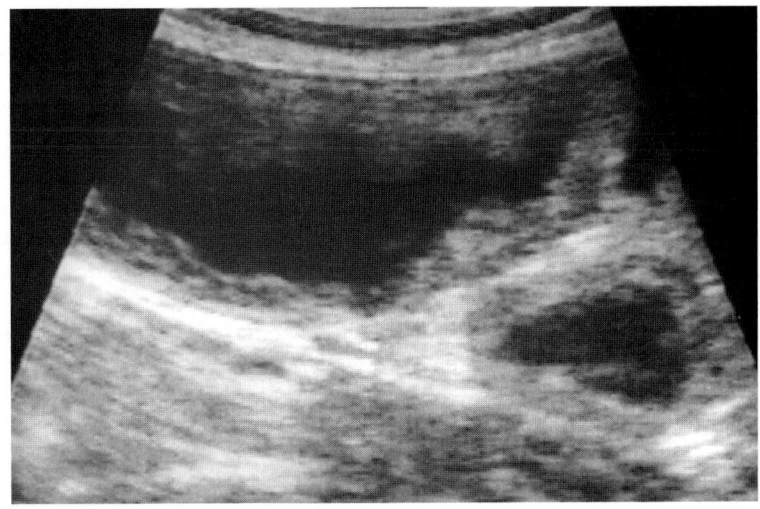

Figure 15-18. Sagittal sonogram of uterine horn of a 4-year-old weimaraner with history of mucopurulent vaginal discharge, fever, and dehydration that began 3 weeks after the bitch was in estrus. The uterus is moderately enlarged (2.7 cm in diameter), because it is distended with anechoic fluid and has a mildly thickened wall. In view of the history, these sonographic findings are highly indicative of pyometra. *Klebsiella* was cultured from the vaginal discharge.

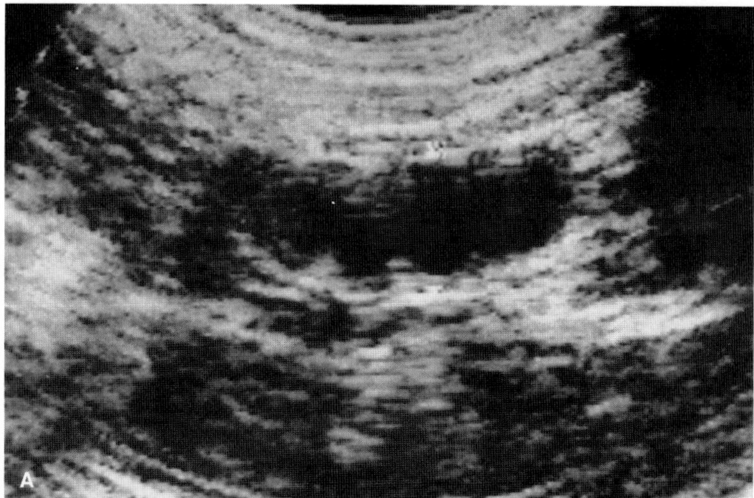

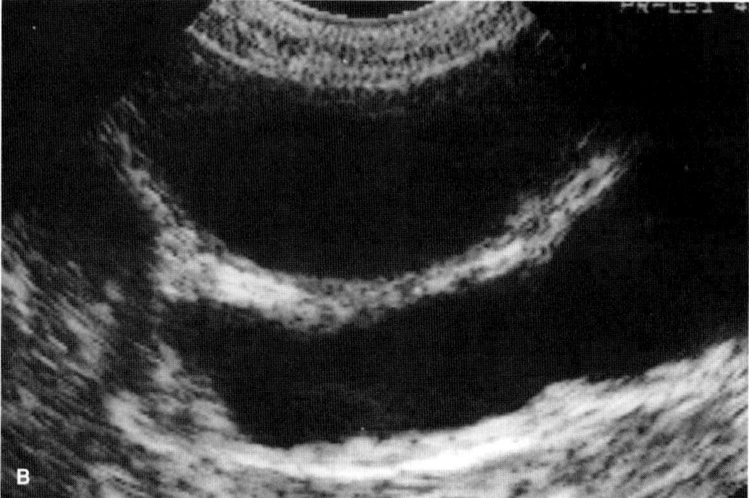

Figure 15-19. Sagittal sonogram of the uterine horn of a middle-aged, asymptomatic beagle with presumptive mucometra. The bitch had been bred, and sonography was initially performed to determine whether she was pregnant. (**A**) On day 25, after the luteinizing hormone peak, the uterine wall is thin (0.2 cm), and the lumen contains a small amount (0.7 cm) of anechoic fluid. (**B**) The uterus was maximally distended on day 44 after the luteinizing hormone peak. The lumen of the uterine horn contains 1.5 cm of fluid. One week later, the accumulation of uterine fluid spontaneously resolved. The bitch remained healthy, and the following year whelped a litter of four pups.

When mummification of the fetus occurs, the fetus decreases in size and anatomic definition and increases in echogenicity. The placenta and fetal membranes associated with the dead fetus persist, and the volume of fluid contained within the gestational sac may continue to enlarge as the pregnancy advances. This is more common in cats than in dogs (Fig. 15-22).

Sonography does not necessarily detect fetal distress unless there is serious cardiovascular distress. In this case, there may be persistent bradycardia of less than 120 to 150 beats per minute despite stimulation of the fetus by gently tapping it with the transducer. The normal heart rate for a beagle fetus is initially 214 ±13.3 beats per minute. Heart rate slowly increases until 40 days of gestation. From 40 to 60 days of gestation, the heart rate stabilizes at 238.2 ±16.1 beats per minute. Five days before parturition, the heart rate decreases to 218 ±6.7 beats per minute. The fetal heart rate of cats is stable throughout gestation at 228.2 ±35.5 beats per minute.[10]

Certain maternal or fetal systemic diseases or congenital defects may be recognized by the sonographic detection of hydrops fetalis, polyhydramnios, or oligohydramnios. Hydrops fetalis may be a familial condition of bulldogs, schnauzers, and chow chows.[14] Doppler examination of placental, umbilical, and fetal blood

(text continues on p. 287)

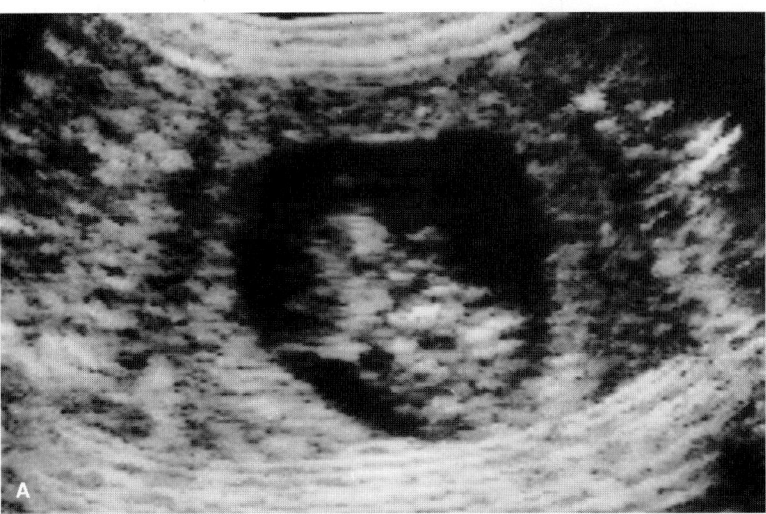

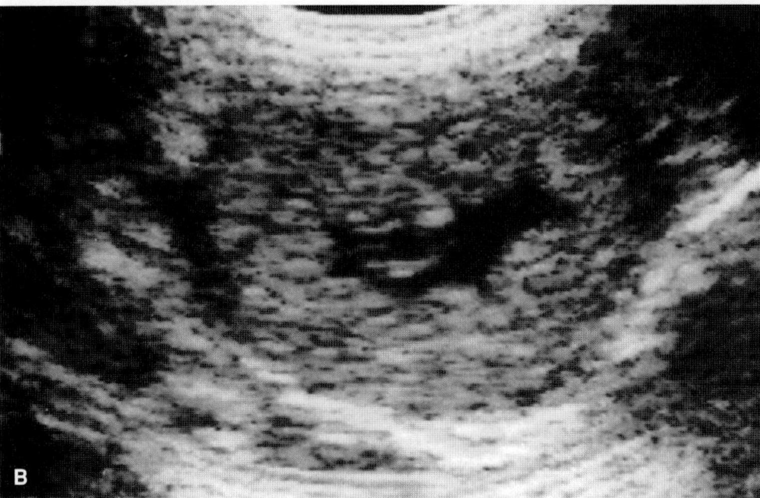

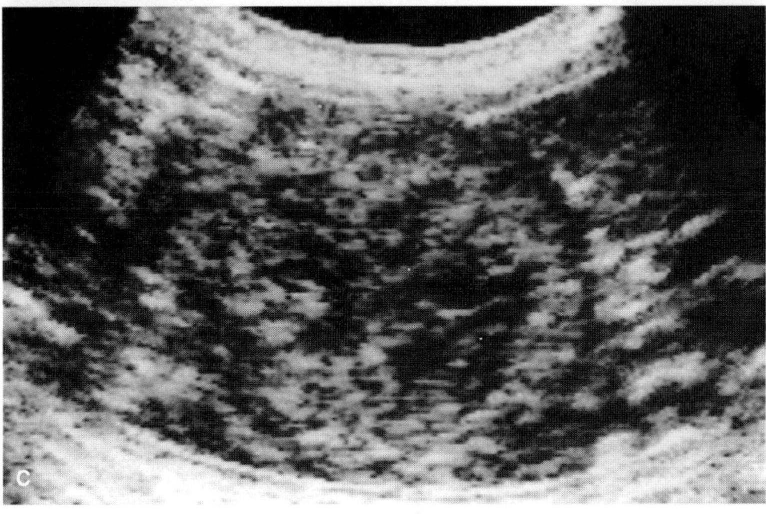

Figure 15-20. Transverse sonograms of one viable and two resorbing gestational sacs from a pregnant beagle at day 33 after the luteinizing hormone peak. Eventually, the bitch resorbed or aborted all of her embryos. Embryonic death was iatrogenic. The bitch was receiving an antiprogestin. Spontaneous resorptions of partial or entire litters between days 28 to 35 after the luteinizing hormone peak can have similar sonographic appearance. (**A**) This image shows a bipolar-shaped embryo contained in a gestational sac that is of appropriate size (2 cm in diameter) for the stage of pregnancy. In real-time ultrasound, the embryo had a heartbeat, confirming that it was viable. (**B**) This image shows a nonviable gestational sac that contains very little fluid and a circular yolk sac membrane. An embryo was not detected. (**C**) This image shows a nonviable gestational sac that contains echogenic fluid. An embryo was not detected.

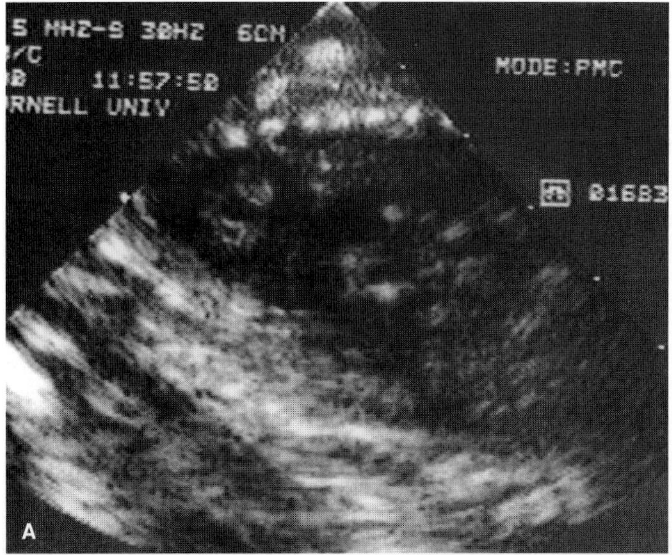

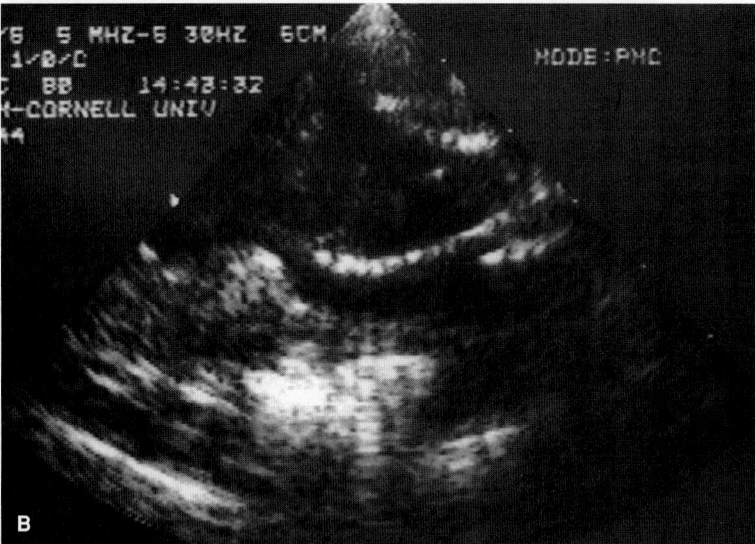

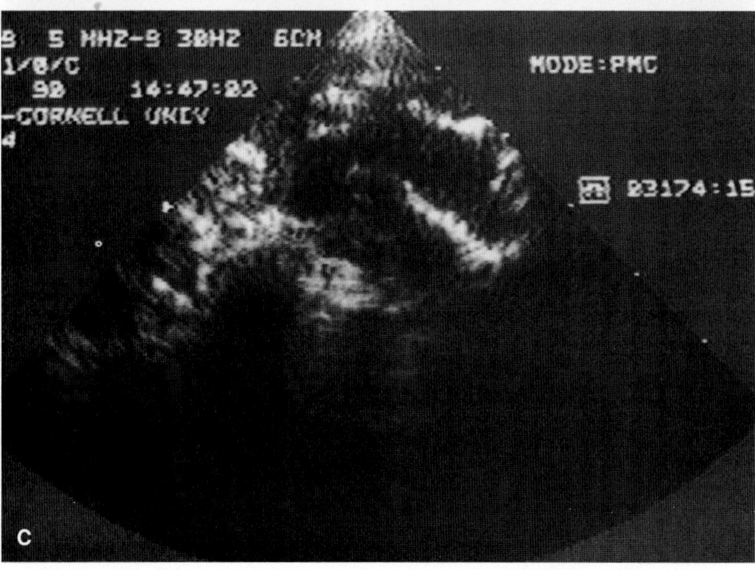

Figure 15-21. Sagittal sonograms of beagle fetuses that died and became macerated in the third trimester. The cause of death was iatrogenic. Serial collections of allantoic fluid were obtained from these fetuses in the second and third trimesters. (**A**) This is the 3.5-cm-diameter body of a day-54 fetus that has been dead for 1 day. The heart, lung, and liver are difficult to detect, because all of these structures are abnormally hypoechoic due to autolysis. The hyperechoic rib cage is obvious, and the fetus is an appropriate size for the stage of gestation. Cranial is to the left in the photograph. (**B**) This is the 2.6-cm-diameter body of a day-55 fetus that has been dead for 2 days. The soft tissues are extremely hypoechoic, and the viscera cannot be distinguished. The hyperechoic rib cage and skeletal structures of one front leg are obvious. The fetus is smaller than expected for the stage of gestation because of resorption of fluid from the soft tissues. Cranial is to the right in the photograph. (**C**) At day 57, the body of this 1.5-cm-diameter fetus that has been dead for 4 days is much smaller than expected. The viscera are not detectable, and although the rib cage is detectable, it is not obvious because its shape is distorted.

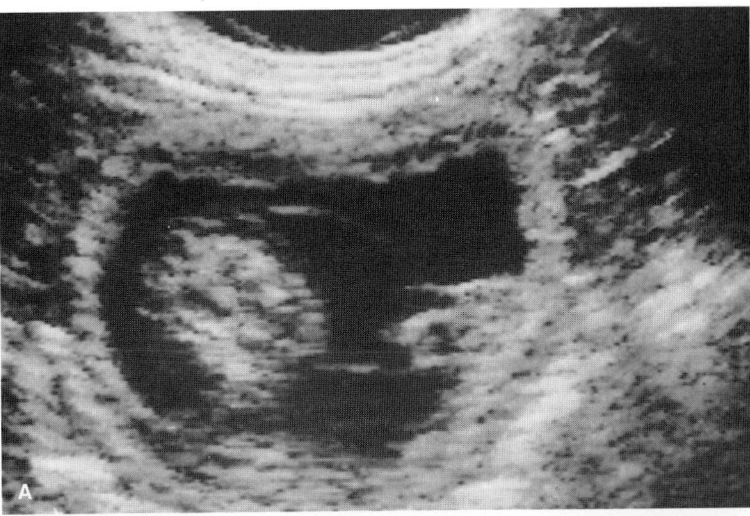

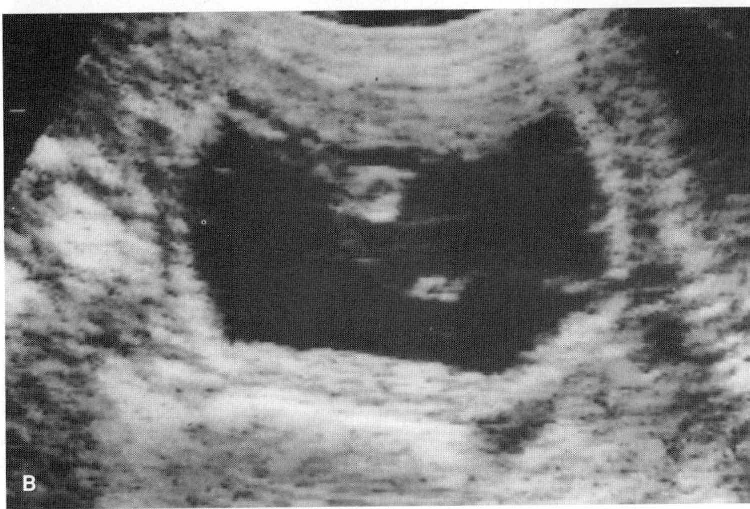

Figure 15-22. Transverse sonograms of a live fetus and a mummified fetus from the same pregnant queen at day 35 after coitus. (**A**) Body diameter of the live fetus is 1.3 cm, which is appropriate for the stage of gestation. Structures of the yolk sac and allantoic membranes are normal. (**B**) Although the mummified fetus is quite small (0.6 cm), it is contained in a gestational sac that is comparable in size to the one containing the viable fetus. A distorted fetal membrane is visible. The fetus had been dead for 2 weeks.

vessels can detect altered blood flow in some states of fetal distress. The acquisition and interpretation of this information can be time consuming and requires Doppler instrumentation and technical expertise by the sonographer.

In women, sonography is useful for the detection of many categories of fetal malformation. Presumably, it is also useful for detection of fetal malformations of small animals, but little information is available. Many fetal malformations probably are undetected in small animals because most of these species are multiparous. It is time consuming to meticulously examine each fetus in a litter, and in many instances, the consequences of detection or failure to detect fetal malformation may not warrant such an extensive evaluation.

LESS COMMON DISEASES

The less common diseases of the uterus may be categorized as mass lesions and miscellaneous conditions affecting reproduction. One of the reasons that mass lesions of the uterus are rare in pet dogs, cats, and ferrets is that most of these animals are neutered. Rabbits and rodents are usually not neutered, and mass lesions of the uterus are more common in these species. Sonography is an accurate method for detecting

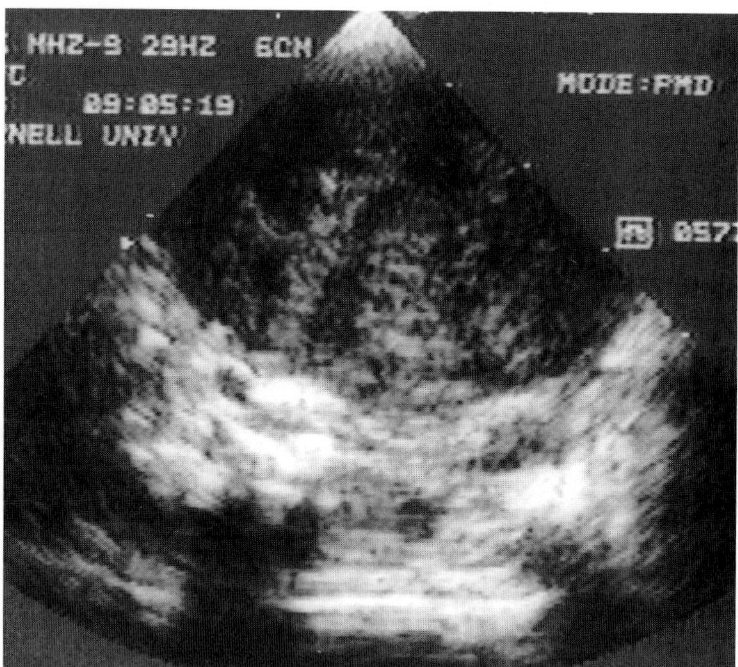

Figure 15-23. Transverse sonogram of a mass lesion located in the uterine body of an adult guinea pig that had hematuria and a palpable abdominal mass. The 3.5-cm mass is well demarcated and of mixed echogenicity. Sonographic findings suggest that the mass is probably composed of solid tissue, and it is more likely to be a neoplasm or a granuloma and less likely to be a hematoma or an abscess. The histologic diagnosis was uterine leiomyoma.

abdominal mass lesions, and the procedure is indicated whenever a uterine mass is suspected based on abdominal palpation, radiography, problem of vaginal discharge, complications after ovariohysterectomy, or problems associated with urination or defecation. The differential diagnosis for mass lesions of the uterus includes neoplasm, abscess, granuloma, scar tissue, hematoma, hyperplastic endometrial polyp, retained fetus, and segmental fluid distention.

Neoplasms of the Uterus

Leiomyoma is the most common neoplasm of the dog and cat uterus (Fig. 15-23), followed by leiomyosarcomas in dogs and endometrial adenocarcinomas in cats. Most common in rabbits, affecting virtually all older intact females, is endometrial adenocarcinoma (Fig. 15-24). Fibroma, fibrosarcoma, lipoma, lymphoma, and squamous cell carcinoma of the uterus have also been reported in dogs and cats.

The sonographic appearance of these neoplasms is not well described in small animals. There is probably no sonographic feature that

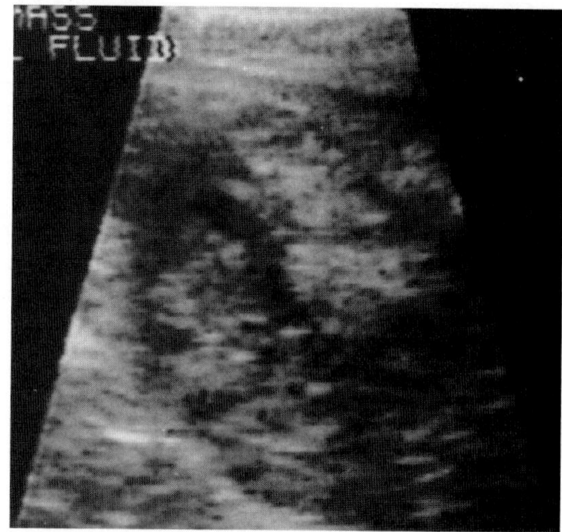

Figure 15-24. Transverse sonogram of a mass lesion located in the uterine horn of an adult mixed-breed rabbit that had a hemorrhagic genitourinary discharge. It is a well-demarcated, 2.7-cm diameter mass with a lobulated, hyperechoic center and a thin hypoechoic rim. The sonographic findings suggest that the mass is probably composed of solid tissue. The *sonographic* diagnosis for this mass lesion of the uterus is the same as the diagnosis for the uterine mass shown in Figure 15-23. Histologic diagnosis is necessary to differentiate between the two. The *histologic* diagnosis was uterine adenocarcinoma.

can accurately differentiate a neoplasm of the uterus from a granuloma, hematoma, scar tissue, or abscess. Neoplasms may have a well-demarcated or poorly demarcated margin, and they may be homogeneous or heterogenous in echogenicity. Typically, abscesses are fluid-filled lesions with well-demarcated, thick walls (Fig. 15-25). Scar tissue is poorly demarcated hyperechoic tissue (Fig. 15-26). Hematomas may be solid, or they may be multiloculated fluid-filled cavities that contain fibrin. However, the sonographic appearance of these masses is not highly reliable. Any uterine mass may have variable echogenicity and appear solid or cavitated (Fig. 15-27). Benign mass lesions cannot necessarily be differentiated from neoplasms solely on the basis of sonographic appearance.

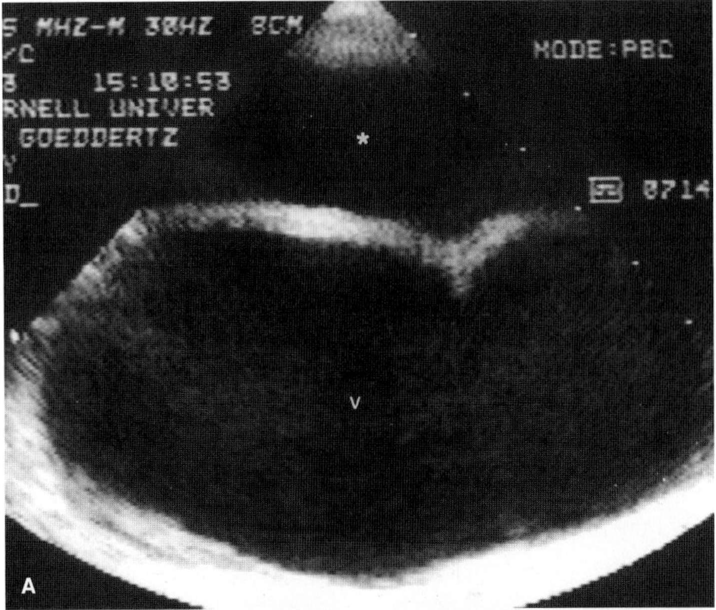

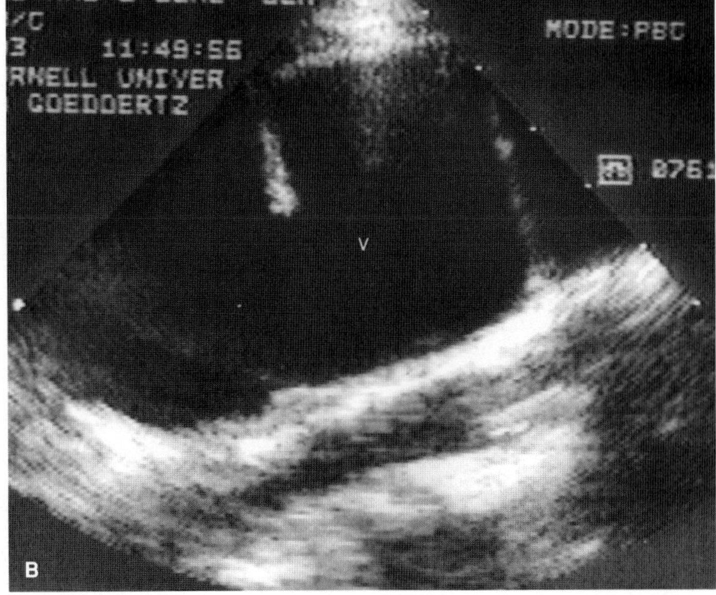

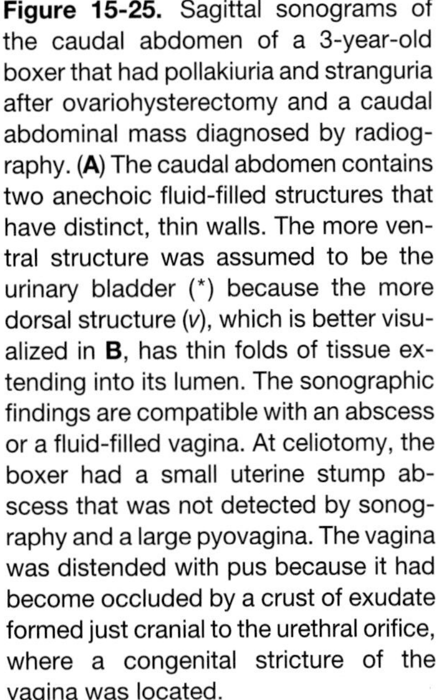
Figure 15-25. Sagittal sonograms of the caudal abdomen of a 3-year-old boxer that had pollakiuria and stranguria after ovariohysterectomy and a caudal abdominal mass diagnosed by radiography. (**A**) The caudal abdomen contains two anechoic fluid-filled structures that have distinct, thin walls. The more ventral structure was assumed to be the urinary bladder (*) because the more dorsal structure (*v*), which is better visualized in **B**, has thin folds of tissue extending into its lumen. The sonographic findings are compatible with an abscess or a fluid-filled vagina. At celiotomy, the boxer had a small uterine stump abscess that was not detected by sonography and a large pyovagina. The vagina was distended with pus because it had become occluded by a crust of exudate formed just cranial to the urethral orifice, where a congenital stricture of the vagina was located.

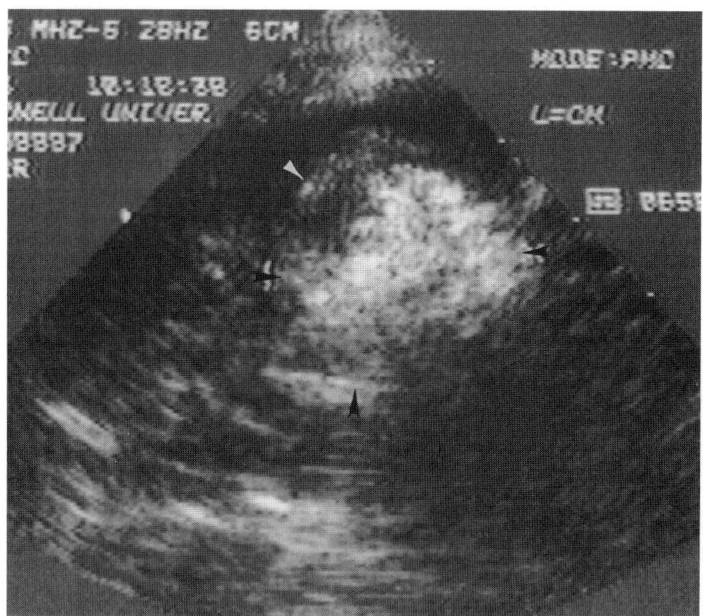

Figure 15-26. Transverse sonogram of the uterine stump of a Jack Russell terrier that had pollakiuria and a palpable small caudal abdominal mass after ovariohysterectomy. A normal-appearing uterine stump (*white arrowhead*) that is uniformly hypoechoic and 0.5 cm in diameter is visible dorsal to the anechoic urinary bladder. The caudal abdominal mass is a 2.5-cm, poorly marginated, hyperechoic area (*black arrowheads*) dorsal to and perhaps adhered to the uterine stump. The mass has the typical appearance of scar tissue or steatitis. A uterine stump abscess is not likely because a focal hypoechoic or anechoic area is not visible within the mass. The terrier recovered uneventfully without therapy.

Hyperplastic Endometrial Polyps

Hyperplastic endometrial polyps are benign and are usually detected as incidental findings in asymptomatic older bitches and queens, or they may protrude into the vagina. They may be associated with infertility. In bitches, the sonographic appearance of these polyps is quite characteristic. They contain numerous, small, anechoic cysts (Fig. 15-28). They may be present for several years without a change in their appearance.

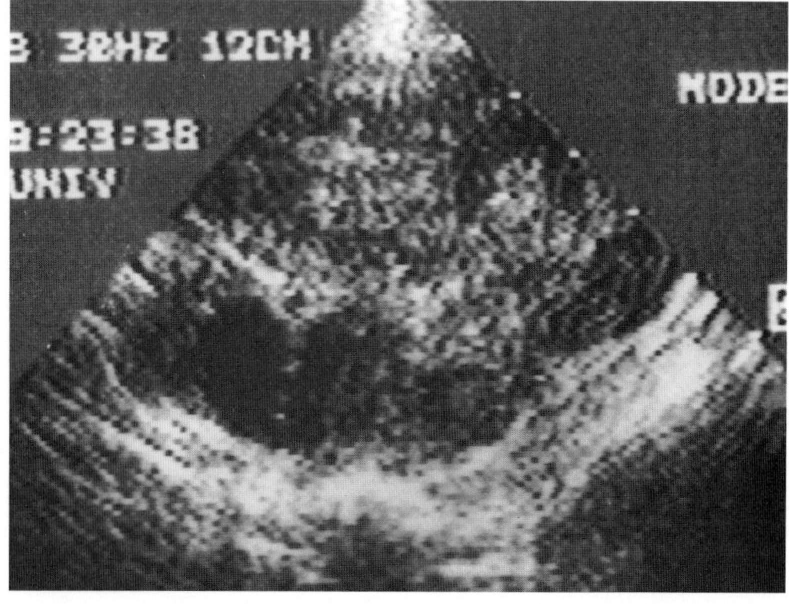

Figure 15-27. Sagittal sonogram of a solid-appearing, 8 × 5 cm uterine stump mass in a German shepherd that had anemia 1 day after ovariohysterectomy. The mass was confirmed to be a hematoma at celiotomy. Notice that the sonographic appearance of the mass is misleading. It appears to be mostly composed of solid tissue of mixed echogenicity and two small anechoic fluid cavities. Commonly, hematomas appear as complex fluid-filled cavities. In the acute stage, a hematoma may form a solid clot. Under these circumstances, the sonographic appearance is that of a solid mass.

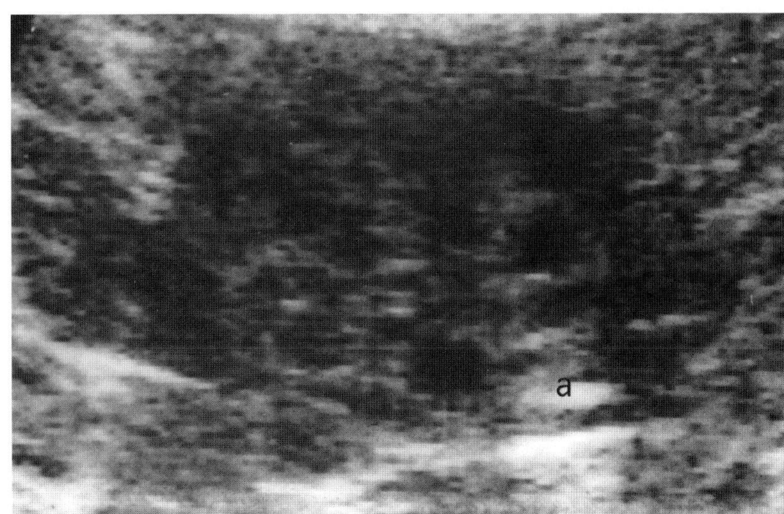

Figure 15-28. Sagittal sonogram of a 3.8 × 2.1 cm hyperplastic endometrial polyp located in the uterine horn of an 8-year-old beagle. The mass contains multiple, 3- to 5-mm diameter anechoic cysts. There is acoustic enhancement deep to the image of one of the cysts (*a*). The polyp was present in the bitch for at least 1 year. During this time, it caused no health problems, although, it is unknown whether the bitch had a problem of infertility because of the polyp. When the bitch was in estrus, the polyp increased slightly.

Miscellaneous Conditions Affecting Reproduction

Sonography may be indicated for evaluation of some of the less common uterine diseases that cause reproductive problems. Part or all of the uterine horns are undetectable in cases of infertility secondary to congenital aplasia, hermaphrodism, and hysterectomy. There are inadequate numbers of reports pertaining to sonography of retained placenta, subinvolution of placental sites, and ectopic pregnancy to determine the accuracy of their sonographic diagnosis or characterize their sonographic appearance.

REFERENCES

1. England GCW, Yeager AE. Ultrasonographic appearance of the ovary and uterus of the bitch during oestrus, ovulation and pregnancy. J Reprod Fertil 1993;47:107.
2. Taverne MAM, van Oord HA. Accuracy of pregnancy diagnosis in dogs by means of linear-array ultrasound scanning. In: Taverne MM, Willemse AH, eds. Diagnostic ultrasound and animal reproduction. Boston: Kluwer Academia, 1989; 105.
3. Spaulding K. Ultrasound evaluation of the gravid uterus in the bitch. In: Syllabus of the second annual meeting of the American Institute of Ultrasound in Medicine, 1990:67.
4. Yeager AE, Concannon PW. Association between the preovulatory luteinizing hormone surge and the early ultrasonographic detection of pregnancy and fetal heartbeats in beagle dogs. Theriogenology 1990;34:655.
5. Yeager AE, Mohammed HO, Meyers-Wallen V, et al. Ultrasonographic appearance of the uterus, placenta, fetus, and fetal membranes throughout accurately timed pregnancy in beagles. Am J Vet Res 1992;53:342.
6. Davidson AP, Nyland TG, Tsutsui T. Pregnancy diagnosis with ultrasound in the domestic cat. Vet Radiol 1986;27:109.
7. Beck KA, Baldwin CJ, Bosu WTK. Ultrasound prediction of parturition in queens. Vet Radiol 1990;31:32.
8. England GCW, Allen WE. Studies on canine pregnancy using B-mode ultrasound: diagnosis of early pregnancy and the number of conceptuses. J Small Anim Pract 1990;31:321.
9. Shille VM, Gonterek J. The use of ultrasonography for pregnancy diagnosis in the bitch. J Am Vet Med Assoc 1985;187: 1021.

10. Verstegen JP, Silva LDM, Onclin K, Donnay I. Echocardiographic study of heart rate in dog and cat fetuses in utero. J Reprod Fertil Suppl 1993;47:175.
11. Yeager AE, Concannon PW. Serial ultrasonographic appearance of postpartum uterine involution in beagle dogs. Theriogenology 1990;34:523.
12. England GCW. Ultrasound evaluation of pregnancy and spontaneous embryonic resorption in the bitch. J Small Anim Pract 1992;33:430.
13. Muller K, Arbeiter K. Ultrasound and clinical signs of fetal resorption in the bitch. J Reprod Fertil Suppl 1993; 47:558.
14. Allen WE, England GCW, White KB. Hydrops fetalis diagnosed by real-time ultrasonography in a bichon frise bitch. J Small Anim Pract 1989;30:465.

Small Animal Ultrasound, edited by Ronald W. Green.
Lippincott-Raven Publishers, Philadelphia © 1996.

OVARIES

Amy E. Yeager and Patrick W. Concannon

The ovaries of dogs and other small animals can be difficult to detect because of their small size. They are difficult to resolve from the surrounding tissues, and they are easily obscured by intestinal gas. This is especially true during the anestrus phase of the reproductive cycle, when ovaries are smallest and most uniform in shape and echogenicity. Because of these difficulties, it is important to use excellent scanning technique for sonographic examination of the ovaries, similar to the technique used to scan the uterus (see Chap. 15). The same transducers used to scan the uterus (5 to 10 MHz) are appropriate for scanning the ovaries.

SCANNING TECHNIQUES

In most small animal species, the ovaries are located directly caudal to the kidneys. Primates are an exception; their ovaries are located adjacent to the pelvis and dorsolateral to the urinary bladder. To visualize the right ovary of dogs and cats, the examiner first positions the animal in dorsal recumbency; oblique or lateral positions may also be used, in which case the right side of the animal is positioned up. The sonographer uses a sagittal scan plane and locates the right kidney. Placing the kidney on the cranial edge of the sonographic image, the examiner searches for the ovary in the area just caudal to the kidney. This is done by pointing or sliding the transducer medial and lateral to the scan plane that contains the kidney (Fig. 16-1). It may be necessary to apply some degree of abdominal compression with the transducer to visualize the ovary. The left ovary is located by the same method, using the left kidney as a landmark.

SONOGRAPHIC ANATOMY OF THE OVARY

The size, shape, and echogenicity of the ovary vary throughout the estrous cycle because of the development and regression of follicles and corpora lutea (CL). During anestrus, the ovaries have an ellipsoid shape, smooth contour, and uniform echogenicity that is hypoechoic compared with the surrounding fat (Fig. 16-2). During proestrus, both ovaries contain multiple, discrete, anechoic preovulatory follicles. These increase in diameter as the time of ovulation approaches. During estrus and diestrus, CL develop, and anovulatory follicles regress. Mature CL appear as oval hypoechoic structures in the ovary.

Canine Ovary

Detailed studies of changes in the ovary during ovarian cycle have been conducted in dogs but not other small animals.[1–3] The timing of

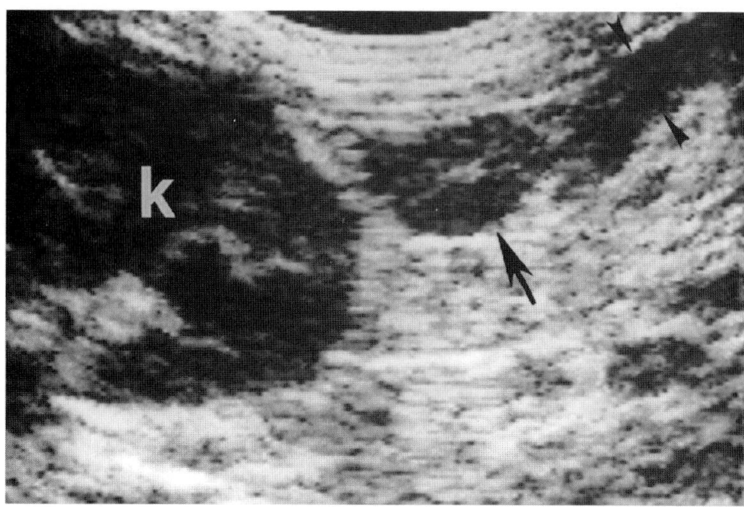

Figure 16-1. Sagittal sonogram of the ovary from a mixed-breed, pregnant cat shows the proximity of the ovary (*arrow*), kidney (*K*), and uterine horn (*arrowheads*). The sonogram was obtained 11 days after mating. Four to six, 3-mm, hypoechoic corpora lutea are faintly visible within the ovary.

changes is preferably related to the time of the preovulatory luteinizing hormone peak (LHP). Ovulation in dogs occurs spontaneously about 40 to 48 hours after the LHP.[4]

Proestrus

At the beginning of proestrus, the ovary is small. Typically, it is 10 to 20 mm long and 5 to 10 mm wide. Multiple, small (1 to 2 mm in diameter), anechoic follicles located in each ovary first appear on proestrus day 1 to 4 (Fig. 16-3*A*). These are oval or circular, and they may or may not have detectable smooth, thin (1 mm) walls (Figs. 16-3*B* and 16-4*A*). Preovulatory follicles gradually increase in size. Usually, three to five follicles develop per ovary, although we have found none in one ovary and as many as 10 in the contralateral ovary. Preovulatory follicles within the same ovary typically have the same diameter. Between bitches, follicle diameter varies and is usually 4 to 8 mm in diameter (range, 3 to 11 mm) on the day after the LHP (Figs. 16-3*C* and 16-4*B*), which is considered to be 1 day before ovulation. At this time, the ovary is somewhat enlarged compared with the onset of proestrus. It is approximately 15 to 25 mm long and 8 to 13 mm wide. During the first part of proestrus, the ovary has a smooth, oval contour. Beginning with the LHP, the ovary may

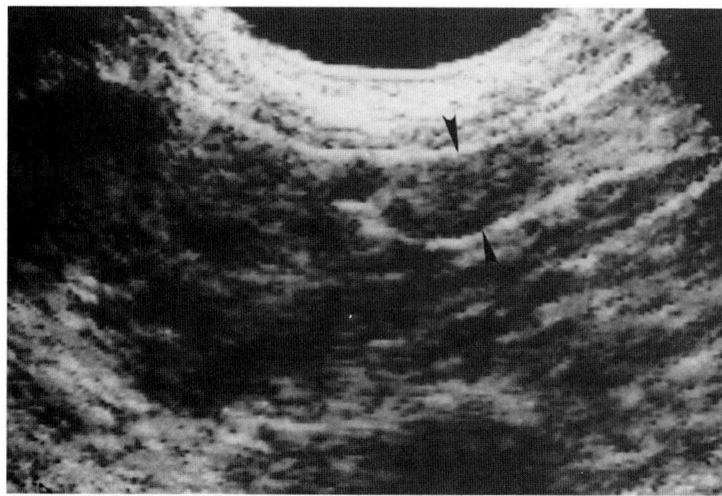

Figure 16-2. Sagittal sonogram of an anestrus beagle ovary (*arrowheads*). The ovary is small (1.2 × 0.6 cm), uniformly hypoechoic, and has a smooth, oval contour.

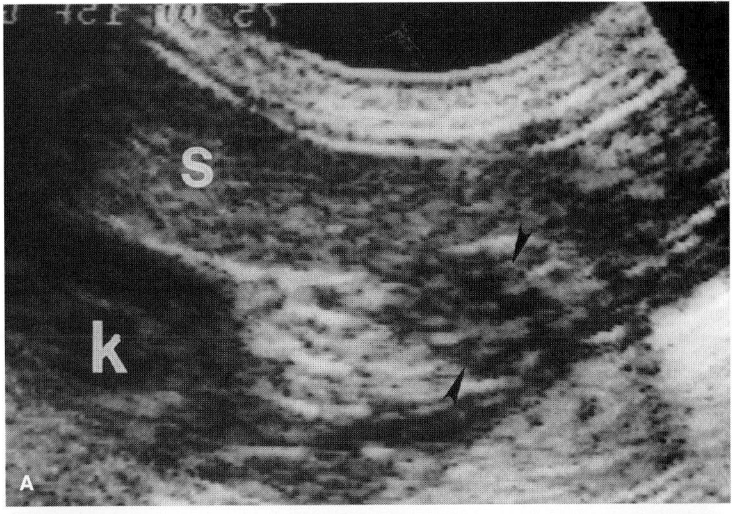

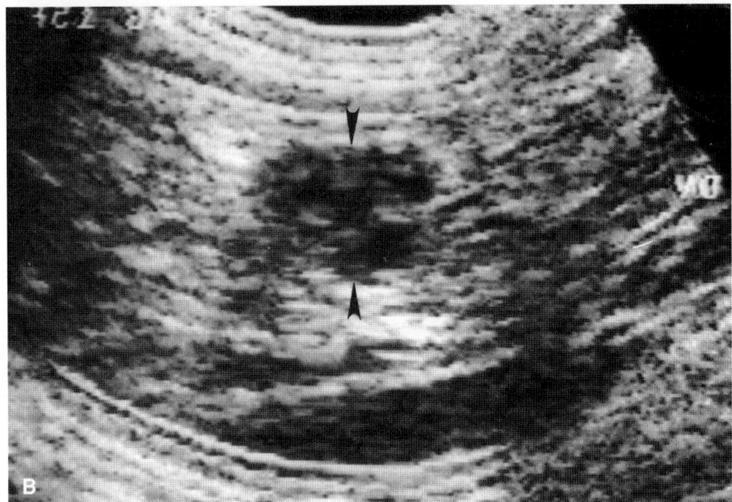

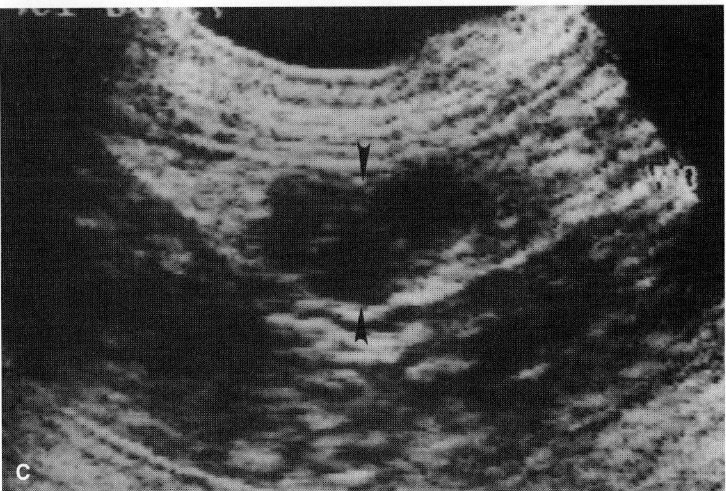

Figure 16-3. Serial sagittal sonograms of a beagle ovary (*arrowheads*) during proestrus and estrus. (**A**) Six days before the luteinizing hormone peak (LHP), the ovary is small and has a smooth, oval contour. Three small anechoic (2-mm-diameter) follicles are visible. The spleen (*S*) and kidney (*K*) are also apparent. (**B**) Two days before the LHP, the ovary is slightly enlarged and four midsized anechoic follicles (3 to 4-mm in diameter) are visible. (**C**) One day after the LHP, the ovary shows continued, gradual enlargement. It appears to consist of three large anechoic follicles (5 to 6 mm in diameter), which cause slight bulges in the ovarian contour and are surrounded by 1-mm-thick walls.

(continued)

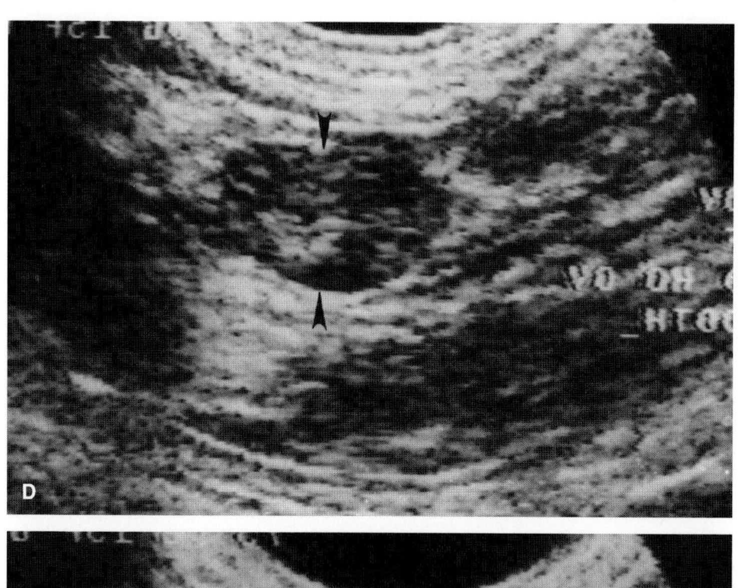

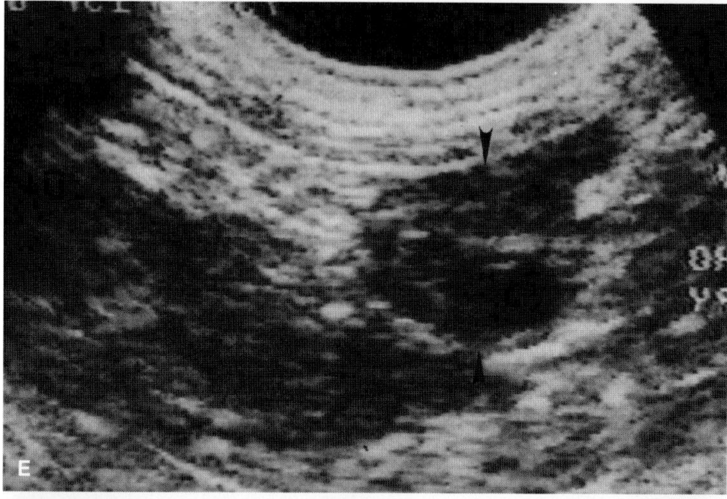

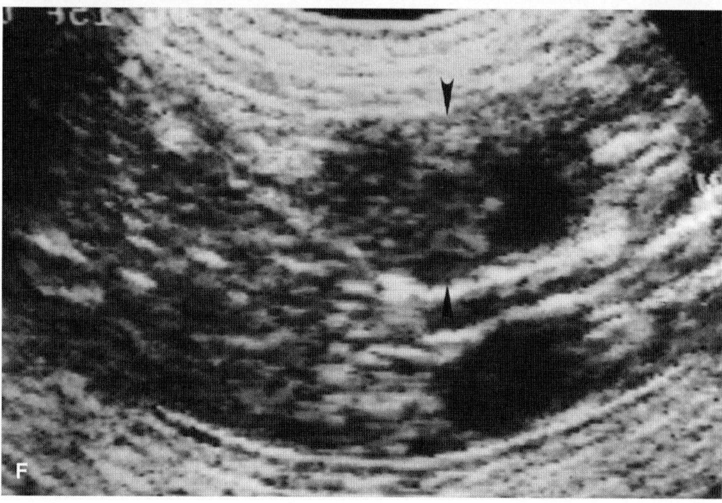

Figure 16-3. *(Continued)* (**D**) Two days after the LHP, on the presumed day of ovulation, the ovary is a smooth, oval shape, and it is not substantially changed in size compared with the day before. The previously detected anechoic follicles appear to be replaced by three oval corpora lutea (CL). The CL are 6 to 8 mm in diameter, and they appear solid (slightly hypoechoic compared with the ovarian stroma). (**E**) Four days after the LHP, a 5-mm-diameter anechoic fluid-filled cavity has formed within one of the three visible CL. (**F**) Seven days after the LHP, the ovary is, for the most part, unchanged in appearance. Both the ovary and the CL with the fluid-filled cavity (6 mm in diameter) are slightly larger than before, and the fluid-filled cavity has a slightly irregular wall. The two solid CL that are visible are unchanged in appearance.

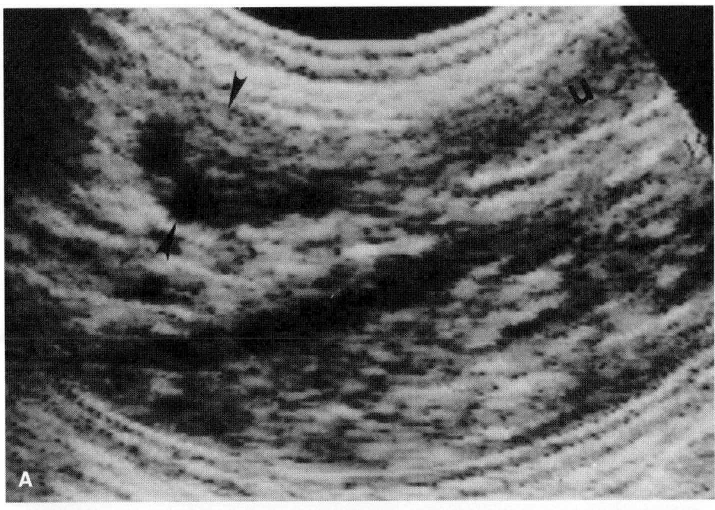

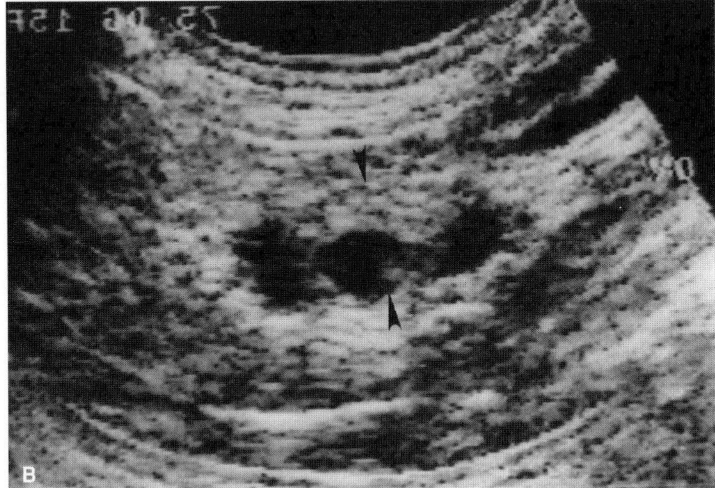

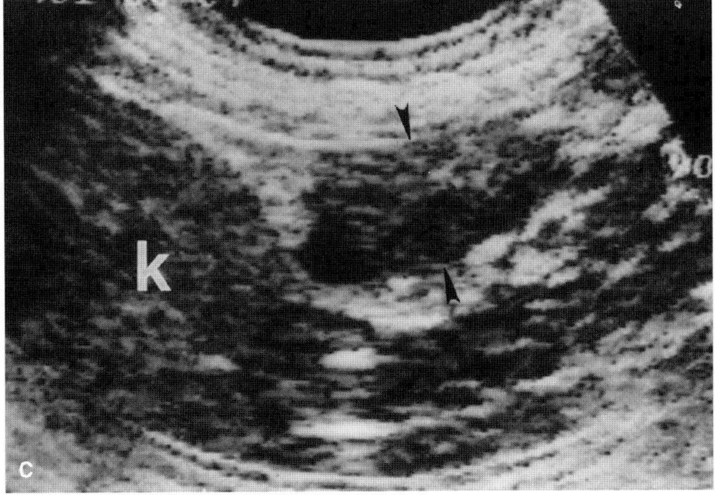

Figure 16-4. Sagittal sonograms of a beagle ovary (*arrowheads*) during proestrus, estrus, and diestrus. (**A**) Two days before the luteinizing hormone peak (LHP), the ovary is small and has a smooth, oval shape. Three, midsized (3-mm-diameter) anechoic follicles are visible. The uterine horn (*u*) is also apparent. (**B**) One day after the LHP, the ovary has smooth contour and it is slightly enlarged. Three midsized (4-mm-diameter) anechoic follicles are visible. (**C**) Two days after the LHP, on the presumed day of evulation, the ovary is unchanged in size and contour. One anechoic and two nearly anechoic, 4-mm-diameter follicles or corpora lutea (CL) are visible. The ovary is in proximity to the kidney (*K*). *(continued)*

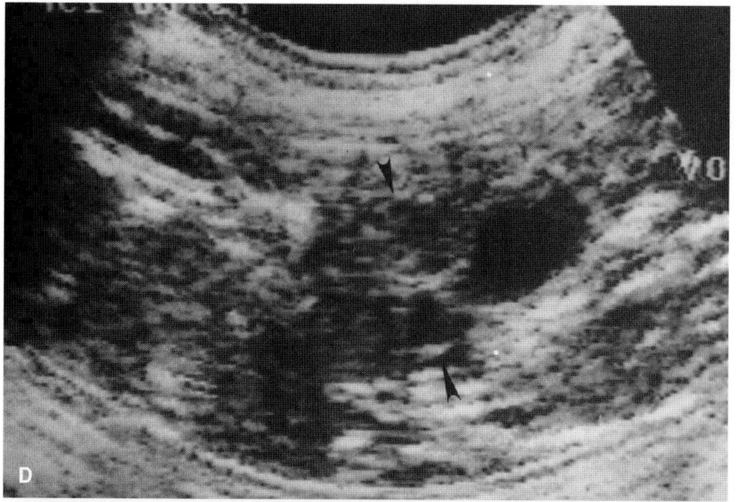

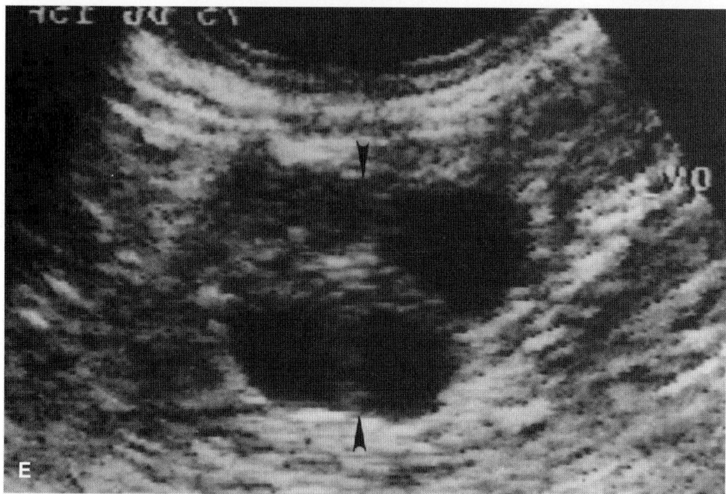

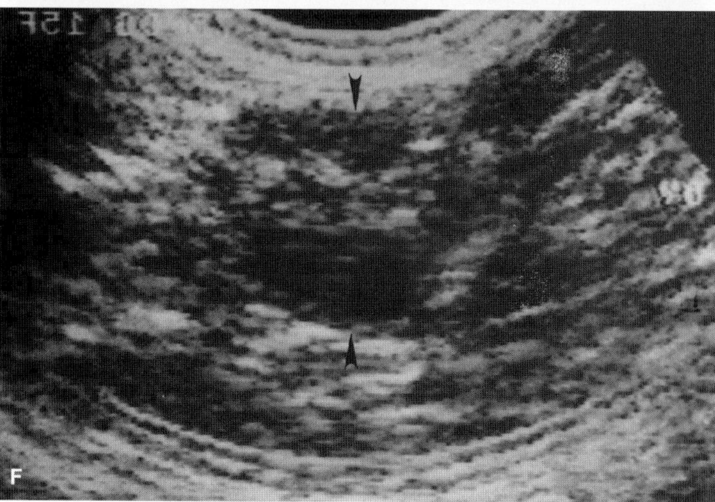

Figure 16-4. *(Continued)* (**D**) Four days after the LHP, the ovary is slightly enlarged compared with the day of ovulation, and it has developed a mildly bumpy contour. Five CL are visible. Two of these have fluid-filled cavities of dissimilar diameter (2 and 7 mm), and three appear solid (slightly hypoechoic compared to the ovarian stroma) and 5 to 8 mm in diameter. (**E**) Seven days after the LHP, the ovary is obviously enlarged, with a bumpy contour. It contains two or three solid CL (5 mm in diameter) and three CL with large, anechoic fluid cavities (6 to 9 mm in diameter). The fluid-filled cavities have thin (1 mm), smooth walls. (**F**) Fifteen days after the LHP, the ovary has decreased in size compared to late estrus primarily because the diameter of the two visible CL fluid-filled cavities (3 to 4 mm) has obviously decreased. These have thicker walls (2 mm) than before. Three solid CL (4 to 6 mm in diameter) are also visible.

develop a slightly bumpy contour because of enlarging follicles.

Ovulation

Sonography is probably not an accurate method for prediction or detection of the day of ovulation in the dog, because ovulation does not appear to cause obvious collapse of the follicles. Neither the ovary nor follicles detected on the day of ovulation are decreased in size compared with their appearance the day before ovulation. Around the time of ovulation, immature CL commonly have thin walls and fluid antra. Such CL appear anechoic and may be indistinguishable from preovulatory follicles, nonovulatory follicles that can persist in the ovary throughout estrus and early diestrus, and ovarian cysts that can be present at all stages of the ovarian cycle.

If daily examination of canine ovaries is performed beginning in proestrus, a decrease (Fig. 16-4*C*) or disappearance (Fig. 16-3*D*) in the number of preovulatory follicles is usually detected on the presumed day of ovulation, 2 days after the LHP. Typically, two, one, or no anechoic structures are visible in each ovary on the day of ovulation. After ovulation, the number of anechoic structures in the ovary increases and may equal the preovulatory number, often in 1 to 2 days. Occasionally, a small amount of anechoic fluid may be detected adjacent to an ovary on the day of ovulation. It is unknown whether this is follicular fluid or hemorrhage, presumably within the bursa.

The detection of solid hypoechoic-appearing CL in the canine ovary is a strong indication that ovulation has occurred (Figs. 16-3*D* and 16-4*C*). Unfortunately, most studies suggest that solid CL may be difficult to detect or infrequent compared with CL with fluid antra. Failure to visualize solid CL using 7.5-MHz transducers may not be a reliable indication that ovulation has not occurred. One study using higher-quality equipment (ie, annular phased-array equipment and a 9.5-MHz transducer) suggested that the ovary is devoid of anechoic follicles when ovulation is complete and that all CL are readily apparent as hypoechoic structures.[5]

Estrus

After ovulation, three to five CL are typically detected per ovary. One (Fig. 16-3*E, F*), several (Fig. 16-4*D, F*), or all of the CL are likely to contain anechoic fluid antra that are 3 to 12 mm in diameter. Within the same ovary, the CL with fluid antra tend to have dissimilar diameters. During estrus, the CL with antra gradually increase in diameter until the eighth day after the LHP. At this time, the ovary generally has a volume four times larger than during early proestrus, and it has a slightly to moderately bumpy contour, resembling a blackberry. Ovaries with three or more CL with fluid antra (Fig. 16-4*E*) are larger and have bumpier contours than ovaries that contain mostly solid CL (Fig. 16-3*F*).

Diestrus

CL with anechoic antra evolve into mature, solid CL during the first part of diestrus. During the first week of diestrus, ovarian size decreases, because there is a decrease in the antral and total diameter of the CL (Fig. 16-4*F*). There is a concurrent increase in CL wall thickness. By 12 to 15 days after the LHP, most CL no longer contain antra. They appear uniformly hypoechoic (solid) and are 5 to 8 mm in diameter (Fig. 16-5).

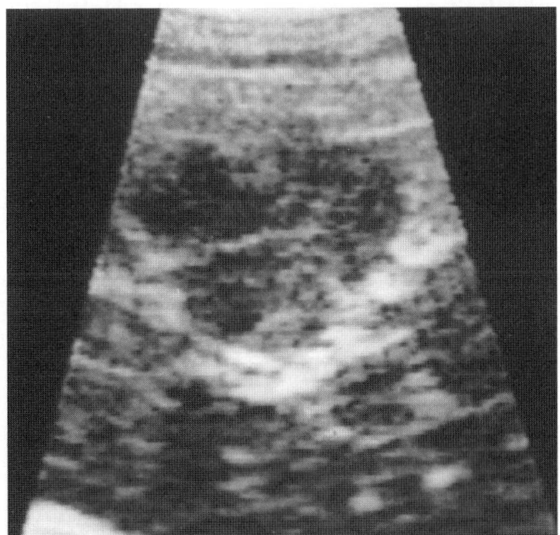

Figure 16-5. Sagittal sonogram of a diestrus beagle ovary 15 days after the luteinizing hormone peak. The ovary is uniformly hypoechoic and has a lobulated structure. It appears to contain three or four 7- to 10-mm-diameter, solid corpora lutea.

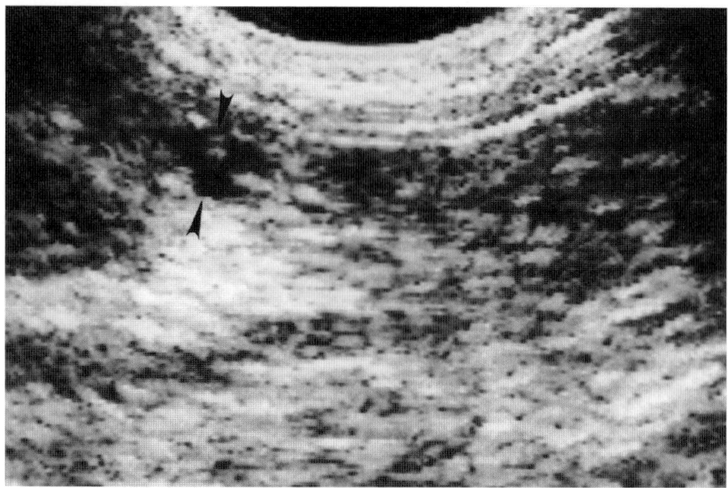

Figure 16-6. Sagittal sonogram of a cat ovary (*arrowheads*) obtained 2 days before mating. Three small (2- to 3-mm), anechoic preovulatory follicles are visible.

Hypoechoic CL are detectable for at least 30 days after the LHP. There is no obvious difference in the appearance of ovaries from pregnant bitches and nonpregnant bitches.

Feline Ovary

Detailed studies of the changes in the ovary during the ovarian cycle have not been reported for domestic cats. We have observed that several oval, 2- to 4-mm-diameter, anechoic preovulatory follicles develop in each ovary before mating (Fig. 16-6). After mating, the follicles do not appear to collapse. During the first part of diestrus, CL may appear anechoic or hypoechoic, and they are 3 to 4 mm in diameter (Fig. 16-7).

OVARIAN DISEASES AND DISORDERS

There are few ovarian diseases of pet dogs, cats, and ferrets, because most of these animals are ovariectomized. Most intact females of these species are maintained for breeding purposes. In these circumstances, diseases of the ovary are not a common cause of infertility.

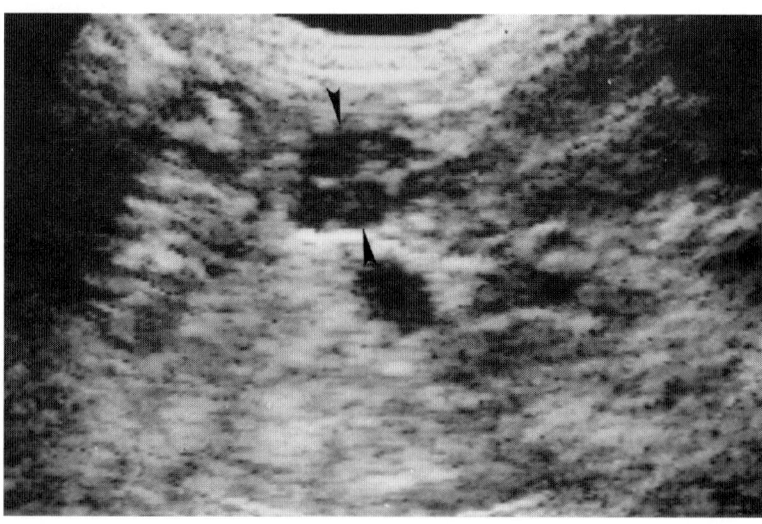

Figure 16-7. Sagittal sonogram of the diestrus ovary (*arrowheads*) of a pregnant domestic cat (30 days after first mating). Five corpora lutea are visible. They are hypoechoic compared with the ovarian stroma and 3 to 4-mm in diameter.

Ovarian and Paraovarian Cysts

Cysts are the most common abnormalities of the dog ovary. Cystic ovarian rete are common in guinea pigs. It is difficult or impossible to differentiate functional cysts (ie, those that produce estrogen or progesterone) from nonfunctional cysts based on their sonographic appearance. In dogs, cysts are frequently nonfunctional and incidental findings. In such cases, the cystic ovary may be large enough to be radiographically apparent, but it is rarely large enough to detect by palpation. Functional follicular cysts or luteinized cysts may cause persistent estrus, decreased interestrus interval, or prolonged anestrus, and the condition may result in infertility.

Benign ovarian cysts (Figs. 16-8 and 16-9) have sonographic features typical of benign cysts in general. A cyst is a discrete oval structure with a thin, smooth wall that may show a specular reflection artifact. It has an anechoic lumen that contains no internal echoes. An acoustic enhancement artifact is detected in association with a cyst.

Ovarian Neoplasms

Clinical signs frequently displayed by bitches with ovarian neoplasms are abdominal distention, palpable abdominal mass, abnormal estrus behavior, or infertility. In the bitch, the most

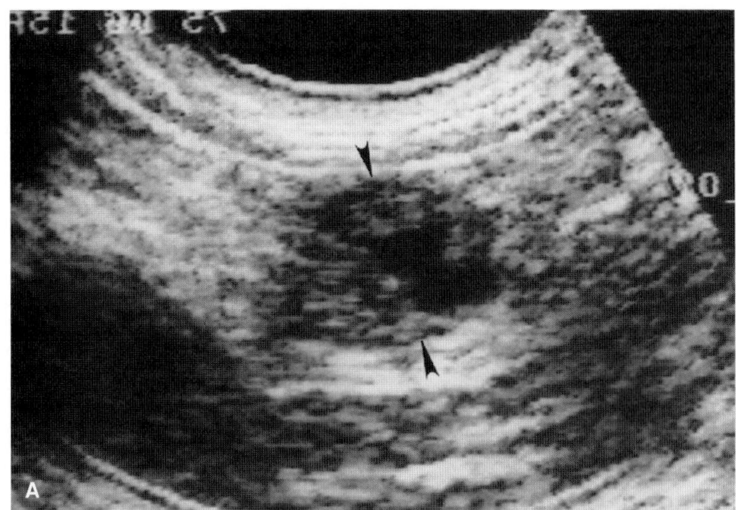

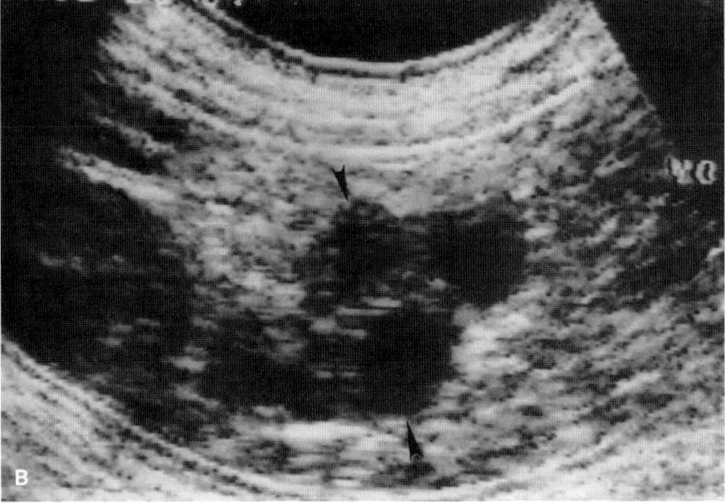

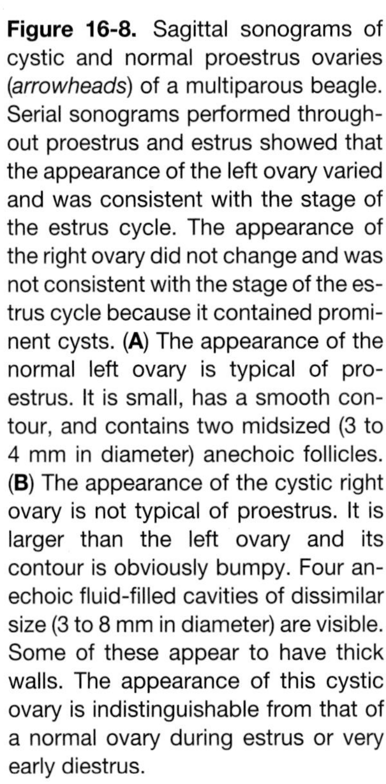
Figure 16-8. Sagittal sonograms of cystic and normal proestrus ovaries (*arrowheads*) of a multiparous beagle. Serial sonograms performed throughout proestrus and estrus showed that the appearance of the left ovary varied and was consistent with the stage of the estrus cycle. The appearance of the right ovary did not change and was not consistent with the stage of the estrus cycle because it contained prominent cysts. (**A**) The appearance of the normal left ovary is typical of proestrus. It is small, has a smooth contour, and contains two midsized (3 to 4 mm in diameter) anechoic follicles. (**B**) The appearance of the cystic right ovary is not typical of proestrus. It is larger than the left ovary and its contour is obviously bumpy. Four anechoic fluid-filled cavities of dissimilar size (3 to 8 mm in diameter) are visible. Some of these appear to have thick walls. The appearance of this cystic ovary is indistinguishable from that of a normal ovary during estrus or very early diestrus.

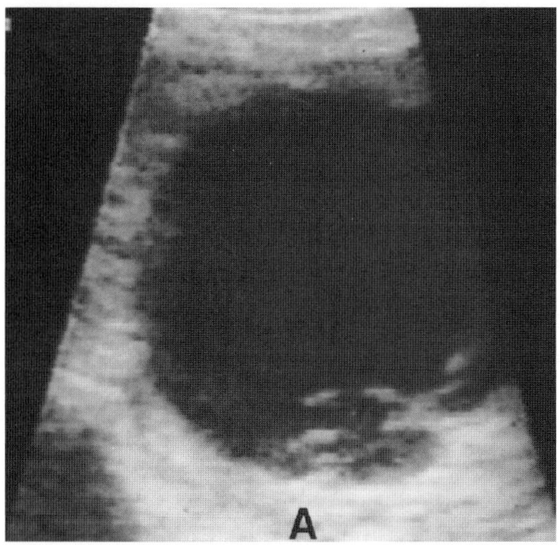

Figure 16-9. Sagittal sonogram of a cystic ovary from a 5-year-old female guinea pig that had a bloody vaginal discharge. The large (2.2 × 2.4 cm) ovarian mass has the appearance of a benign cystic lesion because it has a thin wall, an anechoic cavity with few internal septations, and acoustic enhancement (*A*). Ovariohysterectomy and histologic examination showed that the ovarian mass was cystic ovarian rete, a benign and incidental finding. Both ovaries were affected. Sonography, ovariohysterectomy, and histology also revealed that the cause of the bloody discharge was multifocal endometrial gland adenomas.

common ovarian neoplasms are papillary adenomas or adenocarcinomas and granulosa cell tumor. Teratomas and dysgerminomas occur less frequently, and other tumors are rare.

The sonographic appearance of ovarian tumors of the small animal species has not been reported. Conjecture about their sonographic appearance can be made based on the gross appearance of these tumors. Teratoma and granulosa cell tumor often contain cystic cavities that, in contrast to benign cystic lesions, have thick, irregular walls and contain echoes caused by necrotic debris, tumor tissue, or hemorrhage in the lumen. Hyperechoic foci of fat, bone, or tooth are detectable within a teratoma. The bone and tooth elements of the teratoma cast acoustic shadows. These findings may be indistinguishable from dystrophic mineralization, which can occur in the other types of ovarian tumors. Papillary adenomas and adenocarcinomas are frequently bilateral.

Sonographic evaluation of an animal with potentially neoplastic ovarian mass should include assessment for metastatic tumors. Tumor metastasis is suspected when there is detection of peritoneal fluid or soft tissue nodules involving viscera or peritoneum. Ultrasound-guided biopsy of an ovarian mass may be performed as an additional diagnostic procedure.

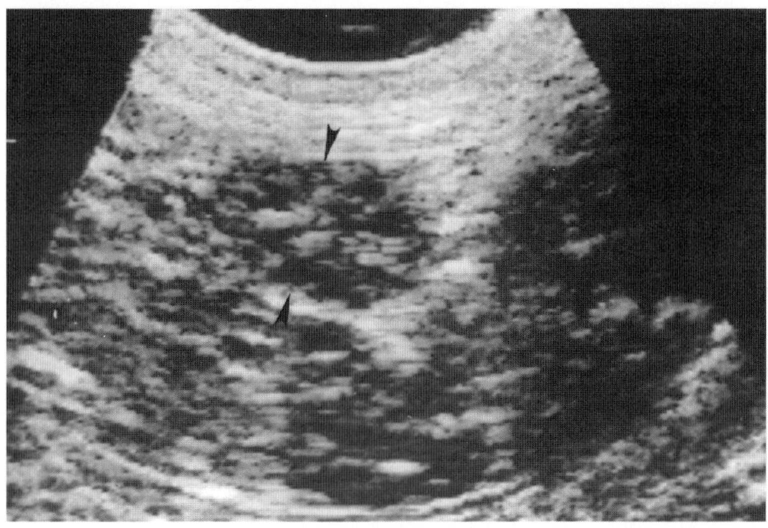

Figure 16-10. Sagittal sonogram of a beagle ovary (*arrowheads*) shows the follicle development that was induced with follicle-stimulating hormone treatment. This treatment failed to induce a fertile ovulation. The appearance of the ovary resembles early proestrus. The ovary is enlarged (1.8 × 1.1 cm) compared with pretreatment images. It has a smooth contour and contains numerous, small (1 to 2 mm) follicles.

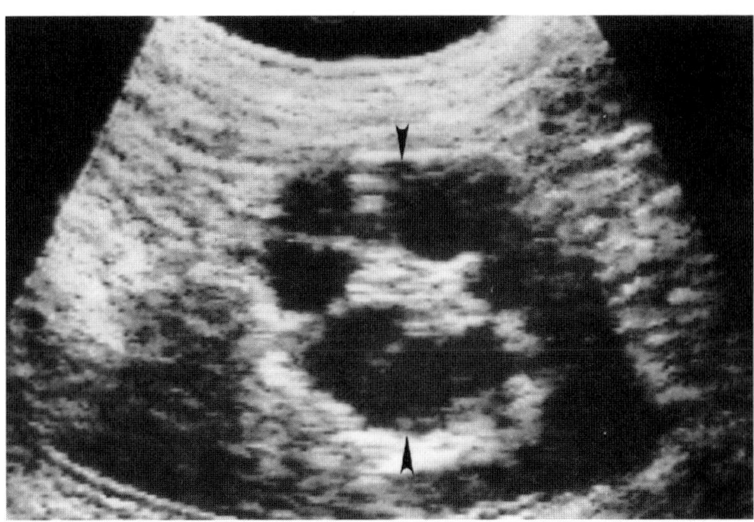

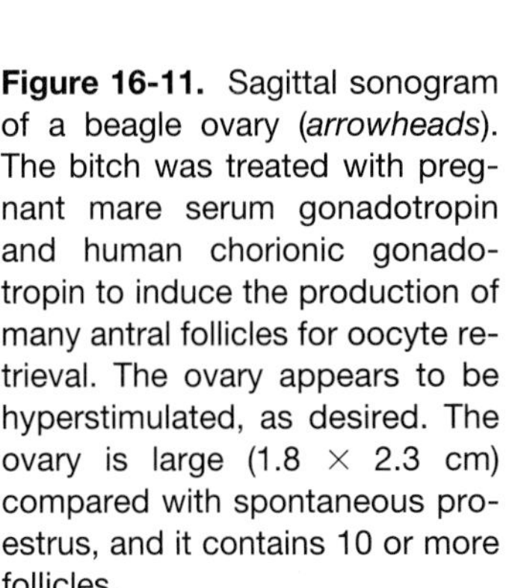
Figure 16-11. Sagittal sonogram of a beagle ovary (*arrowheads*). The bitch was treated with pregnant mare serum gonadotropin and human chorionic gonadotropin to induce the production of many antral follicles for oocyte retrieval. The ovary appears to be hyperstimulated, as desired. The ovary is large (1.8 × 2.3 cm) compared with spontaneous proestrus, and it contains 10 or more follicles.

Complications of Ovariectomy

After ovariectomy, an animal may develop fever, abdominal pain, anemia, uremia, or a distended abdomen. Sonography is a useful diagnostic tool for the detection of a mass lesion at the ovarian pedicle, which may be hematoma, abscess, or a surgical sponge. Hydronephrosis, which can occur secondary to ligation of the ureter, is readily detected by sonography. The sonographic detection of peritoneal fluid can accurately indicate hemoperitoneum, uroperitoneum, or peritonitis.

Conditions Associated With Infertility

Sonographic evaluation of the ovaries is useful in humans for detection of abnormal follicular growth and disturbed ovulation. Sonography may also prove useful for the detection of similar conditions in small animals.

In humans, sonography is used to monitor or guide some treatments of infertility. For example, the ovaries may be evaluated for hyperstimulation or hypostimulation during artificially induced estrous cycles. Sonography may be similarly useful in small animals, especially the dog, because there is no consistently reliable method of estrus induction for this species (Figs. 16-10 and 16-11). Ultrasound-guided needle aspiration techniques are used to harvest oocytes in humans and bovines. These techniques may be impractical for small animals because of the small size of their preovulatory follicles.

REFERENCES

1. Wallace SS, Mahaffey MB, Miller DM, et al. Ultrasonographic appearance of the ovaries of dogs during follicular and luteal phases of the estrous cycle. Am J Vet Res 1992;53:209.
2. Hayer P, Gunzel-Apel AR, Luerssen D, et al. Ultrasonographic monitoring of follicular development, ovulation, and the early luteal phase in the bitch. J Reprod Fertil Suppl 1993;47:93.
3. England GCW, Yeager AE. Ultrasonographic appearance of the ovary and uterus of the bitch during oestrus, ovulation, and early pregnancy. J Reprod Fertil Suppl 1993;47:107.
4. Concannon P, Hansel W, McEntee K. Changes in LH, progesterone and sexual behavior associated with preovulatory luteinization in the bitch. Biol Reprod 1977;17:604.
5. Boyd JS, Renton JP, Harvey MJA, et al. Problems associated with ultrasonography of the canine ovary around the time of ovulation. J Reprod Fertil Suppl 1993; 47:101.

Small Animal Ultrasound, edited by Ronald W. Green.
Lippincott-Raven Publishers, Philadelphia © 1996.

LYMPH NODES

Linda D. Homco

Little information can be found in the veterinary literature describing the sonographic appearance of the normal or diseased lymph nodes in companion animals. Historically, the normal lymph node, because of its limitations in gray scale and the poor transducer resolution of veterinary ultrasound equipment, has not been examined during routine sonography. Lymph nodes change in size and shape in response to disease. Knowledge of the normal sonographic appearance as well as recognition of alterations in the size, shape, or internal architecture of regional lymph nodes provide important information in diagnosing and staging diseases.

NORMAL ANATOMY AND LOCATION

Lymph nodes that can potentially be evaluated with ultrasonography are discussed by anatomic regions. Canine and feline lymph nodes are similar; the cat's lymph nodes are smaller than the dog's. The number of nodes in each group varies in the dog and cat.[1–3]

Lumbar Aortic Lymph Nodes

The lumbar aortic lymph nodes are small nodes that lie along the aorta and caudal vena cava from the diaphragm to the deep circumflex iliac arteries (Fig. 17-1).[4] These nodes may be absent in the dog, but there may be as many as 17.[5,6]

The *left lumbar* lymph node is the largest. It is 1 to 2 cm long and lies between the sublumbar musculature and the left crus of the diaphragm.[5] Lumbar nodes drain the lumbar vertebrae, adrenal glands, and portions of the urogenital system.

The *medial iliac* lymph node, which many refer to as the sublumbar node, lies between the deep circumflex iliac and the external iliac artery (see Fig. 17-1). It may be single or paired and is as large as 4 cm long, 1 cm wide, and 0.5 cm thick in the mature dog.[5] It is bounded on the right side by the vena cava. It drains the dorsal abdomen, pelvis, pelvic limbs, genital system, and the caudal digestive and urinary tracts.

Abdominal Visceral Lymph Nodes

The *hepatic* lymph nodes lie on each side of the portal vein and may be up to 3 cm long in the dog (see Fig. 17-1).[5] They drain the stomach, duodenum, pancreas, and liver.

The *splenic* lymph nodes (sometimes referred to as the gastrosplenic lymph nodes) are a group of three to five nodes that lie in the splenic hilum along the splenic artery and vein (see Fig. 17-1). They may be large, but are usually 1.5 cm long

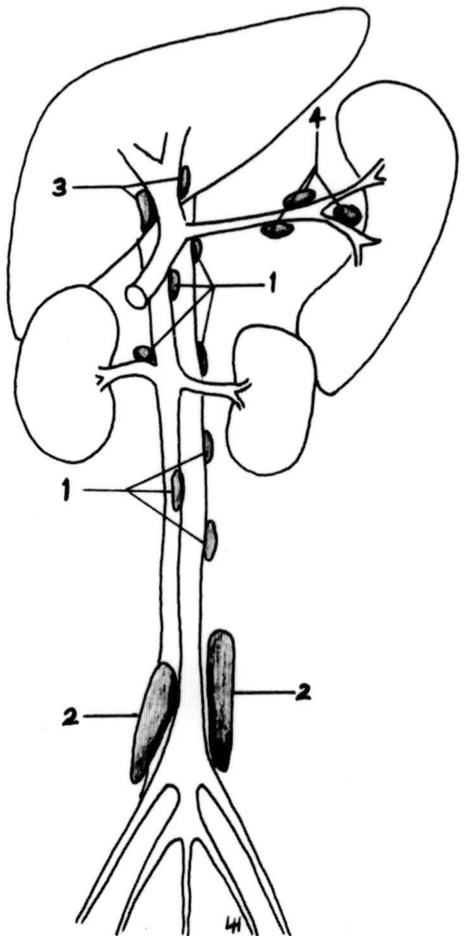

Figure 17-1. Diagram of the normal anatomic locations of various abdominal lymph nodes: lumbar aortic lymph nodes (*1*), medial iliac lymph nodes (*2*), hepatic lymph nodes (*3*), and splenic lymph nodes (*4*).

in the mature dog.[5] These nodes drain the esophagus, stomach, pancreas, spleen, liver, omentum, and diaphragm.

The *cranial mesenteric* lymph nodes are the largest nodes in the abdomen (Fig. 17-2). In medium-sized dogs, they average 6 cm long, 2 cm wide, and 0.5 cm thick.[5] They lie along the cranial mesenteric artery and vein in the jejunal mesentery. Afferent lymphatics to these nodes come from the jejunum, ileum, and pancreas.

The *colic* lymph nodes lie in the mesocolon close to the intestines (see Fig. 17-2). They drain the ileum, cecum, and colon.

Thoracic Lymph Nodes

The *sternal* lymph nodes are usually paired and lie adjacent to the second sternebra or costal cartilages, although a solitary node may occur (Fig. 17-3). When two nodes are present, they are ellipsoid and vary from 2 mm to 2 cm long in the dog.[5] The sternal nodes receive afferent lymphatics from the ribs, sternum, and thymus, and are the major lymphatic drainage from the peritoneal cavity by means of the sternal lymphatics from the diaphragm.[5]

The *mediastinal* lymph nodes in the dog vary in number and lie along the cranial vena cava and the brachiocephalic arteries within the cranial mediastinum (see Fig. 17-3). They are oblong and vary from 1 mm to 3 cm long in the dog.[5] These nodes receive afferents from the muscles of the thorax, vertebrae, ribs, trachea, esophagus, thyroid, thymus, mediastinum, pleura, heart, and aorta, and efferent lymphatics from the deep cervical, sternal, tracheobronchial, and pulmonary lymph nodes.

The *tracheobronchial* lymph nodes include all the nodes that lie near the bronchi at the tracheal bifurcation (see Fig. 17-3). These nodes vary in number and are ellipsoid, measuring 5 mm to 3 cm long.[5] These nodes drain primarily the lungs and bronchi, but they also drain portions of the heart, aorta, esophagus, trachea, mediastinum, and diaphragm.

Superficial Lymph Nodes

Subcutaneous lymph nodes most frequently evaluated for disease are the *superficial inguinal, deep femoral, popliteal, axillary, superficial cervical,* and *submandibular* nodes. The reader may refer to anatomy texts for information on the precise location of numerous, potentially clinically important superficial lymph nodes and the anatomic regions they drain.[1–5]

SCANNING TECHNIQUES

To evaluate abdominal lymph nodes for lymphadenopathy, the entire abdomen must be scanned carefully. The hilus of the spleen, the

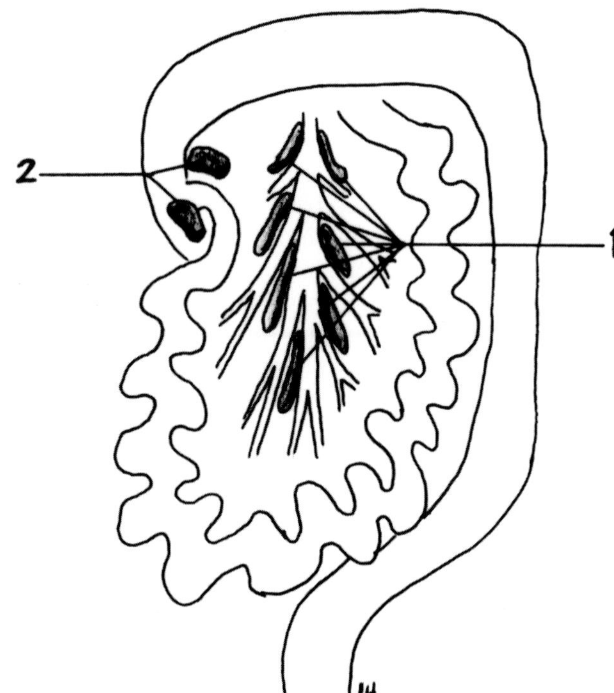

Figure 17-2. Diagram of the locations of the gastrointestinal lymph nodes: cranial mesenteric lymph nodes (*1*), and colic lymph nodes (*2*).

porta hepatis of the liver, and the perirenal area must be scrutinized, because lymphadenopathy can be detected in the area of the cranial mesenteric and celiac arteries, the portal vein, and the kidneys. Many retroperitoneal lymph nodes within the sublumbar region follow the aorta. To evaluate for lymphadenopathy in the iliac or caudal lumbar region, the urinary bladder can

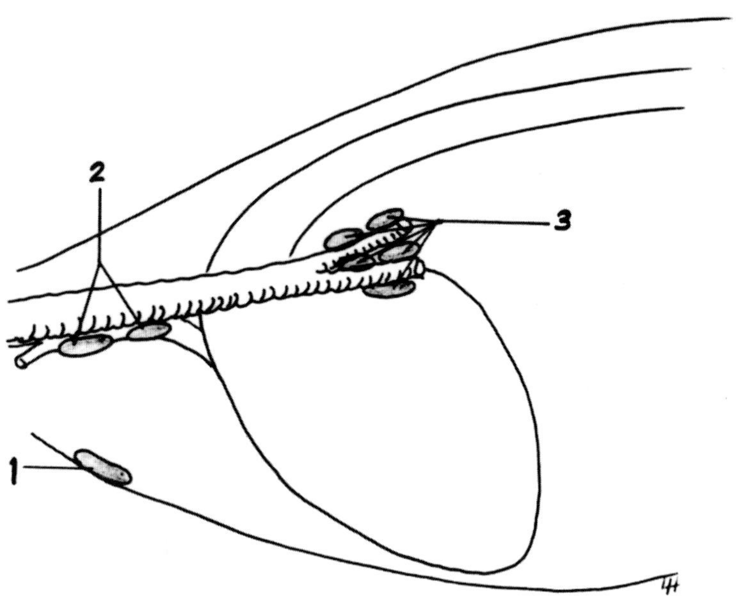

Figure 17-3. Diagram of the normal anatomic locations of the thoracic lymph nodes: sternal lymph nodes (*1*), mediastinal lymph nodes (*2*), and tracheobronchial lymph nodes (*3*).

be used as an imaging window. With the animal in dorsal recumbency, the mesenteric lymph nodes are typically identified in the middorsal abdomen. Excessively enlarged mesenteric lymph nodes can become pendulous when the patient is scanned in lateral recumbency or standing. The identification of colic and other regional intestinal lymph nodes is not always possible and relies on meticulous scanning of the gastrointestinal tract in these regions.

Thoracic lymph nodes are difficult to image unless pleural or mediastinal fluid provides an imaging window, or the lymph nodes become large enough to displace air-filled lung. Because access to the tracheobronchial lymph nodes is limited to transesophageal probes, thoracic lymph node imaging is usually confined to sternal or cranial mediastinal lymphadenopathies. Structures in the cranial thorax can be imaged using an intercostal or thoracic inlet approach when the animal is standing or in sternal or lateral recumbencies.

The use of high-resolution or small-parts transducers is necessary when lymph node imaging is the primary goal. The frequencies of these transducers are 7.5 or 10 MHz in sector or linear configurations. Larger and deeper nodes may be identified with 5.0-MHz transducers, but the success of lymph node evaluation with a lower-frequency transducer is limited. Effective imaging of superficial lymph nodes requires a high-frequency transducer with a short focal zone. Standoff pads may be used with lower-frequency transducers or those for which the focal zone is beyond the depth of the lymph node to be evaluated.

NORMAL SONOGRAPHIC APPEARANCE

Normal lymph nodes appear as ovoid or spindle-shaped, somewhat flattened structures that are usually isoechoic with the surrounding tissues (Fig. 17-4). Microscopically, each node is made up of a central medulla, which contains cords of lymphocytes and small sinuses, and an outer cortex containing lymphatic nodules or follicles.[7] Afferent and efferent lymphatics and blood vessels enter and leave each node at the hilus.[6] The literature describes a central or slightly eccentric echogenic line visible in many histologically normal human lymph nodes, which is thought to represent fat in the hilum and is called the hilar fat sign (Figs. 17-4 and 17-5).[7–9] This hyperechoic line has been reported in the normal canine medial iliac lymph node and histologically appears to represent fat, fascia, and vessels that are probably near the hilus.[10] I have not observed this hilar fat sign in all normal canine lymph nodes, probably because of their extremely small size compared with the human counterparts.

Lumbar Aortic Lymph Nodes

When normal, the lumbar aortic lymph nodes are not recognized on an ultrasound examination unless a higher-frequency transducer is used to provide better resolution. These nodes are discretely hypoechoic structures surrounded by a hyperechoic connective tissue capsule. The medial iliac lymph node is the one most often found, and it has a very thin, elongated spindle shape in most dogs (see Fig. 17-4).

Abdominal Visceral Lymph Nodes

The abdominal visceral nodes are rarely seen because of interference from gas and ingesta in the gastrointestinal tract, and in the normal animal, their typically thin, elongated shape has a maximum thickness of 5 mm.

Thoracic Lymph Nodes

All of the lymph nodes listed in the thoracic cavity are inaccessible in the normal animal because of the lack of an acoustic window.

Superficial Lymph Nodes

Many superficial lymph nodes can be imaged with a high-frequency transducer and a standoff pad. Most of these lymph nodes are flat and

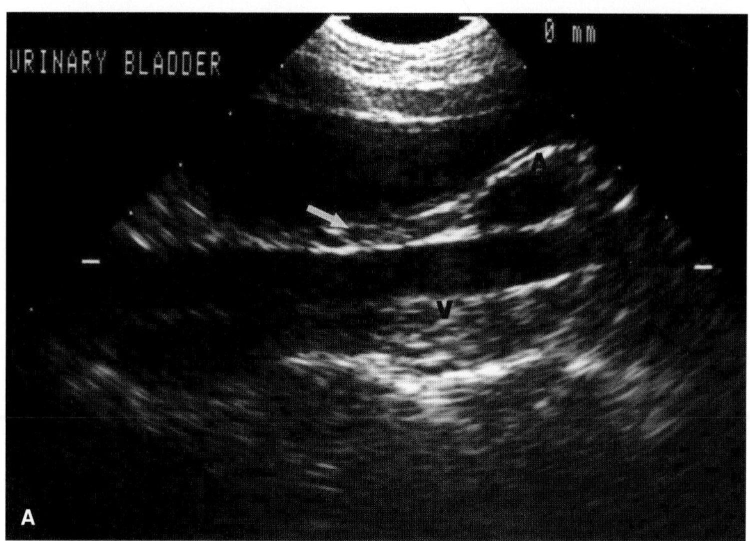

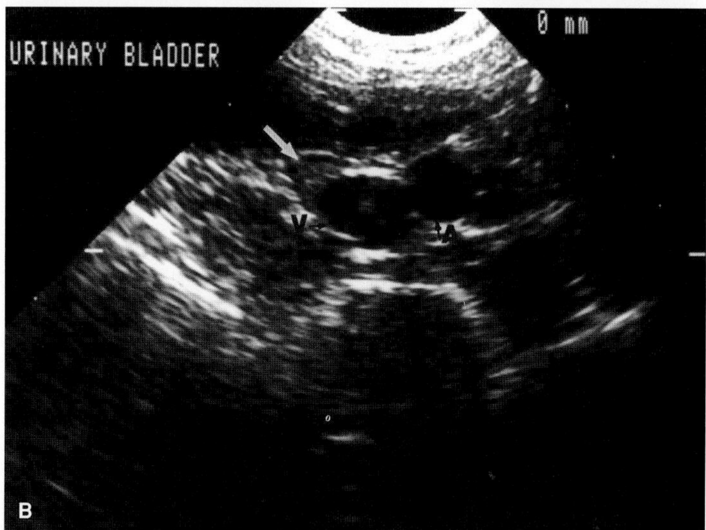

Figure 17-4. (**A**) Sagittal and (**B**) transverse sonograms of the normal medial iliac lymph node (*arrows*) in a dog. The urinary bladder was used as an imaging window. (**A**) Notice the long and nearly flat spindle shape of the node that is ventral to the vena cava. A thin echogenic central line represents the hilar fat sign. (**B**) The node is almost isoechoic with the surrounding fat and fascia. *V*, vena cava; *A*, aorta.

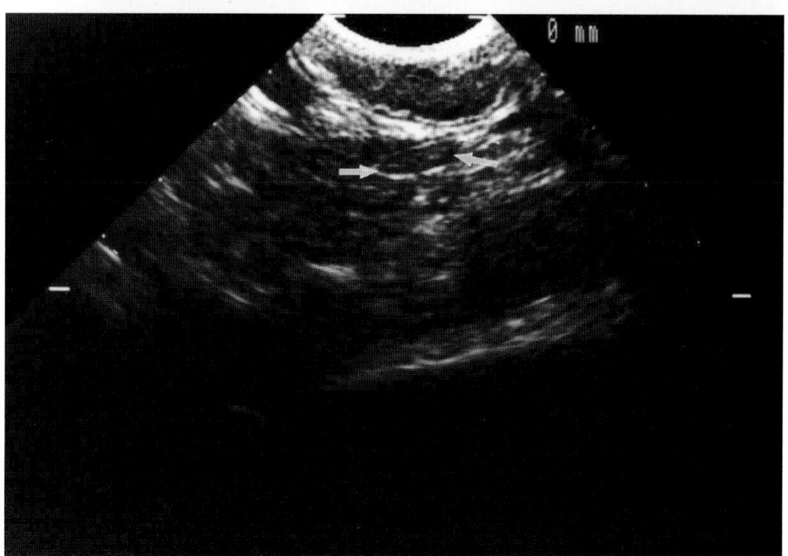

Figure 17-5. Sagittal sonogram of a normal mesenteric lymph node in a dog (*arrows*). Notice the faint echogenic central line, which is the normal hilar fat sign.

oval, homogenous, and hypoechoic to the surrounding fat and fibrous tissue.

DISEASES OF THE LYMPH NODES

Little information describing the sonographic appearance of diseases of the lymph nodes in companion animals is found in the veterinary literature.[11,12] Much of the information presented here is from personal experience and is based on descriptions from the human literature.

Most diseases of the lymph nodes, whether inflammatory or neoplastic, result in some degree of node enlargement. Because most normal lymph nodes are flat and ovoid or spindle shaped, any change in shape toward a rounded appearance should suggest disease.[8] Abnormal lymph nodes generally become hypoechoic as a result of inflammation (Figs. 17-6 through 17-8) or infiltration (Figs. 17-10 through 17-13).[11,12] Hyperechoic or hypoechoic zones may be seen in inflammatory (see Figs. 17-6*B, D*, 17-7*E, F*) and neoplastic (see Figs. 17-10*C*, 17-12, and 17-13*F*) lymph nodes.[13] Tiny micronodules of disease within the parenchyma may create a grainy appearance (see Figs. 17-9 and 17-10*B*).[13] The human literature describes loss of the hilar fat sign as an indicator of malignancy.[8,9,14]

(text continues on p. 316)

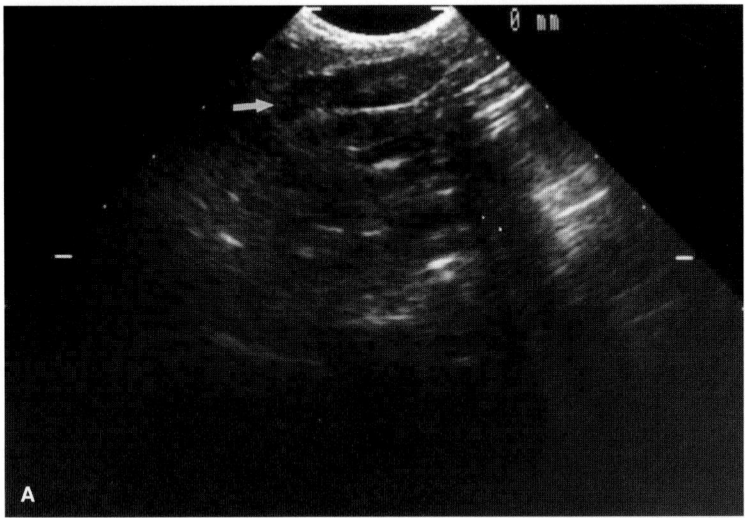

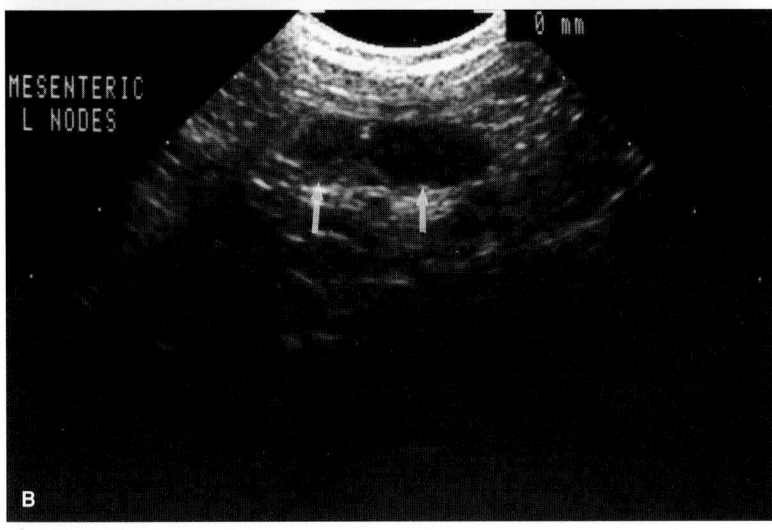

Figure 17-6 Sonograms of reactive mesenteric lymph nodes. Notice how all of these nodes maintain an elliptical or oval shape despite enlargement (**A**) Reactive mesenteric lymph node (*arrow*) in a dog with granulomatous enteritis. The hilar fat sign remains. (**B**) Reactive mesenteric lymph nodes (*arrows*) in a cat with feline infectious peritonitis.

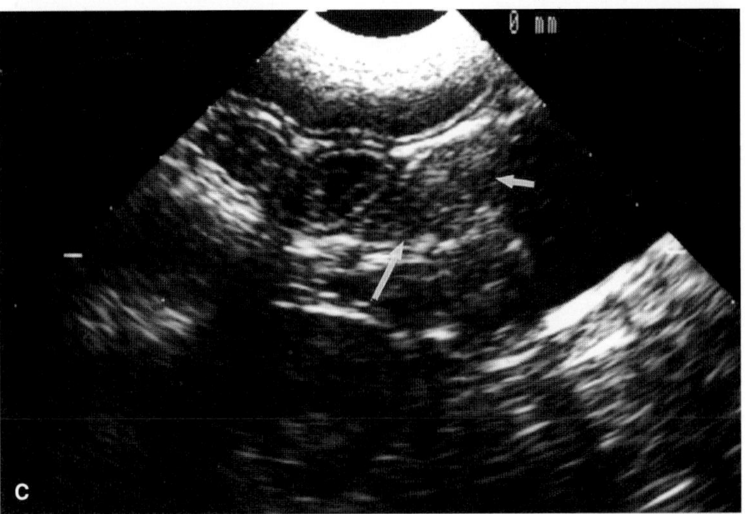

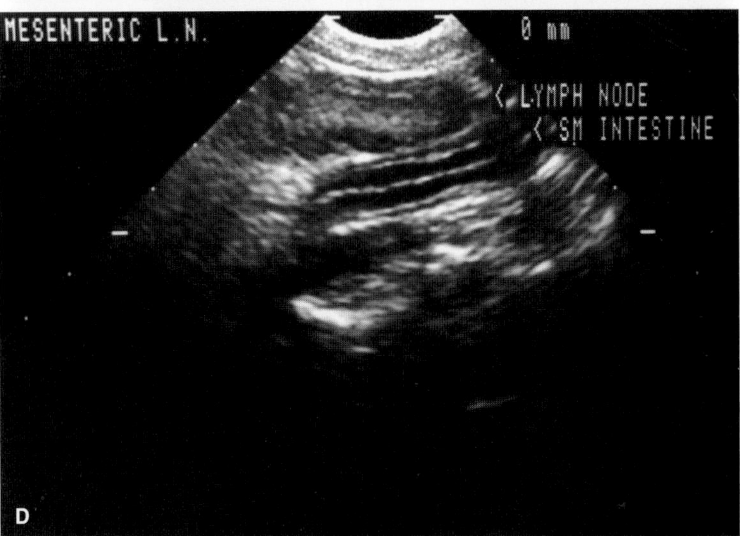

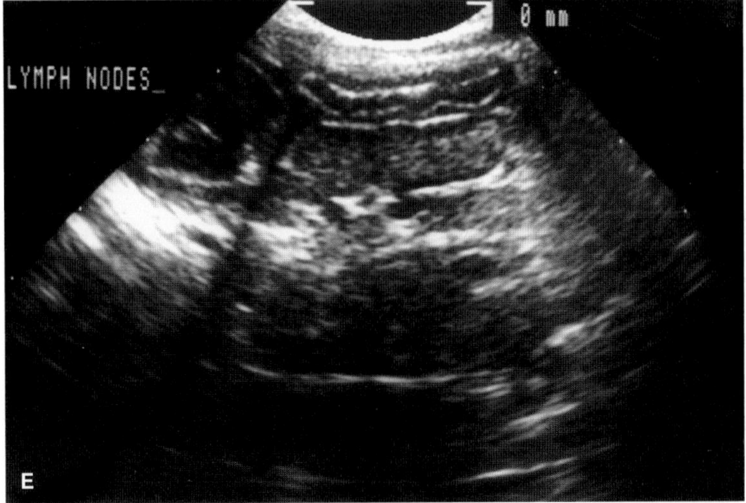

Figure 17-6 *(Continued)* (**C**) Reactive mesenteric lymph node (*arrows*) in a young dog with eosinophilic enteritis. (**D**) Reactive mesenteric lymph node adjacent to a normal segment of small bowel in a dog with intestinal phycomycosis. (**E**) Reactive mesenteric lymph node in a young dog with viral enteritis (parvovirus). (**F**) Reactive mesenteric lymph nodes (*arrows*) in a dog with viral enteritis (coronavirus).

(continued)

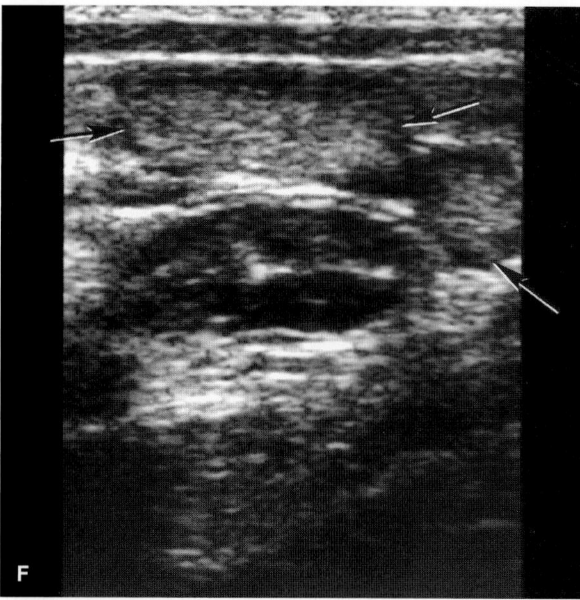

Figure 17-6 *(Continued)*

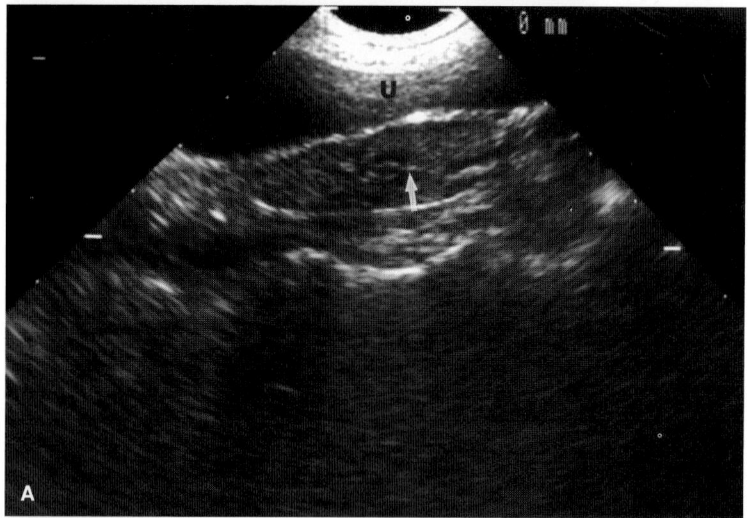

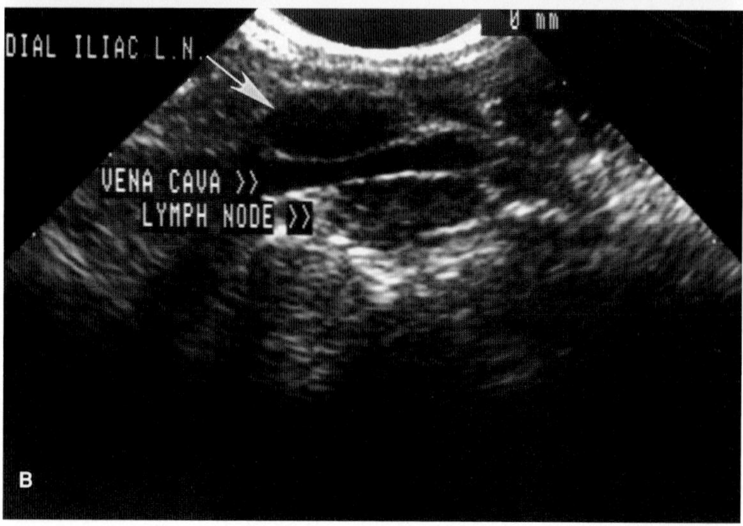

Figure 17-7 Sonograms of reactive medial iliac lymph nodes. The urinary bladder (*U*) serves as an excellent imaging window for most of these lymph nodes. Notice how most of these nodes maintain an oval shape. (**A**) Reactive medial iliac lymph node in a spayed female dog with chronic vaginitis. Notice the persistence of the hilar fat sign (*arrow*). (**B**) Reactive medial iliac lymph nodes (*arrows*) in an intact female dog with ulcerative vaginitis.

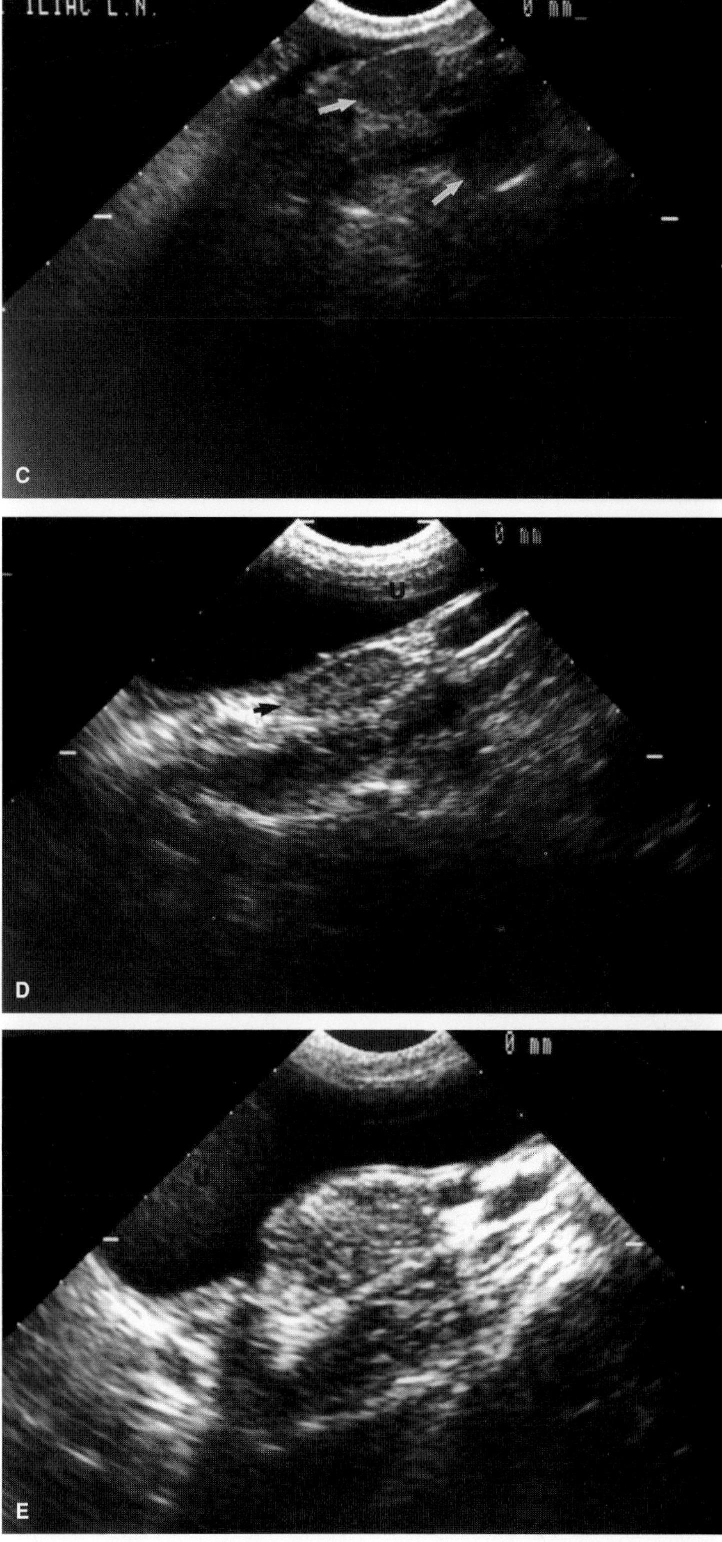

Figure 17-7 *(Continued)* (**C**) Reactive medial iliac lymph node in a dog with chronic ascites (modified transudate) (*arrows*). (**D**) Reactive medial iliac lymph node (*arrow*) in an intact male dog with orchitis (*Nocardia* sp.). (**E**) Sagittal sonogram of reactive medial iliac lymph node in a dog with chronic bacterial prostatitis. *(continued)*

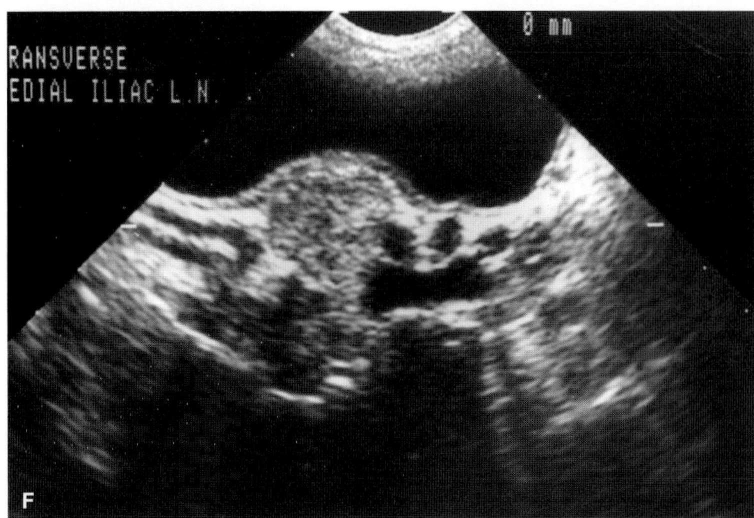

Figure 17-7 *(Continued)* (**F**) Transverse sonogram of the right medial iliac lymph node in a dog with chronic bacterial prostatitis. Anechoic structures adjacent to the lymph node are the iliac vessels.

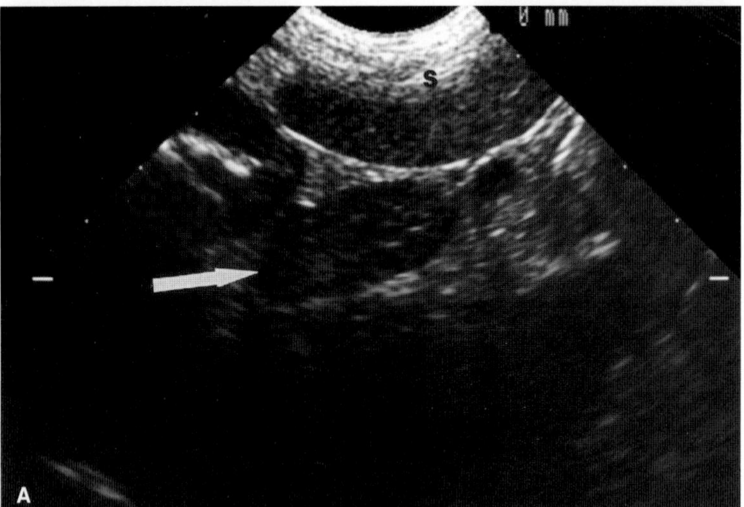

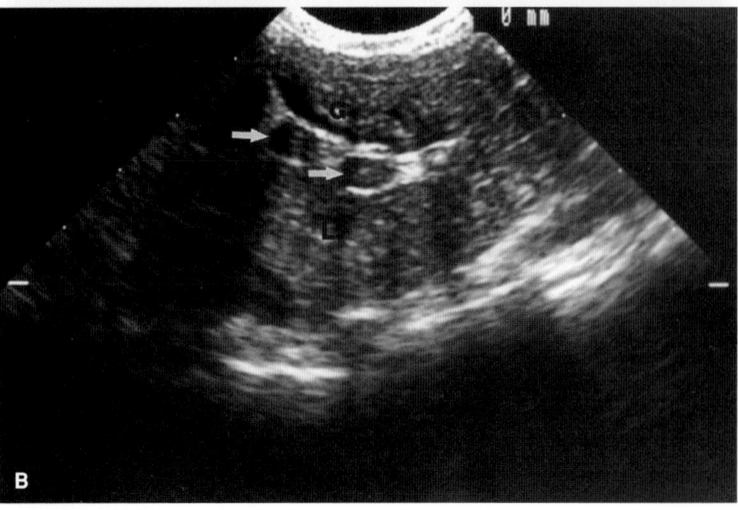

Figure 17-8. (**A**) Reactive splenic lymph node (*arrow*) in a dog with a splenic (S) abscess (*Salmonella* sp.). This node is hypoechoic but does not create distal enhancement, as is typical of lymphosarcoma (see Fig. 17-11*G*, *H*). (**B**) Reactive splenic lymph nodes (*arrows*) in a dog with chronic eosinophilic gastritis. This transverse sonogram of the nodes shows a cross section of the hilar fat sign appearing as a white central dot. *L*, liver; *G*, stomach.

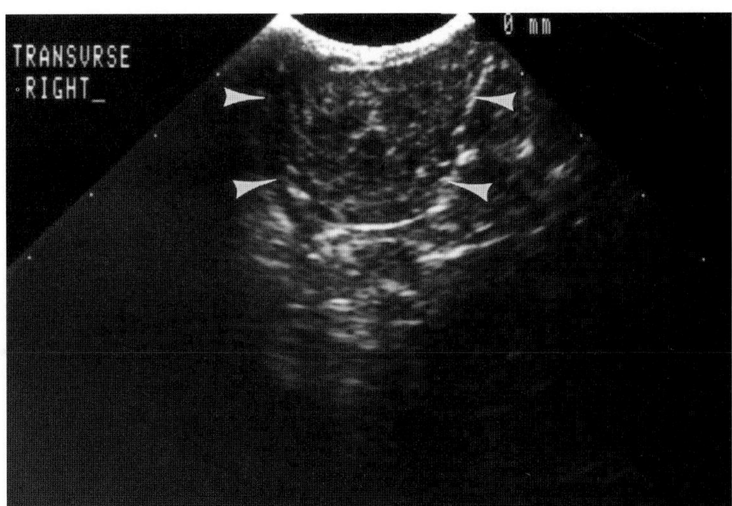

Figure 17-9. Sonogram of reactive lymphoid hyperplasia of the mediastinal lymph node (*arrowheads*) in a cat. The grainy appearance of the parenchyma is most likely caused by micronodules.

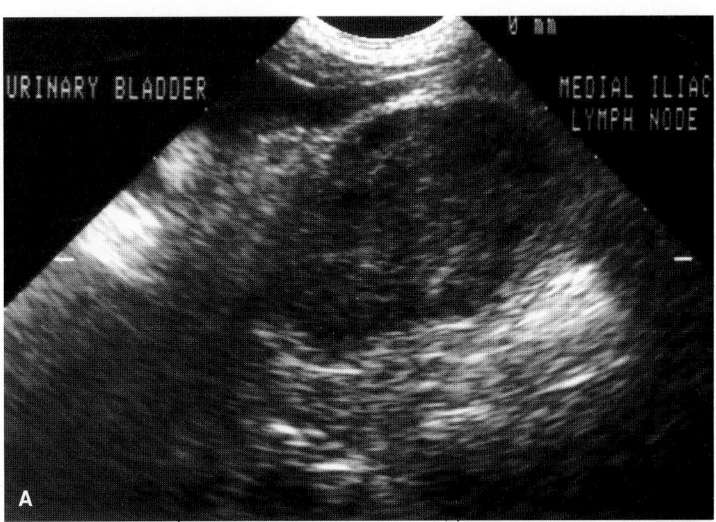

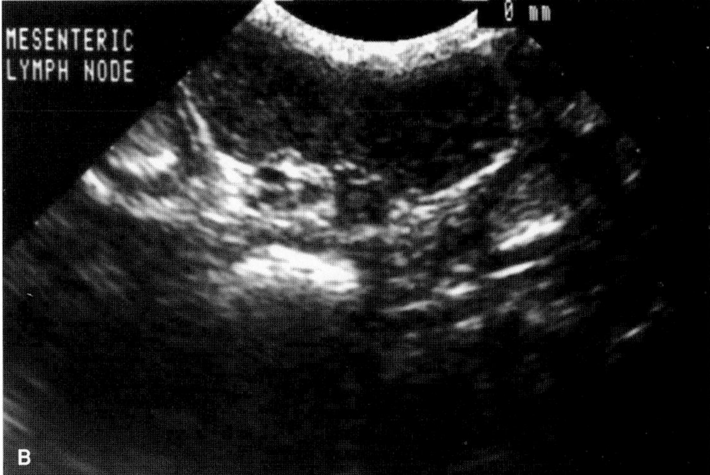

Figure 17-10. Metastatic disease of the abdominal lymph nodes. Notice the plump and rounded appearance of these nodes compared with the reactive nodes seen in Figures 17-6 and 17-7. (**A**) Sagittal sonogram of the medial iliac lymph node in a dog with regional metastasis of a squamous cell carcinoma of the urinary bladder. (**B**) Sonogram of a mesenteric lymph node in a cat with regional metastasis of mast cell neoplasia.

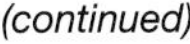
(continued)

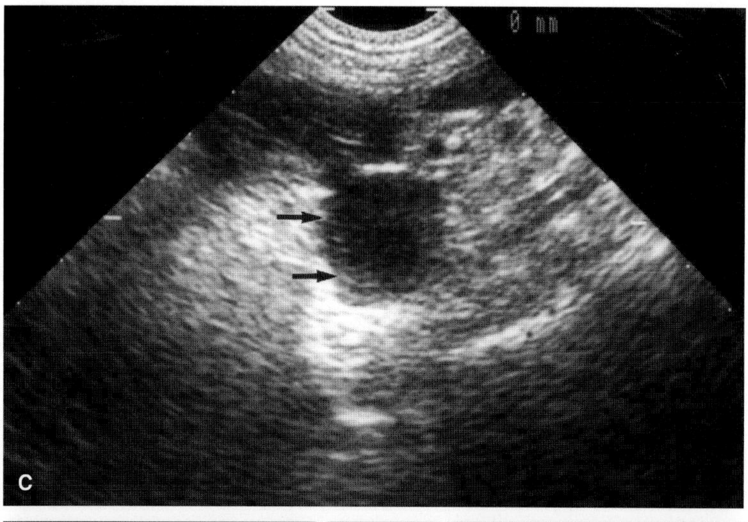

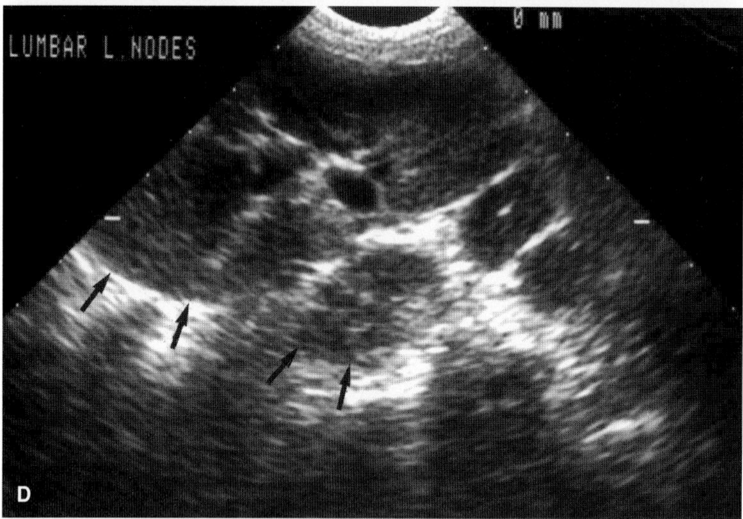

Figure 17-10. *(Continued)* (**C**) Sonogram of the splenic lymph node (*arrows*) in a dog with regional metastasis of a gastric carcinoma. (**D**) Sonogram of the cranial lumbar aortic lymph nodes (*arrows*) in a dog with malignant histiocytosis.

Although ultrasound evaluation of nodes cannot definitely discriminate between malignant and benign neoplasms, there are suggestive patterns. Lymph nodes associated with malignant disease are generally larger and more numerous than in benign diseases (see Fig. 17-11).[8,9] Nodes associated with malignant disease are more hypoechoic than those associated with benign disease.[8] Most nodes involved in malignant disease tend to develop a rounded shape (see Figs. 17-10 through 17-13), but in benign disease, they tend to retain their original oval or spindle shape despite an increase in size (see Figs. 17-6 through 17-8).[8]

The ultrasonographic appearance of lymphoma varies from hypoechoic to anechoic, with very good sound transmission (see Figs. 17-11 and 17-13).[9] This change causes the nodes to appear echo free, with moderate distant enhancement apparent.[9,14]

Metastatic disease can occur by lymphatic or hematogenous spread. Malignant metastases often start in the regional nodes adjacent to the affected organ (see Fig. 17-10).[8] Although the echo patterns of metastatic disease may vary, they are less likely to be hypoechoic and are rarely echo free, as with lymphoma.[9,15]

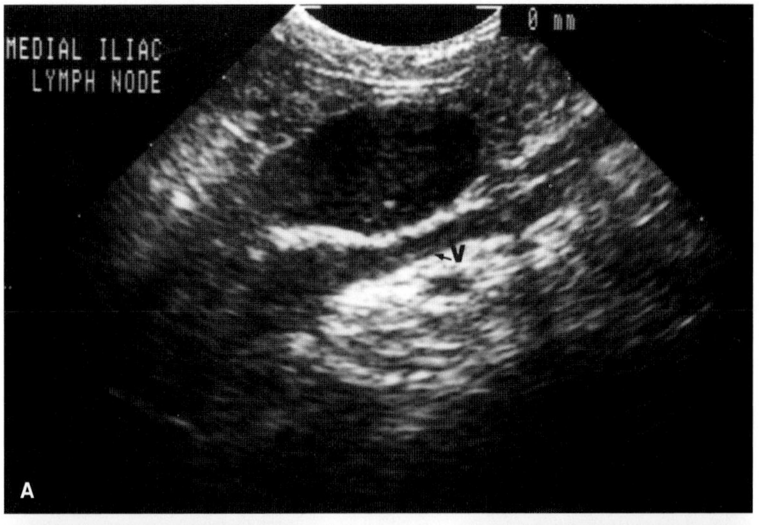

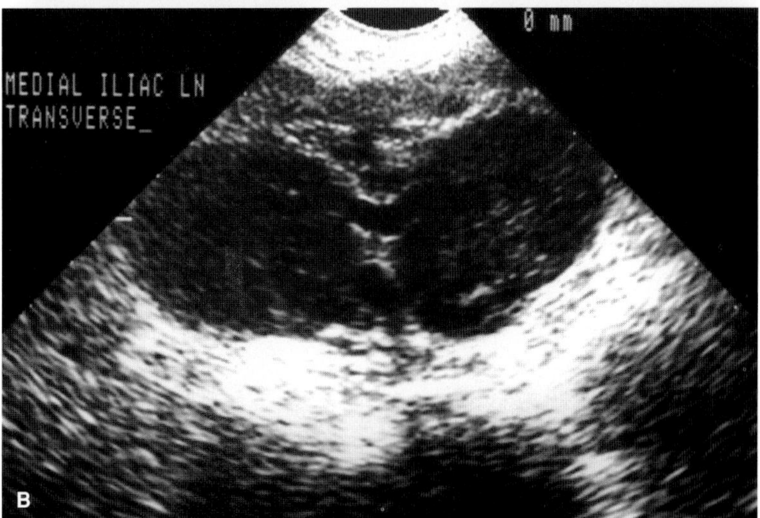

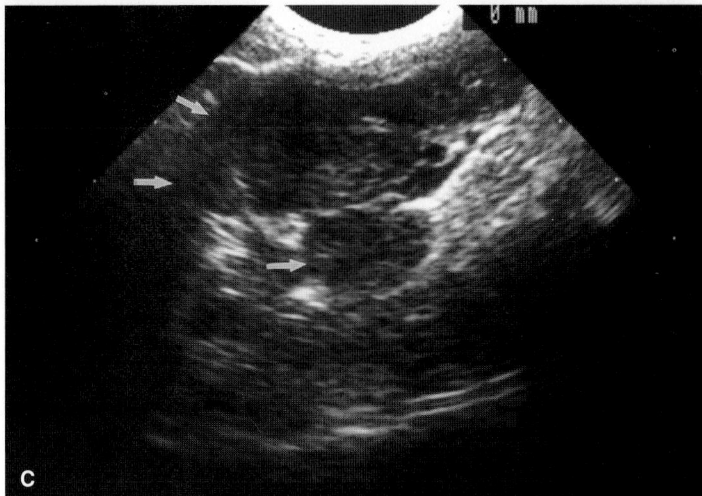

Figure 17-11. Primary neoplasia (lymphosarcoma) of the abdominal lymph nodes. Notice the generally rounded shape with hypoechoic parenchyma and occasional distant enhancement. (**A**) Sagittal sonogram of the medial iliac lymph node of a dog with multicentric lymphosarcoma. *V*, vena cava. (**B**) Transverse sonogram of the enlarged medial iliac lymph nodes in a dog with multicentric lymphosarcoma. The anechoic central structures are the iliac vessels. (**C**) Mesenteric lymph nodes (*arrows*) in a cat with lymphosarcoma.

(continued)

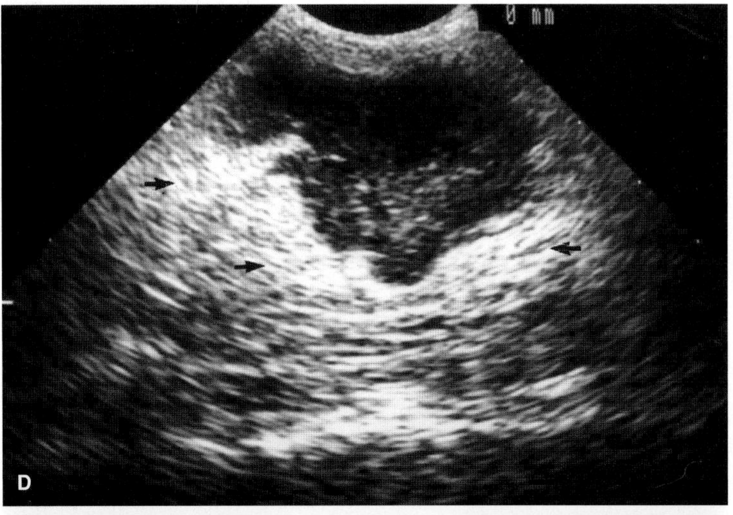

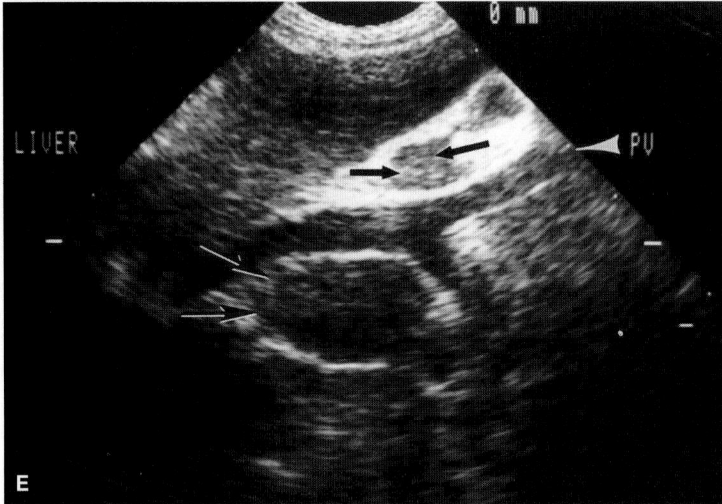

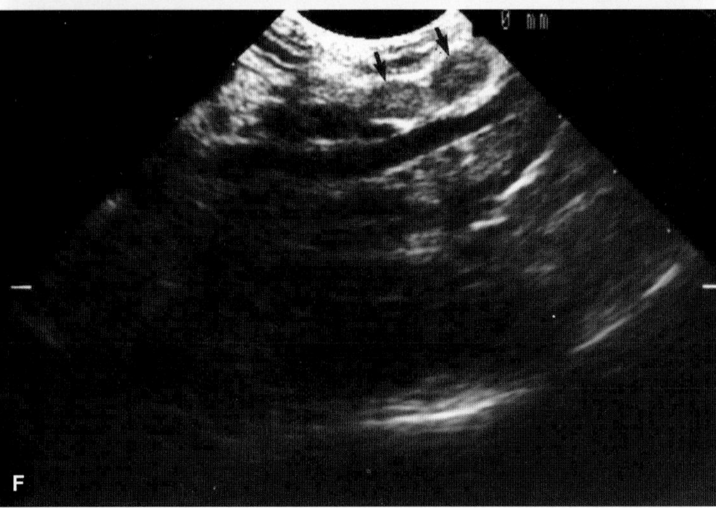

Figure 17-11. *(Continued)* (**D**) Mesenteric lymph node in a cat with lymphosarcoma. Notice the distant enhancement (*arrows*) from this irregularly shaped node. (**E**) Hepatic lymph nodes (*arrows*) in a dog with multicentric lymphosarcoma. *PV*, portal vein. (**F**) Lumbar aortic lymph nodes (*arrows*) adjacent to the aorta in a dog with multicentric lymphosarcoma.

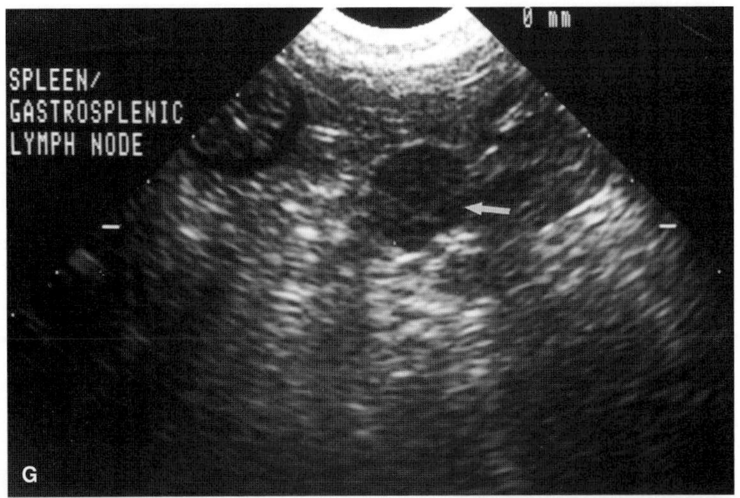

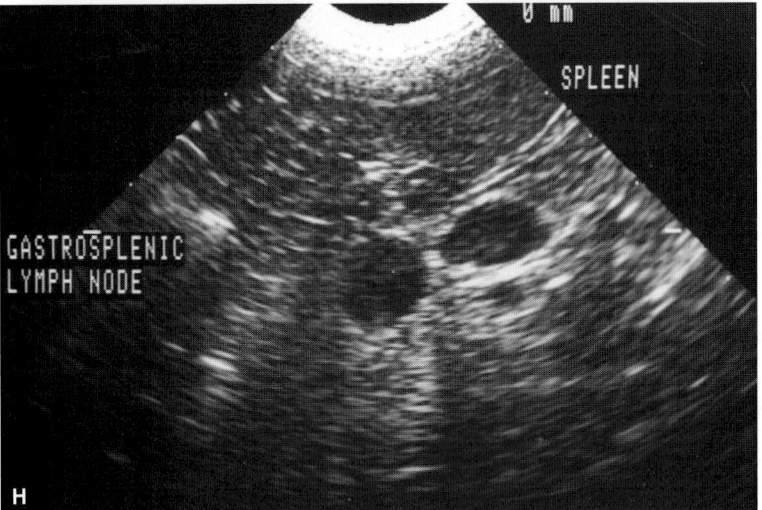

Figure 17-11. *(Continued)* (**G**) Splenic lymph node (*arrow*) in a dog with lymphosarcoma. (**H**) Splenic lymph nodes in a dog with lymphosarcoma.

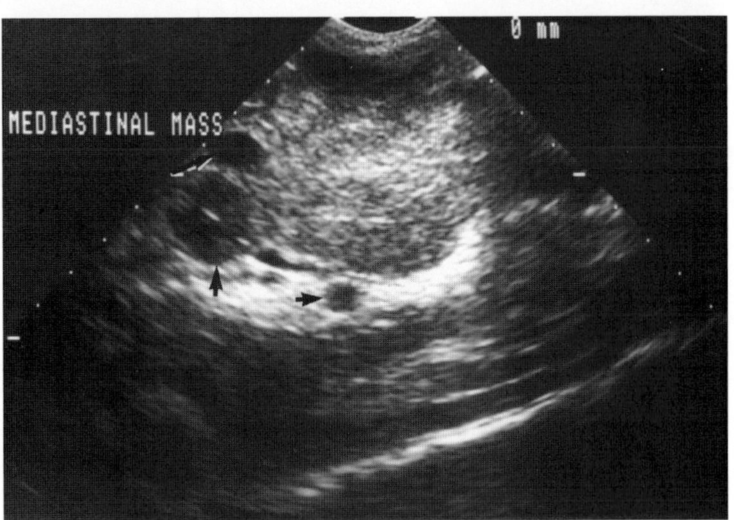

Figure 17-12. Transverse sonogram of the cranial mediastinum in a dog with cranial mediastinal lymphosarcoma. Three mediastinal vessels that are displaced by this mass are seen in cross section (*arrows*).

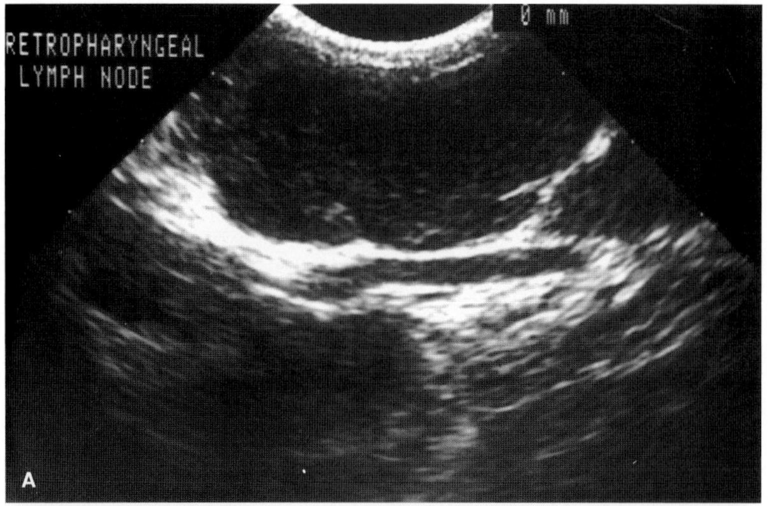

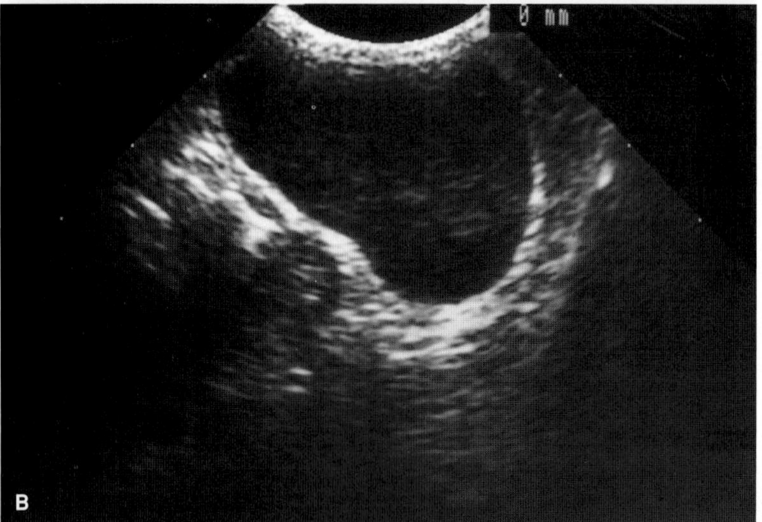

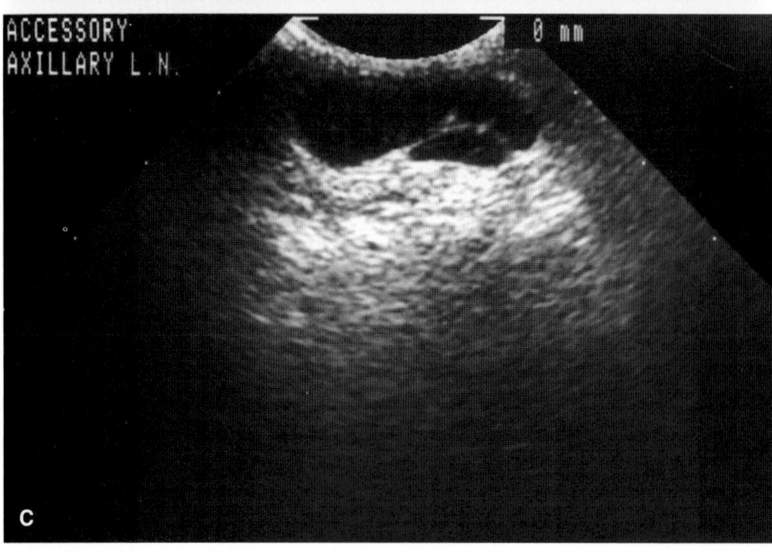

Figure 17-13. Primary neoplasia (lymphosarcoma) of the superficial lymph nodes. Notice the rounded shape, hypoechoic parenchyma, and occasional distant enhancement characteristic of this disease. All of these examples are from dogs with multicentric lymphosarcoma. (**A**) Retropharyngeal lymph node with an irregular shape. (**B**) Superficial cervical lymph node with a nearly anechoic parenchyma. (**C**) Accessory axillary lymph node with an irregular shape and marked enhancement.

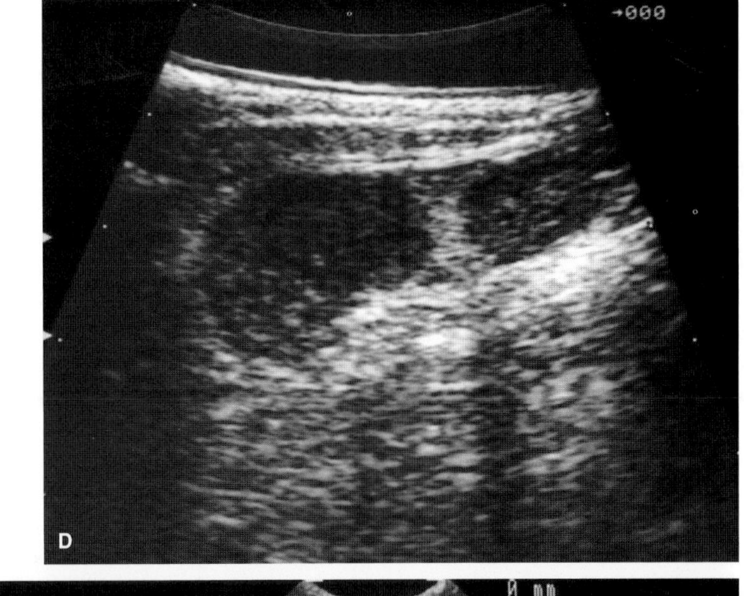

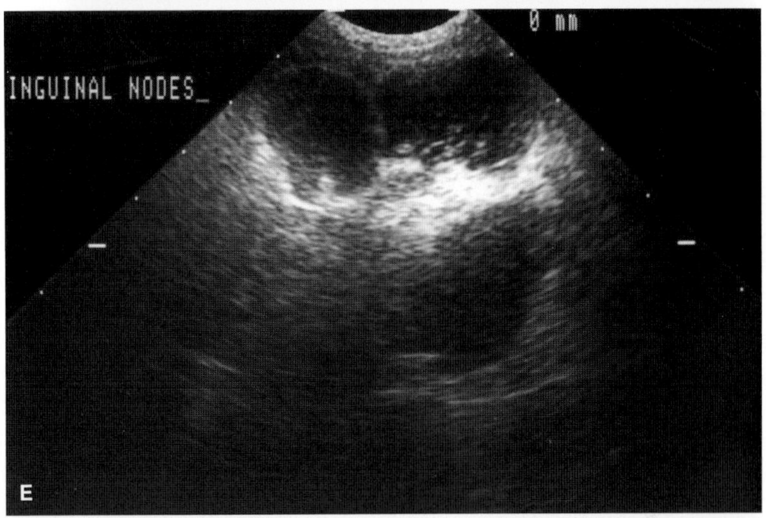

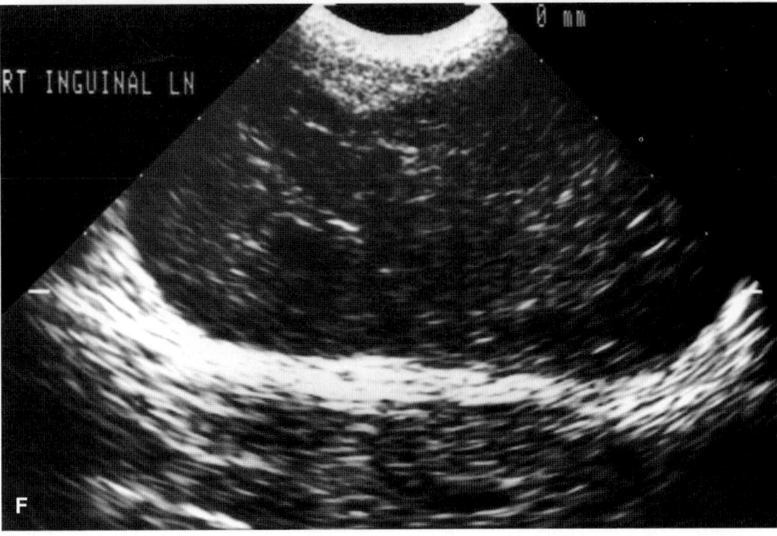

Figure 17-13. *(Continued)* (**D**) Popliteal lymph nodes, showing two adjacent affected nodes rather than a typical solitary node. (**E**) Inguinal lymph nodes with distant enhancement. (**F**) Inguinal lymph node with a mixed-echo pattern throughout.

BIOPSY TECHNIQUES

Ultrasound-guided biopsy and fine-needle aspiration are possible when large lymph nodes are apparent and are recommended if there is a question of regional metastatic disease. The sonographer must remember the proximity of many lymph nodes to large blood vessels. Some risk is encountered when the needle tip is not apparent on the real-time image.

CONCLUSION

Ultrasonography of the normal lymph nodes is not possible because of their small dimensions, interference from gastrointestinal viscera, and limitations of available transducer resolution. Better equipment and improved operator skills may allow occasional detection of normal nodes. Lymph nodes that are easily detected on routine sonography and have a rounded or plump oval shape should be assumed to be abnormal. No characteristic sonographic appearances have been described for the dog and cat.

REFERENCES

1. Adams DR. Lymphatic system. In: Adams DR, ed. Canine anatomy: a systemic study. Ames: The Iowa State University Press, 1986:379.
2. Tompkins MB. Lymphoid system. In: Hudson LC, Hamilton WP, eds. Atlas of feline anatomy for veterinarians. Philadelphia: WB Saunders, 1993:113.
3. Rosenzweig LJ. The circulatory system and the brachial and lumbosacral plexuses. In: Rosenzweig LJ, ed. Anatomy of the cat: text and dissection guide. Dubuque: William C Brown, 1990: 211.
4. Saar LI, Getty R. Carnivore lymphatic system. In: Getty R, ed. Sisson and Grossman's the anatomy of the domestic animals. 5th ed. Philadelphia: WB Saunders, 1975:1652.
5. Evans HE, Christensen GC. The lymphatic system. In: Evans HE, Christensen GC, eds. Miller's anatomy of the dog. 2nd ed. Philadelphia: WB Saunders, 1979:802.
6. Rogers KS, Barton CL, Landis M. Canine and feline lymph nodes. Part I. Anatomy and function. Compend Cont Educ 1993;15:397.
7. Marchal G, Oyen R, Verschakelen J, et al. Sonographic appearance of normal lymph nodes. J Ultrasound Med 1985; 4:417.
8. Smeets AJ, Zonderland HM, van der Voorde F, Lameris JS. Evaluation of abdominal lymph nodes by ultrasound. J Ultrasound Med 1990;9:325.
9. Mittelstaedt CA. Retroperitoneum. In: Mittelstaedt CA, ed. General ultrasound. New York: Churchill Livingstone, 1992: 749.
10. Spaulding KA, Richey J. Determination of the sonographic appearance of normal medial iliac lymph nodes in the dog. Proceedings of the American College of Veterinary Radiology Annual Meeting, scientific program. Chicago, IL, 1993.
11. Saunders HM, Pugh CR, Rhodes WH. Expanding applications of abdominal ultrasonography. J Am Anim Hosp Assoc 1992;28:369.
12. Pugh CR. Ultrasonographic examination of abdominal lymph nodes in the dog. Vet Radiol Ultrasound 1994;35:110.
13. Rubaltelli L, Proto E, Salmaso R, et al. Sonography of abnormal lymph nodes in vitro: correlation of sonographic and histologic findings. Am J Roentgenol 1990; 155:1241.
14. Carroll BA. Ultrasound of lymphoma. Semin Ultrasound 1982;3:114.
15. Hillman BJ, Haber K. Echographic characteristics of malignant lymph nodes. J Clin Ultrasound 1980;8:213.

Small Animal Ultrasound, edited by Ronald W. Green.
Lippincott-Raven Publishers, Philadelphia © 1996.

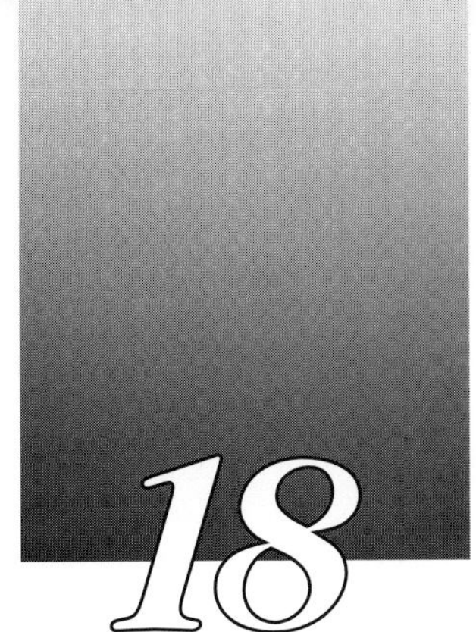

EYE

Phillip F. Steyn

Two-dimensional real-time ultrasound is an excellent way to evaluate the eye and orbit. It supplies a two-dimensional cross section image of the anterior chamber, lens, vitreous chamber, retina, choroid, sclera, and the internal structures of the orbit. Sonography is a relatively simple and quick examination to perform, and it creates little stress for the patient. Sonography allows the clinician to evaluate the internal structures of the eye when the anterior chamber or cornea is opaque and direct visualization with an ophthalmoscope is not possible.[1] Retrobulbar masses can be detected and characterized by ultrasound, and ultrasound-guided fine-needle aspirates can confirm the diagnosis.

SCANNING TECHNIQUES

Transducer Selection

A 7.5- or a 10.0-MHz transducer, using linear, curvilinear, or sector scanning, is required. A 7.5-MHz transducer should be adequate for most ophthalmic studies, although a 10.0-MHz transducer would be beneficial for studies of more superficial structures in smaller patients. Disinfecting the transducer head before the examination helps to prevent infections.

Patient Positioning

Chemical restraint usually is not required, although it should be used when needed to avoid unwarranted damage to the cornea or other parts of the eye. Tranquilization can cause prolapse of the nictitating membrane, which can be inconvenient. Most dogs, cats, and exotic species presented for an ultrasound examination of the orbit are most comfortable in the sitting position or in sternal recumbency. The ultrasonographer can sit or stand next to the patient, with the patient's eyes at approximately the same level as the examiner's chest.

Patient Preparation

A few drops of sterile topical local anesthesia are applied to the surface of the eye, and sterile lubricating jelly (K-Y lubricating jelly, Johnson & Johnson, New Brunswick, NJ) is used as a coupling gel. It is unnecessary to shave the eyelids, because the corneal contact method provides excellent sonographic visualization of the eye. A standoff pad is required to evaluate the anterior segment, but it is unnecessary if the lens, vitreous, or retrobulbar areas are being examined. Because most ocular ultrasound examinations are performed to evaluate the structures behind the lens, standoff pads are seldom indicated.

Imaging through the eyelid results in suboptimal images due to poor acoustic coupling and is not recommended.[2–4]

Performing the Examination

Manual retraction of the eyelids is required to enable accurate transducer-corneal contact. The eyes should be scanned in frontal (ie, horizontal) and sagittal (ie, vertical) planes. Representative images of the entire eye in both planes should be acquired; this amounts to about 12 images per eye. It is prudent to use images of the other eye as a control. The various images are acquired by changing the angle of incidence of the transducer while the transducer is fixed on the anterior surface. This avoids excessive corneal friction and prevents further damage to the eye.

The eyes should be flushed carefully with copious amounts of sterile saline after completion of the study to remove all of the coupling gel. Antibiotic ophthalmic ointment can also be administered after the scan if deemed necessary.

INDICATIONS FOR OPHTHALMIC ULTRASOUND

The most common indication for an ultrasound examination of the eye and periorbital structures is any condition in which the clinician is unable to directly visualize the entire eye because of opacification of the cornea or the lens (Table 18-1). The remainder of the globe and retrobulbar areas can be well visualized sonographically in patients with pannus, hyphema, hypopyon, and cataracts.

TABLE 18-1
Indications for Ultrasonographic Examination of the Eye and Orbit

Corneal opacification
Lens opacification
Decreased retropulsion or nonretropulsion of an eye
Exophthalmos, unilateral or bilateral
Enophthalmos
Displacement of the globe
Foreign body
Painful opening of the mouth
Biometry
Doppler flow evaluation of the vascularity of masses
Needle guidance for aspiration or biopsy

Decreased retropulsion or nonretropulsion of an eye is another important indication, because ultrasound is an effective method for evaluating the retrobulbar structures. Ultrasound can help differentiate retrobulbar masses (eg, neoplasia from abscesses) and soft tissue swelling (eg, cellulitis).

Unilateral or bilateral exophthalmos, ocular tumors, enophthalmos, globe displacement, foreign bodies, and pain on opening the mouth are also indications for orbital ultrasound, especially when these conditions are unexplained or accompanied by opaque ocular media. Biometry of the intraorbital structures is best performed using ultrasound.[5] Ocular ultrasound is not indicated if the ocular media are clear, unless the nature, extent, and size of an intraocular mass must be determined.[2]

Color flow Doppler ultrasound is helpful in evaluating the amount of blood flow to ocular or retrobulbar masses and assisting in differentiating benign from malignant tumors. Fast-growing, aggressive tumors generally have more blood flow than less hostile masses.[6]

Ultrasound-guided biopsy or fine-needle aspiration for cytologic or microbial culture and sensitivity testing should also be considered an important indication. Fine-needle aspirates of abdominal structures using a 20-gauge or smaller needle (ie, outer diameter of <1.0 mm) have not been shown to put the patient at risk of extensive bleeding or sepsis and are therefore regarded safe.[7] Similar principles and risk factors presumably apply to fine-needle aspirates or biopsies of the eye and periorbital structures. The globe should not be pierced.

NORMAL SONOGRAPHIC ANATOMY

Most eyes examined with ultrasound require scanning of structures caudal to the iris. The ciliary body, anterior and posterior lens capsules, lens, vitreous, retina, optic nerve, fundus, and retrobulbar space are structures that should be identified on each scan. These structures can be adequately visualized with the corneal contact technique (Fig. 18-1). A standoff device is necessary to image the structures rostral to the lens.

The anterior and posterior *lens capsules* are seen as parallel reflections of approximately equal amplitudes or intensities. The angle of incidence often has to be changed in small increments to see both lens capsules satisfactorily. The distance between the anterior and posterior lens capsules (ie, intercapsular distance) and the distance from the anterior or the posterior lens capsule to the caudal-most aspect of the eye should always be measured and compared with the other eye.

The normal *lens* should be anechoic; intralenticular echoes are considered consistent with cataracts, which are discussed in a subsequent section. The *ciliary body* should be examined in its entirety, looking for any masses, cysts, or asymmetry. Normally the ciliary body is relatively easy to image and has a homogeneous echo pattern that makes it easily differentiated from the adjacent lens. It is often necessary to direct the ultrasound beam away from midline to the nasal or temporal aspect of the ciliary body for a complete appreciation of it.

The *vitreous* should be anechoic and smoothly concave. An occasional incidental finding is visualization of a remnant of the hyaline artery, seen as a linear reflection extending from the fundus to the posterior lens capsule. Any other reflection from within the vitreous should be regarded with suspicion. Retrobulbar masses can often be seen distorting the smooth concavity of the vitreous; detached retinas are seen as linear reflections; and vitreous hemorrhage is visualized as a diffuse echo pattern that does not disrupt the normal shape of the vitreous unless the hemorrhage is subretinal.

The *retina* and *choroid* cannot be differentiated from each other and are seen as a smooth, echogenic line that follows the shape of the vitreous. Retrobulbar fluid or masses should not normally be seen. The optic nerve is seen as a wedge-shaped retrobulbar structure that terminates at the fundus but does not protrude into the vitreous.

DISEASES AND DISORDERS OF THE EYE

Cataracts

The normal lens is sonographically empty or anechoic; only the anterior and posterior lens capsules are visualized as reflective surfaces. Cataracts are seen as increased intralenticular

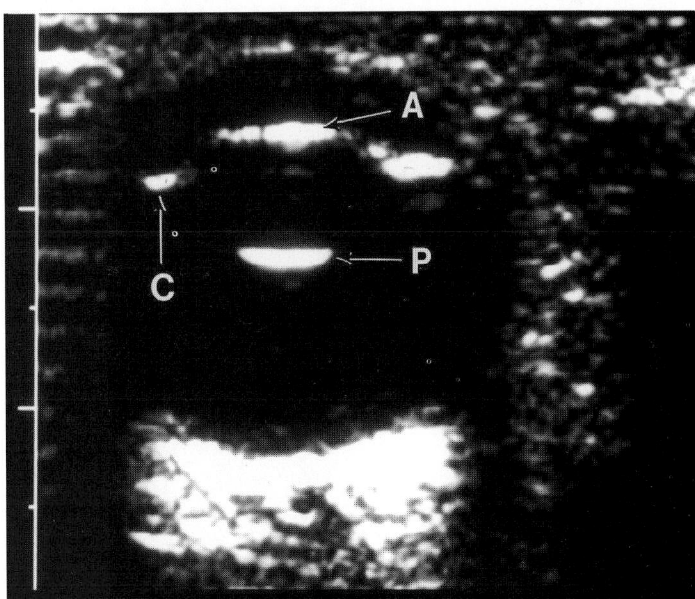

Figure 18-1. A transversely oriented sonogram of a normal eye. The anterior (*A*) and posterior (*P*) lens capsules are well visualized, as is the ciliary body (*C*). The vitreous is anechoic and smoothly concave in the far field. The optic nerve is situated at the 6 o'clock position.

echoes (Fig. 18-2). These echoes originate from abnormal tissue components that have acoustic impedances different from that of normal lens tissue. The anterior and posterior lens capsules are more echogenic and therefore more easily visualized than normal lenses.[2,8] The examiner should take care to evaluate the retinas of patients with cataracts before recommending cataract surgery; an eye with a detached retina is not a good candidate for cataract surgery (Fig. 18-3).

Lens Displacement

Luxation or subluxation of the lens can occur after trauma, as a result of severe inflammatory changes, or secondary to neoplasia. The lens often maintains its normal shape, helping the sonographer in finding a posteriorly luxated lens in the vitreous. A luxated cataractous lens is easily seen with ultrasound (Fig. 18-4).

Ciliary Body Lesions

Tumors and cysts arising from the ciliary body can be visualized with ultrasound. Neoplasia is seen as irregularly shaped masses with a mixed echo pattern. Ciliary body tumors can precipitate cataracts, luxate or subluxate the lens, or cause a retinal detachment. Examples of melanoma (Fig. 18-5) and adenocarcinoma (Fig. 18-6) of the ciliary body are illustrated. Ciliary body cysts tend to be more anechoic.[3,9]

Vitreous Hemorrhage

Head trauma is the most common cause of vitreous hemorrhage. The vitreous is normally anechoic, but hemorrhage into the vitreous changes its acoustic nature by producing multiple, small, nonspecular echoes (see Fig. 18-6). The echo pattern of the hemorrhage can vary considerably, depending on the amount of free blood present and the stage of hematoma formation or resolution. Classically, hematomas have a mixed echo pattern caused by elements with different reflective qualities. Eye or head movement can cause these echoes to move freely, thereby differentiating them from vitreous membranes.[3]

Detached Retina

Most retinal detachments are actually intraretinal in nature, because the separation develops

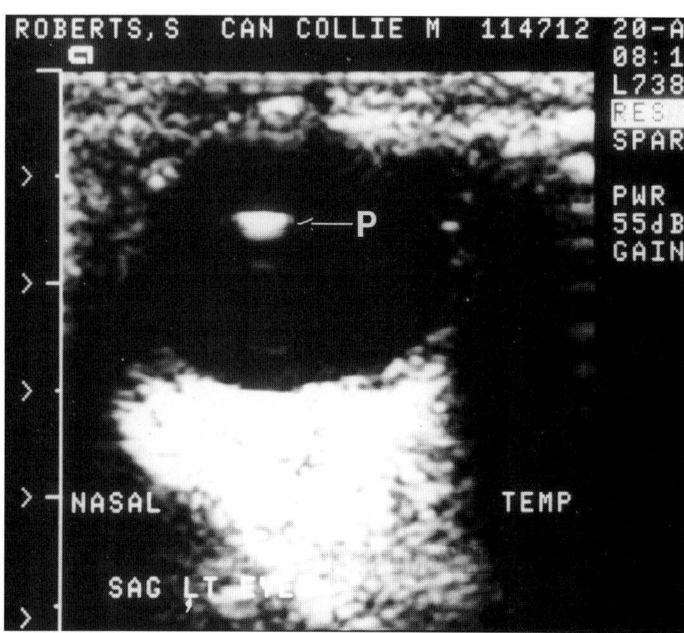

Figure 18-2. A sagittal sonogram of the left eye, demonstrating increased echogenicity of the posterior lens capsule (*P*). The diagnosis was a cataract.

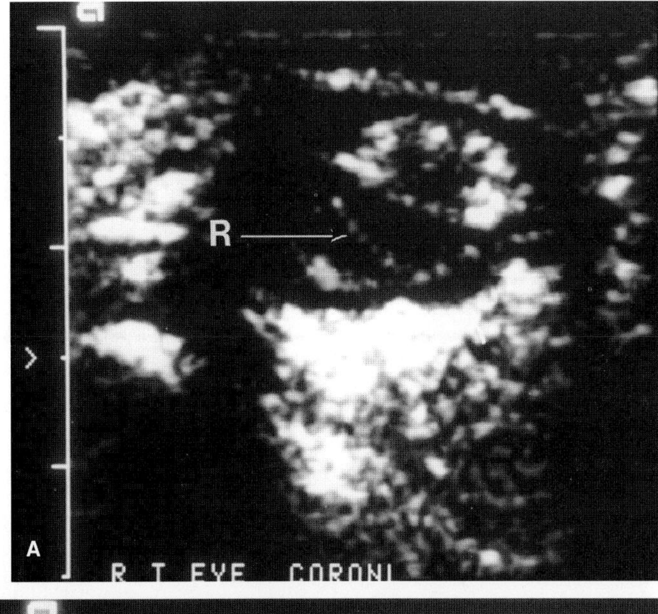

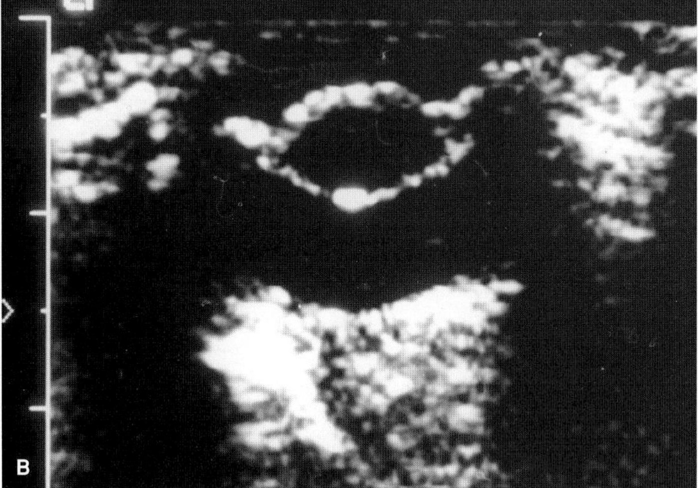

Figure 18-3. This patient presented for bilateral cataract surgery. (**A and B**) Increased echoes from the lens capsules of both eyes are seen, consistent with cataracts. The diagnosis was bilateral cataracts and a detached retina (*R*) in the right eye.

between the sensory retina and the retinal pigment epithelium. Bullous retinal detachments occur when fluid and cells enter this potential space, as in choroiditis, malignancies, hemorrhage, hypertension, and hyperviscosity syndrome. Traction retinal detachments occur after trauma or hemorrhage, when fibrous bands develop between the retina and the vitreous. These fibrous bands can loosen the retina by traction. Rhegmatogenous detachments occur when liquefied vitreous exudes into the subretinal space.[3,10]

A detached retina, often still attached at the fundus (Figs. 18-7 through 18-9), can be visualized as an echogenic linear structure in the vitreous. If the retina is detached on both sides of the fundus, a classic gull-wing–appearing structure may be seen. Increased echoes can be seen

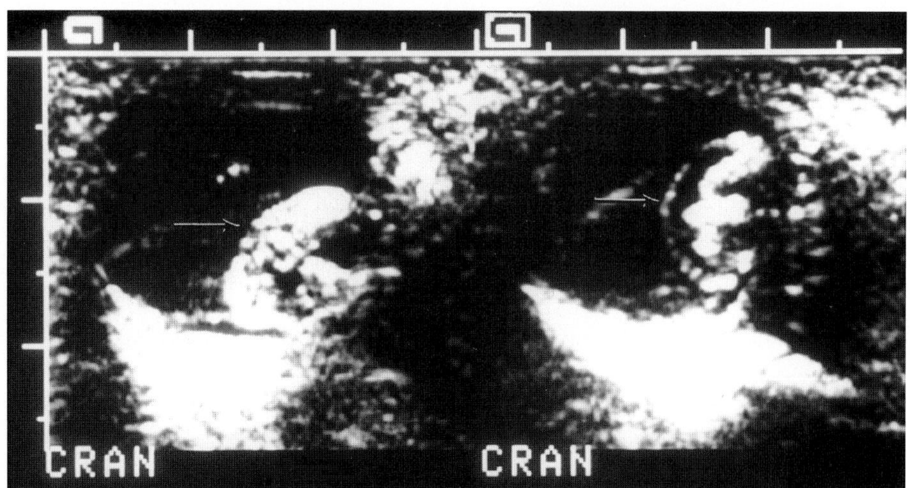

Figure 18-4. Transverse sonograms of both eyes of this dog demonstrate bilateral lens luxations (*arrows*). The lenses also have cataracts, enhancing their visualization.

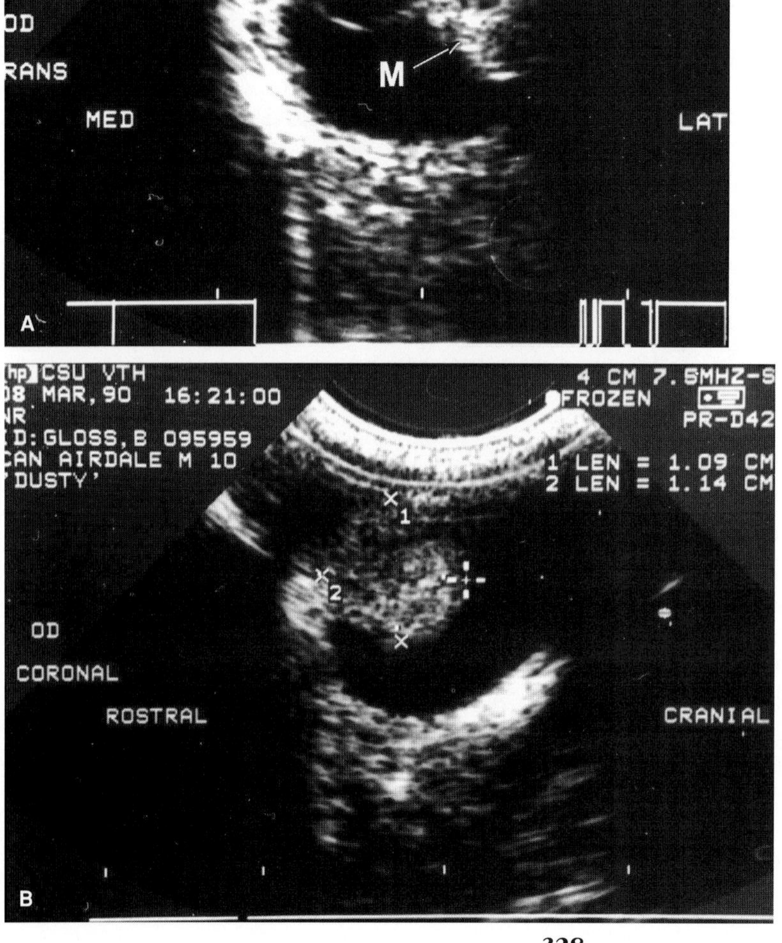

Figure 18-5. A 10-year-old intact male Airedale terrier presents with an intraocular mass in the right eye. The lens has been displaced by the echogenic mass (*M*). (**A**) The lens and the vitreous are within normal sonographic limits. (**B**) On the coronal image, the mass is well defined and measures 1.09 × 1.14 cm. No sonographic evidence is seen of retrobulbar extension of the mass. The diagnosis was ciliary body melanoma.

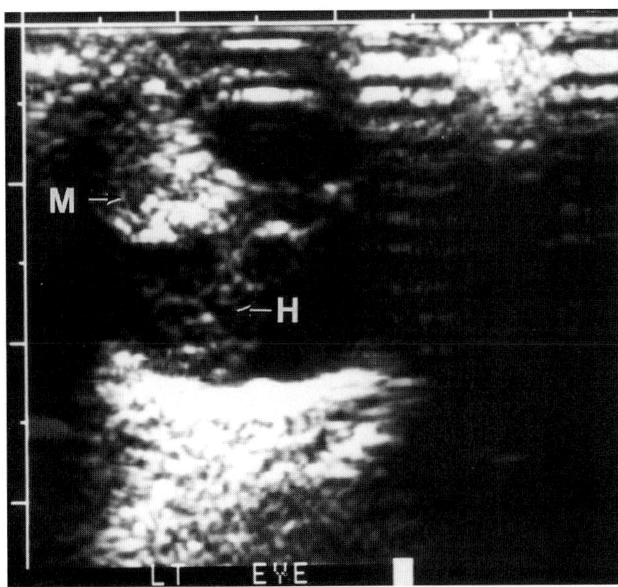

Figure 18-6 A hyperechoic mass (*M*) displacing the lens is seen in the ciliary body. The increased echoes (*H*) in the vitreous are compatible with hemorrhage. The diagnosis was ciliary body adenocarcinoma.

in cases of hemorrhage into or fibrosis of the vitreous.

Surgical intervention is a very important option in the treatment of cataracts. However, the prognosis is less favorable if the patient has a concomitant detached retina. Retinal function can be evaluated under general anesthesia by performing electroretinography, but this technique has been known to give false-negative results. Ultrasound is a noninvasive method of evaluating the integrity of the retina in patients with cataracts without having to use general anesthesia. This method enhances the accuracy of diagnosing a detached retina, thereby enhancing the accuracy of the prognosis for cataract surgery.[8]

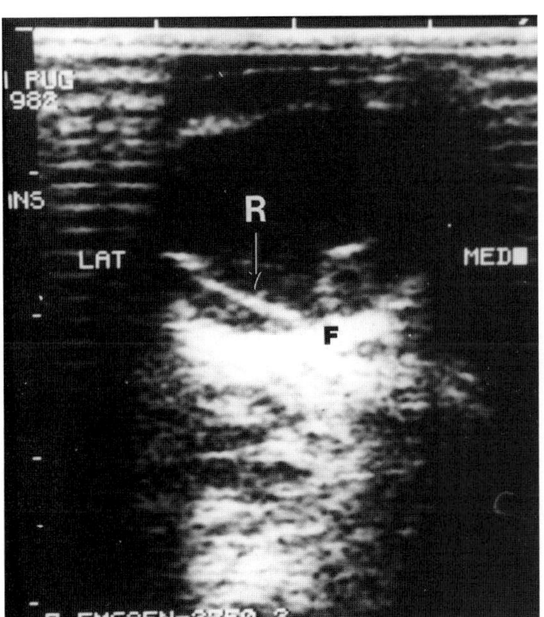

Figure 18-7 The classic sonographic sign of a detached retina is a "gull wing" sign. The retina (*R*) is still attached at the fundus (*F*).

Papilledema and Papillitis

Papilledema and papillitis are seen as a convex protrusion of the intrascleral portion of the optic nerve into the vitreous. These conditions are difficult to differentiate.

Foreign Bodies

Ultrasound is a sensitive method for detecting foreign bodies in the eye (Fig. 18-10). Foreign bodies are often not seen on direct ophthalmic examination because they are surrounded by blood or embedded in the tissue of the iris. Studies using a 10-MHz transducer show that small ($1.0 \times 0.5 \times 0.3$ mm) plastic, metal, and glass foreign bodies can be detected. The metallic and

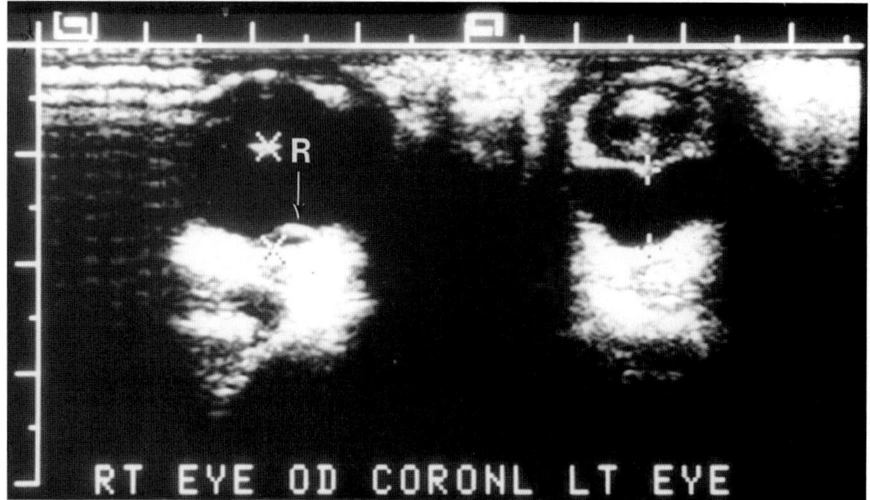

Figure 18-8. This 12-year-old cairn terrier presented with bilateral blindness. The diagnosis was severe cataract in the left eye and a mild detached retina (*R*) in the right eye.

glass foreign bodies demonstrate a reverberation artifact (ie, comet-tail pattern) because they are such strong reflectors and absorb very little sound. Plastic foreign bodies absorb more of the ultrasound beam, which results in an acoustic shadow.[11,12]

Retrobulbar Disease

Patients with retrobulbar disease usually present with exophthalmos, decreased retropulsion, or nonretropulsion, and they may demonstrate some degree of difficulty in opening the mouth.

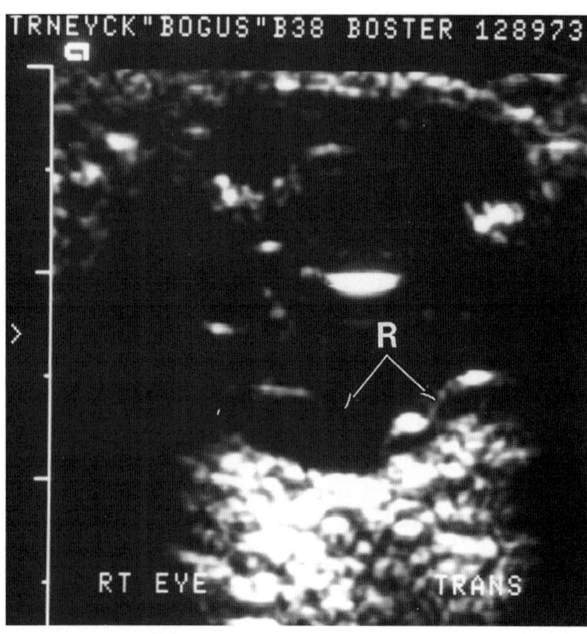

Figure 18-9. The detached retina (*R*) is not seen in its entirety on this image, because the angle of incidence is not optimal for visualization of some portions. The increased echoes of the posterior lens capsule are caused by a cataract.

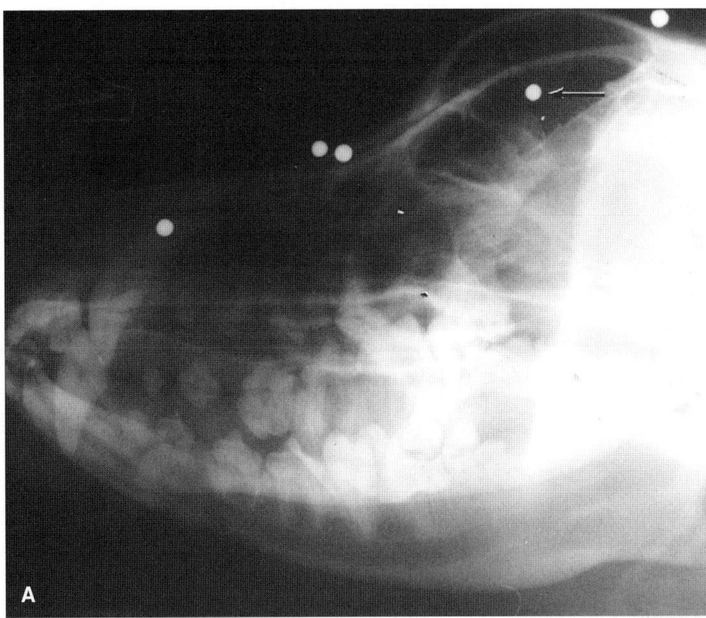

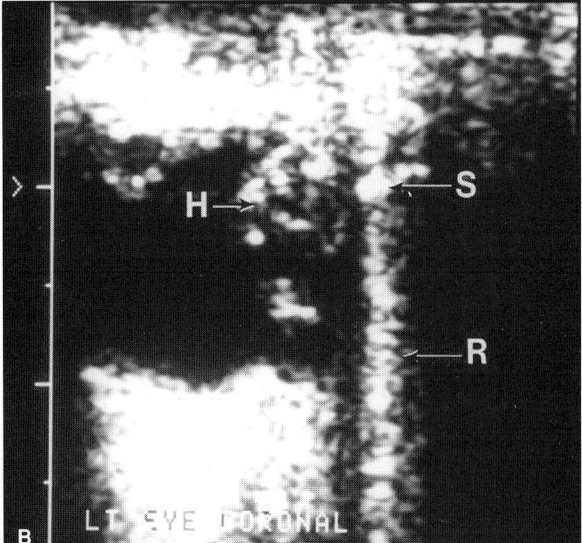

Figure 18-10. (**A**) The lateral radiograph of a dog's skull shows several metal densities (bird shot), one of which (*arrow*) is thought to be potentially within the orbit. (**B**) The sonogram of this dog's left eye shows a hyperechoic structure (*S*) that demonstrates reverberation artifact (*R*) in the far field. The diagnosis was a foreign body (bird shot) and hematoma (*H*).

Sonographic signs of retrobulbar disease include a convex deformity of the caudal aspect of the globe, nonvisualization of the optic nerve that is often associated with increased echogenicity of the retrobulbar region, well-defined hypoechoic masses in the retrobulbar region, and well-defined hyperechoic retrobulbar masses that deform the globe (Figs. 18-11 and 18-12).

Neoplastic masses tend to be well defined and hyperechoic, although much variation exists. Malignancies do not always deform the caudal aspect of the globe. Cellulitis tends to present as a diffuse nondeforming hypoechoic lesion.[5,13] Retrobulbar abscesses are visualized as relatively well-described hypoechoic masses and often result in a convex deformity of the

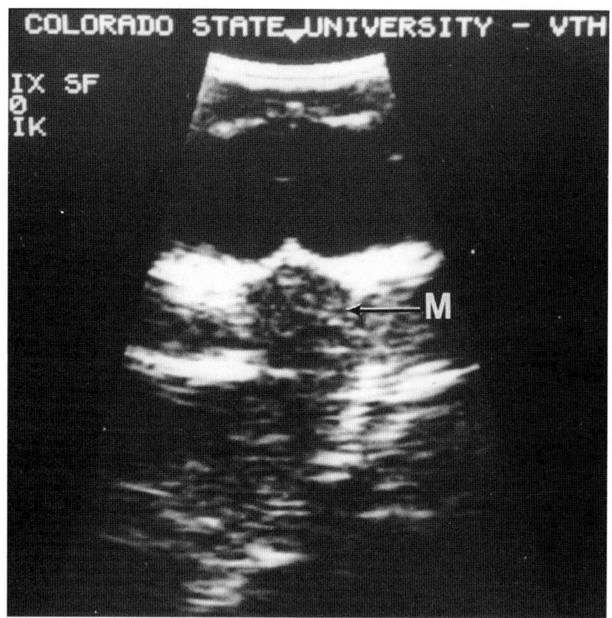

Figure 18-11. A hypoechoic mass (*M*) with a rather homogenous consistency is in the retrobulbar space, displacing the vitreous rostrally. The diagnosis was optic nerve meningioma.

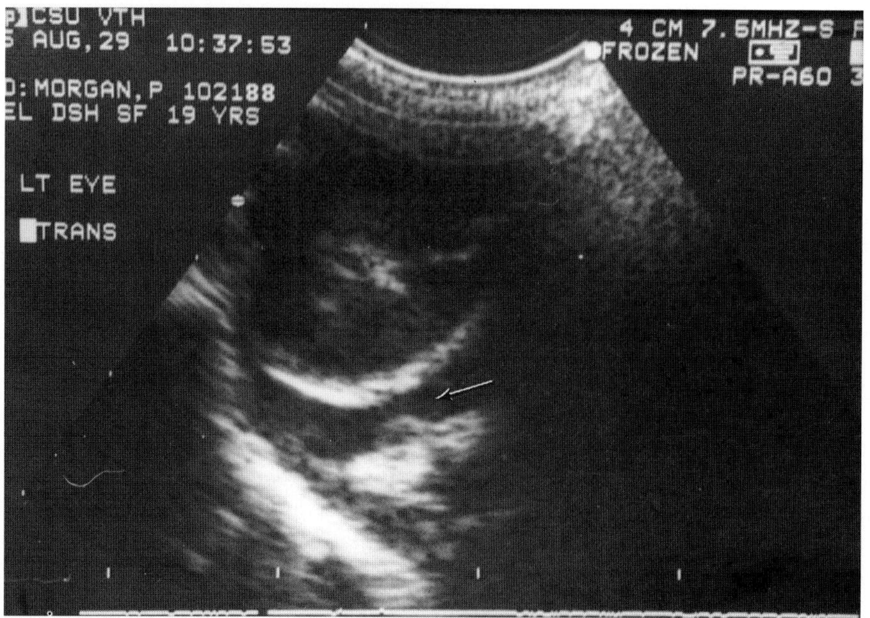

Figure 18-12. A diffuse homogenous retrobulbar echo pattern (*arrow*) and diffuse increased echoes of the vitreous are visualized in this 19-year-old domestic short-hair cat with a pyogranulomatous panophthalmitis.

vitreous.[14] An optic nerve meningioma was described as a well-defined hypoechoic mass that deformed the globe and caused poor visualization of the optic nerve.[15]

SPECIAL IMAGING TECHNIQUES

Doppler Flow Studies

The blood flow to optic masses can be studied with Doppler ultrasound. The velocity of ophthalmic blood flow has been determined in human subjects.[16,17]

Contrast Studies

Contrast agents that have been developed for echocardiographic work have demonstrated contrast enhancement in the orbit, choroid, and ciliary body in dogs' eyes. These agents also permit evaluation of intraocular blood flow. Although most ultrasound contrast studies are still in the experimental stages, their use in ophthalmology should enhance the evaluation of tissues of the uveal tract, which are usually poorly echogenic.[18]

CONCLUSION

The eye is easily accessible for sonography, and the vitreous provides an acoustic window for the observation of the structures in the eye. Ultrasound provides an excellent way to evaluate the internal structures of the eye, especially when direct observation is not possible because of hyphema, hypopyon, or cataracts. Sonography is also a good way to evaluate structures behind the eye, such as retrobulbar abscesses, tumors, and foreign bodies.

REFERENCES

1. Schiffer SP, Rantanen NW, Leary GW, Bryan GM. Biometric study of the canine eye, using A-mode ultrasonography. Am J Vet Res 1982;43:826.
2. Dziezyc J, Hager DA. Ocular ultrasonography in veterinary medicine. Semin Vet Med Surg (Small Anim) 1988;3:1.
3. Dziezyc J, Hager DA, Millichamp NJ. Two-dimensional real-time ocular ultrasonography in the diagnosis of ocular lesions in dogs. J Am Anim Hosp Assoc 1987;23:501.
4. Hager DA, Dziezyc J, Millichamp NJ. Two-dimensional real-time ocular ultrasonography in the dog. Technique and normal anatomy. Vet Radiol 1987;28:60.
5. Bryne SF. Standardized echography of the eye and orbit. Neuroradiology 1986; 28:618.
6. Susal AL, Gaynon W, Walker JT. Linear array multiple transducer examination of the eye. Ophthalmology 1983;90:266.
7. Livragh T, Damascelli B, Lombardi C, Spangnoli I. Risk in fine-needle abdominal biopsy. J Clin Ultrasound 1983;11:77.
8. Van der Woerdt A, Wilkie DA, Myer W. Ultrasonographic abnormalities of dogs with cataracts: 147 cases (1986–1992). J Am Vet Med Assoc 1993;203:838.
9. Coleman DJ, Lizzi FL, Jack RL. Ultrasonography of the eye and orbit. Philadelphia: Lea & Febiger, 1977.
10. Dziezyc J, Wolf D, Barrie KP. Surgical repair of rhegmatogenous retinal detachments in dogs. J Am Vet Med Assoc 1986;188:902.
11. Nouby-Mahmoud G, Silverman RH, Coleman DJ. Ophthalmic surgery 1993; 24:94.
12. Sassani JW, Peart RE, Haak NW, Hodes BL. Combined use of A-scan ultrasound, plain roentgenograms, and computerized axial tomography in the evaluation of a pseudo-intraocular foreign body. J Clin Ultrasound 1984;12:171.
13. Morgan RV. Ultrasonography of retrobulbar diseases of the dog and cat. J Am Anim Hosp Assoc 1989;25:393.
14. Miller WW, Cartee RE. B-scan ultrasonography for the detection of the space-occupying ocular masses. J Am Vet Med Assoc 1985;187:66.
15. Abrams K, Toal R T. What's your diagnosis? J Am Vet Med Assoc 1990;196:951.

16. Williamson TH, Baster G, Paul R, Dutom GN. Colour doppler ultrasound in the management of a case of cranial arteritis. Br J Ophthalmol 1992;76:690.
17. Rojamapongpun P, Drance SM. Velocity of ophthalmic arterial flow recorded by doppler ultrasound in normal subjects. Am J Ophthalmol 1993;115: 174.
18. Miszalok V, Fritsch T, Wollensak J. Contrast echography of the eye and orbit. Ophthalmologica 1986;193:231.

Small Animal Ultrasound, edited by Ronald W. Green.
Lippincott-Raven Publishers, Philadelphia © 1996.

MUSCULOSKELETAL SYSTEM

Charles S. Farrow

The musculoskeletal system is composed of muscle, bone, cartilage, and the specialized connective tissues of tendons, ligaments, fascia, and aponeuroses. The system is maintained, coordinated, and controlled by a complex network of blood vessels and nerves. Individual component parts or the entire system may become diseased, although most injuries typically affect a single region.

Of the various elements that comprise the musculoskeletal system, muscle is the most amenable to sonographic diagnosis. If the part or lesion in question is large enough, tendons, ligaments, joints, and periarticular swellings may also be investigated sonographically. Bone is not well suited to sonographic study.

The objectives of musculoskeletal sonography are to answer the following questions:[1]

- Is a lesion present?
- If so, where is it located?
- How extensive is it?
- What is its nature?
- Does the lesion change with time?

This chapter is divided into four sections: muscle, tendon, ligament, and joint. Muscle-tendon origin tears are included under the heading of muscle avulsion, and muscle-tendon insertion injuries are discussed under the heading of tendon avulsion. This categorization is not entirely accurate, because many muscles possess small but discrete tendons at their origins. Nevertheless, such a scheme lends itself to a clearer functional view of musculotendinous injuries, an important prerequisite to successful sonographic diagnosis.

MUSCLES

Skeletal muscle, also called voluntary muscle, is responsible for skeletal movement and support. It is composed of striped muscle fibers arranged parallel or oblique to the long axis of the muscle. When contraction occurs, the muscle shortens to one half or one third of its original, resting length. Motion is achieved by the application of muscular force to bones and joints; the joints function as levers and fulcra.[2]

Associated dense connective tissues related to muscular form and function include fascia, aponeuroses, and tendons. Fascia are thin sheets of tissue that cover muscles and maintain their shape and position. An aponeurosis is a thin, tendinous tissue used to attach flat muscles. A tendon is an extension of muscle that attaches the muscle to bone. The point at which the muscle and tendon join is called the musculotendinous junction.

After trauma, skeletal muscle compensates for tissue damage and loss by a combination of hypertrophy and, to a lesser extent, regeneration. Muscle also has a large capacity to reabsorb extravasated blood and typically heals with relatively little scar tissue. Muscle tissue is relatively resistant to infection and malignant disease.[3]

Scanning Technique

Of great importance when scanning for a particular muscular disorder, especially an injury, is to thoroughly know the anatomy. It is important to know the origin, insertion, and action of the muscle or muscle group under investigation.[4] Those unfamiliar with the normal muscular anatomy of the region should scan the opposite side first and use it as a basis for comparison.

If possible, the injured or diseased muscles should be scanned in the active and resting states. This is especially true of leg muscles, which may appear very different in standing and in recumbent animals. It is also advisable to flex and extend the damaged muscle as part of the routine examination to expose lesions not detectable in static studies. Scanning an injured muscle or muscle group during flexion and extension often enables an examiner to estimate the extent of functional damage to the associated limb.

A 7.5-MHz transducer (without a standoff device) is preferable for most examinations of the thigh region and brachium. For examining large dogs, a 5-MHz transducer is often necessary to image deeper muscles. For scanning the crus and antebrachium, a standoff may be required, especially for viewing superficially located lesions.

Two of the biggest problems in sonographically examining muscle injuries are animals that do not hold still and chronic lesions. In dogs that refuse to lie still, the musculature is constantly changing because of repeated contraction and relaxation, making imaging difficult. This problem can sometimes be alleviated by performing the examination while the dog stands. If this method is unsuitable, tranquilization or sedation should be used. Analgesia is a necessity when examining most acute injuries.

Many chronic lesions, although clearly debilitating, may be sonographically undetectable. Although probably the result of a combination of factors, this difficulty usually is the result of not looking in the right place or not appreciating abnormal muscular anatomy. These difficulties may be remedied in part by reviewing the relevant muscles with respect to their origins, insertions, size, shape, and function. Questionable lesions should be confirmed by examining the opposite limb or side.

Sonographic Protocol for Muscle Injury

Before Sonography. Before the examination, the practitioner should review regional muscular anatomy and function. It is important to examine radiographs of the injury site, checking for a fracture, dislocation, soft tissue swelling, or deficit. The examiner must be particularly vigilant in looking for small chip fractures that indicate an avulsion-type injury. Positive findings often indicate the injury site. Muscle calcification can indicate chronic injuries.

The clinician must visually examine the injured limb by comparing it with the normal opposite leg. The examiner palpates, flexes, and extends the normal leg and then performs the same examination on the injured limb, paying particular attention to the comparative tension in the individual muscles of each leg and any difference in the range of relative limb movement. An elevation in surface temperature often reflects underlying inflammation.

During Sonography. The sonographer inspects the musculature for edema, hemorrhage, and hematoma. The dependent aspects of all major fascial planes are checked for dispersed hemorrhage and edema. The examiner establishes the integrity of the muscle origin, body, musculotendinous junction, and insertion. If possible, the injury site is examined while the animal is weight bearing. The individual parts of the injured muscles are reexamined during flexion and extension.

Normal Sonographic Anatomy and Indications

Normal skeletal muscle possesses a distinctive sonographic appearance, exhibiting a relatively hypoechoic background with a foreground pattern composed of moderately spaced hyperechoic spindles. The bounding fascia is typically represented by brilliant, broad bands that run parallel to the long axis of the limb, except proximally, where considerable muscular obliquity exists (Fig. 19-1).

Sonographic guidance is potentially useful for locating masses for biopsies, draining abscesses, and obtaining fluid from cavitary lesions. It may also be employed to guide a biopsy needle exactly to a particular location within a muscle. Ultrasound is superior to computed tomography and fluoroscopic guidance with respect to cost, safety, and procedure time. Sonographic localization is preferable to simple palpation because of its greater precision and ability to avoid major vessels. It also results in fewer needle passes and less pain.[5]

Disorders and Diseases

Exercise-Induced Muscle Injury

When a muscle is used in an unusual way, especially if done so repeatedly, soreness often develops 24 to 48 hours afterward. Overuse may also result in a nagging muscle soreness, which is most evident the day after the inciting activity. This type of muscle soreness is usually associated with normal sonographic findings. Stress fractures, although rare in dogs, may result in a similar patient profile.

Atrophy

Muscle atrophy most often results from reduced use or disuse of an injured or diseased limb. Although reduced in volume, the affected muscle is otherwise indistinguishable from normal. Severe osteoarthritis, particularly that caused by hip dysplasia, is often seen in conjunction with atrophy of the thigh muscles. Casting and internal surgical fixation, especially if prolonged, may cause posttraumatic osteoporosis, a generalized demineralization of the bone, at and distal to the injury site.[6]

Atrophy may also stem from a denervating disease or injury, which aside from a reduction in muscle mass, causes no change in sonographic appearance.

Bruise

Muscle bruising (ie, contusion) is a common injury in dogs and cats that have been hit by cars. It is caused by intramuscular bleeding, primarily from capillaries. The increased intramuscular pressure resulting from the hemorrhage,

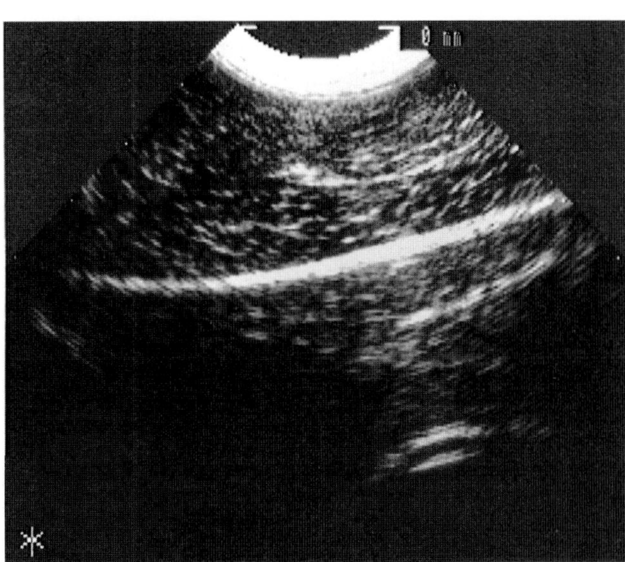

Figure 19-1. Sector scan (long section) of normal canine quadriceps muscle.

combined with the restrictive effect of the fascia, exert a compression effect on the damaged vessels, usually stopping the bleeding within a few minutes. As the hemorrhage subsides, the escaped blood begins to dissipate into the adjacent intercellular space. These events may be observed sonographically, initially as a spreading area of decreased echogenicity and loss of usual echotexture and later as a more generalized reduction in echogenicity.

Hematoma

Hematomas may be intramuscular or intermuscular in nature (Fig. 19-2). The development of an intramuscular hematoma requires a rapid or sustained internal blood loss. The process is accelerated by accompanying tissue cavitation. Residual scarring may cause chronic pain and lead to reinjury.[7] Rarely, if an intramuscular hematoma becomes large enough and if it develops enough pressure, it may cause regional ischemia, anoxia, and eventually necrosis. This is called compartment or compartmental syndrome.[8]

Sonographically observed lesions compatible with hemorrhagic compartmentalization typically appear as discrete, oval or circular, anechoic, hypoechoic or mixed-echoic structures in displaced or damaged muscle. Such lesions are often located adjacent to or surrounding a large artery. In one report, a large fluid-filled capsule, containing a hematoma and characterized sonographically by alternating echoic and anechoic rings radiating outwardly from a blood vessel, was removed from the thigh of a dog with compartment syndrome.[9]

Hematomas may also arise externally near the fascial sheaths or large intermuscular septa (Fig. 19-3). In these locations, the hematoma tends to migrate distally, affording a greater surface area on which the cleanup process may take place. The wider distribution of the extravasated blood also serves to minimize potentially dangerous pressure effects. An intermuscular hematoma usually is a less serious injury than an intramuscular hemorrhage and usually heals more promptly.

Sonographically, a hematoma may assume a variety of appearances. Initially, a hematoma appears anechoic and relatively well circumscribed. In the next few days, the hematoma gradually becomes more echoic and textured (Figs. 19-4 and 19-5). After 1 or 2 weeks, some hematomas become hyperechoic; others disappear. Although the sonographic progression of hematomas is predictable, the rate at which these changes occur varies widely, and it may be difficult to determine the age of a hematoma accurately.

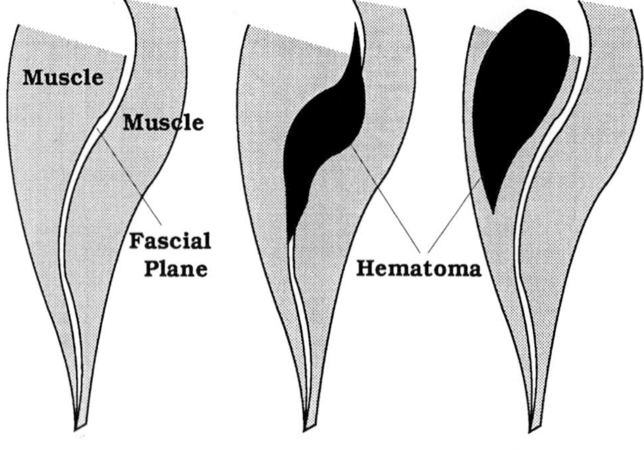

Figure 19-2. Potential distribution of a muscular hemorrhage.

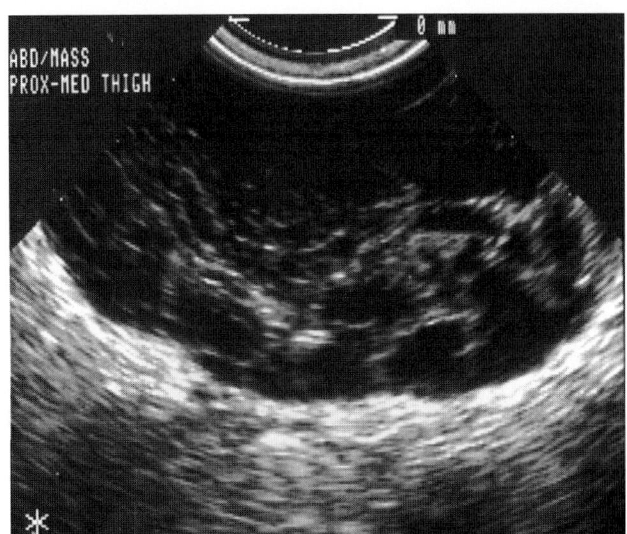

Figure 19-3. Sector scan (cross section) of canine quadriceps shows a 24-hour-old hematoma.

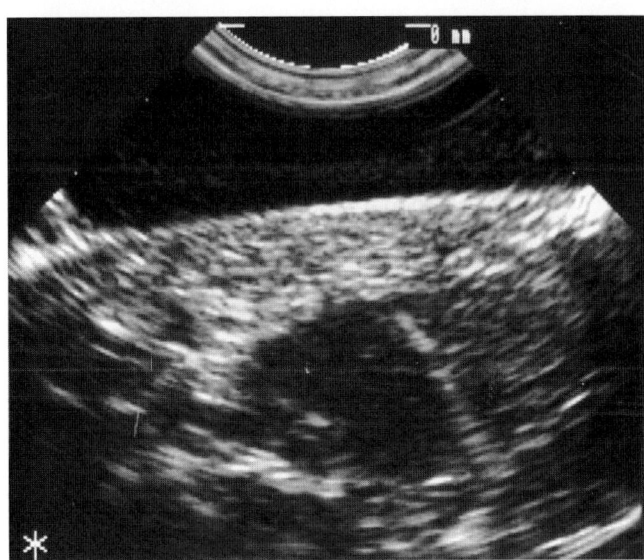

Figure 19-4. Sector scan (long section) of the author's middle inner forearm shows a 10-hour-old hematoma and the artery (lower left) that gave rise to it. The injury was caused by a slash from a hockey stick just above the glove.

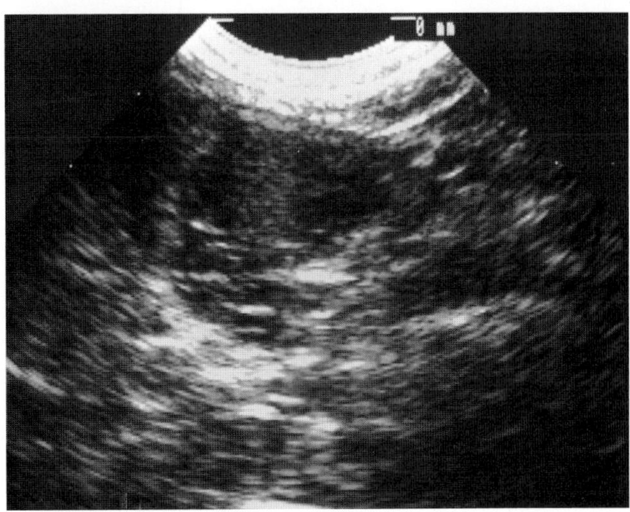

Figure 19-5. One-week recheck of the hematoma shown in Figure 19-3 shows increased, variably structured echogenicity through much of the lesion.

Strain

Muscle tearing is usually described according to severity. Contemporary classification schemes describe muscle tears qualitatively as being mild, moderate, or severe in degree (Fig. 19-6).[10] A complete separation is called a rupture, unless it occurs at the origin or insertion of the muscle, in which case it is called an avulsion. Large impacts often result in a combination of strain and contusion (Fig. 19-7).

Avulsion

Muscle avulsions occur occasionally in nonracing dogs and only rarely in cats. Tearing may occur at the origin or insertion of a muscle-tendon unit, but it tends to be specific (ie, proximal or distal) for an individual muscle. When muscles avulse, they contract toward their uninjured portion, often causing a distinctive bulge and concavity in the leg surface. In a typical quadriceps avulsion, one or more muscle bellies contract proximally, often resulting in a distinctive bulge in the cranial part of the proximal thigh region. When the gastrocnemius muscle pulls free of the calcaneus, the Achilles tendon may "roll up" the caudal part of the crus, much like a sash cord, resulting in proximal bulging and distal thinning.

In the dog, avulsion of the origin of the extensor carpi radialis is associated with reduced flexion of the cubital joint, and depending on the duration of the injury, localized bone deposition on the lateral epicondyle of the humerus. Avulsion of the medial head of the gastrocnemius muscle may be indicated radiographically by a lateral fabellar fracture.[11] Avulsion of the origin of the long digital extensor muscle from the extensor fossa on the lateral epicondyle has been reported, typically in conjunction with a displaced fracture fragment. All of these lesions are detectable sonographically, especially if seen shortly after the injury.

Greyhounds have their own group of race-related avulsion-type injuries. The most common involve the long head of the triceps, the gracilis, and the tensor fasciae latae.[12]

Infection and Abscess

Abscesses are usually localized initially, but they may eventually become regional if their content reaches adjacent fascial planes. *Actinomyces* infection may cause extensive communicating cavitation (Fig. 19-8). Nearby joints may be secondarily infected, or conversely, a hematogenously infected joint may initiate infection in the periarticular tissues, especially in puppies and kittens.

A variety of abscesses have been observed in dogs, cats, horses, and farm animals; some are anechoic, and others display different degrees of

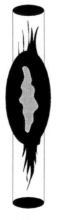

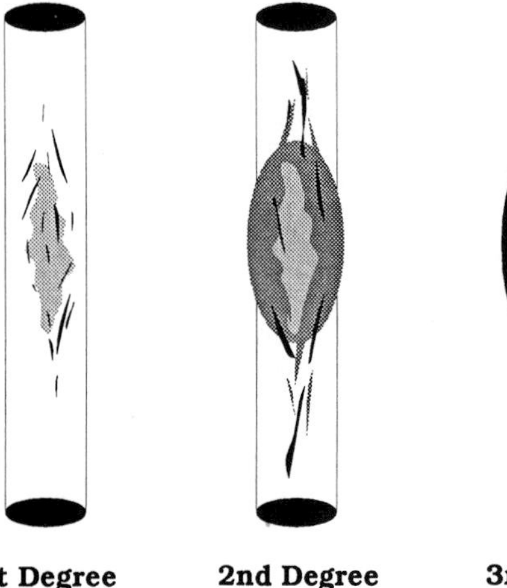

Figure 19-6 Muscle and tendon injuries are called strains and are described qualitatively according to the severity and extent of the injury. A recent first-degree strain is characterized by a slight reduction in echogenicity. A recent second-degree injury results in a moderate drop in echogenicity, accompanied by increased spacing of the spindle-shaped elements that comprise the normal echotexture of the damaged muscle or tendon. Localized or regional swelling and a discrete hematoma may also be present. A recent third-degree injury exhibits the features of a second-degree injury, but on a larger scale. Overt discontinuity often exists, and there are usually secondary hemorrhage and edema in the surrounding deep fascial planes, especially distally.

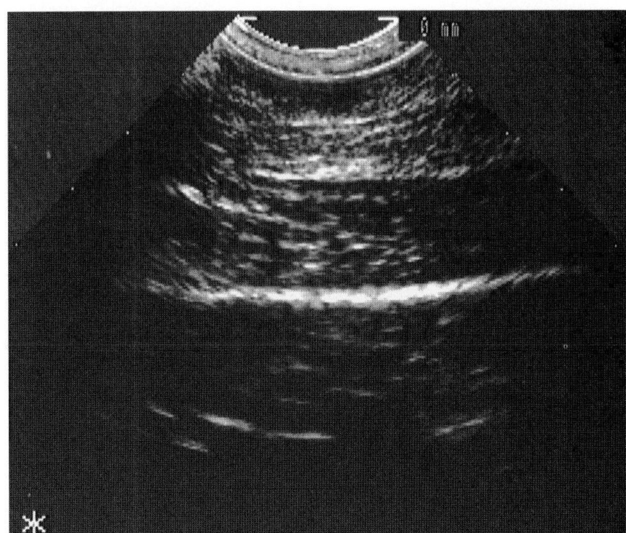

Figure 19-7 Sector scan of canine quadriceps shows the sonographic features of a third-degree strain: enlargement, discontinuity, decreased echogenicity, textural change (spindle spreading), and hematoma. Compare this lesion with the normal canine quadriceps shown in Figure 19-1.

echogenicity. Some have discrete walls and others do not (Fig. 19-9). It appears that the echogenicity increases with the cellular density of the lesion. Published reports of muscle abscessation (principally in horses) have also described variable echogenicity and differences in wall thickness; the latter influences the success or failure of attempted biopsy.[13,14]

Occasionally, entire limbs or limb segments may become swollen. Where there are no external wounds and septicemia is suspected clinically, sonography may be employed to differentiate inflammatory edema from exudate (Fig. 19-10). Inguinal abscesses may be associated with various degrees of subcutaneous edema (Fig. 19-11).

Foreign Body

In some small animal practices, embedded porcupine quills are the most common intramuscular foreign body. Less commonly, foxtails

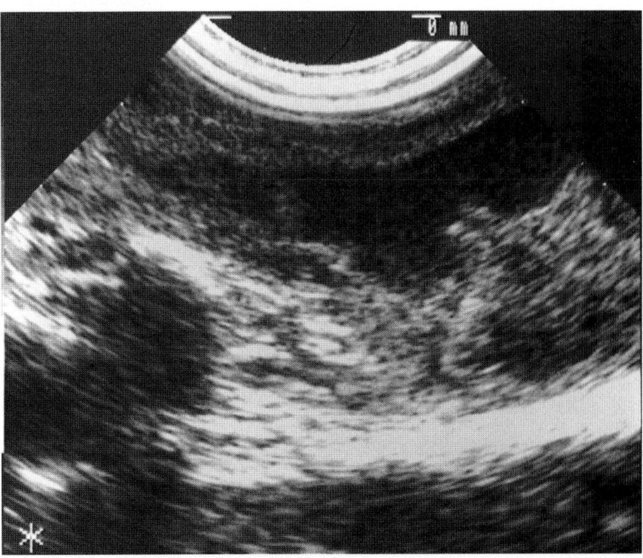

Figure 19-8. Sector scan of a canine lateral thigh region leg shows a granular hypoechoic band extending across the near field, which contains a large, horizontally oriented fluid pocket (ie, pus in necrotic muscle). A thick-walled *Actinomyces* lesion is located in the far right midfield.

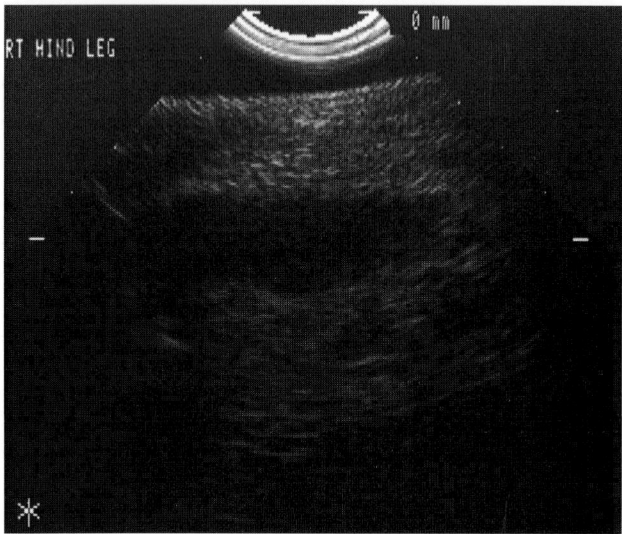

Figure 19-9. Sector scan of a canine caudolateral gastrocnemius muscle shows a deep ovoid hypoechoic abscess secondary to a puncture wound.

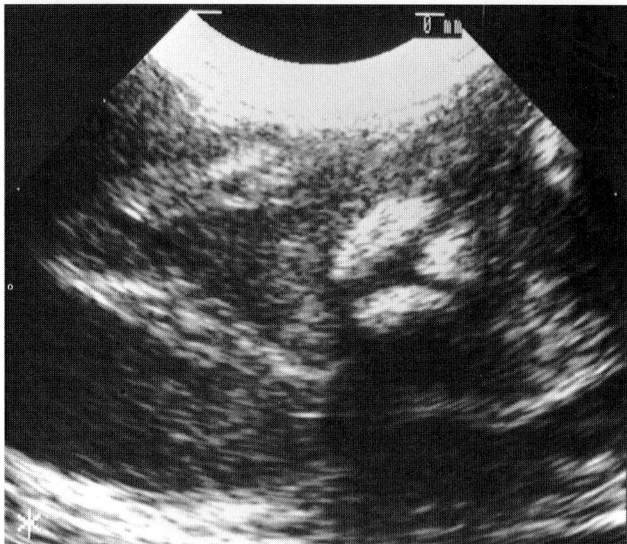

Figure 19-10. Sector scan of a puppy's genual joint in cross section shows intense acoustic shadowing by the hyperechoic ossification centers of the distal femur. Granular-appearing pus, the result of a widespread hematogenous infection, surrounds the bone and joint but does not enter it.

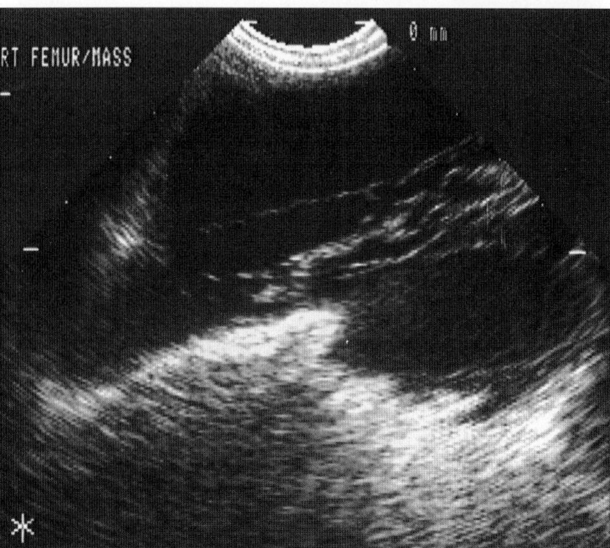

Figure 19-11. Sector scan of a dog's inguinal region shows a large, ovoid, hypoechoic abscess in the right midfield with extensive, overlying subcutaneous edema.

become imbedded in the leg, often entering in the interdigital webs of the toes and then migrating proximally to the antebrachium or crus. Occasionally, a dog is impaled on a stake, which is removed but leaves behind one or two fragments. Bullets and airgun and shotgun pellets are usually suspected by their superficial wound characteristics and verified radiographically. Glass shards have been detected sonographically, which were radiographically invisible.

Foreign bodies located in muscle appear hyperechoic and are focal or linear, depending on their size and shape and on the transducer orientation (Fig. 19-12). Most are associated with artifacts: acoustic shadowing in the case of quills, wood slivers, plastic, and gravel; and reverberation (comet-tail pattern) in the case of metallic foreign bodies.[15] Shadowing is often not detectable when wood fragments, quills, or plant awns are surrounded by fluid, and reverberation is not visible when metallic foreign bodies are lying adjacent to bone (Fig. 19-13).

Fibrosis and Fibrositis

Occasionally, traumatized skeletal muscle undergoes fibrosis or scarring instead of healing. Depending on the extent of involvement, this replacement of muscle by connective tissue may reduce the muscle's ability to contract and the range of motion in the affected leg. Chronic pain associated with muscular fibrosis is called fibrositis.

Calcification

After single or repeated muscular trauma, especially to the thigh region, and sometimes after the formation of an intramuscular hematoma, calcification and later ossification occur within the connective tissue of the muscle. This condition is called myositis ossificans.[16]

Contracture

Contracture is a term used to describe the temporary or permanent shortening of a muscle during relaxation, usually causing reduced flexibility and range of motion in the affected leg. Most contractures seen in animals are the result of long-standing reduced or modified use of an arthritic limb, usually accompanied by marked muscular atrophy. For example, the thigh muscles of older dogs with advanced hip dysplasia and arthritis are often severely shrunken and tightened to the extent that the hind legs cannot be extended during radiography. In such dogs, a generalized increase in echogenicity compatible with fibrotic muscle has been observed.

Contracture of the quadriceps muscle in immature dogs after a midshaft femoral fracture has been theorized to be a form of avascular my-

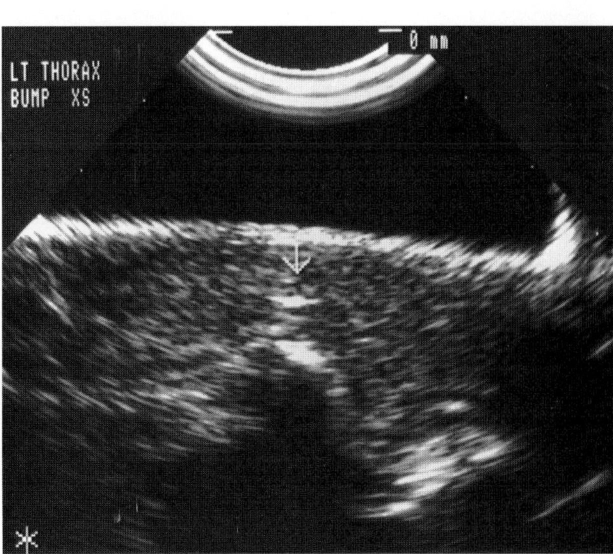

Figure 19-12. Sector scan of a canine thoracic wall shows a focal echogenicity (*arrow*) produced by a porcupine quill fragment embedded in the musculature of the thoracic wall just above a shadowing rib.

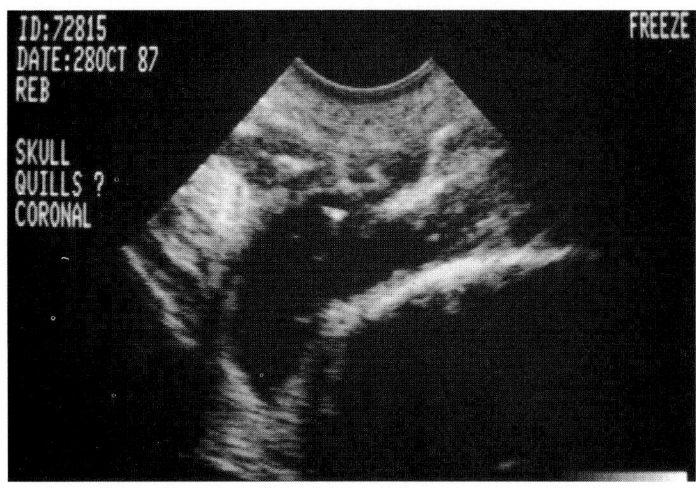

Figure 19-13. Sector scan of a canine cranium shows a small triangular echogenicity (porcupine quill) in the upper part of a crescent-shaped fluid pocket located along the cranial rim. A pair of communicating abscesses lie just above the quill.

opathy caused by injury to the cranial femoral artery.[17] Contractures have also been reported in young dogs that developed infection subsequent to attempted femoral repair.

Contracture of the infraspinatus, supraspinatus, and gracilis muscles have been reported in hunting dogs and pets.[18]

Tumor

Primary striated muscle tumors are rare. Benign muscle tumors are called rhabdomyomas, and malignancies are classified as rhabdomyosarcomas.[19] Local mesenchymal tumors such as fibrosarcoma and myxosarcoma may invade contiguous skeletal muscle (Fig. 19-14). Occasionally, fatty tumors develop deep within the leg between individual muscles and are called lipomas if benign and liposarcomas if cancerous. Metastatic muscular lymphoma and hemangiosarcoma are reported in the dog but are equally rare.[20]

Ultrasound is extremely accurate in determining the presence of medium and large muscular tumors. It can be reliably used to assess their actual size, volume, and configuration.

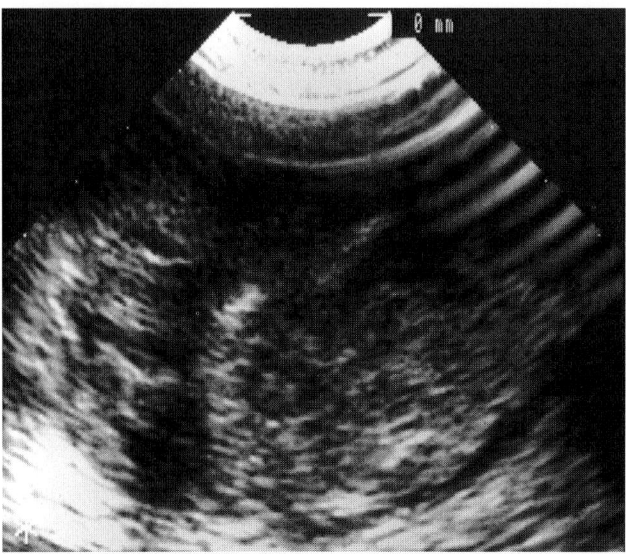

Figure 19-14. Sector scan of a canine caudal thigh region shows a well-circumscribed mass, thought to be a fibrosarcoma.

Most soft tissue tumors, including sarcomas, fibrous tumors, and tumors of neural sheath origin, are hypoechoic relative to surrounding normal tissues. Features suggesting malignancy include marginal irregularity, inhomogeneous echotexture, and evidence of muscle fiber rupture or infiltration of adjacent anatomic structures. Benignity is usually associated with a homogeneous echo pattern, even margination, and displacement or spreading of surrounding muscle tissue.[21]

TENDONS

Scanning Technique

Most tendons are best examined with the animal in a standing position using a 7.5-MHz transducer equipped with a standoff device. Small tendons may be examined with a 10-MHz scanner (with or without a standoff), if the animal remains still. A narrow field should be used wherever possible to improve image resolution.

When a mechanical sector scanner is used to image a tendon longitudinally, the resultant narrow, hyperechoic, vertically oriented artifactual band located centrally at the top of the near field should be reduced to a minimum by using the time-gain compensation controls.

In examining a tendon sonographically, the examiner must check for the size and shape, discontinuity, hemorrhage or edema, variable echotexture, fluid in the tendon sheath, and increased bursal volume.

After carefully examining a particular tendon, the practitioner must also check its muscular and junctional regions for additional lesions. If possible, he or she should gently flex and extend the injured limb and observe the movement of the injured muscle-tendon unit during contraction and relaxation.

Normal Sonographic Anatomy

Normal tendon is characterized sonographically by an internal pattern of fine parallel and linear echoes that become thinner and more numerous as transducer frequency increases. This distinctive echotexture is caused by specular reflections at the interface between collagen bundles and endotendineum septa.[22] Although tendons have a distinct, fluid-containing synovial sheath where they pass through osseous or fibrous groves (especially across joints), these parts are not normally observed sonographically. The same is also true of the peritonea, the connective tissue coat that surrounds the tendon.

Imaging in the longitudinal plane during relaxation may produce a false decrease in echogenicity in the outer thirds of the tendon because of surface concavity.

Disorders and Diseases

Strains

Strains are the most common form of tendinous injury. They are classified qualitatively according to increasing severity: first, second, and third degree. Complete discontinuity is called rupture.

Sonographically, tendon strains in cattle, sheep, and humans are characterized by combinations of changes in the normal fibrillar pattern: increased fibrillar thickness, interruption, fragmentation, and disappearance of echotexture.[17]

Analysis of the sonographic-histologic correlations for horses with tendon injuries of various severities and durations have shown that anechoic tendons represent recent hemorrhage, edema, and cellular infiltration; hypoechoic lesions corresponded to granulation and immature fibrous tissue, and mature fibrous tissue is relatively hyperechoic.[23] Another equine study correlated histologic, ultrasonic, and magnetic resonance imaging data and concluded that ultrasound images remained abnormal until fibrillar realignment occurred and the lesion had healed.[24]

Avulsion

Avulsion of the gastrocnemius tendon from its attachment on the tuber calcis is among the most common small animal tendon injuries. Most are second- or third-degree strains, and some are completely ruptured (Fig. 19-15). Al-

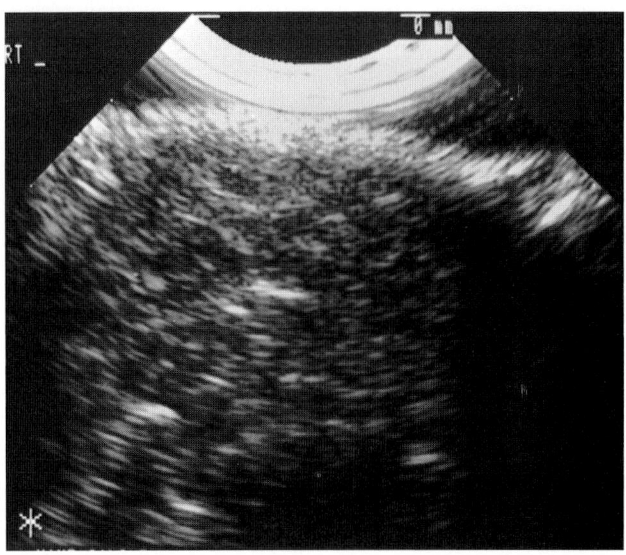

Figure 19-15. Sector scan of the distal aspect of a canine Achilles tendon (cross section) shows enlargement, decreased echogenicity, and altered echotexture (fibrillar spreading and thickening) compatible with a third-degree strain.

though some of these injuries are associated with a proximal calcaneal fracture, most are not. However, many chronic distal Achilles tendon strains are associated with chronic-appearing bone deposition on the proximal part of the tuber calcis.

Calcification

Metaplastic calcification has been reported in the supraspinatus tendon of dogs, and although sonography was not performed, such technology is probably capable of detecting these lesions.[25,26]

Dislocation

Dislocation of the tendon of the superficial digital flexor muscle was reported recently in 10 dogs, four of which were Shetland sheepdogs.[27] The injury was associated with acute lameness and swelling at the proximal aspect of the calcaneus. Eight of the dislocations were lateral, and two were medial. In another report of 12 dogs with a similar condition, the dislocation was thought to be caused by a shallow calcaneal groove, which was demonstrated radiographically.[28] The localized swelling was attributed to distention of the calcaneal bursa, something that could best be assessed sonographically. Although the diagnosis is usually based on the results of palpation, sonography may be used for confirmation (Fig. 19-16).

Bursitis

Bursitis is only infrequently a primary disorder in dogs. In most cases, a bursa becomes inflamed secondary to an associated tendonitis, which is typically brought about by overuse (eg, sled dogs, racing dogs). Bursitis may also be traumatic in origin, particularly when such structures are relatively unprotected because of their subsurface location.

Occasionally, a bursa becomes infected as a result of a puncture wound (including bite wounds) or as the result of the migration of infectious agents from a nearby communicating tendon sheath. Foreign bodies such as porcupine quills and foxtails sometimes find their way into a bursal cavity, where they may precipitate a suppurative bursitis.

Bursal calcification of the greater trochanter of the femur has been described and is usually bilateral.[29] Both the cause and effect (if any) of this finding is speculative.

LIGAMENTS

Scanning Technique

Generally speaking, ligaments, because of their relatively small, flat shape and because of their proximity to bone are difficult to scan in dogs

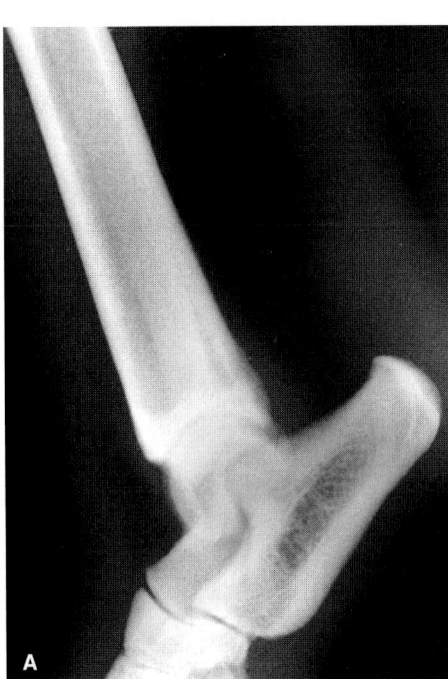

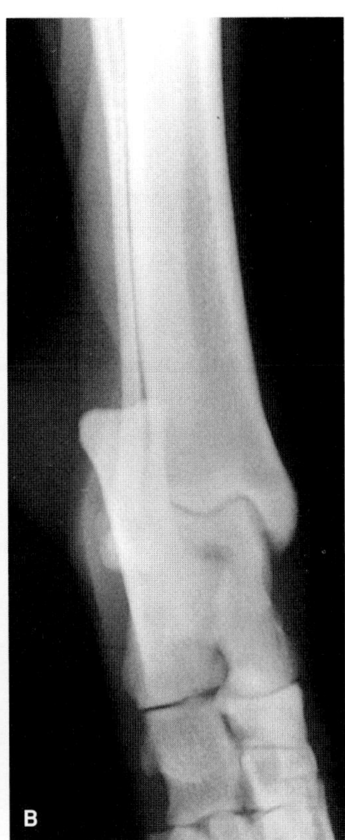

Figure 19-16. (**A**) Lateral projection of a canine tarsocrural joint shows enlargement of the distal aspect of the common calcaneal tendon (Achilles tendon) at the point of tendinous insertion on the calcaneal tuberosity (**B**) Lateral dorsoplantar oblique projection shows the characteristic eccentric soft tissue swelling associated with the proximolateral aspect of the calcaneal tuberosity, typical of lateral displacement of the Achilles tendon.

and cats. Some frequently injured ligaments, such as the cranial and caudal cruciates, are inaccessible sonographically because of their deep intraarticular locations. Others, like the antebrachiocarpal collateral ligaments that appear as little more than thickened areas of the lateral aspects of the joint capsule, lack sufficient anatomic definition to be identified sonographically. Fresh injuries are much more likely to be identified than chronic ones; there is only a small chance of sonographically diagnosing an old sprain. With few exceptions, standard and stress radiography are far more sensitive than ultrasound for identifying damaged ligaments.[30]

When performing a sonographic examination on a dog or cat suspected of having a sprain, it is best to have the animal sedated (ie, pain free and motionless) and lying on its side with the injured limb uppermost. A 10-MHz transducer is best for scanning, but a 7.5-MHz equipped with a standoff device suffices. The scan angle is determined by the suspected location of the injury and the regional anatomy of the individual.

The examination is begun by scanning the swollen, painful, or unstable part of the limb. Radiographs of the suspected injury site should be displayed on a nearby viewbox for reference. The injured joint should then be scanned while performing the five basic stress maneuvers: flexion, extension, axial rotation, traction, and lateral-medial angulation.[31]

Sonographic Anatomy

Normal ligament sonographically resembles normal tendon, because they have similar compositions: dense connective tissue with longitudinally oriented collagen fibrils interspersed with fibroblasts. Unlike tendons, ligaments lack a synovial sheath.

Disorders and Diseases

Sprains are the most commonly encountered ligamentous injury. Like strains, sprains are qualitatively classified according to the severity of the injury as first, second, and third degree (Fig. 19-17).[32] Total discontinuity is called a rupture. Sprains are often accompanied by avulsion fractures, which in some instances serve to incriminate the damaged ligament.[33]

As for tendons, the sonographic appearance of ligamentous sprains reflects the nature of the lesion: an anechoic lesion representing hemorrhage and edema; a hypoechoic lesion depicting cellular infiltration and granulation tissue; normal echogenicity describing tissue restoration, and increased echogenicity indicating scarring. Such lesions change with time and are best assessed serially and in the context of limb function.

As with most musculoskeletal injuries, sonography is best preceded by radiography (Fig. 19-18).

JOINTS

The place of ultrasound in the diagnosis of joint disorders in pet animals has yet to be established. Arthrography, although it appears to be a dying art in veterinary radiology, is still in

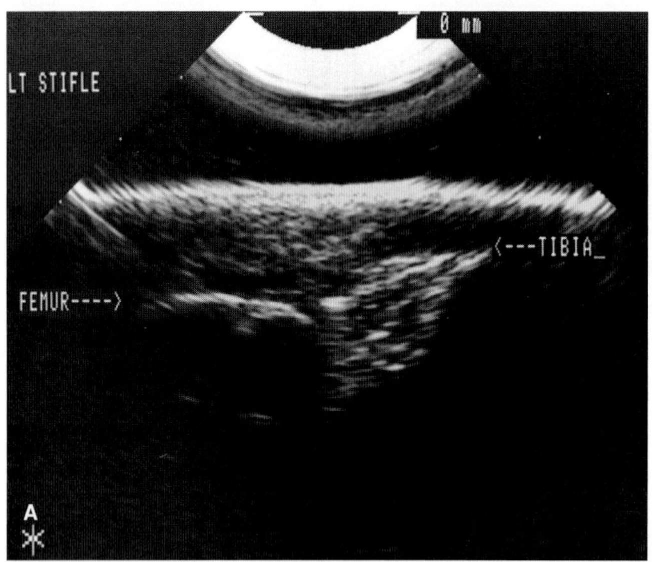

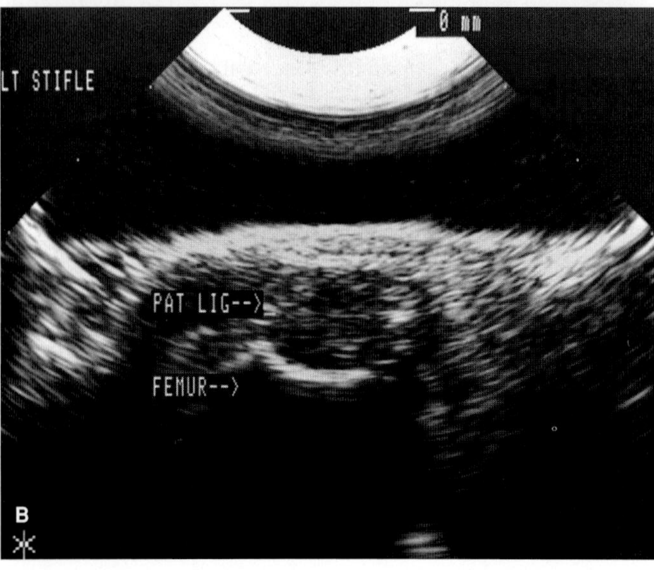

Figure 19-17. (**A**) Long-axis and (**B**) cross-section of a patellar ligament show evidence of a second-degree sprain: reduced echogenicity, enlargement, and an uneven fibrillar pattern.

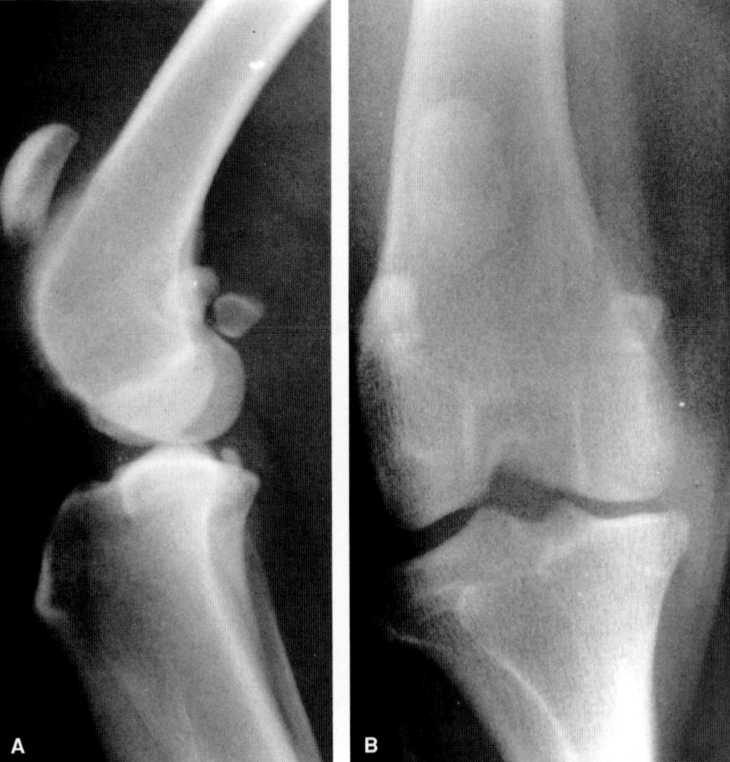

Figure 19-18. (**A**) Lateral and (**B**) craniocaudal projections of a canine genual joint show enlargement of the patellar ligament and proximocranial displacement of the patella, consistent with a third-degree sprain.

many ways a superior method of diagnosis. The few articles published on the sonography of joints appear somewhat less than persuasive about the utility of ultrasound: just how much diagnostic information can be consistently obtained by scanning the joints of dogs and cats? The following discussion represents my limited experience in this area and that published on the subject of hip dysplasia in puppies.

Extraarticular Masses and Mass Effects

Large-breed dogs may develop hygromas over the olecranon and, less frequently, above the calcaneus and greater trochanter. These swellings involve neither the underlying joint or bursa, although they likely exert some degree of indirect pressure on these structures. The significance of such potential compression is conjectural. Hygromas are well suited to sonographic investigation, and it is strongly recommended that sonography be performed before aspiration, biopsy, or surgery of such lesions.

Retrograde femoral pinning may lead to extraarticular scarring as a result of pin-induced inflammation. This scarring may assume the shape of a discrete hyperechoic mass surrounding the pin tip (Fig. 19-19). In some instances, a deep seroma develops around the base of the pin, with or without a cicatrix. In a few cases, a synovial fistula may form.

Neonatal Hip Dysplasia

Sonography of the coxal joint has been reported in babies and puppies.[34,35] Pediatricians have used sonography to diagnose instability, dislocation, and joint effusion of the hip.[34] Veterinarians have employed sonography to examine the coxal joints of normal puppies serially over 12 weeks and have found it feasible up to 8 weeks.[35]

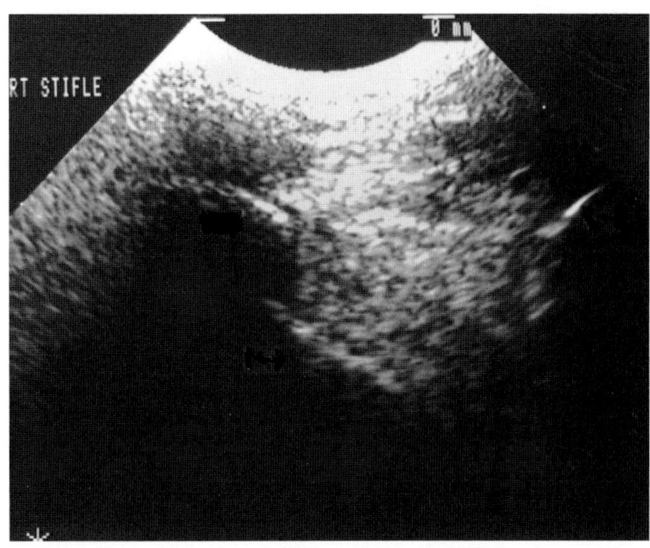

Figure 19-19. Sector scan (long section) of a canine genual joint shows a poorly marginated hyperechoic mass midway between the patella and the tibial crest, deep to patellar ligament.

REFERENCES

1. Fornage BD, Rifkin MD. Ultrasound examination of tendons. Radiol Clin North Am 1988;26:87.
2. Seely RK, Stephens TD, Tate P. Anatomy and physiology. 2nd ed. St. Louis: Mosby-Year Book, 1992:307.
3. Kakulas BA. Muscle trauma. In: Mastaglia FL, Walton JN, eds. Skeletal muscle pathology. 2nd ed. Edinburgh: Churchill Livingstone, 1992:737.
4. Hagen-Ansert SL. Muscular system. In: Hagen-Ansert SL, ed. Textbook of diagnostic ultrasonography. 3rd ed. St. Louis: Mosby-Year Book, 1989:138.
5. Christensen RA, van Sonnenberg E, Casola G, Wittich GR. Interventional ultrasound in the musculoskeletal system. Radiol Clin North Am 1988;26:145.
6. Salter RD. Textbook of disorders and injuries of the musculoskeletal system. Baltimore: Williams & Wilkins, 1983:417.
7. Reid DC. Sports injury assessment and rehabilitation. New York: Churchill Livingstone, 1992:89.
8. deHaan JJ, Beale BS. Compartmental syndrome in the dog: case report and literature review. J Am Anim Hosp Assoc 1993;29:134.
9. Williams J, Bailey MQ, Schertel ER, Valentine A. Compartment syndrome in a Labrador retriever. Vet Radiol Ultrasound 1993;34:244.
10. Brinker WO, Piermattei DL, Flo GW. Handbook of small animal orthopedics and fracture treatment. 2nd ed. Philadelphia: WB Saunders, 1990:323.
11. Houlton JEF, Ness MG. Lateral fabellar fractures in the dog: a review of 8 cases. J Small Anim Pract 1993;34:373.
12. Dee JF, Dee LG, Eaton-Wells RD. Injuries of high performance dogs. In: Whittick WG, ed. Canine orthopedics. 2nd ed. Philadelphia: Lea & Febiger, 1990:519.
13. Love NE, Nickels F. Ultrasonic diagnosis of a deep muscle abscess in a horse. Vet Radiol Ultrasound 1993;34:207.
14. Hager DA. The diagnosis of deep muscle abscesses using two-dimensional real time ultrasound. AAEP Proceedings 1985;32:523.
15. Shah ZR, Crass JR, Oravec DC, Bellon EM. Ultrasonic detection of foreign bodies in soft tissues using turkey muscle as a model. Vet Radiol Ultrasound 1992;33:94.
16. Rogers LF, Crummy AB, Peters ME. The superficial soft tissues. In: Juhl HG, Crummy AB, eds. Essentials of radio-

logic imaging. 6th ed. Philadelphia: JB Lippincott, 1985:841.

17. Butler HC. Surgery of tendinous injuries and muscle as a model. In: Newton CD, Nunamaker DM. Textbook of small animal orthopedics. Philadelphia: JB Lippincott, 1985:841.
18. Vaughan LC. Muscle and tendon injuries in dogs. J Small Anim Pract 1979;20:711.
19. Huges JT. Tumors of striated muscle. In: Mastaglia FL, Walton JN, eds. Skeletal muscle pathology. 2nd ed. Edinburgh; Churchill Livingstone, 1992:725.
20. McGavin MD. Muscular system. In: Thomson RD, ed. Special veterinary pathology. Toronto: BC Decker, 1988: 345.
21. Vincent LM. Ultrasound of soft tissue abnormalities of the extremities. Radiol Clin North Am 1988;26:131.
22. Martinoli C, Derchi LE, Pastorino C. Bertolotto M, Silvestri E. Analysis of echotexture of tendons with US. Radiology 1993;186:839.
23. Reef VB, Martin BB, Stebbins K. Comparison of ultrasonic, gross, and histologic appearance of tendon injuries in performance horses. Proc Am Assoc Equine Pract 1989;35:279.
24. Crass JR, Genovese RL, Render JA, Bellon EM. Magnetic resonance, ultrasound and histopathologic correlation of acute and healing equine tendon injuries. Vet Radiol Ultrasound 1992;33:206.
25. Anderson A, Stead AC, Coughlan AR. Unusual muscle and tendon disorders of the forelimb in the dog. J Small Anim Pract 1993;34:313.
26. Flo GL, Middleton D. Mineralization of the supraspinatus tendon in dogs. J Am Vet Med Assoc 1990;197:95.
27. Mauterer JV, Prata RG, Carberry CC, Schrader SC. Displacement of the tendon of the superficial digital flexor muscle in dogs: 10 cases (1983–1991). J Am Vet Med Assoc 1993;203:1162.
28. Reinke JD, Mughannam AJ. Lateral luxation of the superficial digital flexor tendon in 12 dogs. J Am Anim Hosp Assoc 1993;29:303.
29. Johnston DF. Bursitis/tendinitis. In: Newton CD, Nunamaker DM, eds. Textbook of small animal orthopedics. Philadelphia: JB Lippincott, 1985.
30. Farrow CS. Sprain, strain and contusion. Vet Clin North Am 1978;8:169.
31. Farrow CS. Stress radiography: applications in small animal practice. J Am Vet Med Assoc 1982;181:777.
32. Brinker WO, Piermattei DL, Flo GW. Handbook of small animal orthopedics and fracture treatment. 2nd ed. Philadelphia: WB Saunders 1990:314.
33. Farrow CS. Carpal sprain injury in the dog. JAVRS 1977;18:38.
34. Novick GS. Sonography in pediatric hip disorders. Radiol Clin North Am 1988; 26:29.
35. Greshake RJ, Ackerman N. Ultrasound evaluation of the coxofemoral joints of the canine neonate. Vet Radiol Ultrasound 1993;34:99.

Small Animal Ultrasound, edited by Ronald W. Green.
Lippincott-Raven Publishers, Philadelphia © 1996.

GROSS ANATOMY OF THE ABDOMEN FOR THE ULTRASONOLOGIST

Michael A. Walker

It has been philosophized that in diagnosis we miss more things because we do not think about them than we do because we do not know of them. It is important to perform systematic examinations and not just focus on the obvious, an approach that requires the examiner to be knowledgeable about normal gross anatomy. A sonogram is a two-dimensional representation of the patient's anatomy in a certain plane. This two-dimensional planar anatomy is different from gross anatomy or radiographic anatomy, but it is similar to that seen with computed tomography (CT) and magnetic resonance imaging (MRI).

The purpose of this chapter is to use the noninvasive medium of MRI to demonstrate the anatomy and associations of the various organs in image planes that are used in abdominal sonography. The chapter consists of a review of the abdominal viscera and a discussion of the regionalized anatomy of the abdomen. The illustrations provide MRI presentations of the major abdominal viscera. The MRI images were obtained using a Toshiba 0.35-Tesla superconducting magnet. Images were 3 to 5 mm thick and T1 weighted. Antemortem and immediately postmortem images were made using four dogs.

THE ABDOMINAL VISCERA

The abdomen extends from the diaphragm to the pelvis. The abdominal cavity is continuous with the pelvic cavity and contains the potential peritoneal cavity. The peritoneal cavity is filled with the abdominal viscera and with some fat.

Liver

The liver (see Chap. 6), the largest gland in the body, contains the left, right, quadrate, and caudate lobes; the left lateral, left medial, right lateral, and right medial sublobes; and the papillary and caudate processes (Figs. 20-1 through 20-11, and 20-15). It lies caudal to the diaphragm and cranial to the stomach.

The left hepatic lobe lies almost entirely to the left of the median plane and consists of the left lateral and medial sublobes. The left lateral lobe lies caudolateral to the left medial sublobe. A midsagittal fissure divides the left from the right lobes of the liver. The fissure extends to the porta hepatis or hilus of the liver. The biliary duct lies ventral to the portal vein, which lies ventral to the hepatic artery in the porta hepatis. Four fifths of the blood to the liver is supplied by

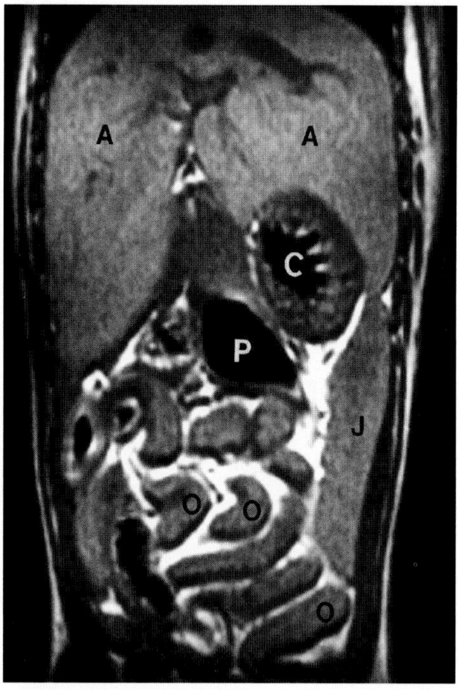

Figure 20-1. Frontal view through the dorsal third of the abdomen. *A*, liver; *C*, fundus of stomach; *J*, spleen; *O*, small intestine; *P*, large intestine.

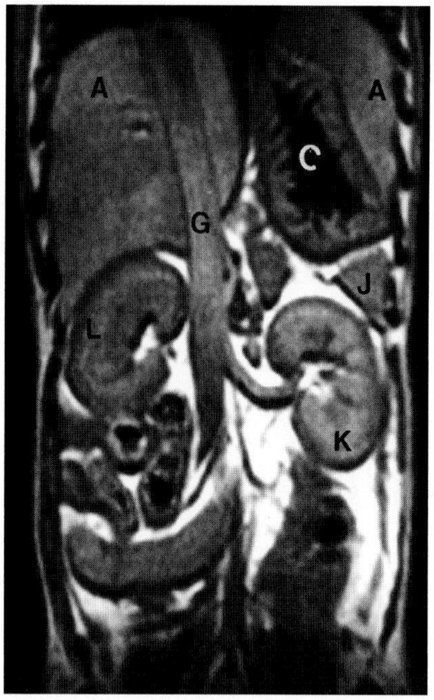

Figure 20-2. Frontal view through the middle and dorsal thirds of the abdomen. *A*, liver; *C*, fundus of stomach; *G*, vena cava; *J*, spleen; *K*, left kidney; *R*, right kidney.

the portal vein, and one fifth is supplied by the hepatic arteries.

The quadrate lobe lies in the median plane, and its right surface forms the left half of the fossa for the gallbladder. The right hepatic lobe lies to the right of the median plane, and it is divided into medial and lateral sublobes. The medial surface of the right medial lobe forms the right half of the fossa for the gallbladder. In part, the right lateral hepatic sublobe lies between the right medial lobe cranially and the caudate process of the caudate lobe caudally.

The caudate lobe lies in an oblique transverse position in the abdomen and has the caudate and papillary processes. The caudate process forms the renal fossa for the right kidney. The papillary process lies in the lesser curvature of the stomach. The left and right medial sublobes form the ventral boundaries for the caudal vena cava and the large hepatic veins that feed into it.

The gallbladder, which stores and concentrates the bile, lies between the quadrate lobe medially and the right medial sublobe laterally and extends to the diaphragm when full (see Figs. 20-3 and 20-7). The hepatic ducts unite with the cystic duct from the gallbladder to form the bile duct. The bile duct extends intramurally in the wall of the duodenum to terminate along with the pancreatic duct on the major duodenal papilla.

Spleen

The dorsal extremity of the elongated spleen (see Chap. 7) usually is found between the fundus of the stomach and the cranial pole of the left kidney (see Figs. 20-1, 20-2, 20-4 through 20-6, 20-8 through 20-12, and 20-15). The position of the ventral extremity of the spleen depends on the size and location of the other abdominal organs. The ventral extremity of the spleen may be found lying along the left lateral wall of the abdomen or coursing toward the right side of the ventral abdomen anywhere caudal to the

(text continues on p. 357)

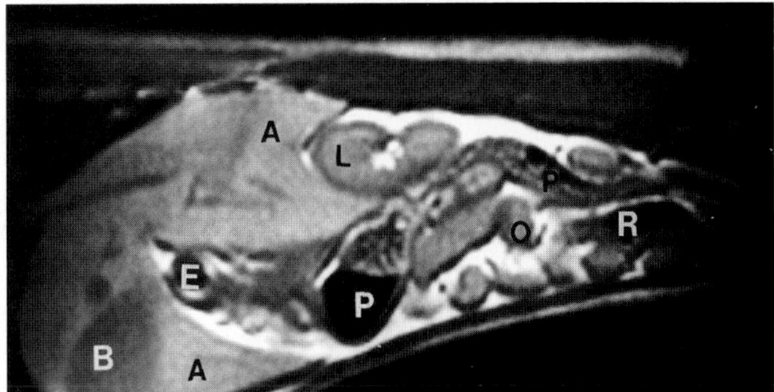

Figure 20-3. Sagittal view through the right side of the abdomen. *A*, liver; *B*, gallbladder; *E*, pylorus of stomach; *L*, right kidney; *O*, small intestine; *P*, large intestine; *R*, urinary bladder.

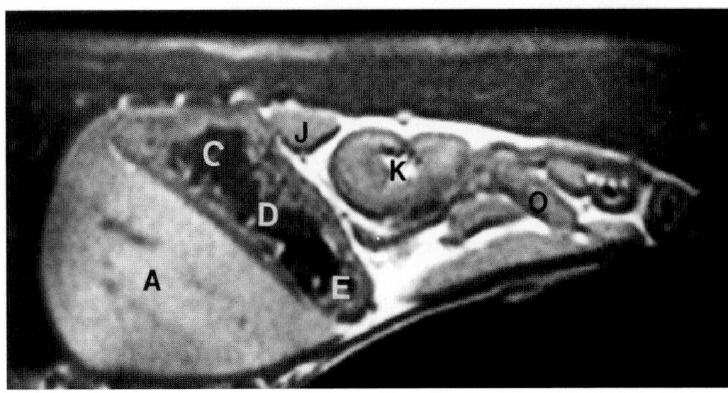

Figure 20-4. Sagittal view through the left side of the abdomen. *A*, liver; *C*, fundus of stomach; *D*, body of stomach; *E*, pylorus of stomach; *J*, spleen; *K*, left kidney; *O*, small intestine.

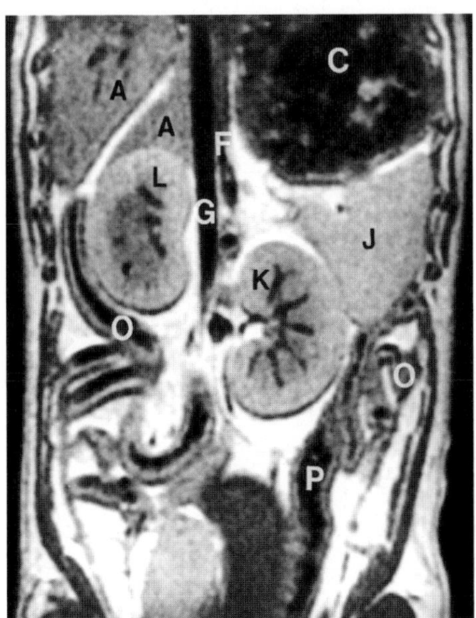

Figure 20-5. Frontal view through the dorsal third of the abdomen. *A*, liver; *C*, fundus of stomach; *F*, aorta; *G*, vena cava; *J*, spleen; *K*, left kidney; *L*, right kidney; *O*, small intestine; *P*, large intestine.

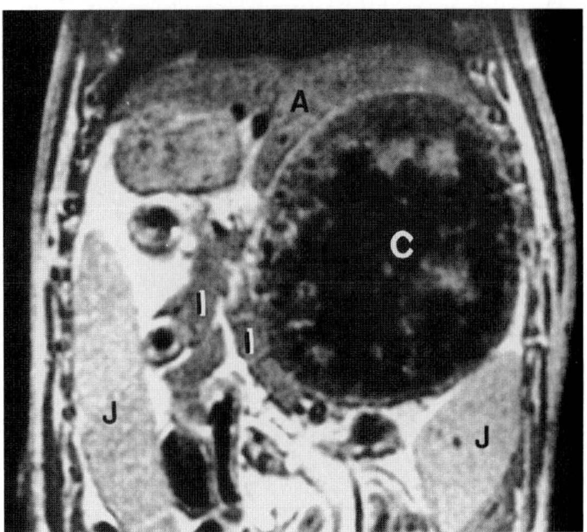

Figure 20-6 Frontal view through the middle third of the abdomen. *A*, liver; *C*, fundus of stomach; *I*, pancreas; *J*, spleen.

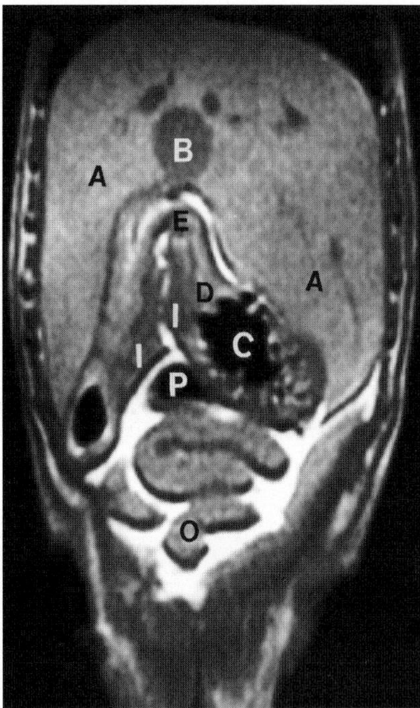

Figure 20-7 Frontal view through the ventral third of the abdomen. *A*, liver; *B*, gallbladder; *C*, fundus of stomach; *D*, body of stomach; *E*, pylorus of stomach; *I*, pancreas; *O*, small intestine; *P*, large intestine.

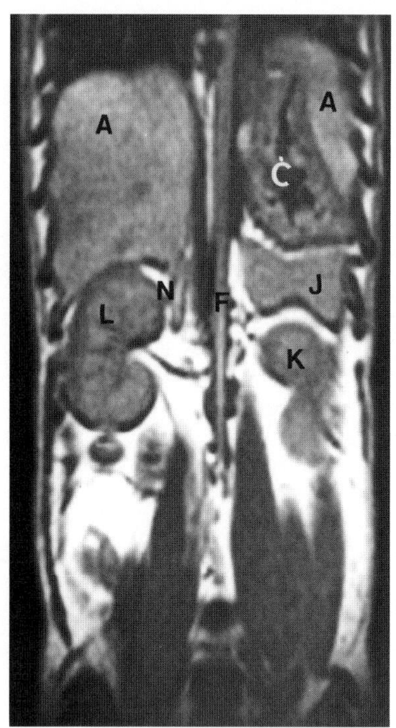

Figure 20-9. Frontal view through the dorsal third of the abdomen. *A*, liver; *C*, fundus of stomach; *F*, aorta; *J*, spleen; *K*, left kidney; *L*, right kidney; *N*, right adrenal gland.

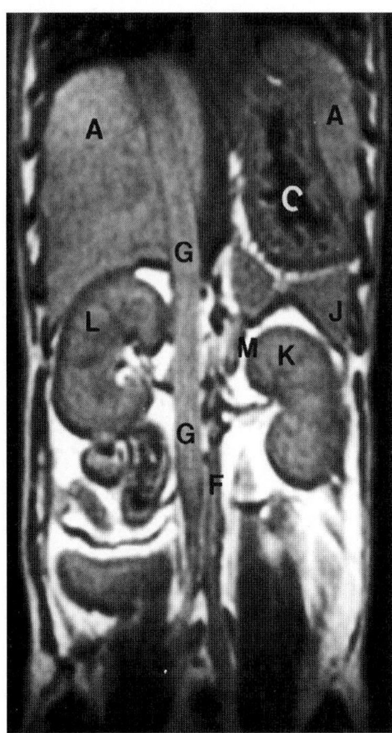

Figure 20-8. Frontal view through the dorsal third of the abdomen. *A*, liver; *C*, fundus of stomach; *F*, aorta; *G*, vena cava; *J*, spleen; *K*, left kidney; *L*, right kidney; *M*, left adrenal gland.

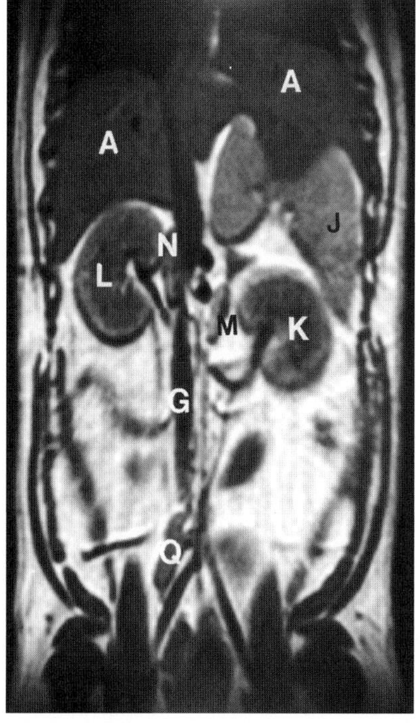

Figure 20-10. Frontal view through the dorsal third of the abdomen. *A*, liver; *G*, vena cava; *J*, spleen; *K*, left kidney; *L*, right kidney; *M*, left adrenal gland; *N*, right adrenal gland; *Q*, lymph nodes.

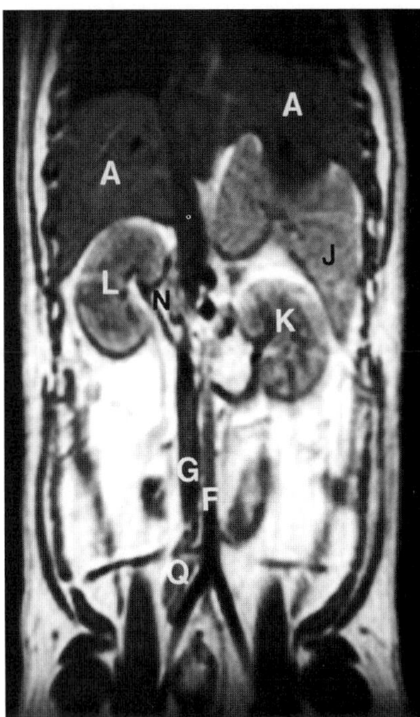

Figure 20-11. Frontal view through the dorsal third of the abdomen. *A*, liver; *F*, aorta; *G*, vena cava; *J*, spleen; *K*, left kidney; *L*, right kidney; *N*, right adrenal gland; *Q*, lymph nodes.

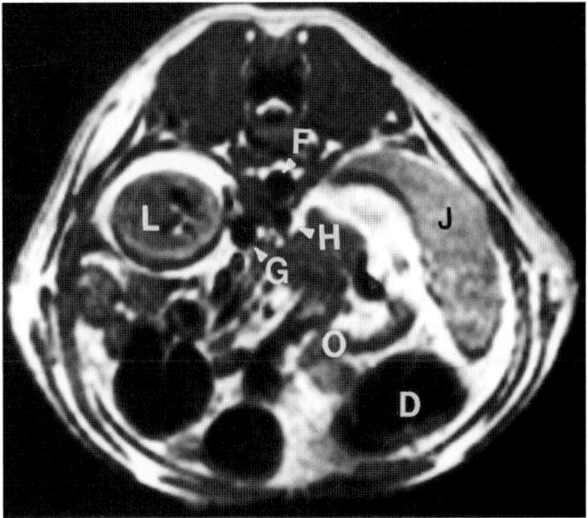

Figure 20-12. Transverse view through the cranial third of the abdomen. *D*, body of stomach; *F*, aorta; *G*, vena cava; *H*, portal vein; *J*, spleen; *L*, right kidney; *O*, small intestine.

liver. The size of the normal spleen varies among individuals and with the administration of certain pharmaceuticals. The spleen is loosely attached to the stomach by a part of the greater omentum, the gastrosplenic ligament. The long hilus of the spleen is located on the spleen's midventral visceral surface and serves as the entrance and exit ports for the splenic arteries and veins.

Pancreas

The pancreas (see Chap. 9) is a lobulated, elongated exocrine and endocrine gland that lies in the form of an inverted V just caudal to the stomach and medial to the duodenum (see Figs. 20-6 and 20-7). The left lobe of the pancreas usually extends from an area close to the cranial pole of the left kidney and the middle portion of the spleen toward the animal's right side. The left lobe lies in the greater omentum between the stomach and the transverse colon. The body of the pancreas lies caudal and to the left of the pylorus of the stomach, forming a 45° angle between the right and left lobes of the pancreas. The portal vein crosses the dorsal portion of the body of the pancreas. The right lobe of the pancreas lies medial to the descending duodenum in the mesoduodenum. The pancreatic ducts vary in number and site of termination but often terminate as two, with the pancreatic duct opening adjacent to the bile duct on the major duodenal papilla and the accessory pancreatic duct opening just a short distance distal on the minor duodenal papilla.

Adrenal Glands

The right and left adrenal glands (see Chap. 11) are located just medial to the cranial pole of their corresponding kidneys (see Figs. 20-8 through 20-11). The left gland is the larger gland, and it is located lateral to the aorta and just caudolateral to the origin of the cranial mesenteric artery. The right adrenal gland is located lateral to the caudal vena cava.

Kidneys

The kidneys (see Chap. 10) are located in the sublumbar retroperitoneal portion of the abdomen (see Figs. 20-2 through 20-5 and 20-8 through 20-12). The left kidney is more loosely attached to the dorsal abdominal wall, and its position varies more than the right kidney. The right kidney lies in contact with the renal fossa of the caudate lobe of the liver and is more cranial than the left. A fibrous capsule envelopes each kidney. The renal sinus is on the medial border of the kidney. The sinus contains the renal pelvis, adipose tissue, and the renal arteries and vein. The parenchyma of the kidney consists of an outer cortex contain-ing the glomeruli and an inner medulla containing the renal tubules. The medulla projects into the renal pelvis as the renal crest. Urine drains from the collecting tubules onto the renal crest. The renal pelvis is elongated craniocaudally to form recesses, from which are about six peripherally extending diverticula.

Ureters

Each of the two tubular ureters (see Chap. 10) begins at its corresponding renal pelvis and extends retroperitoneally along a caudoventral and medial course to terminate obliquely in the neck of the urinary bladder.

Urinary Bladder

The urinary bladder (see Chap. 12) varies in size, shape, and location, depending on how full it is. Generally, it lies just cranial to the brim of the pelvis in the caudoventral abdomen (Figs. 20-13 and 20-14). The bladder lies ventral to the descending colon and lies ventral or ventrolateral to the uterine body. The bladder has a body and a neck; the neck connects with the urethra. The trigone of the bladder is the area of the neck bounded by the urethral orifice caudally and the line connecting the two ureteral openings cranially. The mucosa of the bladder forms irregular folds when the bladder is empty.

Urethra

The female urethra extends caudally from the neck of the urinary bladder and lies in proximity to the ventral wall of the vagina. The male urethra extends caudally from the neck of the urinary bladder, through the pelvic canal, ventrally along the perineum, and then cranially through the penis. The male urethra consists of a prostatic portion, a membranous portion, and a penile portion. The seminal hillock is a small protuberance that may be seen in the lumen of the prostatic urethra.

Uterus and Ovaries

The uterus (see Chap. 15) is a Y-shaped tube consisting of a cervix, a body, and two horns (Figs. 20-13 and 20-15). The length of the normal,

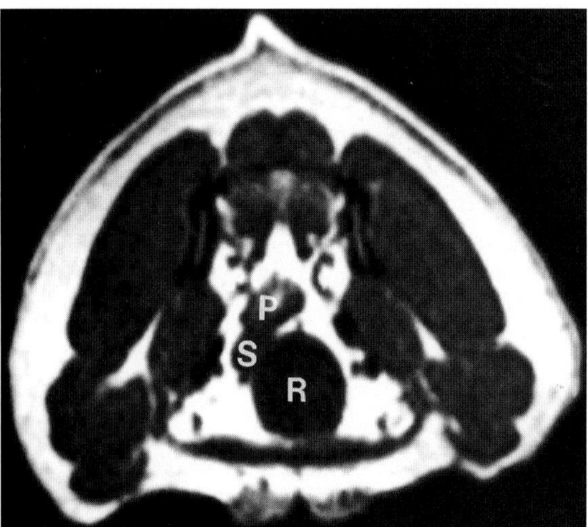

Figure 20-13. Transverse view through the caudal third of the abdomen. *P*, large intestine; *R*, urinary bladder; *S*, uterus.

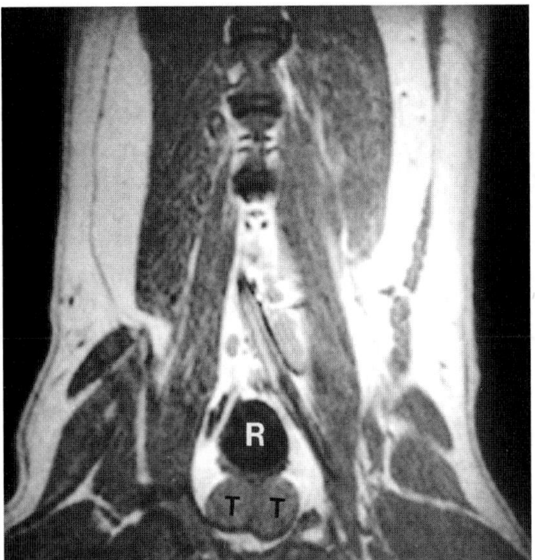

Figure 20-14. Frontal view through the central third of the caudal abdomen. *R*, urinary bladder; *T*, prostate.

nongravid uterus varies with the size of the dog, but it is no more than 1 cm in diameter. The uterus extends from the vagina to the oviducts and ovaries. The uterine body lies ventral to the colon and dorsal or dorsolateral to the urinary bladder. The uterus is made up of three layers: an outer serosal lining, a muscularis, and an inner mucosal lining.

The two ovaries (see Chap. 16) vary slightly in position but usually are located caudal to the kidneys. They are oval and about 1 to 2 cm long.

Prostate

The bilobed prostate gland (see Chap. 13) is the only accessory reproductive gland in the male dog. The size of the normal gland depends on the age, breed, and weight of the dog. It is located near the brim of the pelvic canal, ventral to the rectum and dorsal to the pelvis or the ventral abdominal wall (Figs. 20-14 and 20-16). The middorsal sulcus divides the gland into right and left lobes. Ducts from the many glands within the prostate circumferentially enter the prostatic portion of the urethra.

Testes

Each of the two oval testes (see Chap. 14) are located within the scrotum. A line of connective tissue, called the mediastinum testis, extends lengthwise along the middle of each testis. On the dorsolateral surface of each testis is its epididymis. The epididymis extends from its head at the cranial end of its testis to its body, lying along the dorsolateral surface of the testis, to its tail at the caudal end of the testis. The tail of the

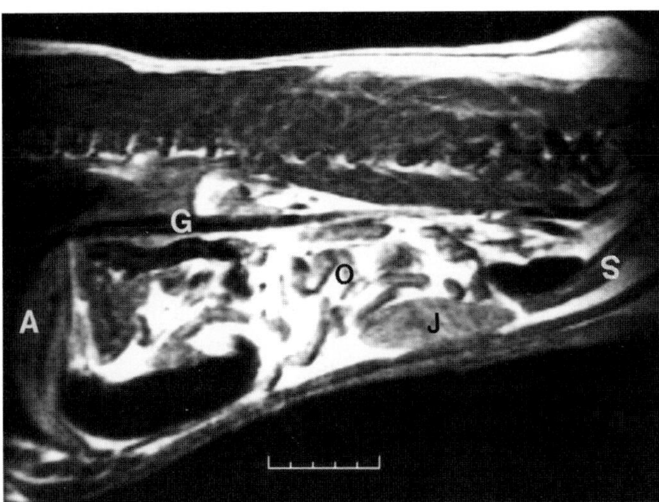

Figure 20-15. Sagittal view through the right side of the abdomen. *A*, liver; *G*, vena cava; *J*, spleen; *O*, small intestine; *S*, uterus.

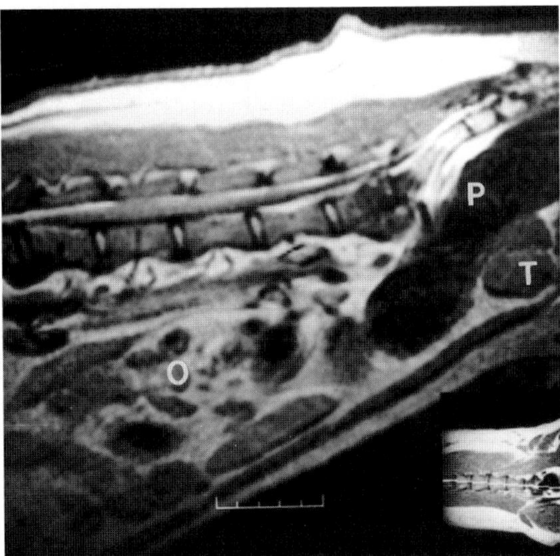

Figure 20-16. Sagittal view through the midabdomen. *O*, small intestine; *P*, large intestine; *T*, prostate.

epididymis continues cranially to the prostatic urethra as the ductus deferens.

Stomach

The stomach (see Chap. 8) consists of a cardia, a fundus, a body, and a pyloric region (see Figs. 20-1 through 20-9, and 20-12). The esophagus enters the cranial side of the stomach at the cardia. The fundus is the large blind pouch of the stomach and, when full, is usually positioned in the left craniodorsal area of the abdomen, just behind the left crus of the diaphragm. The body of the stomach extends from the fundus in an oblique transverse angle across to the right side of the abdomen to become the funnel-shaped pyloric antrum and pyloric canal. The stomach joins the duodenum at the pylorus, which is usually located somewhere in the ventral half of the right side of the abdomen, just caudal to the liver. The acutely angled lesser curvature of the stomach is usually positioned craniodorsal and extends from the cardia to the pylorus. The convex greater curvature is usually positioned caudoventral and also extends from the cardia to the pylorus. The stomach wall consists of serosal, muscular, submucosal, and mucosal tunics.

Small Intestine

The small intestine (see Chap. 8) extends from the stomach to the colon and consists of the duodenum, jejunum, and ileum (see Figs. 20-1, 20-3 through 20-5, 20-7, 20-12, 20-15, and 20-16). The duodenum originates at the pylorus and extends caudally along the right side of the abdomen, where it makes a U-shaped turn cranially and to the left and eventually joins the jejunum at the root of the mesentery. The jejunum forms the second and largest portion of the small intestine; the ileum forms the last and shortest portion. The jejunum and the ileum are suspended by mesentery from the sublumbar region and are relatively mobile within the abdomen. The distinction between the jejunum and the ileum is mucosal, not gross. The ileum ends on the ileal papilla at its junction with the colon. There is a sphincter muscle at the ileocolic orifice. The wall of the small intestine is composed of four tunics: the serosa, muscularis, submucosa, and mucosa.

Cecum, Large Intestine, and Rectum

The cecum (see Chap. 8) is a normal diverticulum of the ascending colon. Associated peritoneal folds cause the cecum to be somewhat spiral. It usually lies in the right side of the abdomen within the duodenal loop. The cecum communicates with the ascending colon through the cecocolic orifice, located about 1 cm distal to the ileocolic orifice. The cecocolic orifice is surrounded by the cecocolic sphincter.

The colon is shaped like a question mark. It has ascending, transverse, and descending portions (Figs. 20-1, 20-3, 20-5, 20-7, 20-13, and 20-16). The right and left colic flexures unite the short ascending with the transverse colon and the transverse with the descending portions of the colon, respectively. The position of the colon may vary somewhat among animals. The ascending and transverse portions lie cranial and usually to the right of the root of the mesentery. The descending colon is located to the left of the root of the mesentery and usually descends down the left side of the abdomen. The rectum is the straight continuation of the colon in the pelvic canal. The rectum lies dorsal to the vagina in the female and dorsal to the urethra in the male.

Aorta, Caudal Vena Cava, and Portal Vein

The abdominal aorta lies along the dorsal midline of the abdominal cavity and extends from the diaphragm to a plane ventral to the seventh lumbar vertebra (see Figs. 20-5, 20-8, 20-9, 20-11, and 20-12). Caudally, it lies to the left of the caudal vena cava. At its termination, it divides into right and left internal iliac and middle sacral arteries. Some of its major abdominal branches include the celiac artery ventral to L1, the cranial mesenteric artery caudal to the celiac and ventral to L1, the phrenicoabdominal arteries ventral to L2, the renal arteries ventral to L3, and the caudal mesenteric artery ventral to the L5–L6 junction.

The caudal vena cava begins in the caudal abdomen, lying just ventral to L7 and to the right side of the aorta (see Figs. 20-2, 20-5, 20-8, 20-10 through 20-12, and 20-15). As the cava extends cranially, it slopes ventrally and to the right, entering the caudate lobe of the liver before reaching the diaphragm.

The portal vein is formed by the cranial and caudal mesenteric veins and the splenic vein (see Fig. 20-12). It terminates in the porta of the liver, where it divides into right and left branches, which then divide and extend throughout the liver.

Lymph Nodes

There are many abdominal parietal and visceral lymph nodes (see Chap. 17). The medial iliac lymph nodes are more commonly evaluated (see Figs. 20-10 and 20-11). They are located alongside the caudal end of the aorta. Even though the normal cranial mesenteric lymph nodes are reported to be the largest lymph nodes of the abdomen, they may be difficult to locate and visualize ultrasonographically. They are located alongside the vessels in the mesentery. There are many other small visceral lymph nodes, such as those adjacent to the kidneys and to the porta hepatis.

REGIONALIZED ANATOMY OF THE ABDOMEN

Left Cranial Region

The left cranial region of the abdomen contains the left half of the liver and the fundus of the stomach (see Fig. 20-1). When the stomach is full, the fundus may extend to the left crus of the diaphragm (see Fig. 20-4). When the stomach is relatively empty, the fundus lies caudal to the left lobe of the liver and contains clearly demarcated rugal folds (see Figs. 20-1 and 20-2).

Right Cranial Region

The right cranial region of the abdomen contains the right half of the liver, the gallbladder, and the porta hepatis with the portal vein and caudal vena cava (see Figs. 20-3, 20-7, and 20-8). The porta hepatis with its contents and the gallbladder can usually be found just to the right of the abdominal midline. The gallbladder may extend obliquely cranial (see Fig. 20-3).

Left Middle Region

The left middle region of the abdomen contains the head and body of the spleen (see Fig. 20-1). The spleen can be found caudal or caudolateral to the fundus of the stomach and cranial or craniolateral to the left kidney (see Figs. 20-1, 20-2, and 20-5). The left kidney lies caudal and slightly medial to the head of the spleen (see Figs. 20-2, 20-4, 20-5, 20-8, and 20-9). The left adrenal gland is located medial to the cranial pole of the left kidney, lateral to the aorta, and cranial to the left renal artery and vein (see Figs. 20-8 and 20-10). The left half of the transverse colon and the descending colon lie in the left middle region of the abdomen (see Fig. 20-5). The small intestine may be found distributed throughout much of this region (see Fig. 20-1). The left lobe of the pancreas lies caudal to the stomach, cranial to the transverse colon, and medial to the body of the spleen (see Figs. 20-6 and 20-7). The left ovary usually lies caudal to the left kidney. The left horn of the uterus extends from the left ovary obliquely caudal toward the midline, where it joins the body of the uterus (see Figs. 20-13 and 20-15).

The body of the spleen may cross from the left to the right middle regions of the abdomen and be found along the ventral abdominal wall anywhere caudal to the liver (see Fig. 20-15).

The right ovary is located caudal to the right kidney. The right horn of the uterus extends from the right ovary obliquely caudal toward the midline, where it joins the body of the uterus (see Figs. 20-13 and 20-15).

Right Middle Region

The right middle region of the abdomen contains the right kidney lying adjacent and caudal to the caudate lobe of the liver (see Figs. 20-2, 20-3, 20-5, 20-8 through 20-12). The right adrenal gland lies medial to the cranial pole of the right kidney, lateral to the caudal vena cava, and cranial to the right renal artery and vein (see Figs. 20-9 through 20-11).

The body of the stomach crosses the abdominal midline from left to right, just caudal to the liver (see Figs. 20-3, 20-4, and 20-7). The duodenum begins at the pylorus and extends caudal in the right side of the abdomen. The body of the pancreas lies caudal to the pylorus (see Figs. 20-6 and 20-7). The right lobe of the pancreas extends caudal along the medial side of the descending duodenum (see Figs. 20-6 and 20-7). The cecum, ascending colon, and right half of the transverse colon usually lie in the right middle abdominal region (see Figs. 20-1, 20-3, and 20-7). The small intestine is distributed throughout much of this abdominal region (see Fig. 20-1).

Left and Right Caudal Regions

The left and right caudal regions of the abdomen converge on the pelvic cavity. The aorta, vena cava, and medial iliac lymph nodes are located near the dorsal midline of the abdomen (see Figs. 20-8, 20-10, and 20-11). The colorectum lies ventral to the aorta and dorsal to the urinary bladder (see Figs. 20-13 and 20-16). The body of the uterus is located between the colon and the urinary bladder or just lateral to the dorsum of the bladder (see Figs. 20-13 and 20-15). The bladder is the ventral-most caudal midline abdominal structure (see Fig. 20-13). The prostate is found just caudal to the neck of the bladder, near the pelvic canal (see Figs. 20-14 and 20-16). The urethra runs caudal from the trigone of the urinary bladder and is located just ventral to the vagina in the female or in the middle of the prostate in the male.

BIBLIOGRAPHY

Evans HE, Christensen GC, eds. Miller's anatomy of the dog. 2nd ed. Philadelphia: WB Saunders, 1979.

Small Animal Ultrasound, edited by Ronald W. Green.
Lippincott-Raven Publishers, Philadelphia © 1996.

GLOSSARY OF ULTRASOUND TERMS

A-mode (amplitude mode) one-dimensional display of the amplitude of the signal strength on the y axis and the depth of the signal from the transducer (time) on the x axis. Rarely in use today.

absorption loss or attenuation of sound as it travels through a medium because of its conversion to thermal energy (ie, heat).

acoustic having to do with sound.

acoustic enhancement *see* distant enhancement.

acoustic impedance measure of how easily acoustic waves can be formed as they pass through a particular medium. Acoustic impedance depends on the density of the medium and is used to determine the amount of sound reflected at an interface.

acoustic shadowing failure of the sound beam to pass through an object because of reflection or absorption of the sound. The result is a black or anechoic zone beyond the reflector or absorber.

acoustic window the best place on the patient's surface or within the patient to allow an unobstructed path for the ultrasound beam.

amplification process of increasing small voltages to larger ones.

amplitude the peak height of a sound wave, which is a measure of its strength.

anechoic without internal echoes or echo free. Such a structure appears black.

annular array type of transducer using several concentric ring-shaped elements that produce a three-dimensional beam that is displayed as a sector image.

aperture transducer width.

artifact a signal that seems to be originating from the tissues being scanned but does not have an anatomic correlation in the tissues.

attenuation reduction in the intensity of an ultrasound beam as it travels through a medium. The ultrasound beam can be attenuated by reflection, absorption, or scattering.

axial resolution ability to image closely spaced interfaces on the axis of the ultrasound beam.

axis sound travel in the direction of the transducer's axis.

B-mode (brightness mode) display mode in which the echo signal is displayed as a dot, with intensity proportional to signal strength and position corresponding to the distance from the transducer.

bandwidth range of frequencies contained in an ultrasound pulse.

beam acoustic field produced by a transducer.

beam width thickness of the ultrasound beam. Beam width influences lateral resolution and varies with depth, particularly with focused transducers.

calipers electronic characters that can be superimposed on the image to measure the size of an object or the distance between objects.

cathode ray tube screen used to display the ultrasound image.

comet tail artifact that appears as a series of closely spaced reverberation echoes, usually created by a small, strong reflector, such as a gas bubble or metal.

complex echo pattern structure or mass displaying fluid-filled and echogenic areas.

convex phased array type of transducer that has a series of stationary crystals in a curved row that transmit and receive sound at right angles to the transducer's surface. The image displayed is wedge or pie shaped (ie, sector).

coupling gel water-soluble medium that is applied to the patient's skin to eliminate an air interface and permit transmission of the ultrasound beam from the transducer into the body.

crystal element of piezoelectric material within the transducer.

cycle per second frequency at which the crystal vibrates. The number of cycles per second determines frequency.

decibel (dB) unit of power or intensity ratio.

depth range variation in depth at which the echoes are optimally displayed. The maximum depth depends on the transducer used.

diagnostic ultrasound ultrasound in the frequency range of 1 to 20 MHz.

distant enhancement artifact that occurs deep to fluid-filled structures. Because sound is barely attenuated in fluid, structures distant (deep) to a cystic lesion appear to have more echoes than adjacent areas at the same depth.

Doppler effect apparent change in frequency of a sound wave if there is relative motion between the wave source and the observer.

Doppler imaging ultrasound imaging using the Doppler effect to noninvasively detect blood flow and motion of body structures.

- **color flow Doppler** presentation of two-dimensional, real-time Doppler information in color, superimposed on a real-time, gray-scale anatomic cross-sectional image. Flow directions toward and away from the transducer are presented as different colors on the display.
- **continuous wave Doppler** mode of Doppler operation in which the ultrasound wave cycles repeat indefinitely, rather than being emitted in pulses.
- **duplex Doppler** combination of B-mode imaging and pulsed-wave Doppler.
- **pulsed-wave Doppler** mode of Doppler operation in which the ultrasound wave is created by pulses of cycles.

dorsal (frontal) plane image plane perpendicular to sagittal and transverse planes, dividing the body or organ into dorsal and ventral halves.

dual image split screen displaying two views of an image, one of which is frozen while the other is displayed in real time. Dual imaging can be used in B-mode to compare normal with abnormal anatomy or to display B- and M-mode images simultaneously.

duty factor fraction of time pulsed ultrasound is on.

dynamic focusing electronic pulse delays used to change the focal length of the transducer from one frame to the next.

dynamic range ratio of the largest to the smallest intensity of a group of echoes that a system can display, expressed in decibels.

echo reflection.

echo dropout areas on the image containing few to no returning echoes, usually because of attenuation. Dropout areas can also be created by scanning too rapidly.

echo free *see* anechoic.

echogenic *see* hyperechoic.

echogenicity term that refers to the brightness of tissues being displayed.

echoic describes a structure that produces echoes.

echo pattern *see* echotexture.

echopenic *see* hypoechoic.

echotexture composition of the echoes within a parenchymal organ.

element piezoelectric crystal.

enhancement *see* distant enhancement.

far field region of the image that is farthest from the transducer face characterized by a divergence of the ultrasound beam, and typically displayed at the bottom of the screen.

far gain amount of amplification applied to only the distant echoes within the far field.

field of view displayed spatial distribution of the ultrasound beam.

focal length distance along the ultrasound beam axis from the center of the transducer to the focal point.

focal point point in a focused ultrasound beam that has the highest intensity. The closer the structure of interest is to this point, the greater the resolution.

focal zone region of the sound beam where the beam is the narrowest and the resolution is the highest.

focusing act of narrowing the beam to a smaller width at a select depth. This can be done mechanically in single-element transducers with a lens or by modification of the crystal shape or done electronically by using time-delay electronics.

footprint shape of the portion of the transducer that is in contact with the patient.

frame single display image produced by one complete scan of the sound beam.
frame rate rate at which the image is updated on a real-time system display. The number of frames displayed per unit of time.
frequency number of times the sound wave is repeated in one second, measured in Hertz.

gain measure of the strength of the ultrasound signal throughout the image. It regulates the degree of echo amplification (ie, image brightness).
graded compression technique whereby gradually increasing pressure is applied with the ultrasound probe while scanning the patient. This technique is useful in displacing gas-filled viscera to improve the acoustic window or to identify compressible structures such as veins.
grating lobes additional minor beams of sound traveling out in directions different from the primary beam, which result from the multielement structure of transducer arrays.
gray scale range of brightness between white and black.
gray-scale ultrasound type of ultrasound where each echo is displayed with an intensity proportional to its amplitude, the basis of B-mode ultrasound.

Hertz (Hz) standard unit of frequency, equal to one cycle per second.
homogeneous of uniform composition. A mass, organ, or fluid that contains acoustically similar echoes.
hyperechoic relative term describing a structure with more echoes (brighter) compared with the echogenicity of other structures.
hypoechoic relative term describing a structure with less echoes (darker) compared with the echogenicity of other structures.

interface reflection that occurs whenever two tissues of different acoustic impedance are in contact.
isoechoic term used to describe structures with the same echogenicity.

lateral resolution ability to image closely spaced interfaces perpendicular to the axis of the ultrasound beam.
linear array type of transducer that consists of a series of stationary crystals in a flat row, which results in a rectangular image on the screen.

M-mode (motion mode) display mode in which a B-mode trace is formed and moved as a function of time to represent motion of the echo sources.
main bang near-field artifact created by high level echoes at the skin's surface.
mechanical transducer type of transducer with a small curved surface that typically contains a single oscillating or rotating crystal and a motor drive and displays a pie-shaped (sector) image.
medium material through which an ultrasound wave travels.
megahertz (MHz) 1,000,000 Hertz. The usable frequencies for diagnostic ultrasound range from 2 to 10 MHz.
memory capacity to store information.
mirror image artifactual image appearing on the opposite side of a strong reflector. This artifact is the result of multiple internal reverberations between the object and the reflector, creating a time delay in the return of these internal echoes to the transducer.
mixed echogenicity *see* complex echo pattern.
monitor *see* cathode ray tube.

near field region of the image that is nearest the transducer face and is typically displayed at the top of the screen.
near gain amount of amplification applied to the closest echoes within the near field.
noise artifactual echoes resulting from too much gain rather than echoes from true anatomic structures.
nonspecular type of reflection that occurs when the reflecting surface is smaller than the incident sound beam (eg, parenchyma).
normoechoic term used to describe an organ or tissue that is normal in echogenicity.

operating frequency maximum effective frequency of operation of a transducer.
output power *see* gain.

phantom tissue-equivalent material that has some characteristics representative of tissues.
phased array electronically steered system in which many small elements are coordinated with electronic time delays to produce a focused wave front.
piezoelectric effect ability of certain crystals, when subjected to mechanical pressure, to produce an electrical pulse and vice versa.
postprocessing signal processing done after memory.

power quantity of energy generated by the transducer, expressed in watts.

preprocessing signal processing (eg, gain, time-gain compensation) done before memory.

probe *see* transducer.

propagation speed velocity at which sound travels through a given medium.

pulse burst of ultrasound consisting of several cycles.

pulse repetition frequency number of pulses emitted per second.

pulse-echo principle technique employed in diagnostic ultrasound in which short pulses of ultrasound are emitted and spaced far enough apart in time to give distant echoes enough time to return to the transducer before the next pulse. Most diagnostic ultrasound procedures are pulsed.

real time imaging technique in which the image is created by a rapid succession of B-mode images to produce a cinematic view.

real-time display display that continuously images moving structures or a changing scan plane.

reflection loss or attenuation of sound by the redirection of the sound beam from a boundary back toward its source.

refraction change in direction of an ultrasound beam as it crosses a boundary. An artifact created by the bending of the sound wave as it passes from one medium to another or as it encounters a rounded structure, creating an area of echo dropout mimicking an acoustic shadow.

rejection Elimination of small-amplitude noise signals and unimportant echoes from the image.

resolution ability of a system to differentiate closely spaced tissue interfaces lying along or perpendicular to the axis of the ultrasound beam.

reverberation artifact that is the result of sound bouncing back and forth between two interfaces, resulting in repeated time delays and the display of parallel lines at regular intervals deep to the actual returning echo.

ring-down reverberation artifact that appears as a long series of closely spaced echoes and is caused by a very strong interface, such as gas bubbles.

sagittal (longitudinal) plane image plane parallel to the long axis of the body or organ. The midsagittal plane divides the patient or organ into equal right and left halves.

scan an ultrasound examination; to perform an ultrasound examination.

scanhead transducer assembly.

scanner *see* transducer.

scattering loss or attenuation of sound due to redirection or diffusion when a rough surface or particle suspension is encountered.

screen *see* cathode ray tube.

sector scanner mechanical or phased-array transducer that produces a wedge- or pie-shaped image.

side lobes minor beams of sound traveling out from a transducer in a direction different from that of the primary beam.

slope delay depth at which the time-gain compensation slope begins, used to suppress the artifactual echoes in the near field.

slope rate rate at which echoes are suppressed or amplified as the depth varies.

sonogram static image produced to record an ultrasound examination; an ultrasound examination.

sonographer one who is skilled in performing ultrasound examinations.

sonography production of a sonogram.

sonologist specialist in the interpretation of ultrasound examinations.

sonolucent *see* anechoic.

sound traveling wave of acoustic variables; ultrasound.

sound beam *see* beam.

speckle granular appearance of images caused by the interference of echoes from the distribution of scatterers in tissue.

specular reflector structure that creates a strong echo because the reflecting surface is at right angles to the sound beam and because it has different acoustic impedance from the adjacent structure.

through transmission amount of sound passing through a structure.

time-gain compensation (TGC) change of signal amplification to compensate for ultrasound beam attenuation, transducer focusing, and pulse frequency. The purpose of TGC is to permit display images of equal brightness regardless of depth.

transabdominal scanning of abdominal viscera through the abdominal wall.

transducer any device that converts energy from one form to another. A device containing the piezoelectric crystal within a protective housing that is placed in contact with the patient's skin to produce an ultrasound image.

transducer assembly transducer elements with damping materials assembled in a case.

transrectal probe type of transducer that is introduced into the rectum to evaluate the prostate gland, the urinary bladder, or the rectum.

transverse (cross-sectional) plane image plane perpendicular to the long axis of the body or organ, dividing the body or organ into cranial and caudal sections.

ultrasonic of or pertaining to the frequencies above the audible range.

ultrasonography *see* sonography.

ultrasound any sound above the audible range (>20,000 Hertz).

ultrasound beam *see* beam.

velocity speed of a wave. The velocity of ultrasound in tissues is standardized at 1540 meters per second on all current systems.

wave front pulse configuration of diagnostic ultrasound emitted from the face of the transducer.

wavelength distance a wave travels in a single cycle.

zoom box electronically placed on the screen that allows the material within the box to be expanded to fill the screen. The image is magnified, but because the number of scan lines within the image is unchanged, the resolution is reduced.

INDEX

Page numbers followed by *f* indicate figures.

A

Abdominal sonography, 43–48
  anatomy, gross, 353–362, 354*f*, 355*f*, 356*f*, 357*f*, 358*f*, 359*f*
  clipping the patient for, 36*f*
Abscesses
  hepatic, 116–117, 118*f*
  muscular, 340–341, 342*f*
  pancreatic, 191*f*, 191, 192*f*
  prostatic, 244–245, 245*f*, 246*f*
  renal, 202
  splenic, 145, 146*f*
Absorption, 8
Acoustic power, 9
Acoustic shadowing, 21*f*, 21
Acoustic standoff pads, 41, 42*f*
Acoustic window, 3
Actinomyces infection, 340
Acute renal failure (ARF), 199
Adenocarcinoma
  gastric, 158, 162*f*, 170*f*, 172*f*
  ocular, 326, 329
  prostatic, 245, 246*f*, 247*f*
  pulmonary, 96*f*, 99*f*
  renal, 206, 208
  uterine, 288*f*
Adenomas, adrenal, 223–224*f*
Adrenal-dependent hyperadrenocorticism, 218
Adrenal glands, 48, 50, 211–225
  anatomy
    gross, 357
    normal/location, 211, 212*f*, 213
    sonographic, 213*f*, 213, 214*f*, 215*f*, 215, 216*f*
  biopsy techniques, 225
  diseases of, 215–224
    adrenal-dependent hyperadrenocorticism, 217*f*, 218*f*, 218, 220*f*, 221*f*
    enlargement of gland, 223, 224
    neoplasia, 218–219, 223
    pituitary-dependent hyperadrenocorticism, 217, 218, 219–220*f*, 219
  scanning techniques, 50*f*, 213
Anatomy, gross abdominal, 353–362. *See also* specific organ
  adrenal glands, 357
  aorta, 361
  bladder, urinary, 358
  caudal regions (left and right), 362
  caudal vena cava, 361
  cecum, 360
  kidneys, 357–358
  large intestine, 360–361
  left cranial region, 361
  left middle region, 361–362
  liver, 353–354
  lymph nodes, 361
  ovaries, 359
  pancreas, 357
  portal vein, 361
  prostate, 359
  rectum, 360–361
  right cranial region, 361
  right middle region, 362
  small intestine, 360
  spleen, 354, 357
  stomach, 360
  testes, 359–360
  ureters, 358
  urethra, 358
  uterus, 358–359
Anatomy, normal
  adrenal, 211–213
  bladder, urinary, 227
  GI tract, 149–150
  lymph nodes, 305–306
  prostate gland, 237
  renal, 197
Anatomy, sonographic, 3
  adrenal, 213–215, 216
  bladder, urinary, 227–228

Anatomy, sonographic (*continued*)
heart, 64–65
normal cat, 70–72
normal dog, 65–68
of ligaments, 347
liver, 106–111
lymph nodes, 308–310
muscle, 336–337
ocular, 324–325
ovarian (canine), 293–300
diestrus, 299–300
estrus, 299
ovulation, 299
proestrus, 294–299
ovarian (feline), 300
renal, 198
spleen, 132–135
tendons, 345
testes, 251–254
thorax, 89–90, 93, 95, 97–100
uterus, 268–272
gravid, and fetus, 269–270, 271
nongravid, 268–279
postpartum, 270, 272
Anesthesia, 37, 56
Aorta, 361
Aortic stenosis, 66–67
Arteriovenous malformations, hepatic, 128
Arthrography, 348–349
Artifacts, 19–25
beam-width, 23–24, 25*f*
comet tail, 21, 23–24*f*
edge shadow, 21
grating lobe, 25, 26*f*, 26
mirror-image, 21, 24*f*, 91, 93
gallbladder, 24*f*, 109–110
liver, 111*f*
ring-down, 21, 22*f*
side-lobe, 24–25, 26*f*
Ascites, 20*f*, 128, 181
Aspiration, fine-needle, 55*f*, 56
of the bladder (urinary), 234
splenic, 147
Atrial clot, 85, 86*f*
Atrial septal defect, 69–70
Atrophy, muscular, 337
Avulsion
muscular, 340
tendinous, 345–346

B

Barium sulfate, 151
Biliary system, 107–108
disease of, 119–124
obstruction, 123–124
extrahepatic, 192
Bilomas, 116, 117*f*
Biopsy techniques, 2
adrenal, 225
automated devices, 52, 54*f*, 56, 56*f*
of the urinary bladder, 234
gastric, 173
hepatic, 128–129
lymph nodes, 322
needle-core, 147
pancreatic, 193–195
prostatic, 248, 249*f*
renal, 209
splenic, 147
testicular, 261
ultrasound-guided, 52, 53*f*, 54*f*, 56
thoracic, 100, 101–103*f*, 102
Bladder, urinary, 47*f*, 47, 227–234
anatomy
gross 358
normal 227
sonographic, 157*f*, 227–228, 228*f*
aspirates, fine-needle, 234
biopsy, 234
diseases/abnormalities, 228–233
calculi, 230*f*, 231*f*
cellular debris/crystalline matrix, 230–231
cystitis, 228, 229*f*, 230*f*, 230
ectopic ureters, 233
hemorrhage/blood clots, 233, 234*f*
neoplasia, 231, 232*f*, 233*f*
rupture, 233
urolithiasis, 230
scanning technique, 228, 229*f*
Blood clots (urinary bladder), 233, 234*f*
Bone, 7, 8
Bowel, 7
anatomy, sonographic, 153, 155
inflammatory bowel disease, 166, 168
obstruction, 163*f*, 164*f*
Brain sonography, 52*f*, 52
Brucella canis, 258
Bruise, 337–338
Bursitis, tendinous, 346

C

Calcification
muscular, 343
tendinous, 346
Calculi
prostatic, 247, 249*f*
renal, 204, 206*f*, 206
of the urinary bladder, 230*f*, 231*f*
Carcinomas
adrenocortical, 222*f*
anaplastic, 143*f*
of the bladder, 233*f*
cholangiocellular, 122, 123*f*
pancreatic, 192, 193, 195*f*
Cardiac imaging, 39*f*, 48
sectional. *See* Echocardiography
Cardiomyopathy
canine dilated, 81–82
canine hypertrophic, 80, 81*f*, 82*f*, 83*f*
feline dilated, 81–82
feline hypertrophic, 78, 81*f*, 82*f*, 83*f*
Cataracts, 325–326, 326*f*, 327, 330*f*
Caudal vena cava, 361
Cecum, 149, 155
anatomy, gross, 360
Cholecystitis, 121*f*
Cholecystogram, transhepatic, 124, 125*f*, 126*f*
Choleliths, 121–122, 123*f*
Choroid, 325

Chronic renal failure (CRF), 199, 200
Ciliary body, 325
  lesions, 326, 328*f*, 329*f*
Cirrhosis, 112*t*, 112, 113*f*, 114
Colon, 149, 150, 155–156, 156*f*
Comet tail, 21, 23–24*f*
Congestion, hepatic, 114*t*, 127*f*
Contracture, muscular, 343–344
Contrast studies, 333
Cost of ultrasound equipment, 2
  cost effectiveness, 4
Cranial mediastinum, 40*f*, 48–49, 50*f*
Crystalline matrix, 230–231
Cystic hyperplasia
  benign, 122
  endometrial, 277, 282*f*, 283*f*, 291*f*
Cystitis, 228, 229*f*, 230*f*, 230
Cysts
  hepatic, 116, 117*f*, 121*f*
  ovarian, 301*f*, 301, 302*f*, 302
  paraovarian, 301, 302
  paraprostatic, 247, 248*f*
  renal, 202–203, 204
  splenic, 145–146, 146*f*
  uterine, 277

D

Default settings, 11
Depth controls, 13–15
Diabetes mellitus, 112
Diaphragm, 90, 91*f*, 92*f*, 93, 94
Dislocation, tendinous, 346, 347*f*
Distant enhancement, 20*f*, 20, 23*f*
Donald, Ian, 1
Doppler flow studies, 333
Doppler ultrasound, 19, 59
  color flow, 19
  hepatic use, 125, 128
Duodenum, 149, 155
Duty factor, 9
Dysplasia
  mitral/tricuspid, 70–71, 77*f*, 78*f*
  neonatal, of the hip, 349

E

Ebstein's anomaly, 71, 78*f*
Echocardiography, 39*f*, 59
  patient preparation, 36–37
  radiographic imperative, 59, 61
  worksheet, 60*f*
Echoes, 8, 19
Echogenicities, 41, 43, 44*f*
Echotextures, 41, 43
Elbow joint, ligaments of, 51*f*
Endocardiosis, 73–74, 76, 79*f*
Endocarditis, 76–77, 80*f*, 81*f*
Endoscopic ultrasonography, 151, 153
Epididymis, canine, 252–253
Equipment. *See* Ultrasound machine
Ethylene glycol toxicity, 199, 201*f*, 201
Exercise-induced muscle injury, 337
Eyes, 51*f*, 52, 323–333
  anatomy, sonographic, 324–325, 325*f*
  diseases/disorders, 325–333
    cataracts, 325–326, 326*f*, 327, 330*f*
    ciliary body lesions, 326, 328*f*, 329*f*
    detached retina, 326–327, 327*f*, 329, 330*f*
    foreign bodies, 329–330, 331*f*
    lens displacement, 326, 328
    papilledema and papillitis, 329
    retrobulbar disease, 330–331, 332*f*, 333
    vitreous hemorrhage, 326
  examining, 324
  imaging techniques, special, 333
  indications for ultrasound, 324*t*, 324
  scanning techniques, 323–324

F

Far gain, 13
Fatty liver, 112*t*, 114
Feline infectious peritonitis (FIP), 206, 208, 224*f*
Fetuses, 2
  death, distress/malformation, 2, 281, 283–284, 285*f*, 286*f*, 287*f*
  head diameters, 273*t*, 274*f*
  number of, 270
  scanning for, 269–270
  serial sonograms of, 278–279*f*
Fibrosarcoma, 208*f*, 344*f*
Fibrosis and fibrositis, 343
Fluid
  accumulation, extratesticular, 258
  free, 1–2
Follicle-stimulating hormone treatment, 302*f*
Foreign bodies
  gastric, 157, 159*f*
  intestinal, 163–164, 165*f*, 166*f*
  muscular, 341, 343*f*
  ocular, 329–330, 331*f*

G

Gallbladder, 108–110, 192
  disease of, 119–124
  duplication, 111*f*
  mirror-image artifact, 109–110
  sludge, 119
  volume, measurement of, 124
  wall, 121
Gases, 2
Gastritis, 157, 160, 314*f*
Gastrointestinal (GI) tract, 48, 49, 149–173. *See also* Large intestine; Small intestine; Stomach
  anatomy
    normal/location, 149–150
    sonographic, 151–156
  biopsy of, 173
  diseases, 156–173
    foreign bodies, 157, 159
    gastric abnormalities, 156–162
    gastritis, 157, 160
    hypertrophic pyloric stenosis, 156–157, 158

Gastrointestinal (GI) tract (*continued*)
neoplasia, 158–159, 162
ulcers, 157, 160
uremic gastropathy, 157–158, 161
scanning techniques, 49*f*, 150–151
Gel, 37*f*, 37, 56*f*
Glossary of terms, 363–367
Granulomatous/infiltrative disease, 170
Gull wing sign, 329*f*

H

Halo sign, 201
Heart, 59–87, 301. *See also* Cardiac imaging; Echocardiography
anatomy, sonographic, 64–65, 72*f*
cat (normal), 70–72*f*
dog (normal), 65–69*f*
conceptualization, functional, 61
two-pump, 61*f*
contractility of, 64
diseases
acquired, common, 73–83
canine dilated cardiomopathy, 81–82
canine hypertrophic cardiomyopathy, 81–82, 83
endocardiosis, 73–74, 76, 79
endocarditis, 76–77, 81, 81*f*
feline dilated cardiomopathy, 81–82
feline hypertrophic cardiomyopathy, 78, 82, 83
pericardial fluid, 82, 84
acquired, uncommon, 84–86
atrial clot, 85
hypertrophy secondary to systemic hypertension, 85
pericardial mass/mass effect, 84–85, 85*f*
traumatic pericardial rupture, cardiac herniation, entrapment, 85–86
congenital, common, 65–69
aortic stenosis, 66–67
patent ductus arteriosus, 65–66, 73, 74
pulmonic stenosis, 67
ventricular septal defect, 68–69, 74, 75, 76, 77
congenital, uncommon, 69–73
atrial septal defect, 69–70
Ebstein's anomaly, 71
mitral/tricuspid dysplasia, 70–71, 77, 78
tetralogy of Fallot, 71, 73
flow regions, 62*f*
scanning
beginners, note to, 64–65
positions, 63*f*
preliminary procedures, 59, 61
protocol, simplified, 62–64
technique, 61–62
Hemangiosarcoma
hepatic, 118, 119*f*
splenic, 141, 142*f*, 143*f*
Hematomas
hepatic, 116
muscular, 338*f*, 338, 339*f*
ocular, 331*f*
pericardial, 85*f*
splenic, 144–145, 145*f*
uterine, 290*f*
Hemorrhage
of the urinary bladder, 233
vitreous, 326
Hepatic ultrasound. *See* Liver
Hepatitis, suppurative, 114*t*
Hernia, 92*f*, 93*f*, 93, 94*f*
Hydrocele, 258
Hydronephrosis, 203–204, 205*f*
Hydrops fetalis, 284, 287*f*
Hyperadrenocorticism, 217*f*, 217, 218, 219–220*f*, 219, 221*f*
Hypercalcemia, 207*f*
Hyperechoic, 41
Hyperechoic liver disease, 112*t*, 112–114, 113*f*
Hyperplasia
cystic endometrial, 277, 282*f*, 283*f*
hepatic, benign, 122*f*
prostatic, benign, 240, 241*f*, 241, 242*f*
reactive lymphoid, 315*f*
splenic, 139
Hypertension
portal, 125
systemic, 86*f*
Hypertrophic pyloric stenosis, 156–157, 158*f*
Hypertrophy secondary to systemic hypertension, 86*f*, 86
Hypoechoic, 41
Hypoechoic liver disease, 114, 115*f* 118

I

Ileum, 149
Image
dual, 15–16
recording, 17
television monitors, 10–11
adjusting, 17–18
measuring, 18
video invert, 16–17
Infarction
renal, 206, 207
splenic, 138*f*
testicular, 260
Infection, muscular, 340–341, 342*f*
Infertility; association conditions, 303*f*, 303
Infiltrative disease. *See* Granulomatous/infiltrative disease
Inflammatory bowel disease, 166, 168–169*f*
Insulinomas, pancreatic, 193, 194*f*
Interstitial cell tumor, 255
Intestines. *See* Large intestine; Small intestine

Intussusception, 164, 166–167*f*
Ischemia, splenic, 137, 139
Islet cell tumors, 192, 193

J
Jejunum, 149
Joints, 348–349, 349*f*, 350*f*
  masses (extraarticular) and mass effects, 349
  neonatal hip dysplasia, 349

K
Kidneys, 43, 44*f*, 45, 46*f*, 47, 197–209, 267. *See also* Renal diseases
  anatomy
    gross, 358
    normal, 197
    sonographic, 198*f*, 198
  biopsies, 209
  polycystic, 202–203
  scanning techniques, 199

L
Large intestine, 149. *See also* Cecum; Colon; Rectum
  abnormalities, 170, 172–173
  anatomy
    gross, 360–361
    sonographic, 155–156, 157
Leiomyomas, 158, 161*f*, 288*f*
Leiomyosarcomas, gastric, 162, 170, 171*f*
Lens capsules, 325
Lens displacement, 326, 328
Ligaments, 346–348
  anatomy, sonographic, 347
  disorders/diseases, 347–348, 349
  scanning technique, 51*f*, 346–347
Lipidosis, hepatic, 112, 114*f*
Liver, 43, 45*f*, 105–129
  abnormalities/disease states, 112–128. *See also* specific diseases, eg, Cirrhosis
    abscesses, 116–117, 118*f*
    bilomas, 116, 117*f*
    cirrhosis, 112*t*, 112, 113*f*, 114
    cysts, 116, 117*f*, 121*f*
    diffuse disease, 112–116, 113*f*
      biopsy of, 128
    fatty liver, 112*t*, 114
    focal disease, 116–119, 124*f*, 125*f*
      biopsy, 128–129
    hemangiosarcoma, 118, 119*f*
    hematomas, 116
    hepatic congestion, 114
    lipidosis, 112, 114*f*
    lymphoma, 114*t*
    lymphosarcoma, 114, 115*f*, 116
    neoplasia, 117, 118*f*, 118–119, 120*f*
    nodules, 117–118
    steroid hepatopathy, 112–114
    suppurative hepatitis, 114
  anatomy
    gross, 353–354
    sonographic, 106–111
      approaches/normal landmarks, 106*f*, 106–110, 107*f*, 108*f*, 109*f*, 110*f*, 111*f*
      size of liver, 110–111
  biopsy, 128–129
  scanning techniques, 105–106
  vasculature, 107
    abnormalities, 124–128
Lungs, 7, 8, 49, 95, 96*f*, 97*f*, 97–98, 98*f*, 99–100*f*
Lupus erythematosus, systemic, 200*f*
Luteinizing hormone peak (LHP), 294, 295–296, 297–298*f*
Lymph nodes, 48, 50, 305–322
  abdominal visceral, 305–306, 307, 308
  anatomy
    gross, 361
    normal/location, 305–306, 306*f*, 307*f*
    sonographic, 308–310, 309*f*
  biopsy techniques, 322
  diseases, 310–312*f*, 310–322, 312–314*f*
    metastatic, 315–316*f*
    neoplasia, 317–319*f*, 320–321*f*
  lumbar aortic, 305, 308
  scanning techniques, 50*f*, 306–308
  superficial, 306, 308, 310
  thoracic, 306, 307, 308
Lymphoma, 85*f*, 114*t*
Lymphosarcoma, 100
  cranial mediastinal, 319
  gastric, 162, 163*f*, 170, 171*f*, 172*f*, 173*f*
  hepatic, 114, 115*f*, 116
  of the lymph nodes, 319*f*, 320–321*f*
  renal, 208, 209*f*
  splenic, 135, 136*f*, 137*f*, 141

M
Magnetic resonance imaging (MRI), 353
Mastocytosis, splenic, 137*f*
Mediastinum, 98–100, 101–103
Medullary rim sign, 201, 207
Melanoma, ocular, 326
Meningioma, optic nerve, 332*f*
Mode selection, 16
Monitors, 10–11, 17–18
Motion-mode sonography, 19
Mucometra, 279, 284*f*
Muscle, 335–345
  anatomy, sonographic, 336–337, 337*f*
  disorders/diseases, 337–345
    abscess, 340–341, 342*f*
    atrophy, 337
    avulsion, 340
    bruise, 337–338
    calcification, 343
    classification of injuries, 340*f*
    contracture, 343–344

Muscle, disorders/diseases (*continued*)
  exercise-induced injury, 337
  fibrosis and fibrositis, 343
  foreign body, 341, 343*f*
  hematoma, 338*f*, 338, 339*f*
  infection, 340–341, 342*f*
  injury; sonographic protocol, 336
  strain, 340, 341*f*
  tumors, 344–345
 scanning technique, 336
Musculoskeletal system, 335–349. *See also* Joints; Ligaments; Muscle; Tendons
 imaging, 51, 52

N

Near gain control, 11
Needles, 2. *See also* Aspiration, fine-needle
 type/size of, 54*f*, 56
Neoplasia
 of the adrenal glands, 218–219, 223
 adrenocortical, primary, 218, 221–222
 of the bladder (urinary), 231, 232*f*, 233*f*
 focal splenic, 141, 142
 gastric, 158–159, 162, 170
 hepatic, 117, 118*f*, 118–119, 120*f*
 of the lymph nodes, 317–319*f*, 320*f*
 ocular, 326
 ovarian, 301–302
 pancreatic, 192–193
 prostatic, 245–247, 247*f*
 renal, 206, 208
 testicular, 254–257
  sonography of, 255–257, 258
 uterine, 288–289, 289*f*, 290*f*
Nephrocalcinosis, 206
Nephropathy, 200*f*, 203
Nodules
 hepatic, 117–118
 splenic regenerative, 144*f*

O

Ocular sonography, 52. *See also* Eyes
 transpalpebral technique, 51*f*
Ovariectomy, complications of, 303
Ovaries, 48, 293–303
 anatomy
  canine, sonographic, 293–294, 294*f*, 299–300
   diestrus, 299*f*, 299–300
   estrus, 295–296*f*, 299
   ovulation, 299
   proestrus, 295–296*f*, 301*f*
  feline, sonographic, 300*f*, 300
  gross, 359
 diseases/disorders, 300–303
  cysts, 301*f*, 301, 302*f*, 302
  neoplasms, 301–302
 scanning techniques, 293, 294*f*

P

Pancreas, 48, 49, 177–195
 anatomy
  gross, 357
  normal/location, 177, 178*f*
  sonographic, 179, 180*f*, 181*f*, 182*f*
 biopsy techniques, 193–195
 diseases, 181–193
  neoplasia, 192–193
  pancreatitis, 181, 182*f*, 183*f*, 184*f*, 185*f*, 186*f*, 186, 187*f*, 188*f*, 188, 189*f*, 190*f*, 191–192, 192*f*
 scanning techniques, 49*f*, 179
Pancreatitis, 159*f*, 169, 182*f*, 183*f*
 acute edematous, 181–186, 184*f*
 acute hemorrhagic, 186*f*, 186–187, 187*f*, 188*f*
 chronic, 188, 189*f*, 190*f*
 complications of, 188, 191–192, 192*f*
Papilledema, 329
Papillitis, 329
Paralytic ileus, 163, 164*f*
Patent ductus arteriosus, 65–66, 73*f*, 74*f*
Patient preparation
 for biopsy procedures, 56–57
 for echocardiography, 36–37
 positioning, ultrasound approaches, 37–41
  for the eye, 323
 for scanning, 33, 36–37
  ocular, 323–324
Pericardial fluid, 81–82, 84*f*
Pericardial mass/mass effect, 84, 85
Pericardial rupture (traumatic), cardiac herniation, entrapment, 86–87
Perirenal pseudocyst, 204, 205*f*
Peristalsis, 156
Peritonitis
 infectious, 169
  feline, 206, 208*f*, 224*f*
Pheochromocytoma, 222*f*, 223*f*, 223
Phlegmon, pancreatic, 191–192, 194*f*
Phycomycosis, 169
Pituitary-dependent hyperadrenocorticism, 217, 218
Pleura, 49, 95*f*, 95
Polyps, 158, 161*f*
 hyperplastic endometrial, 290, 291*f*
Portal veins, 107, 361
Power controls, 13–15
Pregnancy, scanning for, 269–270, 272, 274–276
 beagle pregnancy, 282*f*
  fetal head, 280–281*f*
  gestation length, estimation of, 272*f*
  postpartum, 282*f*
  serial sonograms, 274–277*f*, 278–279*f*, 280–281
 domestic cat pregnancy, serial sonograms, 271*f*
Proestrus (canine), 294–299
Prostate gland, 47, 48, 151, 237–249

anatomy
gross, 359
normal/location, 237
sonographic, 238, 239*f*, 240*f*, 240
biopsy techniques, 248, 249*f*
diseases of, 240–247
abscess, 244–245, 245*f*, 246*f*
benign prostatic hyperplasia, 240, 241*f*, 242*f*
calculi, 247, 249*f*
cysts, paraprostatic, 247, 248*f*
neoplasia, 245–247, 246*f*, 247*f*
prostatitis, 241, 243*f*, 243–245, 244*f*
scanning techniques, 48*f*, 237–238
Prostatitis, 241, 243–245
abscess, 244–245, 246
acute bacterial, 241, 243*f*
chronic bacterial, 243*f*, 243, 244*f*
granulomatous, 243–244
Pseudocholecystitis, 122*f*
Pseudocysts, 192*f*, 204, 205*f*
Pulmonic stenosis, 67, 75*f*
Pulser, 9
Pulse repetition frequency (PRF), 9
Purchase considerations, 2–4
cost/cost effectiveness, 2, 4
interpreting the sonogram, 3–4
scanning the patient, 3
training time, 3–4
used equipment, 2
Pyelonephritis, 201–202, 202*f*, 203*f*
Pyometra, 279, 283*f*, 284*f*

R

Radiography
characteristic features
aortic stenosis, 66
atrial clot, 85
atrial septal defect, 69
canine dilated cardiomyopathy, 81–82
canine hypertrophic cardiomyopathy, 80–81
Ebstein's anomaly, 71
endocardiosis, 73–74
endocarditis, 76–77
feline dilated cardiomyopathy, 81–82
feline hypertrophic cardiomyopathy, 78
hypertrophy secondary to systemic hypertension, 85
mitral/tricuspid dysplasia, 70–71
patent ductus arteriosus, 65
pericardial fluid, 82
pericardial mass/mass effect, 84–85
pericardial rupture (traumatic), cardiac herniation, entrapment, 85–86
pulmonic stenosis, 67
tetralogy of Fallot, 71, 73
ventricular septal defect, 68
thoracic, 59, 61
Real-time ultrasound, 18–19
Receiver, 9–10
Rectum, 149, 150
anatomy, gross, 361
Recumbency
dorsal, 38*f*, 38
lateral, 38–39, 39*f*
sternal, 39–40, 40*f*
Reflection, 8
Refraction, 8, 21, 23*f*
Renal diseases, 199–208
abscess, 202
acute renal failure, 199*f*, 199
calculi, 204, 206*f*, 206
chronic renal failure, 199, 200*f*, 200
ethylene glycol toxicity, 199, 201
feline infectious peritonitis, 206, 208*f*
hydronephrosis, 203–204, 205
infarct, 206, 207
neoplasia, 206, 208
nephrocalcinosis, 206
perirenal pseudocyst, 204, 205
polycystic kidneys, 202–203, 204*f*
pyelonephritis, 201–202, 203
urinoma, 204
Reproduction, uterine conditions affecting, 291
Reticuloendothelial system (RES) hyperplasia, 139
Retina, 325
detached, 326–327, 327*f*, 329, 330*f*
Retrobulbar disease, 330–331, 332*f*, 333
Reverberation, 21, 22*f*

S

Scanner, 8–9, 19
Scanning the patient, 3, 43
heart
preliminary procedures, 59, 61
protocol, simplified, 62–64
technique, 61–62
intracavitary, 40–41
patient preparation, 33, 36–37
planes and image orientation, 31–33, 34*f*, 35–36*f*, 36
techniques. *See* Scanning techniques
Scanning techniques, 29–56
adrenal glands, 213
bladder, urinary, 228
GI tract, 150–151
hepatic, 105–106
ligaments, 346–347
lymph nodes, 306–308
muscle, 336
ovarian, 293, 294*f*
pancreatic, 179
prostate gland, 237–238
renal, 199
splenic, 131–132
tendons, 345
testes, 251

Scanning techniques (*continued*)
  thoracic, 89
  uterine, 265–268
Scrotal enlargement, 258
Scrotal wall, 253
Scrotum
  scanning technique, manual stabilization, 49*f*
Seminoma, 255
Sertoli cell tumor, 254–255
Shunts
  extrahepatic, 127–128, 128*f*
  intrahepatic, 127*f*, 127
  portosystemic, 126, 128
Signal conversion/processing, 10
Slope delay, 11
Slope rate, 11, 13
Small intestine, 149, 268–269. *See also* Duodenum; Ileum; Jejunum
  abnormalities, 162–170
    foreign bodies, 163–164, 165*f*, 166*f*
    granulomatous/infiltrative disease, 170
    inflammatory disease, 166, 168
    intussusception, 164, 166–167
    neoplasia, 170
    obstruction/dilatation, 162–163
  anatomy
    gross, 360
    sonographic, 151, 153–155*f*
  empty, sagittal sonogram, 270*f*
  layers of, 153
  scanning techniques, 150–151
Sonographers
  beginners, note to, 64–65
  role of, 29
  scanning abilities, 3
Sonography. *See* Ultrasound; Ultrasound machine; *and specific organs, eg, Pancreas*
Sound waves, behavior inside the body, 7–8
Spleen, 43, 44*f*, 46*f*, 131–147
  abnormalities/disease states, 135–147
    diffuse disease, 135–140, 147
      congestive, 135, 137, 139
      infiltrative, 135, 136, 137, 138
    focal disease, 140–141, 144–146, 147
      neoplasia, 141, 142
      nonmalignant, 141, 144–146
    hyperplasia, 139
    splenomegaly, 134*f*, 135, 138*f*, 139–140
  anatomy
    gross, 354, 357
    sonographic, 132–135
      abnormal, 134–135
      approaches/landmarks, 132*f*, 132–133, 133*f*, 134*f*
      size of spleen, 133–134
    aspiration, fine-needle, 147
    biopsy of, 147
    scanning techniques, 131–132
Splenitis
  emphysematous, 139*f*
  gangrenous, 140*f*
Splenomegaly, 134*f*
  congestive, 135, 137, 138*f*
  infectious/inflammatory, 139–140
  infiltrative, 135
Standing, 40*f*, 40
Steroid hepatopathy, 112*t*
Stomach, 7, 149, 160*f*
  anatomy
    gross, 360
    sonographic, 151*f*, 151, 152*f*, 153*f*
  layers of, 153
  scanning techniques, 150
Strains
  muscular, 340, 341*f*
  tendinous, 345

T

Tendons, 345–346
  anatomy, sonographic, 345
  disorders/diseases, 345–346
    avulsion, 345–346
    bursitis, 346
    calcification, 346
    classification of injuries, 340*f*
    dislocation, 346, 347*f*
    strains, 345, 346*f*
  scanning technique, 345
Terminology, 363–367
Testes, 48, 49, 251–262
  anatomy
    gross, 359–360
    normal sonographic, 251–254, 252*f*, 253*f*
  atrophic, 257, 260
  biopsy techniques, 261
  diseases/abnormalities
    infectious disorders, 257–258, 259*f*
    interstitial cell tumor, 255
    neoplasia, 254–257
    nonneoplastic, noninfectious, 258, 260*f*, 260–261, 261*f*
    seminoma, 255
    Sertoli cell tumor, 254–255
    ultrasonography of, 254
  nondescended (retained), 257, 258*f*, 258, 260–261
  palpation, 251
  scanning technique, 251
    manual stabilization, 49*f*
  sonography of tumors, 255, 256*f*, 257*f*, 257, 258
  vascular compromise, 260, 261
Tetralogy of Fallot, 71, 73
Thoracic wall, 90–91*f*, 90
Thorax, 48–49, 89–102. *See also specific organ*
  anatomy (ultrasound), 89–90, 90*f*, 93, 95, 97–100
  biopsy of, 100, 102
  scanning techniques, 89
Time-gain compensation, 11–13, 14

Tissue
  abnormalities, 3–4
  reflection and, 8
Torsion, splenic, 139, 140*f*
Training
  time required, 3–4
  understanding ultrasound, 3
Transducers, 8–9, 19, 41*f*
  disinfecting, 56*f*, 56
  movements, 29–30, 31, 32, 33
    fanning, 29–30, 32*f*
    rocking/rolling, 30, 33*f*
    rotating, 29, 31*f*
    sliding, 29, 30*f*
  selection
    control of, 15
    ocular, 323
Transrectal ultrasound, 41*f*, 151
Trauma, splenic, 146*f*, 146–147
Tumors
  muscular, 344–345
  testicular, 255, 256*f*, 257, 258

U

Ulcers, gastric, 157, 160
Ultrasound
  advantages of, 1–2
  beam characteristics, 7
  how it works, 7–26
  images, production of, 1–2
Ultrasound machine, 8–11. *See also main entries for specific types, eg, Doppler ultrasound*
  controls, 11–18
    power, depth, zoom controls, 13, 14*f*, 15*f*, 15, 16*f*
    secondary, 15–18, 16*f*, 17*f*, 18*f*
    time-gain compensation, 10*f*, 11*f*, 11, 12*f*, 13*f*, 13, 14
  image viewing/recording, 10–11
  interior, 8–11
    diagram, 9*f*
  keyboard, 4*f*
  memory storage, 10
  portable, 2*f*, 3*f*
  pulser, 9
  receiver, 9–10
  scanner, 8–9
  signal conversion/processing, 10
  types of, 18–19
  used equipment, 2
Uremic gastropathy, 157–158, 161*f*
Ureters
  anatomy, gross, 358
  ectopic, 233
Urethra, anatomy, gross, 358
Urinary bladder. *See* Bladder, urinary
Urinoma, 204
Urolithiasis, 230
Uterine horns, 48*f*, 268*f*, 269*f*, 283*f*
Uterus, 47, 265–291
  anatomy
    gross, 358–359
    sonographic, 268–272
      gravid, and fetus, 269–270, 271
      nongravid uterus, 268–269
      postpartum, 270, 272
  diseases of
    common, 272, 277–287
      cystic endometrial hyperplasia, 277, 282*f*, 283*f*
      endometritis, 277, 282*f*, 283*f*
      fetal death, distress/malformation, 281, 283–284, 285*f*, 286*f*, 287
      hydrops fetalis, 284, 287*f*
      pyometra, 279, 283*f*, 284*f*
    less common, 287–291
      hyperplastic endometrial polyps, 290, 291*f*
      neoplasms, 288–289, 289*f*, 290*f*
      reproduction, conditions affecting, 291
  scanning technique, 265, 266*f*, 267*f*, 267–268
  sonographic evaluation, 265, 266

V

Vasculature
  hepatic, 107
    abnormalities, 124–128
  testicular, compromised, 260, 261
Veins, hepatic, 107
Ventricular septal defect, 68–69, 74*f*, 75*f*, 76*f*, 77*f*
Veterinary Radiology & Ultrasound, 1
Video invert, 16–17
Vitreous, 325
  hemorrhage, 326

X

X-ray films, 1

Z

Zoom controls, 13–15